CRASH COURSE
General Medicine
SECOND EDITION

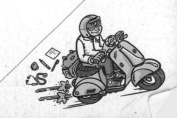

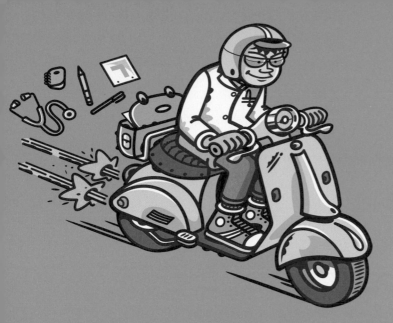

Series editor
Daniel Horton-Szar
BSc (Hons), MB, BS (Hons)
Northgate Medical Practice
Canterbury
Kent

Faculty Advisors
P John Rees
Senior Lecturer in Medicine, Consultant
Physician, Dean of Undergraduate
Education
Guy's, Kings and St Thomas's School
of Medicine
Guy's Hospital
London

Wilf Yeo
Senior Lecturer in Pharmacology and
Therapeutics
Royal Hallamshire Hospital
Sheffield

General Medicine

SECOND EDITION

Robert Parker
BSc, MSc, MRCP
Specialist Registrar in Respiratory and General Internal Medicine,
Oxford Radcliffe Hospitals NHS Trust, Oxford

Asheesh Sharma
MA, MRCP
Specialist Registrar in Nephrology and General Internal Medicine,
Royal Liverpool and Broadgreen University Hospitals NHS Trust, Liverpool

First edition authors
Rachael Hough and Iftikhar Ul Haq

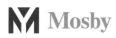 Mosby

Edinburgh • London • New York • Oxford • Philadelphia • St Louis • Sydney • Toronto 2005

MOSBY
An imprint of Elsevier Limited

Commissioning Editor: Fiona Conn
Project Development Manager: Fiona Conn & The Partnership Publishing Solutions Ltd
Project Manager: Cheryl Brant
Designer: Andy Chapman
Illustration Management: Bruce Hogarth

First edition 1999
This edition 2005

ISBN 0723433313

British Library Cataloguing in Publication Data
A catalogue record for this book is available from the British Library

Library of Congress Cataloging in Publication Data
A catalog record for this book is available from the Library of Congress

Note
Medical knowledge is constantly changing. Standard safety precautions must be followed, but as new research and clinical experience broaden our knowledge, changes in treatment and drug therapy may become necessary or appropriate. Readers are advised to check the most current product information provided by the manufacturer of each drug to be administered to verify the recommended dose, the method and duration of administration, and contraindications. It is the responsibility of the practitioner, relying on experience and knowledge of the patient, to determine dosages and the best treatment for each individual patient. Neither the Publisher nor the authors assume any liability for any injury and/or damage to persons or property arising from this publication.

The Publisher

Printed in Italy

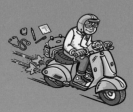

Author preface

General or internal medicine comprises a wide range of medical sub specialities. Despite the increasing fragmentation of general medicine there remains a need to train general physicians able to provide acute and chronic care to medical patients. Therefore the subject remains an integral part of medical school training and examinations.

This updated second edition endeavours to build on the tried and trusted format of the Crash Course series. The first section is designed to provide the student with a structure on how to approach the common clinical scenarios. The second explains examination, investigation and provides an example on how to integrate this in a clerking. The third section covers more didactic material on various specialities. This cannot be exhaustive and should be used in conjunction with other textbooks both from the Crash Course range and otherwise. The final section provides questions to reinforce the knowledge acquired.

Clinical medicine can be daunting at first but with practise can be a rewarding and enjoyable subject. We hope this book will be used by clinical students from tentative beginnings on the wards to final examinations to gain confidence with patients and continue to help them as their skills develop and examinations approach.

Robert Parker
Asheesh Sharma

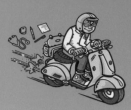

Preface

Over the last six years since the first editions were published, there have been many changes in medicine, and in the way it is taught. These second editions have been largely rewritten to take these changes into account, and to keep *Crash Course* up to date for the twenty-first century. New material has been added to include recent research, and all pharmacological and disease management information has been updated in line with current best practice. We have listened to feedback from hundreds of medical students who have been using *Crash Course* and have improved the structure and layout of the books accordingly: pathology and disease management material has been moved closer to the diagnostic skills chapters; there are more MCQs and now we have Extended Matching Questions as well, with explanations of each answer. We have also included `Further Reading' sections, where appropriate, to highlight important papers and studies that you should be aware of, and the clarity of text and figures is better than ever.

However, the principles on which we developed the series remain the same. Clinical medicine is a huge subject, and teaching on the wards can sometimes be sporadic because of the competing demands of patient care. The last thing a student needs when finals are approaching is to waste time assembling information from different sources, or wading through pages of irrelevant detail. As before, *Crash Course* brings you all the information you need in compact, manageable volumes that integrate an approach to common patient presentations with clinical skills, pathology and management of the relevant diseases. We still tread the fine line between producing clear, concise text and providing enough detail for those aiming at distinction. The series is still written by junior doctors with recent examination experience, in partnership with senior faculty members from across the UK.

I wish you the best of luck in your future careers!

Dr Dan Horton-Szar
Series Editor

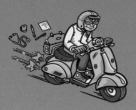

Acknowledgement

To Clare for her patience and good humour.

RP

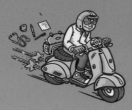

Dedications

To Mum, Dad, Sheetal and Neelima – thank you for your endless support and love.

AS

For my parents, missed always...

RP

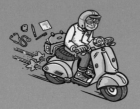

Contents

Author preface v
Preface vi
Acknowledgement vii
Dedications .viii

Part I: The Patient Presents With 1

1. **Chest Pain** 3
   Introduction 3
   Differential diagnosis of chest pain 3
   History in the patient with chest pain 3
   Examining the patient with chest pain 4
   Investigating the patient with
      chest pain 4

2. **Shortness of Breath** 9
   Introduction 9
   History in the patient with
      breathlessness 9
   Examining the patient with
      breathlessness 10
   Investigating the patient with
      breathlessness 12

3. **Palpitations** 15
   Introduction 15
   Differential diagnosis by description
      of the rhythm 15
   History 16
   Consequences of palpitations 16
   Examining the patient with
      palpitations 17
   Investigating the patient with
      palpitations 18

4. **Heart Murmurs** 21
   Introduction 21
   Differential diagnosis of heart
      murmurs 21
   History in the patient with heart
      murmurs 22
   Examining the patient with heart
      murmurs 22

5. **Cough and Haemoptysis** 29
   Introduction 29
   Differential diagnosis of cough
      and haemoptysis 29
   History in the patient with cough
      and haemoptysis 29
   Examining the patient with cough
      and haemoptysis 30
   Investigating the patient with cough
      and haemoptysis 32

6. **Pyrexia of Unknown Origin** 33
   Introduction 33
   Causes of PUO 33
   History in the patient with PUO 33
   Examining the patient with PUO 33
   Investigating the patient with PUO 33

7. **Dyspepsia** 37
   Introduction 37
   Causes of dyspepsia 37
   History and examination in the
      patient with dyspepsia 37
   Investigating the patient with
      dyspepsia 38

8. **Haematemesis and Melaena** 41
   Introduction 41
   Differential diagnosis of haematemesis
      and melaena 41
   History in the patient with
      haematemesis and melaena 41
   Examining the patient with
      haematemesis and melaena 42
   Investigating the patient with
      haematemesis and melaena 43

9. **Change in Bowel Habit** 45
   Introduction 45
   Differential diagnosis of a change in
      bowel habit 45
   History in the patient with a change in
      bowel habit 45
   Examining the patient with a change in
      bowel habit 45
   Investigating the patient with a change
      in bowel habit 45

10. **Weight Loss** **51**
   Introduction 51
   Differential diagnosis of weight loss 51
   History in the patient with weight loss . . .51
   Examining the patient with weight
      loss 52
   Investigating the patient with
      weight loss .54

11. **Jaundice** **57**
   Introduction 57
   Differential diagnosis of jaundice 57
   History in the patient with jaundice 57
   Examining the patient with jaundice 57
   Investigating the patient with jaundice . . .59

12. **Abdominal Pain** **63**
   Introduction 63
   Differential diagnosis of abdominal
      pain 63
   History in the patient with
      abdominal pain 63
   Examining the patient with
      abdominal pain 65
   Investigating the patient with
      abdominal pain 66

13. **Polyuria and Polydipsia** **69**
   Introduction 69
   Differential diagnosis of polyuria 69
   History in the patient with polyuria
      and polydipsia 70
   Examining the patient with polyuria
      and polydipsia 71
   Investigating the patient with polyuria
      and polydipsia 72

14. **Haematuria and Proteinuria** **75**
   Introduction 75
   Differential diagnosis of haematuria
      and proteinuria 75
   History in the patient with haematuria
      and proteinuria 77
   Examining the patient with haematuria
      and proteinuria 77
   Investigating the patient with
      haematuria and proteinuria 78

15. **Hypertension** **81**
   Introduction 81
   Differential diagnosis of
      hypertension 81
   History in the patient with
      hypertension 81
   Examining the patient with
      hypertension 82
   Investigating the patient with
      hypertension 83

16. **Headache and Facial Pain** **87**
   Introduction 87
   Differential diagnosis of headache
      and facial pain 87
   History in the patient with headache
      and facial pain 87
   Examining the patient with headache
      and facial pain 89
   Investigating the patient with
      headache and facial pain 89

17. **Joint Disease** **93**
   Differential diagnosis of joint disease 93
   History in the patient with joint
      disease 93
   Examining the patient with joint
      disease 94
   Investigating the patient with joint
      disease 96

18. **Skin Diseases** **99**
   Differential diagnosis by appearance 99
   History in the patient with skin
      rashes 101
   Examining the patient with a skin
      rash 101
   Investigating the patient with
      skin rashes 102

19. **Loss of Consciousness** **105**
   Introduction 105
   Differential diagnosis of loss of
      consciousness 105
   History in the patient with loss of
      consciousness 105
   Examining the patient with loss of
      consciousness 107
   Investigating the patient with loss of
      consciousness 109

20. Confusional States **113**
Introduction 113
Differential diagnosis of confusion 113
History in the confused patient 113
Examining the confused patient 114
Investigating the confused patient 115

21. Acute Neurological Deficit **119**
Introduction 119
Differential diagnosis of stroke 119
History in the stroke patient 120
Examining the stroke patient 121
Investigating the stroke patient 123

22. Lymphadenopathy and Splenomegaly . .**125**
Introduction 125
Differential diagnosis of
lymphadenopathy and
splenomegaly 125
History in the patient with
lymphadenopathy and
splenomegaly 125
Examining the patient with
lymphadenopathy and
splenomegaly 126
Investigating the patient with
lymphadenopathy and
splenomegaly 128

**23. Sensory and Motor Neurological
Deficits** **131**
Introduction 131
Differential diagnosis of sensory and/or
motor neurological deficits 131
History in the patient with sensory
and/or motor neurological deficits . . .131
Examining the patient with sensory
and/or motor neurological deficits . . .133
Investigating the patient with sensory
and/or motor neurological deficits . . .136

24. Bruising and Bleeding **139**
Introduction 139
Differential diagnosis of bruising or
bleeding .139
History in the patient with bruising
and bleeding 140
Examining the patient with bruising
and bleeding 140
Investigating the patient with bruising
and bleeding 141

25. Vertigo and Dizziness **145**
Introduction 145
Differential diagnosis in the patient
with vertigo or dizziness 145
History in the patient with vertigo 145
Examining the patient with vertigo 147
Investigating the patient with vertigo . . .147

26. Anaemia **149**
Introduction 149
Differential diagnosis of anaemia 149
History in the anaemic patient 150
Examining the anaemic patient 150
Investigating the anaemic patient 152

Part II: Diseases and Disorders **155**

27. Cardiovascular System **157**
Ischaemic heart disease 157
Acute myocardial infarction 162
Arrhythmias 169
Heart failure 174
Hypertension 179
Valvular heart disease 184
Miscellaneous cardiovascular
conditions 186

28. Respiratory Disease **195**
Asthma 195
Chronic obstructive pulmonary
disease .198
Tuberculosis 201
Lung cancer 204
Pneumonia 208
Respiratory failure 210
Miscellaneous respiratory conditions . . .213

29. Gastrointestinal and Liver Disease **221**
Oesophageal disorders 221
Gastroduodenal disorders 222
Small bowel disorders 225
Inflammatory bowel disease 228
Colorectal disease 232
Irritable bowel syndrome and
non-ulcer dyspepsia 234
Diseases of the gallbladder 235
Diseases of the pancreas 236
Acute viral hepatitis 238
Chronic liver disease 240

30. **Genitourinary Disease** **245**
    Glomerular disease 245
    Acute renal failure 247
    Chronic renal failure 250
    Urinary tract infection 252
    Miscellaneous genitourinary
        conditions 254
    Fluid and electrolyte balance 256

31. **Central Nervous System** **261**
    Cerebrovascular disease 261
    Management of conditions
        causing headache 265
    Parkinsonism 268
    Multiple sclerosis 270
    Meningitis .272
    Encephalitis 274
    Epilepsy 274
    Intracranial tumours 277
    Miscellaneous neurological disorders . . .278

32. **Metabolic and Endocrine Disorders** **283**
    Diabetes mellitus 283
    Obesity 289
    Lipid disorders 290
    How to use the cardiovascular
        disease risk prediction charts for
        primary prevention 293
    Metabolic bone disease 294
    Hypercalcaemia 297
    Hyperparathyroidism 298
    Hypoparathyroidism 299
    Crystal arthropathy 299
    Pituitary disorders 301
    Thyroid disorders 305
    Disorders of the adrenal glands 310
    Miscellaneous endocrine conditions 313

33. **Musculoskeletal and Skin Disorders** . . .**315**
    Arthritis 315
    Rheumatoid arthritis 315
    Osteoarthritis 317
    Spondyloarthropathies 318
    Systemic lupus erythematosus 320
    Polymyalgia rheumatica 322
    Other connective tissue disorders 323
    Primary skin diseases 326
    Skin manifestations of systemic
        disease .329
    Malignant skin tumours 331

34. **Haematological Disorders** **333**
    Anaemia 333
    Leukaemias 341
    Multiple myeloma 344
    Malignant lymphomas 346
    Bleeding disorders 349
    Disseminated intravascular
        coagulation 350
    Thrombotic disorders 351
    Thrombotic thrombocytopenic
        purpura .352

35. **Infectious Diseases** **355**
    Introduction 355
    HIV and AIDS 355
    Malaria 359
    Methicillin resistant *Staphylococcus*
        aureus (MRSA) 362

36. **Drug Overdose** **363**
    Epidemiology 363
    Aetiology 363
    Presentation 363
    Investigations 364
    Management 364

**Part III: History, Examination and
Common Investigations** **367**

37. **Taking a History** **369**
    General principles–the bedside
        manner .369
    The history .369
    Presenting complaint 369
    History of the presenting complaint 370
    Past medical history 370
    Family history 371
    Social history 371
    Systems review 371

38. **Examination of the Patient** **379**
    Introduction 379
    First things first 379
    General inspection 379
    The face and body habitus 381
    The neck 381
    The hands .382
    The cardiovascular system 384
    The respiratory system 387
    The abdomen 390
    The nervous system 393

The joints 402
The skin 404

39. The Clerking **405**
Introduction 405
Medical sample clerking 406

40. Common Investigations **409**
Introduction 409
The cardiovascular system 409
The respiratory system 414
The gastrointestinal system 417
The urinary system 419
The nervous system 420
Metabolic and endocrine disorders 420

Musculoskeletal and skin disease 425
Haematological disorders 425
Miscellaneous tests 427

Part IV: Self-assessment **429**

Multiple-choice Questions 431
Short-answer Questions 441
Extended-matching Questions 443
Patient-management Problems 449
MCQ Answers 451
SAQ Answers 461
EMQ Answers 465

Index 467

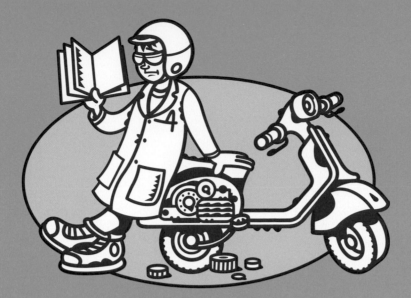

THE PATIENT PRESENTS WITH

1. Chest Pain — 3

2. Shortness of Breath — 9

3. Palpitations — 15

4. Heart Murmurs — 21

5. Cough and Haemoptysis — 29

6. Pyrexia of Unknown Origin — 33

7. Dyspepsia — 37

8. Haematemesis and Melaena — 41

9. Change in Bowel Habit — 45

10. Weight Loss — 51

11. Jaundice — 57

12. Abdominal Pain — 63

13. Polyuria and Polydipsia — 69

14. Haematuria and Proteinuria — 75

15. Hypertension — 81

16. Headache and Facial Pain — 87

17. Joint Disease — 93

18. Skin Diseases — 99

19. Loss of Consciousness — 105

20. Confusional States — 113

21. Acute Neurological Deficit — 119

22. Lymphadenopathy and Splenomegaly — 125

23. Sensory and Motor Neurological Deficits — 131

24. Bruising and Bleeding — 139

25. Vertigo and Dizziness — 145

26. Anaemia — 149

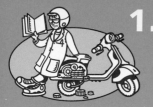

1. Chest Pain

Introduction

Chest pain is a common cause for both referral and admission to hospital. It has many possible aetiologies that need to be elucidated. Taking a clear history is essential in making the correct diagnosis.

Differential diagnosis of chest pain

Pleuritic chest pain

This is a sharp pain that is worse on deep inspiration, coughing, or movement. The differential diagnosis includes the following:

- Pneumothorax.
- Pneumonia.
- Pulmonary embolus.
- Pericarditis: retrosternal.

Central chest pain

The differential diagnosis of central pain includes the following:

- Angina: crushing/tightness.
- Myocardial infarction : angina-like but more severe, long lasting and with associated symptoms.
- Dissecting aortic aneurysm: tearing interscapular pain.
- Oesophagitis: burning.
- Oesophageal spasm.

Chest wall tenderness

The differential diagnosis of chest wall tenderness includes the following:

- Rib fracture.
- Shingles (herpes zoster): pain precedes rash.
- Costochondritis (Tietze's syndrome).

Atypical presentations

The differential diagnosis in atypical presentations (or in any of the above) includes anxiety and referred pain from vertebral collapse causing nerve root irritation or intra-abdominal pathology (e.g. pancreatitis, peptic ulcer, or biliary tree disorders).

History in the patient with chest pain

A careful history of the chest pain will generally be suggestive of the likely underlying problem. The focus should then turn to any associated symptoms and risk factors.

What type of chest pain does the patient have?
Onset and progression of pain

Cardiac ischaemic pain typically builds up over a few minutes and may be brought on by exercise, emotion, or cold weather. In angina, the pain resolves on resting or with nitrate usage (GTN). It is often reproducible with consistent effort. In unstable angina, the pain may come on at rest or be of increasing frequency or severity. In myocardial infarction (MI), the pain is severe, often associated with systemic symptoms such as nausea, vomiting, and sweating, and lasts for at least 30 minutes and is not usually fully relieved by GTN. Spontaneous pneumothorax and pulmonary embolism usually cause sudden onset of pleuritic pain and dyspnoea (the patient often remembers exactly what they were doing at the time).

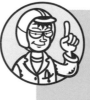 Always be aware of the patient with chronic stable angina whose symptoms are more frequent or occurring at rest. This is a medical emergency

Site and radiation of pain

Cardiac ischaemia and pericarditis cause retrosternal pain. With ischaemia, the pain is tight and 'crushing' and often radiates to the jaw or arms. Pericarditis is pleuritic and it may be worse on lying flat but relieved by sitting forward, while a dissecting aortic aneurysm causes tearing pain radiating through to the back. Pulmonary disease may cause unilateral pain, which the patient can often localise specifically. Oesophageal disease can also cause retrosternal pain and may mimic cardiac pain. Referred pain from vertebral collapse or shingles will follow a dermatomal pattern.

Nature of pain
The precise nature of the pain gives important clues as to the underlying diagnosis (see above).

Are there any associated symptoms?
Important associated symptoms include:
- Dyspnoea: pulmonary embolism, pneumonia, pneumothorax, pulmonary oedema in cardiac ischaemia, hyperventilation in anxiety.
- Cough: purulent sputum in pneumonia, haemoptysis in pulmonary embolism, frothy pink sputum in pulmonary oedema.
- Rigors: pneumonia (particularly lobar pneumonia).
- Calf swelling: has a pulmonary embolism (PE) arisen from deep vein thrombosis?
- Palpitations: arrhythmia can cause angina or result from cardiac ischaemia, PE, or pneumonia.
- Clamminess, nausea, vomiting, and sweating are features of myocardial infarction or massive pulmonary embolism.

Are risk factors present?
Important risk factors include:
- Ischaemic heart disease: smoking, family history, hypercholesterolaemia, hypertension, diabetes.
- PE: recent travel, immobility, or surgery, family history, pregnancy, malignancy.
- Pneumothorax: spontaneous (young, thin men), trauma, emphysema, asthma, malignancy.

Examining the patient with chest pain

The examination should focus on determining the cause of the pain then looking for risk factors and consequences of the underlying problem. A schematic guide to examining the patient with chest pain is given in Fig. 1.1.

What is the cause of the pain?
Pay particular attention to:
- Pulse: tachycardia/bradycardia or arrhythmia.
- Blood pressure: discrepancy between left and right arms in aortic dissection (the pulse volumes may also be unequal).

- Chest wall tenderness: rib fracture, costochondritis, anxiety, shingles.
- Chest examination: pneumothorax, consolidation, pleural rub, pulmonary oedema.
- Cardiac examination: rub (pericarditis), murmur of aortic regurgitation in aortic dissection.

Are there risk factors?
The following risk factors may be present:
- Abnormal lipids: xanthelasma, tendon xanthoma.
- Tar stained fingers: predisposition to ischaemic heart disease.
- Hot, oedematous, tender calf suggesting deep vein thrombosis.
- Hypertension: ischaemic heart disease.

What are the complications?
Complications may include:
- Pulse: arrhythmia, tachycardia / bradycardia.
- Blood pressure: shock in tension pneumothorax, massive pulmonary embolism, MI.
- Cardiac failure: pulmonary oedema and third heart sound.
- Murmurs: acute mitral regurgitation and ventricular septal defect after MI.

Investigating the patient with chest pain

All patients with chest pain should have an electrocardiogram (ECG) and chest radiograph (CXR). Further investigation will be directed by findings in these tests in conjunction with the history and clinical examination. An algorithm for the investigation of the patient with chest pain is given in Fig. 1.2.

Blood tests
Patients will have a full blood count, urea and electrolytes and glucose performed as routine. Other tests may include cardiac enzymes, Troponin I or T (see Chapter 40) at 6–12 hours after symptom onset, inflammatory markers or D-dimers as guided by history and examination. Aspartate transaminase and lactate dehydrogenase are now largely redundant in acute ischaemic chest pain.

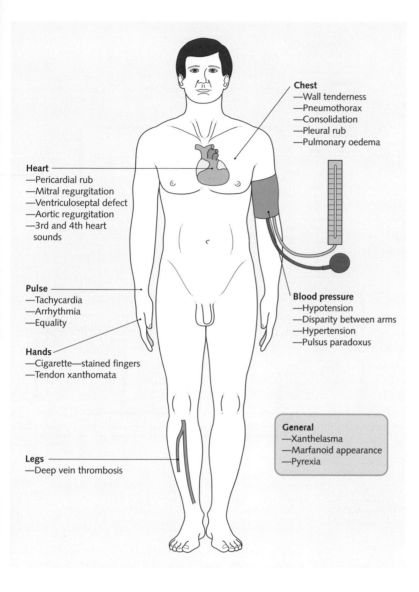

Chest
—Wall tenderness
—Pneumothorax
—Consolidation
—Pleural rub
—Pulmonary oedema

Heart
—Pericardial rub
—Mitral regurgitation
—Ventriculoseptal defect
—Aortic regurgitation
—3rd and 4th heart
   sounds

Pulse
—Tachycardia
—Arrhythmia
—Equality

Hands
—Cigarette—stained fingers
—Tendon xanthomata

Legs
—Deep vein thrombosis

Blood pressure
—Hypotension
—Disparity between arms
—Hypertension
—Pulsus paradoxus

General
—Xanthelasma
—Marfanoid appearance
—Pyrexia

Fig. 1.1 Examining the patient with chest pain.

 Whilst cardiac enzymes have been largely replaced by troponin measurements, they remain useful, especially after MI, to assess reinfarction as troponins remain raised for 2 weeks and creatine kinase should return to normal after 2–3 days

 Remember that cocaine use may be a cause of ischaemic chest pain in young patients with no obvious risk factors

Electrocardiogram

New onset left bundle branch block, T wave changes, ST depression and elevation (Fig. 1.3) on ECG are suggestive of an acute coronary syndrome. It is vital to recognise those patients who would benefit from thrombolysis or angioplasty as soon as possible. The management of myocardial infarction with and without ST segment elevation is discussed later (see Chapter 27). Changes suggestive of PE are shown in Fig. 1.4. Arrhythmia may also be detected on ECG. Serial or continuous ECGs may be needed as all the disease processes can be dynamic.

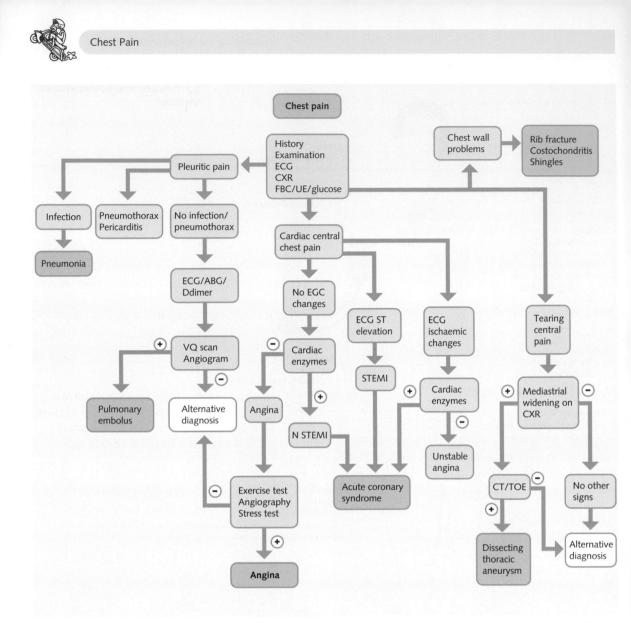

Fig. 1.2 Algorithm for the investigation of the patient with chest pain. (CXR, chest X-ray; ECG, electrocardiogram; FBC, full blood count; U&Es, urea and electrolytes, STEMI, ST segment elevation myocardial infarction; NSTEMI, non STEMI; CT, computerised tomography; TOE, transoesophageal echocardiography; V/Q scan, ventilation-perfusion scan.)

Fig. 1.3 Causes of ST elevation on ECG.

Causes of ST elevation	
Cause	**Distribution of ST elevation**
Myocardial infarction	Inferior AV_F, II, III Anteroseptal V_{1-4} Lateral I, Av_L, V_{4-6}
Pericarditis	Across all leads (saddle-shaped ST change)
Prinzmetal's angina	Leads of affected coronary artery (spasm)
Aortic dissection	Only if coronary artery involved
Left ventricular aneurysm	Persistent changes following infarct

ECG changes associated with pulmonary embolus

- Sinus tachycardia
- Atrial arrhythmia, e.g. atrial fibrillation
- Right heart strain
- Right axis deviation
- Right bundle branch block
- $S_1 Q_3 T_3$, i.e. deep S wave in I, Q wave in III, T wave inversion in III

Fig. 1.4 Electrocardiogram (ECG) changes associated with pulmonary embolus. Note that sinus tachycardia may be the only abnormality present.

Chest X-ray

Pneumothorax, consolidation (pneumonia), widened mediastinum (aortic dissection), pulmonary oedema (myocardial ischaemia/infarction) and fractured ribs may be detected on CXR.

Arterial blood gases

The assessment of arterial blood gases is useful in determining the severity of PE, pneumonia, or pulmonary oedema, showing hypoxia and occasionally hypocapnia. In hyperventilation related to anxiety, the pO_2 may be mildly elevated whilst there will be hypocapnia and a respiratory alkalosis.

Echocardiogram

Echocardiography can be used acutely to demonstrate cardiac dysfunction, valvular pathology, pericardial effusions and aortic dissection (particularly transoesophageal echocardiography). Computerised tomography (CT) is an alternative in aortic dissection.

Percutaneous coronary intervention

Angioplasty and coronary artery stenting can be used to reopen occluded arteries in acute myocardial infarction instead of thrombolysis. Coronary angiography allows direct visualisation of the coronary arterial anatomy. It is used in angina to determine whether elective angioplasty or coronary artery bypass grafting might be beneficial.

Ventilation-perfusion scan

Ventilation-perfusion (V/Q) scan is used to diagnose PE. In some circumstances (e.g. when there is pre-existing obstructive airways disease) interpretation of this test can be difficult, so pulmonary angiography should then be performed. A CT pulmonary angiogram is preferred to a V/Q scan especially if underlying lung disease is present.

Exercise test

An exercise test may be diagnostic when angina is suspected. It is mainly used in risk stratification post MI or in the outpatient clinic when investigating chest pain. It is CONTRAINDICATED in acute coronary syndromes.

Upper gastrointestinal endoscopy

Upper gastrointestinal endoscopy will confirm oesophagitis and should be considered when the cause of chest pain is unclear.

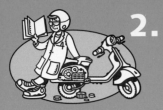

2. Shortness of Breath

Introduction

Shortness of breath (dyspnoea) is the subjective sensation of breathlessness which is excessive for any given level of activity. Dyspnoea may be due to any of the following:

- Pulmonary disease: disorders of the airways, lung parenchyma, pleura, respiratory muscles, or chest wall.
- Cardiac disease (e.g. the rise in left atrial pressure associated with cardiac dysfunction causing pulmonary oedema).
- Metabolic disease (e.g. thyrotoxicosis, ketoacidosis).
- Anaemia.
- Psychogenic causes [e.g. anxiety or hyperventilation (psychogenic dyspnoea)].

History in the patient with breathlessness

How breathless is the patient?
Try to quantify the severity by exercise tolerance (e.g. distance walked on the flat or on hills, whilst dressing or climbing stairs). How does it affect daily activities?

Specific types of dyspnoea
Orthopnoea is breathlessness on lying down. It is characteristic of heart failure but can occur with other conditions such as diaphragmatic paralysis. Paroxysmal nocturnal dyspnoea is breathlessness that wakes the patient from sleep, and is generally a symptom of cardiac disease.

Onset of dyspnoea
The onset of breathlessness and rate of decline will often give a clue to its aetiology:

- Acute onset may be due to a foreign body, pneumothorax, pulmonary embolism, asthma, or acute pulmonary oedema.
- Subacute onset is more suggestive of parenchymal disease (e.g. alveolitis, pleural effusion, pneumonia and carcinoma of the bronchus or trachea).

- Chronic onset and progressive decline is associated with chronic obstructive pulmonary disease (COPD), cryptogenic fibrosing alveolitis; occupational fibrotic lung disease, non-respiratory causes (e.g. heart failure, anaemia, or hyperthyroidism).

Determining the patient's exercise tolerance gives a useful marker of the progression of symptoms

Other factors in the history
In addition to the above, the following should be assessed when taking a history from a patient with breathlessness:

- Is the breathlessness associated with a cough? A chronic persistent cough may be due to smoking, asthma, COPD, drugs [especially angiotensin-converting enzyme (ACE) inhibitors], occupational agents, cardiac failure, or psychogenic factors.
- How long has the cough been present?
- Is the cough worse at any particular time of day?
- Are there any precipitating factors?
- If there is sputum, what does it looks like?
- Does the patient have haemoptysis? This is coughing up blood, either frank blood or blood-tinged sputum. It needs to be distinguished from haematemesis and nasopharyngeal bleeding (see Chapter 5 for the causes of cough and haemoptysis.)
- Ask about stridor (a harsh sound caused by turbulent airflow through a narrowed airway). Inspiratory stridor suggests extrathoracic obstruction, expiratory stridor suggests intrathoracic obstruction, and inspiratory and expiratory stridor suggests a fixed obstruction.
- Does the patient wheeze? These are whistling noises caused by turbulent airflow through narrowed intrathoracic airways. The commonest cause is asthma.
- Does the breathlessness affect the activities of daily living and quality of life?

- Occupational history, including exposure to asbestos and dusts. Occupational lung disease is important as improving the working environment may improve symptoms or the patient may benefit from financial compensation.
- Dyspnoea that improves at weekends may imply a response to a trigger at work.
- Is there any known lung disease either present such as asthma or previously (e.g. tuberculosis)?
- Ask if any history of atopy (e.g. childhood asthma, rhinitis or eczema).
- Does the patient own a pet? This can exacerbate asthma or cause a chronic progressive lung disease (e.g. the extrinsic allergic alveolitis of 'pigeon fanciers' lung').
- What medications is the patient taking? Non-cardioselective beta blockers may exacerbate wheeze; however, concerns over the cardioselective agents are probably exaggerated.
- What medications has the patient taken in the past (e.g. pulmonary fibrosis associated with amiodarone use)?
- Inquire about general health (e.g. weight loss, appetite, etc., for a non respiratory cause for the dyspnoea.
- Full smoking history.

Examining the patient with breathlessness

The findings on examination of common respiratory conditions are listed in Fig. 2.1, and the examination approach in the patient with breathlessness is summarised in Fig. 2.2. A more detailed description showing examination findings in respiratory disease can be found in Chapter 38.

Inspection

Note the respiratory rate from the end of the bed, or whilst feeling the pulse. Assess ease of breathing, use of accessory muscles and any audible sounds.

Look for central cyanosis (a blue colour in the mouth and tongue due to excess deoxygenated haemoglobin, i.e. >5 g reduced haemoglobin per 100 ml of blood). It is commonly associated with lung disease and cardiac disease.

Note, however, that cyanosis is an unreliable guide to the degree of hypoxaemia. Peripheral cyanosis is due to poor peripheral circulation (e.g. in cardiac failure, peripheral vascular disease, or arterial obstruction, and physiological when due to cold). Cyanosis is rarely seen in anaemic patients.

The following factors should also be looked for when assessing the patient with breathlessness:

- Anaemia.
- Tar staining of the fingers.
- Clubbing: respiratory causes include carcinoma of the bronchus; pus in any part of the respiratory tract (e.g. empyema, lung abscess, bronchiectasis, cystic fibrosis); fibrosing alveolitis; chronic suppurative pulmonary tuberculosis and mesothelioma.
- Chest movements on inspiration and expiration: pathology is normally found on the side of diminished movements.
- Barrel-shaped chest: emphysema.
- Kyphoscoliosis: can decrease chest size and expansion.
- Ankylosing spondylitis: can 'fix' the chest.
- Use of accessory muscles of respiration.
- Paradoxical abdominal movements in diaphragmatic weakness.

Findings on examination of common respiratory conditions					
Condition	Movement on side of lesion	Position of trachea	Percussion	Tactile vocal fremitus	Breath sounds
Pleural effusion	↓	Central or deviated away from effusion if massive	↓ ('stony dull')	↓	↓ with bronchial breathing at top of effusion
Pneumothorax	↓	Central or deviated away	↑	↓	↓
Pneumonia	↓	Central or deviated towards if associated with collapse	↓	↑	Increased vocal resonance bronchial breathing (absent if obstruction of bronchus) coarse crepitations
Pulmonary fibrosis	↓	Central or deviated towards if upper lobe involvement	↓	↑	Bronchial breathing Fine crepitations

Fig. 2.1 Findings on examination of common respiratory conditions.

Fig. 2.2 Examining the patient with breathlessness.

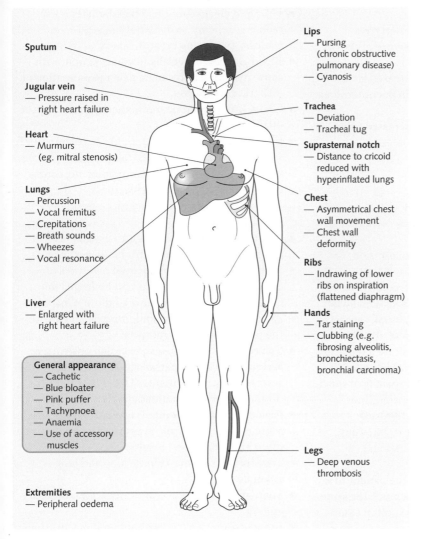

Sputum

Jugular vein
— Pressure raised in right heart failure

Heart
— Murmurs (eg. mitral stenosis)

Lungs
— Percussion
— Vocal fremitus
— Crepitations
— Breath sounds
— Wheezes
— Vocal resonance

Liver
— Enlarged with right heart failure

General appearance
— Cachetic
— Blue bloater
— Pink puffer
— Tachypnoea
— Anaemia
— Use of accessory muscles

Extremities
— Peripheral oedema

Lips
— Pursing (chronic obstructive pulmonary disease)
— Cyanosis

Trachea
— Deviation
— Tracheal tug

Suprasternal notch
— Distance to cricoid reduced with hyperinflated lungs

Chest
— Asymmetrical chest wall movement
— Chest wall deformity

Ribs
— Indrawing of lower ribs on inspiration (flattened diaphragm)

Hands
— Tar staining
— Clubbing (e.g. fibrosing alveolitis, bronchiectasis, bronchial carcinoma)

Legs
— Deep venous thrombosis

- Rhythm of respiration: Cheyne–Stokes respiration describes periods of fast and deep inspiration followed by periods of apnoea due to depression of the central respiratory centre in the medulla. It is seen in neurological disease, severe left ventricular failure and normal people when at high altitude.

Palpation

- Feel for lymphadenopathy secondary to malignant disease or infections.
- Palpate the trachea: displacement may indicate underlying chest disease or cardiac disease.
- Assess the expansion of the rib cage.
- Feel for tactile vocal fremitus.
- Compare both sides anteriorly and posteriorly.

Do not forget to look at the sputum pot:
- Purulent, moderate quantity–bronchitis or pneumonia.
- Purulent, copious quantity–bronchiectasis or pneumonia.
- Pink and frothy–pulmonary oedema.
- Blood stained–causes of haemoptysis.
- Rust-coloured–pneumococcal lobar pneumonia.

Percussion

- Percuss both anteriorly and posteriorly in a systematic manner to assess the nature of the underlying lung.
- Increased resonance indicates increased air beneath and can be seen acutely in pneumothorax or chronically in emphysema.
- Decreased resonance indicates increased solid matter beneath which could be infection or effusion (classically 'stony' dull).

Auscultation

- Expiration: may be prolonged in COPD.
- Bronchial breathing: consolidation, cavitation, or at the top of an effusion.
- Breath sounds: diminished over an effusion, pneumothorax, and in the obese.
- Rhonchi or wheeze: partially obstructed bronchi; found in asthma, bronchitis, and occasionally left ventricular failure. If polyphonic, usually suggests multiple small airway narrowing and, if monophonic and fixed, it may indicate a fixed single obstruction e.g. a central malignant lesion.
- Crepitations or crackles (sudden opening of small closed airways): pulmonary congestion (fine crepitations in early inspiration); fibrosing alveolitis (fine crepitations in late inspiration); bronchial secretions (coarse crepitations).
- Friction rub: pleural disease.
- Assess vocal resonance by asking the patient to say and then whisper '99'. It provides much the same information as vocal fremitus but is often easier to detect. Consolidation leads to increased and easily heard speech due to solid lung tissue conducting the sounds to the chest wall.

To simulate the sound of bronchial breathing, place the stethoscope over your own trachea and listen

Investigating the patient with breathlessness

An algorithm for the investigation of the patient with breathlessness is given in Fig. 2.3. The following investigations should be performed:

- Full blood count: anaemia leading to breathlessness, leucocytosis in pneumonia.

- Urea and electrolytes, and bicarbonate: renal failure secondary to dehydration, sepsis, or acidosis, producing breathlessness.
- Blood glucose: especially in young people with acute dyspnoea as it can be a first presentation of diabetic ketoacidosis.
- Chest X-ray: examine methodically (see Chapter 40).
- Electrocardiogram (ECG): $S_1 Q_3 T_3$ pattern in PE (see Fig. 1.4), p pulmonale (tall p waves >2.5 mm in lead II) in COPD with cor pulmonale; cardiac conditions leading to breathlessness (e.g. myocardial infarction with consequent pulmonary oedema).
- Arterial oxygen saturations are easy to perform and may obviate the need for blood gas analysis.
- Arterial blood gases: pH, partial pressures of oxygen and carbon dioxide, and hydrogen ion concentration (see respiratory failure, Chapter 28). If possible, these should first be taken with the patient breathing room air.
- Spirometry: to distinguish between obstructive and restrictive lung pathology, and to test reversibility to treatments. This is best done for diagnosis when the patient is well.
- Peak expiratory flow rate is useful for assessing acute decline especially in asthmatic patients who often know their best results.
- Transfer factor, flow-volume loop and lung volumes.
- Ventilation-perfusion scan: suspected pulmonary emboli.
- Bronchoscopy with or without washing, brushings or biopsies.
- Computerised tomography scanning can be used to assess both acute and chronic dyspnoea (e.g. to investigate pulmonary emboli and to diagnose and quantify pulmonary fibrosis and bronchiectasis).

Metabolic acidosis leads to a 'deep sighing' pattern of breathing (Kussmaul respiration). Causes include uraemia, diabetic ketoacidosis, salicylate ingestion, methanol ingestion, and lactic acidosis

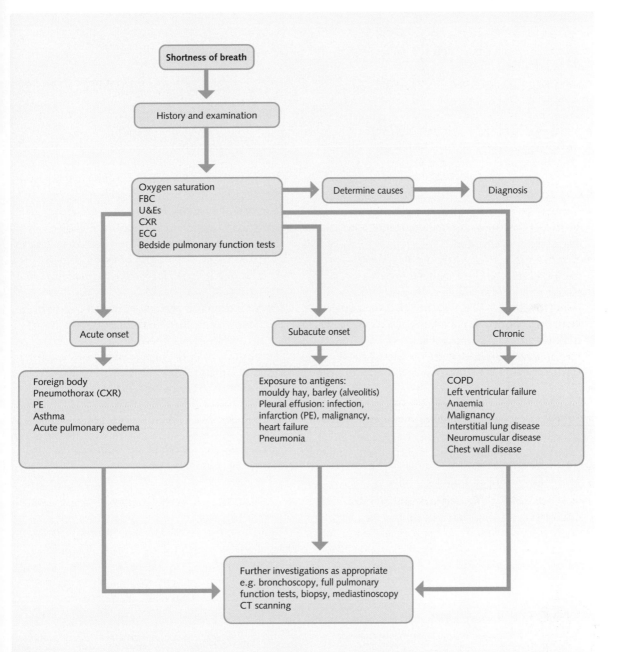

Fig. 2.3 Algorithm for the investigation and differential diagnosis of the breathless patient. Note that more than one cause of shortness of breath may be apparent. (COPD, chronic obstructive pulmonary disease; CXR, chest X-ray; ECG, electrocardiogram; FBC, full blood count; U&Es, urea and electrolytes; PE, pulmonary embolus; V/Q, ventilation-perfusion scan.)

Remember the upper lobes of the lungs are best heard on the anterior chest wall

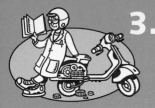

3. Palpitations

Introduction

Always check what the patient means by 'palpitations', or clarify what you mean by them, because the word means different things to different people. It is usually understood as an awareness of the heartbeat. The most common cause is an arrhythmia although other causes include conditions causing an increase in stroke volume (e.g. regurgitant valvular disease) or conditions causing an increase in cardiac output, often non-cardiac causes (e.g. exercise, thyrotoxicosis, anaemia, or anxiety). If an arrhythmia is suspected determine whether there is an underlying cause.

Differential diagnosis by description of the rhythm

Regular rhythm

The differential diagnosis of regular palpitations (Fig. 3.1) includes the following:

- Heavy heart beats with normal rate: most often cardiac consciousness with sinus rhythm. It tends to be worse at rest, especially when in bed at night and during periods of stress.
- Fast heart rate: sinus tachycardia, atrial flutter with block, or ventricular tachycardia.
- Bursts of fast beats: paroxysmal atrial tachycardia. There is often a very long history dating back years with a single attack followed by a long interval before the next attack. Other causes include atrial flutter, junctional rhythm, or ventricular tachycardia.
- Slow heart rate: sinus bradycardia , atrioventricular block.

Irregular rhythm

The differential diagnosis of irregular palpitations (Fig. 3.1) includes the following:

- Missed beats, 'thumps': multiple ectopics from the atrium or ventricle. The symptoms are more troublesome at rest and may disappear during exercise.

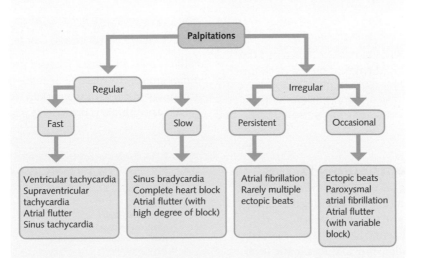

Fig. 3.1 Differential diagnosis of palpitations.

- Fast (or normal if treated): atrial flutter with variable block, atrial fibrillation (persistent irregularity with exercise), and multiple premature beats with sinus tachycardia.

History

A careful history of the palpitations will often lead to the correct diagnosis, especially as between episodes examination and investigations may be unremarkable. Are they continuous or intermittent? Are they fast, normal rate, or slow? Are they regular or irregular? When did the palpitations start? This can vary from a few minutes to decades. Generally, if the onset dates back years and there have been no serious complications (e.g. syncope) the palpitations are usually benign.

How often do the palpitations occur and how long do they last for? They may last for days or seconds, with intervals between episodes of a few hours to years. Has the patient learnt any manoeuvres to terminate the attacks? Enquire about the patient's concerns as they may fear serious underlying cardiac disease, although there is often a benign cause. Are there any associated features? These may be related to the underlying cause (e.g. angina, features of hyperthyroidism) or a consequence of the palpitations (e.g. dizziness or syncope).

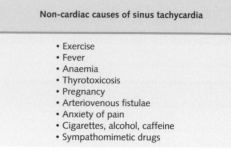

Non-cardiac causes of sinus tachycardia

- Exercise
- Fever
- Anaemia
- Thyrotoxicosis
- Pregnancy
- Arteriovenous fistulae
- Anxiety of pain
- Cigarettes, alcohol, caffeine
- Sympathomimetic drugs

Fig. 3.2 Non-cardiac causes of sinus tachycardia.

hypertrophic obstructive cardiomyopathy or long QT syndromes).

A full drug history of both prescribed and over the counter medications is essential. Remember many drugs both cardiac and non-cardiac can promote palpitations. Most anti-arrhythmic drugs are also potentially pro-arrhythmic.

Non-cardiac causes of sinus tachycardia and causes of sinus bradycardia are outlined in Figs 3.2 and 3.3, respectively.

Non-cardiac causes of palpitations include the following:

- Thyrotoxicosis: may cause sinus tachycardia, paroxysmal atrial tachycardia, and atrial flutter/fibrillation.
- Myxoedema: may be responsible for sinus bradycardia.
- Anxiety: a very common cause of palpitations.

Ask the patient to tap out the heart rhythm on the desk top. This will often give a good guide to diagnosis

Consequences of palpitations

Palpitations can cause a range of problems, from minor anxiety to syncope or sudden death. This accounts for much of the patient's concern. If a benign arrhythmia is present, reassurance that the

Causal and contributory factors

Ask about smoking, alcohol, work, stress, caffeine (tea, coffee, cola) intake and any illegal drug use. These may contribute to extrasystoles.

A history of ischaemic heart disease, valvular heart disease including previous rheumatic fever should be sought, as structural heart problems will predispose to pathological arrhythmias.

A family history of palpitations or sudden cardiac death may be important (e.g.

Causes of sinus bradycardia

- Athletes
- Hypothyroidism
- Obstructive jaundice
- Raised intracranial pressure
- Hypopituitarism
- Hypothermia
- Cardiac causes include ischaemia, drugs (e.g. digoxin and β-blockers), inflammation, degeneration/fibrosis

Fig. 3.3 Causes of sinus bradycardia.

condition is not serious is often all that is required. Changes in rate may be more serious, compromising coronary blood supply and leading to symptoms of myocardial ischaemia or cardiac failure.

Tachycardia or bradycardia may lead to a reduction in cardiac output and cause dizziness or collapse (e.g. Stokes–Adams attacks in complete heart block). Ventricular tachycardia is potentially life threatening and as there exist several effective treatments it should be considered especially in patients with structurally abnormal hearts.

Examining the patient with palpitations

A guide to examining the patient with palpitations is given in Fig. 3.4. Look for signs of systemic diseases. Next feel the pulse. Note the following:

- Rate: beats per minute.
- Rhythm: regular, regularly irregular (e.g. Wenkebach second degree heart block), irregularly irregular (e.g. multiple ectopic beats or atrial fibrillation).
- Volume/character (e.g. a collapsing pulse of hyperdynamic circulation or a low volume pulse of shock or aortic stenosis).

If the patient is symptom free at the time of examination, the pulse may be normal.

The blood pressure will be low if the arrhythmia leads to a reduction in cardiac output. Hypertension may predispose to atrial fibrillation.

The jugular venous pressure may be elevated if cardiac failure is present. 'Cannon' a waves are visible with complete heart block, and a waves are absent in atrial fibrillation.

A displaced apex may point towards cardiomyopathy. Feel for heaves and thrills with

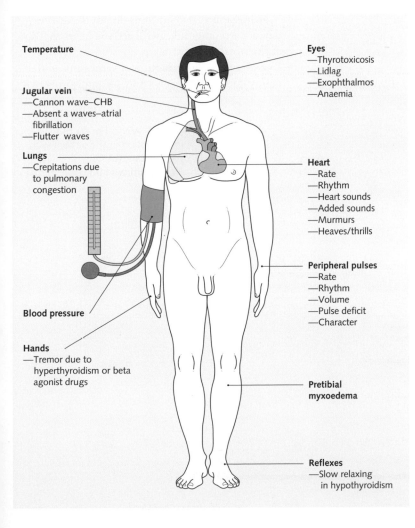

Fig. 3.4 Examining the patient with palpitations. (CHB, complete heart block.)

Temperature

Jugular vein
—Cannon wave–CHB
—Absent a waves–atrial fibrillation
—Flutter waves

Lungs
—Crepitations due to pulmonary congestion

Blood pressure

Hands
—Tremor due to hyperthyroidism or beta agonist drugs

Eyes
—Thyrotoxicosis
—Lidlag
—Exophthalmos
—Anaemia

Heart
—Rate
—Rhythm
—Heart sounds
—Added sounds
—Murmurs
—Heaves/thrills

Peripheral pulses
—Rate
—Rhythm
—Volume
—Pulse deficit
—Character

Pretibial myxoedema

Reflexes
—Slow relaxing in hypothyroidism

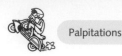

associated right ventricular enlargement and valvular heart disease. Assess the rate and rhythm by auscultation. The peripheral pulse rate may be slower than the apical rate in atrial fibrillation (pulse deficit). Listen for cardiac murmurs (e.g. evidence of mitral valve disease, mitral valve prolapse). Focus on any abnormal findings (see Chapter 4).

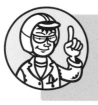 An irregularly irregular pulse (e.g. in atrial fibrillation) is irregular in both rhythm AND volume

Investigating the patient with palpitations

An algorithm for the investigation of the patient with palpitations is given in Fig. 3.5. The following tests should be performed:

Blood tests
- Full blood count: anaemia.
- Urea and electrolytes: especially disturbances of potassium or less commonly magnesium and

calcium may contribute to refractory arrhythmias.
- Thyroid function tests: hypo/hyperthyroidism.
- Drug concentration if appropriate (e.g. digoxin levels).

Other tests
- 12-lead electrocardiogram (ECG): though mandatory for everyone with palpitations rarely provides the diagnosis as it is unlikely that they will be caught on a resting 12-lead ECG. Wolff-Parkinson–White syndrome will be seen at rest, as will AF. Careful analysis of the QRS morphology and QT interval, etc., may be important.
- 24-hour ECG: for intermittent symptoms. It should be carried out with a diary of symptoms to see if they correlate with any rhythm disturbances found.
- Echocardiogram: to exclude any underlying structural heart disease.
- 'Cardiomemo': if symptoms do not occur every day, a 'cardiomemo' can record the heart rhythm at the press of a button.
- Exercise test: the induction of symptoms under controlled conditions with ECG monitoring may be appropriate.

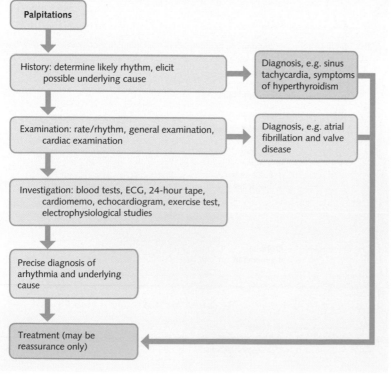

Fig. 3.5 Algorithm for the investigation of the patient with palpitations. (ECG, electrocardiogram.)

- Electrophysiological studies: more rarely, patients may be referred for specialised studies. These can be used to induce arrhythmias, locate the origin of any arrhythmic foci, to assess the response to drug treatment or destroy any aberrant pathway via radiofrequency ablation.

Fast atrial fibrillation is easily confused with a regular tachycardia when assessing the pulse

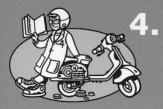

Introduction

Heart murmurs are due to vibration caused by turbulent blood flow within the heart. The commonest causes in examinations and real clinical practice are due to left-sided valvular heart disease and tricuspid regurgitation. Non-valvular causes include:

- Innocent 'flow' murmurs, especially in children.
- High cardiac output states (e.g. pregnancy, thyrotoxicosis, and fever).
- Congenital heart disease, e.g. atrial septal defects (ASD), ventricular septal defects (VSD), patent ductus arteriosus (PDA), and coarctation of the aorta.

Differential diagnosis of heart murmurs

The classification of heart murmurs includes ejection systolic murmurs, pansystolic murmurs, diastolic murmurs, and continuous murmurs.

Ejection systolic murmurs

These usually originate in the right or left ventricular outflow tracts. They reach a crescendo in mid-systole and die down before the second heart sound.

Causes of ejection systolic murmurs in the aortic area (second right intercostal space) include the following:

- Supravalvular (e.g. supra-aortic stenosis or coarctation of the aorta).
- Valvular (e.g. aortic stenosis or aortic sclerosis).
- Subvalvular (e.g. hypertrophic obstructive cardiomyopathy).
- Hyperkinetic high cardiac output states.

Causes of ejection systolic murmurs in the pulmonary area (second left intercostal space) include the following:

- Supravalvular (e.g. pulmonary arterial stenosis).
- Valvular (e.g. pulmonary valve stenosis).
- Subvalvular (e.g. infundibular stenosis).
- Flow murmurs, hyperkinetic states, and left-to-right shunts (e.g. ASD).

Causes of ejection systolic murmurs at the apex include flow murmurs and aortic stenosis (radiation from the aortic area).

Pansystolic murmurs

These murmurs are of uniform intensity and are heard throughout systole, merging with the second heart sound.

Causes of pansystolic murmurs at the lower left sternal edge include:

- Tricuspid regurgitation.
- Ventricular septal defects.

Causes heard best at the apex include:

- Mitral regurgitation.
- Mitral valve prolapse.

Diastolic murmurs

Causes of early diastolic murmurs at the left sternal edge include:

- Aortic regurgitation.
- Pulmonary regurgitation.

Causes of diastolic murmurs at the apex include the following:

- Mitral stenosis.
- Carey Coombs murmur (due to thickening of mitral valve leaflets in acute rheumatic fever).
- Austin Flint murmur (due to fluttering of the anterior mitral valve cusp in aortic regurgitation by the regurgitant stream).
- Graham Steell murmur: pulmonary regurgitation secondary to pulmonary hypertension (also heard at left sternal edge).

Continuous murmurs

Continuous murmurs are heard during systole and diastole, such as patent ductus arteriosus, coronary arteriovenous fistula, ruptured aneurysm of the sinus of Valsalva, cervical venous hum, or ASD with mitral stenosis. These are rare in adult medical practice.

 Pure diastolic murmurs are ALWAYS pathological

History in the patient with heart murmurs

There are no symptoms of cardiac murmurs *per se* and so the history should focus on possible causes of the murmur or consequences of the responsible lesion. Ask about the following:

- Rheumatic fever: particularly affecting the mitral valve.
- Ischaemic heart disease (e.g. mitral regurgitation).
- Congenital heart disease.
- Hypertension: flow murmurs.
- Intravenous drug use use, especially in young people and new right-sided heart murmurs.
- Family history: hypertrophic cardiomyopathy is inherited as an autosomal dominant condition.
- Aortic regurgitation may be associated with rheumatoid arthritis or seronegative arthropathies (e.g. ankylosing spondylitis, Reiter's syndrome, enteropathic or psoriatic arthropathy, Marfan's syndrome, syphilitic aortitis, or coarctation of the aorta). If you suspect any of these, question further about joint symptoms, gastrointestinal symptoms and neurological symptoms as indicated.
- Mitral regurgitation may be caused by connective tissue disorders (e.g. systemic lupus erythematosus, rheumatoid arthritis), ankylosing spondylitis, or by congenital conditions (e.g. Marfan's syndrome, Ehlcrs–Danlos syndrome, pseudoxanthoma elasticum, or osteogenesis imperfecta).

Consequences

The following consequences of a heart murmur may be noted:

- None: aortic valve disease and mitral regurgitation may remain asymptomatic.
- Fatigue and weakness: low cardiac output.
- Palpitations: especially atrial fibrillation.
- Angina: especially in aortic stenosis.
- Symptoms of right ventricular failure: intestinal mucosal congestion, anorexia, ankle and leg oedema plus hepatic pain.
- Symptoms of left ventricular failure: breathlessness on exertion, cough and haemoptysis (especially mitral stenosis), orthopnoea, and paroxysmal nocturnal dyspnoea (PND).

- Syncope due to poor cardiac output in conditions obstructing the outflow tract (e.g. severe aortic stenosis).
- Symptoms of systemic emboli (e.g. transient ischaemic attacks or stroke); often a complication in mitral stenosis.
- Symptoms of an enlarged left atrium pressing on other structures, especially in mitral stenosis [e.g. the recurrent laryngeal nerve leading to hoarseness (Ortner's syndrome), the oesophagus leading to dysphagia, or the left main bronchus leading to left lung collapse].
- Symptoms of infective endocarditis.

Remember that mixed valve disease is common. The clinical skill is to diagnose the dominant valvular lesion

Examining the patient with heart murmurs

Always follow the examination routine–inspection, palpation, then auscultation. Many clues can be gained about the nature of the murmur before the stethoscope is placed on the chest.

Mitral stenosis
Clinical symptoms

Dyspnoea on exertion is an early symptom, and may progress to orthopnoea and PND. Breathlessness often worsens considerably with the onset of atrial fibrillation (loss of atrial systole), and is often accompanied by palpitations. Cough and haemoptysis may occur because of bronchitis, pulmonary infarction, pulmonary congestion, and bronchial vein rupture. Systemic emboli may occur in patients, particularly in atrial fibrillation. Fatigue and cold extremities are late symptoms, probably secondary to a low cardiac output. Chest pain occurs in a few people and may be due to coronary artery embolism or severe pulmonary hypertension. The patient may have coexistent coronary artery disease.

Clinical signs

The clinical signs of mitral stenosis are given in Fig. 4.1.

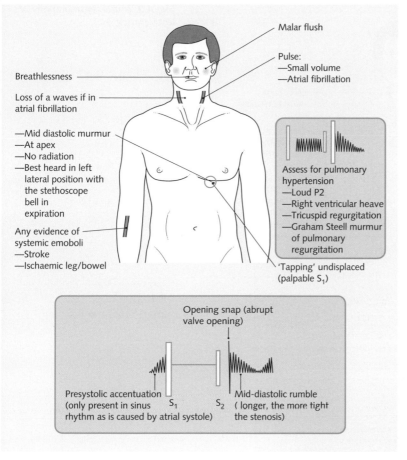

Fig. 4.1 Mitral stenosis. (AF, atrial fibrillation.)

Malar flush

Pulse:
—Small volume
—Atrial fibrillation

Breathlessness

Loss of a waves if in atrial fibrillation

—Mid diastolic murmur
—At apex
—No radiation
—Best heard in left lateral position with the stethoscope bell in expiration

Any evidence of systemic emoboli
—Stroke
—Ischaemic leg/bowel

Assess for pulmonary hypertension
—Loud P2
—Right ventricular heave
—Tricuspid regurgitation
—Graham Steell murmur of pulmonary regurgitation

'Tapping' undisplaced (palpable S_1)

Opening snap (abrupt valve opening)

Presystolic accentuation (only present in sinus rhythm as is caused by atrial systole)

S_1 S_2

Mid-diastolic rumble (longer, the more tight the stenosis)

Differential diagnosis

The differential diagnosis of mitral stenosis includes the following:

- Inflow obstruction (e.g. hypertrophic cardiomyopathy or left atrial myxoma).
- Aortic regurgitation.
- Tricuspid stenosis.

Investigations

The electrocardiogram (ECG) may show atrial fibrillation or 'p' mitrale in sinus rhythm.

The chest radiograph (CXR) shows left atrial enlargement visible as a double shadow behind the heart or widened carina. Valve calcification may be seen in lateral projections.

Echocardiography can be used to assess the area of the mitral valve orifice, and the gradient across the mitral valve. It can also be used to assess left ventricular function and measure the size of the left atrium, and the right-sided heart chambers.

Cardiac catheterisation is usually reserved for patients with suspected coronary artery disease but can be used to measure the pulmonary artery occlusion pressure as an indirect value of left atrial pressure and the left ventricular end diastolic pressure, and hence the gradient across the mitral valve. The measurements should be repeated after exercise if the right-sided heart pressures are normal.

Mitral regurgitation
Clinical symptoms

Progressive exertional dyspnoea, palpitations, and fatigue are common, with symptoms of pulmonary oedema if severe. Atrial fibrillation, systemic emboli, and chest pain are less common than in mitral stenosis.

Clinical signs

The clinical signs of mitral regurgitation are given in Fig. 4.2.

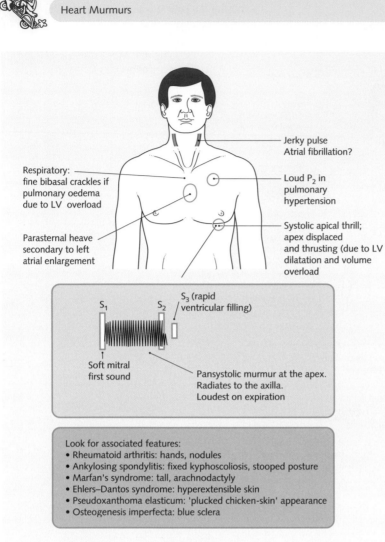

Fig. 4.2 Mitral regurgitation (LV, left ventricle.)

Jerky pulse
Atrial fibrillation?

Respiratory:
fine bibasal crackles if
pulmonary oedema
due to LV overload

Loud P$_2$ in
pulmonary
hypertension

Parasternal heave
secondary to left
atrial enlargement

Systolic apical thrill;
apex displaced
and thrusting (due to LV
dilatation and volume
overload

S$_1$ S$_2$ S$_3$ (rapid
ventricular filling)

Soft mitral
first sound

Pansystolic murmur at the apex.
Radiates to the axilla.
Loudest on expiration

Look for associated features:
• Rheumatoid arthritis: hands, nodules
• Ankylosing spondylitis: fixed kyphoscoliosis, stooped posture
• Marfan's syndrome: tall, arachnodactyly
• Ehlers–Dantos syndrome: hyperextensible skin
• Pseudoxanthoma elasticum: 'plucked chicken-skin' appearance
• Osteogenesis imperfecta: blue sclera

Differential diagnosis

The differential diagnosis of mitral regurgitation includes the following:

- Aortic stenosis.
- Hypertrophic cardiomyopathy.
- VSD.
- Tricuspid regurgitation.

Investigations

The CXR shows cardiomegaly with enlargement of the left ventricle and left atrium. In acute mitral regurgitation the heart size is normal with signs of pulmonary oedema.

The ECG may show signs of previous ischaemic heart disease, left ventricular hypertrophy (LVH), 'p' mitrale associated with left atrial hypertrophy, and occasionally atrial fibrillation.

Echocardiography may reveal a cause for the regurgitation and can be used to assess the degree of left ventricular dilatation and function, which is useful for following the progress of the regurgitation.

Aortic stenosis
Clinical symptoms

Initially the patient may be asymptomatic. Classically late symptoms are angina pectoris, exertional dyspnoea, and syncope. Sudden death may occur, probably secondary to ventricular dysrhythmias.

Clinical signs

Clinical signs in aortic stenosis are given in Fig. 4.3.

Fig. 4.3 Aortic stenosis. (LVH, left ventricular hypertrophy.)

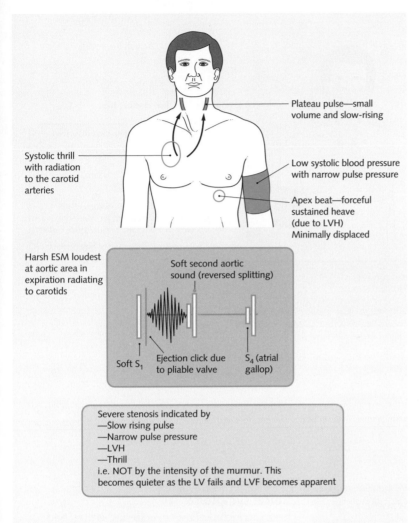

Plateau pulse—small volume and slow-rising

Systolic thrill with radiation to the carotid arteries

Low systolic blood pressure with narrow pulse pressure

Apex beat—forceful sustained heave (due to LVH) Minimally displaced

Harsh ESM loudest at aortic area in expiration radiating to carotids

Soft second aortic sound (reversed splitting)

Soft S₁

Ejection click due to pliable valve

S₄ (atrial gallop)

Severe stenosis indicated by
—Slow rising pulse
—Narrow pulse pressure
—LVH
—Thrill
i.e. NOT by the intensity of the murmur. This becomes quieter as the LV fails and LVF becomes apparent

Investigations

The ECG shows signs of LVH with increased QRS voltages and lateral ST/T segment changes.

The CXR usually shows a normal heart size. The ascending aorta may be prominent due to poststenotic dilatation, and the valve may be calcified.

Echocardiography may show a calcified valve and can be used to estimate the valve area. Cardiac chamber dimensions can be assessed, and doppler studies can be used to assess the gradient across the valve.

Cardiac catheterisation is usually only necessary prior to surgery to exclude coexisting coronary disease but can determine the systolic gradient across the valve.

Aortic regurgitation

Clinical symptoms

The patient is usually asymptomatic until the ventricle fails, giving rise to symptoms of heart failure. Angina rarely occurs.

Clinical signs

Clinical signs in aortic regurgitation are given in Fig. 4.4. The pulse has a sharp rise and fall ('collapsing' or 'water hammer') with a wide pulse pressure. Other manifestations of this are visible pulsation in the nail bed (Quincke's sign), visible arterial pulsation in the neck (Corrigan's sign), head bobbing (de Musset's sign), 'pistol shot' femoral artery sound (Traube's sign), and a diastolic murmur following distal compression of the artery (Duroziez's sign).

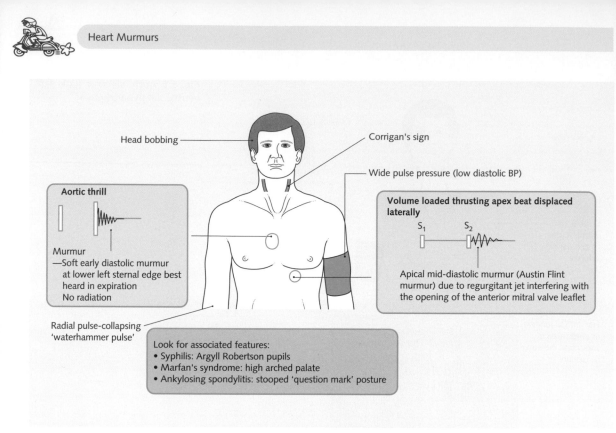

Head bobbing

Corrigan's sign

Wide pulse pressure (low diastolic BP)

Aortic thrill

Murmur
—Soft early diastolic murmur
at lower left sternal edge best
heard in expiration
No radiation

Volume loaded thrusting apex beat displaced laterally

S_1 S_2

Apical mid-diastolic murmur (Austin Flint murmur) due to regurgitant jet interfering with the opening of the anterior mitral valve leaflet

Radial pulse-collapsing 'waterhammer pulse'

Look for associated features:
• Syphilis: Argyll Robertson pupils
• Marfan's syndrome: high arched palate
• Ankylosing spondylitis: stooped 'question mark' posture

Fig. 4.4 Aortic regurgitation.

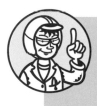

When listening for aortic regurgitation, ask the patient to sit up and hold his or her breath in expiration. Remember 'the absence of silence'

Differential diagnosis

The differential diagnosis of aortic regurgitation includes the following:

• Pulmonary regurgitation.
• PDA.
• VSD and aortic regurgitation.
• Ruptured aneurysm of the sinus of Valsalva.

Investigations

The ECG may show signs of LVH and the CXR reveals cardiomegaly. Echocardiography can assess chamber size severity of regurgitation and may give a clue to the aetiology. Cardiac catheterisation can be used to assess the severity of the regurgitation, assess ventricular function, and for coronary angiography.

Tricuspid regurgitation
Clinical symptoms

These can include fatigue, oedema, ascites, and hepatic pain as the liver capsule is stretched.

Clinical signs

These are shown in Fig. 4.5.

ECG and CXR are both non specific and may show signs of dilatation and failure of the right ventricle.

Echocardiography will diagnose and quantify the tricuspid regurgitation.

Left-sided heart murmurs are loudest in expiration and right-sided heart murmurs in inspiration due to increased blood flow across the valves

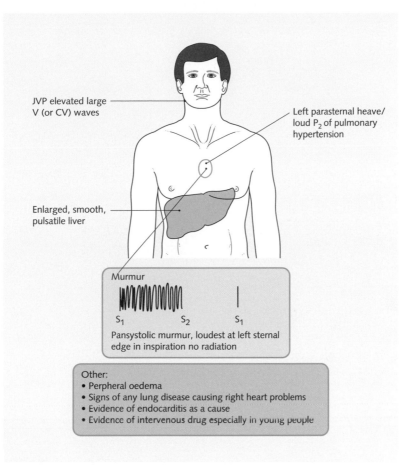

JVP elevated large V (or CV) waves

Left parasternal heave/ loud P_2 of pulmonary hypertension

Enlarged, smooth, pulsatile liver

Murmur

S_1 S_2 S_1

Pansystolic murmur, loudest at left sternal edge in inspiration no radiation

Other:
- Perpheral oedema
- Signs of any lung disease causing right heart problems
- Evidence of endocarditis as a cause
- Evidence of intervenous drug especially in young people

Fig. 4.5 Tricuspid regurgitation.

There are four things to remember when describing a murmur. (i) Where is it loudest on the praecordium? (ii) Where is it in the cardiac cycle? (iii) What happens on inspiration and expiration? (iv) Where does it radiate to?

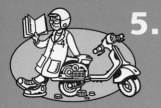

5. Cough and Haemoptysis

Introduction

Coughing is a non-specific reaction to irritation anywhere in the respiratory tract from the pharynx to the alveolus, and it is the commonest manifestation of lower respiratory tract disease. Although most commonly caused by infection, it can herald more serious pathology. Any cough that persists for over 3 weeks merits further investigation in the absence of an obvious cause.

Differential diagnosis of cough and haemoptysis

Cough

The differential diagnosis of cough includes:
- Postnasal drip: sinusitis.
- Upper respiratory tract infections (c.g. pharyngitis, laryngitis, tracheobronchitis).
- Pressure on the trachea (e.g. from a goitre): this may be associated with stridor.
- Lower respiratory tract causes: almost any lung pathology may be associated with cough, in particular asthma (suspect if there is a nocturnal cough), chronic obstructive pulmonary disease (COPD), bronchiectasis, interstitial lung disease and carcinoma.
- Left ventricular failure.
- Drugs [e.g. angiotensin-converting enzyme (ACE) inhibitors] and irritants, especially occupational agents.
- Psychogenic cough.
- Non-respiratory causes (e.g. pericardial irritation, gastro-oesophageal reflux).
- Causes of haemoptysis.

Haemoptysis

Common causes of haemoptysis include the following:
- Acute infections (e.g. exacerbations of COPD).
- Bronchiectasis: can be responsible for massive haemoptysis.
- Bronchial carcinoma: secondary deposits and benign tumours can also lead to haemoptysis but are less common.
- Pulmonary tuberculosis: a common cause worldwide.
- Pulmonary embolus with infarction.
- Left ventricular failure can lead to the production of pink, frothy sputum.
- Vasculitis (e.g. Goodpasture's syndrome and Wegener's granulomatosis).
- Other infections, such as lobar pneumonia ('rusty' sputum) or, less commonly, lung abscess.
- Trauma (e.g. contusions to the chest, inhalation of foreign bodies, or after intubation).

Rare causes of haemoptysis include the following:
- Bleeding diatheses.
- Interstitial lung disease.
- Mitral stenosis.
- Idiopathic pulmonary haemosiderosis.
- Arteriovenous malformations (Osler–Weber–Rendu disease (hereditary haemorrhagic telangiectasia), a favourite in exams but rare in practice).
- Eisenmenger's syndrome.
- Sarcoidosis and amyloidosis.
- Primary pulmonary hypertension.
- Cystic fibrosis.

Note that in up to 15% of cases, no cause for haemoptysis is found.

History in the patient with cough and haemoptysis

The nature of the cough may help in the diagnosis (Fig. 5.1). The following factors should be assessed in the patient with cough or haemoptysis:
- How long has the cough been present? The longer the cough is present, the less likely it is to be the consequence of infection.
- Has the patient been in contact with any person with an infection? Always think of tuberculosis especially in at risk patient groups.
- Has the patient recently been or ever lived abroad?
- How severe is the cough? Complications include worsening of bronchospasm, vomiting, rib fractures, urinary incontinence, and syncope.

Fig. 5.1 Details regarding the nature of the cough that may be important for diagnosis.

Details of coughs that may be important for diagnosis
• If the cough is productive, look at the sputum (see Chapter 2) • A 'brassy' cough, described as hard and metallic, may be associated with pressure on the trachea • A cough associated with retrosternal pain, 'like a hot poker', occurs in tracheitis • A bovine cough results from laryngeal paralysis, usually from bronchial carcinoma infiltrating the left recurrent laryngeal nerve. The voice may have become more hoarse • Croup is a hard and hoarse cough of laryngitis • Associations with stridor may occur with whooping cough and in the presence of laryngeal or tracheal obstruction • Ask about other associated symptoms, e.g. a wheeze may occur with asthma or left ventricular function; there may be orthopnoea or paroxysmal nocturnal dyspnoea (see Chapter 2) • If associated with pleuritic pain, suspect pulmonary embolus • A hacking, irritating frequent cough occurs in pharyngitis • Associations with haemoptysis should trigger the differential diagnosis of haemoptysis

- Is the cough worse at night? Cough can be the only symptom of asthma.
- Does the patient smoke? This can often cause a cough in its own right by acting as an irritant, but is also associated with malignancy.
- Ask about drug history, in particular treatment with ACE inhibitors. Of people on ACE inhibitors, 10–20% will have a dry, tickly cough. It is thought to be related to increased levels of bradykinin. It is more common in women than men. The patient may find the cough tolerable once reassured that there is no serious underlying condition, and the ACE inhibitor may be continued if needed. Newer angiotensin receptor antagonists are often better tolerated because they do not interact with the bradykinin activation pathway.
- Are there any occupational agents or exposure to dust which might account for the cough?
- Has there been any weight loss? Think of carcinoma or lung abscess. Ask about other features of malignancy if suspected, such as change in bowel habit.
- Has there been a history of trauma to the chest?
- Is there a family history of bleeding disorders?
- Ask about a past history of rheumatic fever–haemoptysis in mitral stenosis.
- If a diagnosis is suspected, ask more leading questions.
- Do not overlook non-respiratory causes (e.g. are there any symptoms suggestive of gastro-oesophageal reflux disease?)

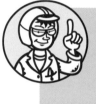

Always be sure what the patient means by 'coughing up blood'. It is confused with epistaxis and haematemesis more times than you would believe!

Examining the patient with cough and haemoptysis

A full general and respiratory examination should be carried out (Fig. 5.2, and see Chapters 2 and 38) Assess the following:

- If the patient appears breathless, assess the severity and count the respiratory rate.
- Check for anaemia: if present think of malignancy, connective tissue diseases, or chronic infection.
- If there is clubbing, suspect bronchial carcinoma, lung abscess, mesothelioma, bronchiectasis, cystic fibrosis, or fibrosing alveolitis.
- If the patient is cyanosed, there may be COPD, or Eisenmenger's syndrome.
- Examine for lymphadenopathy, caused by infections or malignancy.
- Look at the sputum pot if the cough is productive.
- Examine for a goitre. Is there retrosternal extension?

Fig. 5.2 Examining the patient with cough and haemoptysis.

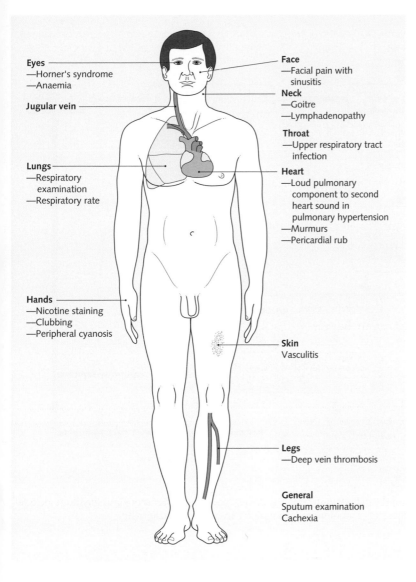

Eyes
—Horner's syndrome
—Anaemia

Jugular vein

Lungs
—Respiratory examination
—Respiratory rate

Hands
—Nicotine staining
—Clubbing
—Peripheral cyanosis

Face
—Facial pain with sinusitis

Neck
—Goitre
—Lymphadenopathy

Throat
—Upper respiratory tract infection

Heart
—Loud pulmonary component to second heart sound in pulmonary hypertension
—Murmurs
—Pericardial rub

Skin
Vasculitis

Legs
—Deep vein thrombosis

General
Sputum examination
Cachexia

- Examine specifically for signs of bronchial carcinoma, (e.g. Horner's syndrome, paraneoplastic syndromes).
- Examine the legs for deep vein thromboses with pulmonary embolus as a cause for haemoptysis.
- Look at the skin. Vasculitides may have skin manifestations.
- Check for facial pain in sinusitis.
- Proceed to a full respiratory examination, including auscultation for bronchial breathing in lobar consolidation, fine crepitations with left ventricular failure and fibrosing alveolitis, and the coarser crepitations of bronchiectasis.
- Auscultate the heart for the murmur of mitral stenosis or a pericardial rub.
- Listen for the pleural rub of pulmonary infarction.

- In pulmonary hypertension, there will be a loud pulmonary component of the second heart sound, a right ventricular heave, a pulmonary systolic murmur, and prominent a waves in the jugular venous pressure.
- A localised wheeze, not disappearing on coughing, suggests a blocked major airway from a carcinoma or a foreign body.

Never forget tuberculosis; it is not a historical disease and is easily overlooked

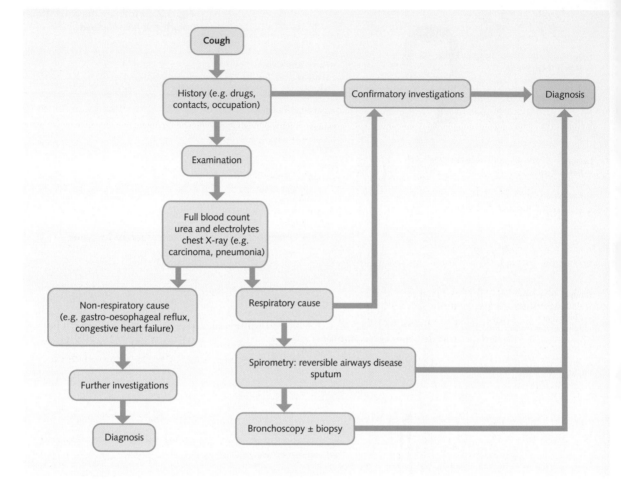

Fig. 5.3 Algorithm for the investigation of the patient with cough and haemoptysis. Confirmatory investigations include sputum and blood cultures for pneumonia, and computerised tomography scanning for malignancy.

Investigating the patient with cough and haemoptysis

An algorithm for the investigation of the patient with cough and haemoptysis is given in Fig. 5.3. The following investigations should be considered in the patient with cough or haemoptysis:

- Full blood count: anaemia with malignancies.
- Urea and electrolytes.
- Chest radiograph: this may reveal the pulmonary cause of the cough (e.g. pneumonia, carcinoma, interstitial lung diseases, bronchiectasis, bilateral hilar lymphadenopathy in sarcoidosis or tuberculosis).
- Sputum: microscopy, culture and cytology.
- Oxygen saturations or arterial blood gas analysis.

- Pharyngoscopy: if an upper respiratory cause is suspected.
- Ventilation/perfusion scan: if a pulmonary embolus is suspected.
- Bronchoscopy with or without washings, brushings or biopsies.
- Peak flow diary for asthma.
- Simple spirometry: if airways disease is suspected.
- Specific lung function tests: if the cause has not been found after the above tests have been carried out (see Chapter 40).
- High-resolution computed tomography: to confirm the presence and degree of interstitial lung disease and bronchiectasis.
- Gastroscopy or barium meal: to investigate possible gastro-oesophageal reflux disease.

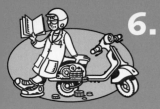

6. Pyrexia of Unknown Origin

Introduction

Most fevers are due to viral illnesses and are self-limiting. Pyrexia of unknown origin (PUO) is a persistent and unexplained fever lasting longer than 3 weeks where a diagnosis is not apparent despite a week of investigation in hospital.

Causes of PUO

The causes of PUO are shown in Fig. 6.1. The commonest malignancy to cause a fever is lymphoma although solid tumours may also be implicated (especially renal cell and gastrointestinal carcinoma).

History in the patient with PUO

This should be thorough as the diagnosis may be difficult to obtain. Note especially:
- Foreign travel: the incubation period of many tropical diseases may mean that the fever starts some time after arrival back home.
- Contact with animals (zoonoses) (e.g. leptospirosis, Q fever, salmonellosis, cat-scratch fever, psittacoses and ornathoses, toxoplasmosis, hydatid disease, toxocariasis, meningitis, anthrax).
- Contact with infected people.
- Sexual history and any history of intravenous drug use.
- Alcohol intake.

- Previous illnesses, particularly recurrent infections and/or a history of immunosuppression.
- Previous surgery or accidents.
- Rashes.
- Diarrhoea.
- A full history of medication, including over-the-counter drugs.
- Immunization history.
- Symptoms such as sweats, weight loss, and itching.
- Lumps.
- Familial disorders (e.g. familial Mediterranean fever).

Every symptom should be explored in detail. The diagnosis should be made by going over the history repeatedly to look for additional or missed clues.

Examining the patient with PUO

The examination of a patient with PUO is shown in Fig. 6.2. It should be especially thorough and may need to be repeated several times. Particular attention should be given to:
- Teeth and throat.
- Temporal artery tenderness and joints.
- Eye signs (e.g. conjunctival petechiae).
- Skin lesions [e.g. rashes, petechiae, and (vasculitic) infarctions].
- Lymphadenopathy and organomegaly.
- Cardiac murmurs and other stigmata of endocarditis.
- Rectal and vaginal examinations.

 The temperature and pulse should be recorded at least 4-hourly when a patient is admitted with PUO

Investigating the patient with PUO

An algorithm for the investigation of the patient with PUO is given in Fig. 6.3. Investigations are

The causes of PUO	
Infections (20-40%)	See Chapter 35
Connective tissue disorders (20%)	See Chapter 33
Malignancy (10-20%)	See Chapter 34
Undiagnosed (20%)	
Drugs [e.g. phenytoin (rare)]	

Fig. 6.1 The causes of pyrexia of unknown origin (PUO).

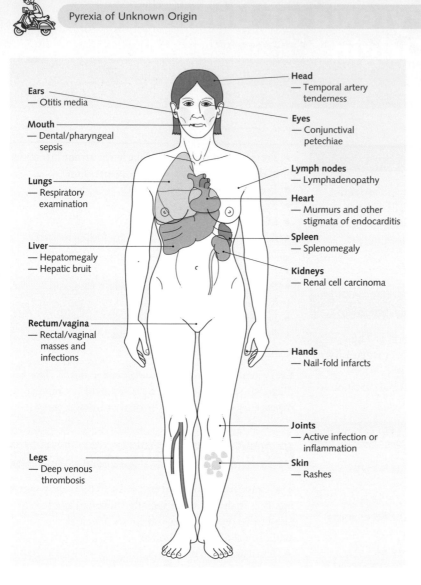

Fig 6.2 Examining the patient with pyrexia of unknown origin (PUO).

Ears
— Otitis media

Mouth
— Dental/pharyngeal sepsis

Lungs
— Respiratory examination

Liver
— Hepatomegaly
— Hepatic bruit

Rectum/vagina
— Rectal/vaginal masses and infections

Legs
— Deep venous thrombosis

Head
— Temporal artery tenderness

Eyes
— Conjunctival petechiae

Lymph nodes
— Lymphadenopathy

Heart
— Murmurs and other stigmata of endocarditis

Spleen
— Splenomegaly

Kidneys
— Renal cell carcinoma

Hands
— Nail-fold infarcts

Joints
— Active infection or inflammation

Skin
— Rashes

best directed from the history and examination. For example, if the patient has just returned from a part of the world where malaria is endemic, thick and thin blood films should be requested. Often there will be no clue, and the best way to proceed is to ask for general non-specific screening tests, which may then suggest an area to focus on.

Full blood count and differential white cell count

Full blood count and differential white cell count may yield information on the following:

- Neutrophil leucocytosis: bacterial infections, myeloproliferative disease, malignancy (e.g. hepatic metastases), collagen vascular diseases.
- Leucopenia: viral infections, lymphoma, systemic lupus erythematosus, brucellosis, disseminated tuberculosis, drugs.

- Monocytosis: subacute bacterial endocarditis, inflammatory bowel disease, Hodgkin's disease, brucellosis, tuberculosis.
- Abnormal mononuclear cells: glandular fever, cytomegalovirus infection, toxoplasmosis.
- Eosinophilia: parasitic infections (e.g. trichiasis, hydatid disease), malignancy (especially Hodgkin's disease), drug reaction, pulmonary eosinophilia.

Inflammatory markers

A very high erythrocyte sedimentation rate suggests the following:

- Multiple myeloma.
- Systemic lupus erythematosus.
- Temporal arteritis.
- Polymyalgia rheumatica.
- Still's disease.

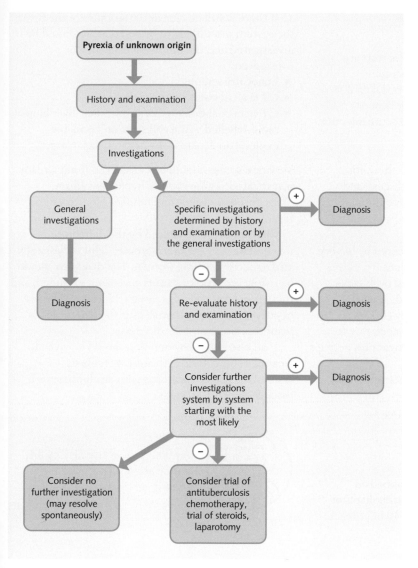

Fig 6.3 Investigation of the patient with pyrexia of unknown origin (PUO).

- Rheumatic fever.
- Lymphoma.
- Subacute bacterial endocarditis.

C-reactive protein is an acute phase reactant and is useful for monitoring disease progress as it has a short half life, and therefore varies more rapidly than the erythrocyte sedimentation rate.

Urea and electrolytes

Assessment of urea and electrolytes may reveal, for example, renal impairment or hyponatraemia due to pneumonia.

Liver function tests

Abnormal results may lead to more detailed investigations of the liver. Note, however, that

alkaline phosphatase may also be raised in metabolic bone disease, Hodgkin's disease, Still's disease, polymyalgia rheumatica and in patients with bony metastases.

Bacteriology and serology

Microscopy and culture from every site possible:
- Urine: bacteria (infections), haematuria (may suggest subacute bacterial endocarditis or hypernephroma).
- Blood cultures: several samples are needed from different veins at different times of the day.
- Faeces' microscopy for ova, cysts and parasites.
- Vaginal and cervical swabs.
- Urethral swabs in men.

- Sputum microscopy and culture.
- Throat swab cultures.

With regard to serology, many specific tests are available (e.g. glandular fever, psittacosis, brucellosis). A second sample must be taken 2–3 weeks later to show a rising antibody titre or immunoglobulin M titres may signal acute infection.

Chest X-ray

Chest X-ray should be performed to show, for example, tuberculosis, subphrenic abscess, and bilateral hilar lymphadenopathy (sarcoidosis).

Further investigations

Further investigations should be directed by history, examination and the results of previous investigations. For example, if a renal problem is suspected, further tests might include a renal ultrasound or computed tomography (CT) scan. If there are no specific clues it may be necessary to proceed 'blindly' with further investigations, perhaps commencing with the following:

- Immunoglobulins and protein electrophoresis.
- Rheumatoid factor, autoantibodies, anti-streptolysin titre and tumour markers.
- Mantoux test for tuberculosis.
- Bone marrow aspiration.
- Lumbar puncture.

All non-essential drugs should be stopped on admission. It may be necessary to withhold other drugs at this stage, one at a time for 48 hours each.

If there is still no clue as to the cause of the fever, the system most likely to be responsible should be investigated and the following tests may be considered:

- Echocardiography.
- CT scan of chest and bronchoscopy.
- CT scan of abdomen, barium studies, liver biopsy, radio-labelled white cell scan, and possibly exploratory laparoscopy or rarely laparotomy.

Very rare causes should be considered if not already investigated. These include hyperthyroidism, phaeochromocytoma, and familial Mediterranean fever.

Factitious fever is caused by the deliberate manipulation of the thermometer. This is classically said to occur in young women. The diagnosis should be suspected if other causes have been excluded, and there is no evidence of a chronic illness, no increase in pulse rate when pyrexial, or if the patient looks inappropriately well despite fever.

If all else fails, consideration should be given to treating tuberculosis with antituberculosis chemotherapy, endocarditis with antibiotics, and vasculitides with steroids.

Always go over the history and examination repeatedly, even when investigations are in progress

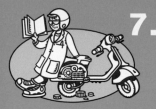

7. Dyspepsia

Introduction

Dyspepsia describes a group of symptoms that relate to the upper gastrointestinal (GI) tract. These symptoms include upper abdominal discomfort, retrosternal pain, anorexia, nausea, vomiting, bloating, fullness, heartburn, and early satiety.

These symptoms are very common and it is neither desirable nor possible to investigate everyone with dyspepsia.

Therefore, the approach to this common presenting complaint involves directing investigations towards those most likely to benefit (e.g. those at risk of cancer where a firm endoscopic/histological diagnosis must be made) as opposed to those in whom empirical therapy is safe and a firm diagnosis would not significantly alter their management (e.g. a young, otherwise well, patient with dyspepsia and no *Helicobacter pylori* infection).

The prevalence of dyspepsia has been estimated to be 23–31%

Causes of dyspepsia

This chapter emphasises that it is not always essential to make a firm diagnosis in the dyspeptic patient in order to treat them appropriately. However, a definitive diagnosis may be reached following investigation or if further investigations are performed at the discretion of the clinician, perhaps due to persistent, uncontrolled symptoms. The causes of dyspepsia are shown in Fig. 7.1.

History and examination in the patient with dyspepsia

The following features should be enquired about, although the precise symptoms correlate poorly with the underlying cause:

Causes of dyspepsia (see Chapter 29)
Duodenal ulcer**
Gastric ulcer**
Oesophageal/gastric cancer*
Oesophagitis/GORD
Gastritis/duodenitis**
Non-ulcer dyspepsia**
Hiatus hernia
Oesophageal motility disorders
Biliary pathology

Fig. 7.1 The causes of dyspepsia. * or ** indicates the conditions associated with *Helicobacter pylori* infection. It is unclear whether it is causative in all these conditions, but some (marked **) have been shown to respond favourably to its eradication. (GORD, gastro-oesophageal reflux disease)

- Heartburn: usually retrosternal and often worse with leaning forward or lying down. Suggestive of acid reflux and may be associated with 'waterbrash', a flood of saliva in the mouth as a reflex response to acid in the lower oesophagus.
- Chest pain: burning retrosternal pain, not related to exertion (unlike angina), which may radiate between the shoulder blades. This can relate to acid-provoked oesophageal spasm which, like angina, is also relieved by nitrates.
- Nocturnal cough/asthma: occasionally due to acid reflux.
- Aggravating factors for reflux:
  - Increased intra-abdominal pressure: stooping/bending/obesity/pregnancy
  - Spicy or fatty foods
  - Alcohol ingestion: also causes gastritis
  - Cigarettes, caffeine, theophylline, anticholinergic drugs: reduce lower oesophageal sphincter tone
  - Non-steroidal anti-inflammatory drugs (NSAIDs): interfere with prostaglandin cytoprotection
  - Hiatus hernia
- Epigastric pain: feature of peptic ulcer disease. Aggravated by food (gastric ulcer) or fasting (duodenal ulcer).

The most important part of the assessment in these patients is to identify those who require endoscopic investigation (see below). This depends on the presence of the 'alarm symptoms or signs' in Fig. 7.2 which MUST be looked for specifically. These features all suggest an elevated risk of cancer and help to ensure that endoscopy is not denied to those at risk of cancer.

Investigating the patient with dyspepsia

An approach to the dyspeptic patient is outlined in Fig. 7.3. The management of specific conditions is further explained in Chapter 29.

The investigations used are explained below. Specialised investigations are used predominantly in cases such as persistent symptoms not responding to the approach in Fig. 7.3 or atypical symptoms (e.g. laryngeal discomfort or atypical chest pain that may result from acid reflux or oesophageal dysmotility). It is important to remember that the majority of patients with dyspepsia can be managed safely without extensive investigations provided the above algorithm is adhered to.

Common investigations
- Full blood count: microcytic anaemia and/or thrombocytosis may suggest gastrointestinal blood loss.
- Electrocardiography (ECG): if considering the diagnosis of angina in cases of atypical chest pain.

Acid reflux can cause non-specific ECG changes and therefore further investigations such as exercise tolerance testing may be necessary.
- *Helicobacter pylori* testing: several tests are available. Carbon tagged breath tests (depend on urease breakdown of urea) are the most accurate and can confirm eradication following treatment (but cannot be used by inpatients taking proton pump inhibitors, bismuth or within 4 weeks of antibiotic use). Immunoglobulin G serological tests confirm previous infection but cannot provide information on eradication. Urease tests can be used on endoscopic specimens and histology/culture can confirm these findings.
- Endoscopy (oesophagogastroduodenoscopy or OGD): very safe but not totally risk free (death rate between 1 in 2000 to 10 000). Allows visualisation of the upper gastrointestinal tract to the second part of the duodenum and biopsy and therapeutic manoeuvres if required (see Chapter 29).
- Barium meal: alternative for patients in whom endoscopy is not possible e.g. elderly frail patients in whom sedation is dangerous.

Specialised investigations
- Oesophageal motility studies: manometry demonstrates motility disorders (e.g. achalasia, systemic sclerosis, diffuse oesophageal spasm).
- 24-hour intraluminal pH monitoring: confirms acid reflux in difficult cases.
- Abdominal ultrasound: if a mass or biliary pathology is suspected (see Chapter 29).

Dyspeptic patients in whom diagnostic endoscopy is indicated	
Unintentional weight loss >3 kg	Unexplained iron deficiency anaemia
Gastrointestinal bleeding	Dysphagia/odynophagia
Previous gastric surgery	Persistent vomiting
Epigastric mass	Suspicious barium meal
Previous gastric ulcer	Age >55 years with recent onset dyspepsia lasting more than 4 weeks.

Fig. 7.2 Patients with dyspepsia in whom diagnostic endoscopy is indicated.

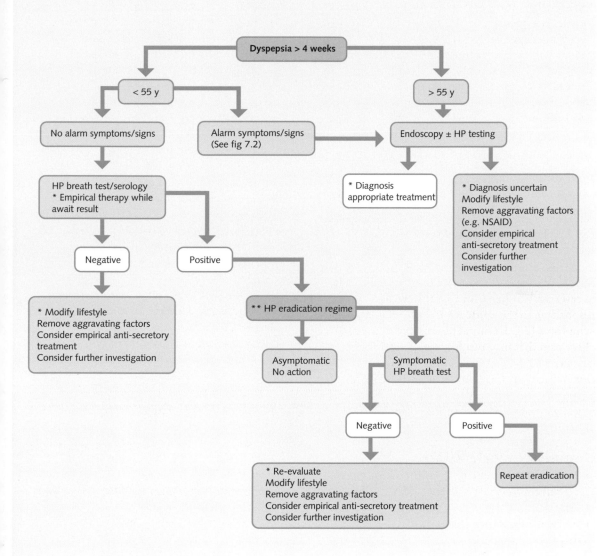

Fig. 7.3 Algorithm for the investigation and management of patients with dyspepsia. *See Chapter 29. **Seek local microbiological advice. (HP, *Helicobacter pylori*; NSAID, non-steroidal anti-inflammatory drug).

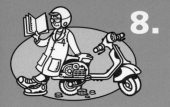

8. Haematemesis and Melaena

Introduction

Haematemesis is the vomiting of fresh (bright red) or altered ('coffee ground') blood. Melaena is the production of black, tarry stools, and is due to bleeding in the gastrointestinal (GI) tract above the splenic flexure. Both are typical signs of an upper GI bleed. GI bleeding is an emergency, and treatment may need to be initiated before a diagnosis has been made (see Chapter 29).

Differential diagnosis of haematemesis and melaena

Figure 8.1 gives the differential diagnosis of haematemaesis and melaena. It is important to note that melaena alone may be caused by pathology in the small bowel or ascending colon.

History in the patient with haematemesis and melaena

The history may have to be taken after initial resuscitation procedures. It is important to determine whether the blood has been vomited or coughed. In cases of difficulty, the presence of food mixed with the blood or an acid pH is suggestive of haematemesis, although the vomitus may not be acidic in patients with carcinoma of the stomach.

Haematemesis may be due to blood swallowed from the nasopharynx or mouth.

You must ask about the following:

- Non-specific symptoms of hypovolaemia: faintness, weakness, dizziness, sweating, palpitations, dyspnoea, pallor, collapse. These symptoms may precede the actual haematemesis/melaena.
- Weight loss and anorexia: carcinoma.
- Current drugs: aspirin, nonsteroidal anti-inflammatory drugs, or excessive alcohol are suggestive of gastric erosions; iron therapy causes black stools but this is not melaena; anticoagulation will exacerbate bleeding.
- Symptoms of chronic blood loss: suggests gastric carcinoma if associated with anorexia and weight loss.
- Heartburn: oesophagitis.
- Intermittent epigastric pain relieved with antacids: peptic ulceration.

The differential diagnosis of haematemesis and melaena	
Cause	**Notes**
Peptic ulcer disease	Cause 50% of major upper GI bleeds. 10% mortality
Erosive gastritis	Causes 20% of upper GI bleeds, rarely severe.
Mallory-Weiss tear	Causes 10% of upper GI bleeds. Laceration in GOJ mucosa, often following retching (e.g. after alcohol binge)
Oesophagitis	Due to GORD
Ruptured oesophageal varices	Cause 10-20% of upper GI bleeds. Mortality up to 40%. Due to portal hypertension.
Vascular abnormalities	Vascular ectasias or angiodysplasias. Also cause of lower GI bleeding.
Gastric neoplasm	Causes 5% of upper GI bleeds.
Rare causes	Oesophageal ulcers or tumours, aortoenteric fistula after abdominal aortic surgery, pancreatic tumour, biliary bleeding, blood dyscrasias.

Fig. 8.1 The differential diagnosis of haematemesis and melaena. (GI, gastrointestinal; GOJ, gastro-oesophageal junction; GORD, gastro-oesophageal reflux disease.)

- Sudden severe abdominal pain: perforation.
- Dysphagia or odynophagia (pain on swallowing): oesophageal carcinoma.
- Chronic excessive alcohol intake: oesophageal varices.
- Enquiry into the causes of liver failure (see Chapter 11): oesophageal varices.
- Retching especially after an alcohol binge: Mallory–Weiss tear.
- Family history: inherited bleeding disorders.
- A past history of GI bleeds and their cause.

Examining the patient with haematemesis and melaena

The approach to examining the patient with haematemesis and melaena is given in Fig. 8.2. Step back from the patient for a few seconds. Do they look well, or pale and clammy? An initial common-sense impression affects the immediacy of subsequent management.

General examination

The general examination should assess the following:

- Anaemia: mucous membranes. If clinically anaemic, this may indicate chronic blood loss.
- Jaundice: may indicate portal hypertension.
- Clubbing: inflammatory bowel disease, cirrhosis.
- Lymphadenopathy: especially Virchow's node (left supraclavicular lymph node) associated with gastric carcinoma (Troisier's sign).
- Pulse and blood pressure: tachycardia is a reflex response to hypovolaemia (due to bleeding) and usually precedes a blood pressure fall. A young and healthy patient may lose more than 500 mL of blood before a rise in heart rate

Fig 8.2 Examining the patient with haematemesis and melaena.

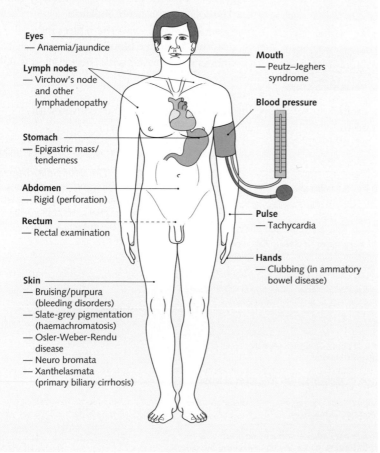

or fall in blood pressure occurs. If the patient is hypotensive, intravenous fluid resuscitation is imperative, as is frequent monitoring of pulse and blood pressure to assess haemodynamic trends.

- Skin: bruises, purpura (bleeding disorders); telangiectasia [Osler–Weber–Rendu disease (hereditary haemorrhagic telangiectasia-autosomal dominant)]; neurofibromata.
- Mouth: pharyngeal lesions; pigmented macules (Peutz–Jeghers syndrome).
- Cachexia.

Specific examination

This includes a search for signs related to the differential diagnosis:

- A rigid abdomen suggests perforation.
- Epigastric tenderness suggests peptic ulcer disease, oesophagitis, hiatus hernia, or gastric carcinoma.
- Epigastric mass: gastric carcinoma.
- If malignancy is suspected, examine for metastases.
- Signs of chronic liver disease and portal hypertension support the possibility of oesophageal varices (see Chapter 11)

Investigating the patient with haematemesis and melaena

 A large upper GI bleed may cause the passage of fresh blood per rectum rather than melaena

An algorithm for the investigation of the patient with haematemesis and melaena is given in Fig. 8.3. The following investigations should be carried out:

- A full blood count should be performed. The haemoglobin may be normal in the acute phase, despite a large GI bleed, as it takes some hours for haemodilution to occur. A low haemoglobin on initial presentation suggests chronic blood loss, and the white cell count may be raised after a GI bleed. Platelet count may be reduced after an acute bleed, or increased after chronic blood loss. A very low platelet count should raise suspicion of a bleeding diathesis.

- Group and save even if there is only a small GI bleed, and the patient is haemodynamically stable. Blood should be cross-matched for more significant bleeding.
- A clotting screen should also be performed as the prothrombin time is raised in liver disease. More specific investigations may be indicated (e.g. in patients with haemophilia or von Willebrand's disease).
- Urea is raised due to the absorption and subsequent breakdown of protein when blood reaches the small bowel. Chronic renal failure can be associated with GI bleeding.
- On erect chest X-ray, the presence of gas under the right hemidiaphragm indicates perforation.

Further investigations are performed to confirm the site of the bleeding, and to make a definitive diagnosis:

- Fibre-optic endoscopy is usually performed within 24 hours if the patient is shocked or has significant co-morbidity, immediately if variceal bleeding is suspected. It allows direct visualization of the pathology and provides a diagnosis in around 90% of cases. This will determine the most appropriate form of medical therapy. The risk of rebleeding (the major cause of mortality) may be estimated. Treatment may be given endoscopically (e.g. banding or sclerosing a bleeding varix, or adrenaline injection of a bleeding vessel).
- Barium examinations are becoming less common as endoscopy is becoming more widely available, though they may be useful when endoscopy is contraindicated (e.g. in patients with an unstable cervical spine).

Most patients do not require further tests but, occasionally, these are performed under the guidance of a specialist when the diagnosis remains uncertain (see Fig. 8.3):

- Isotope studies: abdominal gamma scanning can detect extravasation of radioisotope-labelled red blood cells if active bleeding is present.
- Mesenteric angiography again requires active bleeding to localise the source. It can also be used to visualise the portal venous system.
- Enteroscopy may be used to further investigate the small bowel, and in particularly difficult cases may be combined with laparotomy.
- In the presence of deranged liver function tests or an abdominal mass, ultrasound examination should be performed. Computed tomography of the abdomen can also help in assessment of a mass.

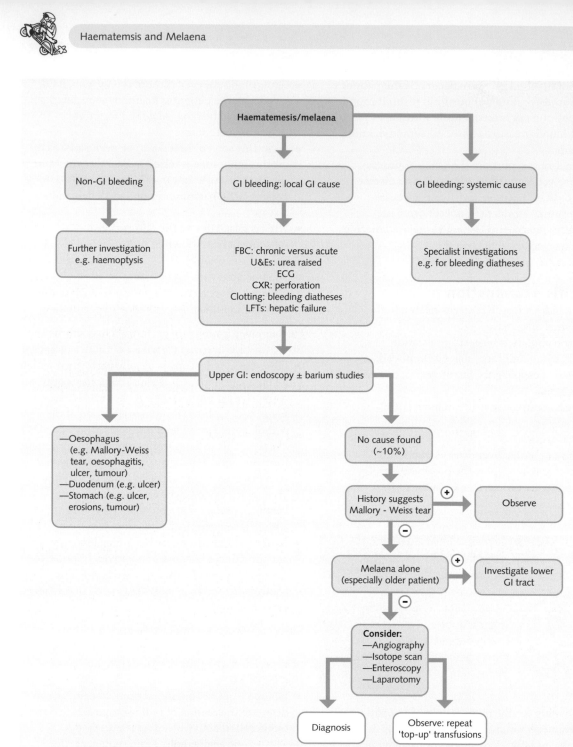

Fig. 8.3 Algorithm for the investigation of the patient with haematemesis and melaena. (ECG, electrocardiogram; CXR, chest X-ray; FBC, full blood count; GI, gastrointestinal; LFTs, liver function tests; U&Es, urea and electrolytes.)

Despite extensive investigation, a small minority of patients will remain undiagnosed. If bleeding is severe laparotomy may be required, but if it is not severe the patient may attend for repeat 'top-up' transfusions as required.

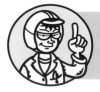

Elevated blood urea with normal serum creatinine suggests gastrointestinal blood loss

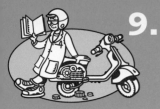

9. Change in Bowel Habit

Introduction

Always ask about the patient's normal bowel habit because there are considerable differences between people, usually varying from three times a day to once every 3 days. It is important to note a change in bowel habit because this is more commonly associated with pathology.

Differential diagnosis of a change in bowel habit

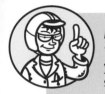

Make sure that by 'constipation' and 'diarrhoea', you and the patient mean the same thing

Diarrhoea

This means an increase in stool water content so that the volume and frequency of defecation increase and the consistency becomes liquid.

Fig. 9.1 summarises the causes of diarrhoea.

Constipation

Ask what is meant by constipation. It usually means that the bowels are only opened infrequently, and that the faeces are hard, with pain on defecation.

Fig. 9.2 summarises the causes of constipation.

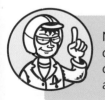

Note the features of acute GI obstruction: absolute constipation, vomiting, pain, and abdominal distension

History in the patient with a change in bowel habit

Ask about the following:
- Normal bowel habit and diet (note variation between individuals).

- Onset: sudden or chronic. Infectious diarrhoea is usually of acute onset.
- Frequency of defecation.
- Stool appearance: formed, loose or watery; colour-normal, red (blood from low in the gastrointestinal (GI) tract), black (melaena), yellow (mucus and slime), 'redcurrant jelly' (intussusception), putty-coloured (obstructive jaundice); volume; do the stools float? (high fat content–think of malabsorption).
- Drugs: antacids, laxatives, cimetidine, digoxin, antibiotics, alcohol.
- Tenesmus (a sense of incomplete voiding).
- Smell: offensively malodorous in malabsorption; characteristic smell of melaena.
- Foreign travel.
- Contact with diarrhoea sufferers.
- Relationship to food.
- Stress.
- Associated features (e.g. pain, fever, vomiting, weight loss, extraintestinal manifestations of inflammatory bowel disease) (see Chapter 29).
- Symptoms of thyrotoxicosis.
- Nocturnal symptoms: these go against a functional disorder.
- Surgical history (e.g. multiple bowel resections for Crohn's disease can result in malabsorption).
- Sexual history: gay bowel syndrome. Suspect this if multiple or unusual organisms are cultured.

Examining the patient with a change in bowel habit

The examination approach in the patient with a change in bowel habit is given in Fig. 9.3.

Investigating the patient with a change in bowel habit

An algorithm for the investigation of the patient with change in bowel habit is given in Fig. 9.4. The wide range of possible diagnoses in patients with altered bowel habit is reflected by the large number of tests that may be performed. Some of

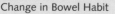

Differential diagnosis of diarrhoea	
Causes	**Examples**
Infective	Bacterial—*Campylobacter* (poultry), *Salmonella* (meat, poultry and dairy), *Shigella* (faecal-oral transmission)
	Viral—rotavirus, Norwalk virus, cytomegalovirus
	Protozoa—*Giardia lamblia, Cryptosporidium, Entamoeba histolytica*
Inflammatory	Inflammatory bowel disease
	Malignancy
	Radiation enteritis
Ischaemic	Emboli or mesenteric atheromatous disease
Functional	Irritable bowel syndrome
Secretory	Infection (e.g. cholera)
	VIPoma/Zollinger Ellison/carcinoid
	Villous adenoma
	Factitious diarrhoea (e.g. laxative abuse)
	Bile salt malabsorption (disruption of enterohepatic circulation)
Osmotic	Medications (e.g. antacids and lactulose)
	Disaccharidase deficiency
	Factitious diarrhoea
Malabsorption	See Chapter 29 for causes
Systemic illness	Hyperthyroidism, diabetes mellitus, Addison's (see Chapter 32)
Overflow diarrhoea	Faecal impaction in elderly
Drugs	Alcohol, digoxin, metformin, neomycin

Fig. 9.1 The differential diagnosis of diarrhoea (see Chapter 29).

these are used commonly whereas others are used much less frequently and only under the guidance of specialists.

Common investigations
- Full blood count.
- Urea and electrolytes, including calcium.
- Thyroid function tests.
- Blood glucose: diabetes.
- Liver function tests.
- Albumin: decreased in malabsorption, protein-losing enteropathies, inflammatory diseases.
- In malabsorption: anaemia-vitamin B_{12}, folate, iron; hyponatraemia in profound secretory diarrhoea; reduced absorption of fat soluble vitamins—prolonged prothrombin time (vitamin K), hypocalcaemia (vitamin D), visual impairment rarely (vitamin A).
- Anti-endomyseal, anti-reticulin and alpha-gliadin antibodies if suspect coeliac disease.
- Inflammatory markers (erythrocyte sedimentation rate and C-reactive protein)—raised in infection/inflammation.
- Stool microscopy, culture and detection of *Clostridium difficile* toxin if suspect infection.
- Abdominal X-ray: pancreatic calcification suggests chronic pancreatitis, distended intestinal loops and fluid levels suggest obstruction, and gross dilatation of the colon suggests Hirschsprung's disease.

Fig. 9.2 The differential diagnosis of constipation (see Chapter 29).

Differential diagnosis of constipation	
Causes	**Examples**
Congenital	Hirschprung's disease
Mechanical obstruction	Inflammatory stricture (e.g. Crohn's disease, diverticulitis) Neoplasm Extra-luminal mass (e.g. pelvic) Rectocele
Lifestyle	Diet Dehydration Immobility Lack of privacy (e.g. hospital ward)
Pain	Fissure-in-ano Thrombosed haemorrhoids Post-operative
Metabolic/endocrine	Hypothyroidism (see Chapter 32) Hypercalcaemia Diabetic neuropathy
Drugs	Opiates, anticholinergics, diuretics
Neurological	Paraplegia (see Chapter 31) Multiple sclerosis
Functional Idiopathic megacolon/rectum	Irritable bowel syndrome

- Rigid sigmoidoscopy—performed without sedation (e.g. in outpatients) and allows inspection and/or biopsy of rectal mucosa.
- Flexible sigmoidoscopy/colonoscopy/barium enema—examination of the large bowel.
- Oesophagogastroduodenoscopy and/or D2 biopsy for malabsorption.
- Abdominal ultrasound and/or computed tomography for suspected masses and pancreatitis.
- Endoscopic retrograde cholangiopancreatography, magnetic resonance cholangiopancreatography and/or endoscopic ultrasound for suspected biliary and pancreatic pathology.
- Small bowel meal/enema or enteroscopy for small bowel pathology.

Specialised investigations
- Faecal fat estimation or ^{14}C trioleate breath test if suspect fat malabsorption.
- Pancrealauryl (measure urinary excretion of molecule cleaved by pancreatic enzymes) and secretin (assessment of aspirated duodenal juice following pancreatic stimulation) tests for pancreatic exocrine function.
- Xylose absorption test for mucosal function.
- Assessment of bile salt absorption using radioisotope-labelled bile acids.
- Lactose hydrogen breath test for bacterial overgrowth.
- Faecal clearance of alpha 1 antitrypsin to investigate protein-losing enteropathy.
- Laxative screen.
- Colonic transit study: to confirm constipation and measure the transit time.
- Studies of pelvic floor function: defaecography and anal manometry.
- Serum vasoactive intestinal polypeptide (VIPoma); serum gastrin (Zollinger–Ellison syndrome); calcitonin (medullary thyroid carcinoma); cortisol (Addison's disease); urinary 5-hydroxyindoleacetic acid (carcinoid syndrome).

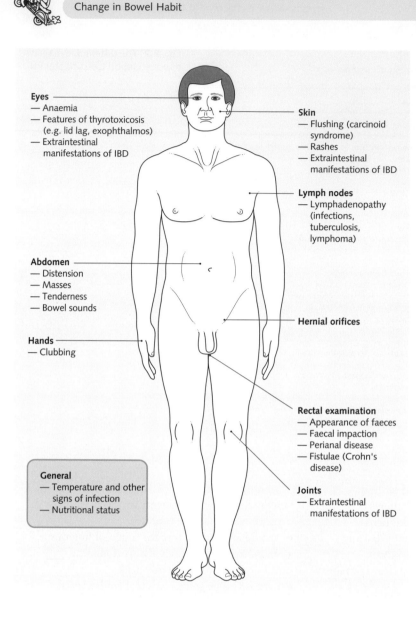

Fig 9.3 Examining the patient with a change in bowel habit. (IBD, inflammatory bowel disease.)

Eyes
— Anaemia
— Features of thyrotoxicosis (e.g. lid lag, exophthalmos)
— Extraintestinal manifestations of IBD

Skin
— Flushing (carcinoid syndrome)
— Rashes
— Extraintestinal manifestations of IBD

Lymph nodes
— Lymphadenopathy (infections, tuberculosis, lymphoma)

Abdomen
— Distension
— Masses
— Tenderness
— Bowel sounds

Hernial orifices

Hands
— Clubbing

Rectal examination
— Appearance of faeces
— Faecal impaction
— Perianal disease
— Fistulae (Crohn's disease)

General
— Temperature and other signs of infection
— Nutritional status

Joints
— Extraintestinal manifestations of IBD

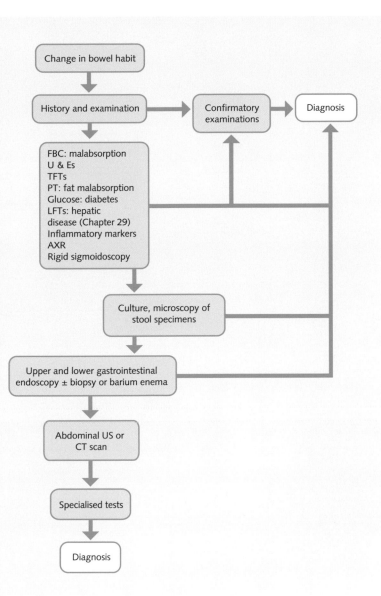

Fig. 9.4 Algorithm for the investigation of the patient with a change of bowel habit. (AXR, abdominal X-ray; CT, computed tomography; FBC, full blood count; LFT, liver function test; U&Es, urea and electrolytes; US, ultrasound; TFTs, thyroid function tests.)

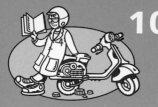

10. Weight Loss

Introduction

Weight loss is due to either a decreased energy intake or increased energy output, or both. Involuntary weight loss is a common manifestation of physical or psychological illness and always warrants further investigation. It should be confirmed objectively with records of previous weights. If this is not possible, a change in clothes size gives a useful clue. Family members may be able to give a more objective history.

Differential diagnosis of weight loss

Distinguish deliberate from involuntary weight loss from the outset. Fig. 10.1 summarises the differential diagnosis of weight loss.

Malignancies anywhere that produce a high metabolic rate or which lead to anorexia or dysphagia (e.g. oesophageal carcinoma) will result in weight loss. Therefore malignancy must be excluded in patients with unexplained weight loss

History in the patient with weight loss

Weight loss can be a complication of disease in any physiological system.

Try to confirm weight loss objectively with records of previous weights. Ask members of the family or friends if they have noticed weight loss. Ask about the amount of weight loss, its duration, and any accompanying symptoms such as anorexia or increased appetite.

Further factors to assess, if the cause is not apparent, include the following:
- Diet: detailed intake and any recent changes in diet history.
- Physical activity: any changes in level.
- Full drug history: including over-the-counter and illegal medicines.
- Alcohol intake: with and without associated liver disease.
- Smoking: if recent onset, this may lead to eating less; if chronic, assess its association with malignancies.
- Symptoms of chronic infection, inflammation or malignancy: fever and sweats, rashes, general malaise, anorexia, change in bowel habit, floating stools (malabsorption), haemoptysis, haematemesis, haematuria, obstructive urinary symptoms (prostate), melaena (or bleeding from any other site), 'lumps and bumps' (including breast), joint or muscle tenderness, contacts with infected people, dysphagia.
- Symptoms of renal insufficiency: anorexia, general malaise and lethargy, bruising, urinary symptoms (e.g. polyuria and nocturia), vomiting, hiccoughs.
- Cardiorespiratory symptoms: cardiac cachexia.
- Neurological symptoms.
- Psychiatric symptoms.

Finally, the symptoms of endocrinopathies include the following:
- Diabetes: polyuria and polydipsia, weakness and fatigue, blurred vision, pruritus or thrush, nocturnal enuresis.
- Adrenal insufficiency: dizziness and collapses, weakness, nausea and diarrhoea, pigmentation.
- Thyrotoxicosis: tremor, diarrhoea, irritability, heat intolerance, palpitations.
- Phaeochromocytoma: paroxysmal (or sustained) hypertension, panic, pain (abdominal or headache), palpitations, perspiration, pallor, paroxysmal thyroid swelling (remember the 'P's), nausea, tremor.
- Panhypopituitarism: pallor, dizziness, loss of body hair, loss of libido, amenorrhoea, visual field defects, symptoms of hypothyroidism.

Fig. 10.1 The differential diagnosis of weight loss.

The differential diagnosis of weight loss	
Causes	**Examples**
Psychiatric/psychological	Anorexia nervosa Depression or agitation Catatonia Schizophrenia Laxative or diuretic abuse Neglect (e.g. 'tea and toast' diet in widowhood) See *Crash Course in Psychiatry*
Physiological	Dieting and exercise Endocrine Uncontrolled diabetes mellitus Hyperthyroidism and rarely hypothyroidism Adrenal insufficiency Phaeochromocytoma Hypopituitarism Severe diabetes insipidus See Chapter 32
Drugs	Alcohol, tobacco, laxatives or diuretics, opiates, amphetamines
Infections	Tuberculosis HIV (human immunodeficiency virus) Other chronic infections and infestations See Chapter 35
Chronic inflammation	Inflammatory bowel disease Connective tissue disease See Chapters 29 and 33
Malignancy	
Chronic illness	Cardiac failure ('cardiac cachexia') Chronic obstructive pulmonary disease Chronic renal failure See Chapters 27, 28 and 30
Gastrointestinal	Peptic ulcer disease Dysphagia Malabsorption Liver disease See Chapter 29
Neurological	Motor neurone disease Myopathies Poliomyelitis See Chapter 31

Examining the patient with weight loss

General observation

The examination approach in the patient with weight loss is given in Fig. 10.2. Does the patient look like they have lost weight (loose skin, loose clothes)? Check the temperature. Does the patient look well or ill? The patient's weight, height and body mass index should be documented.

Hands

The hands should be examined in the patient with weight loss, and the following should be noted:

- Clubbing: malignancy, cirrhosis, inflammatory bowel disease, and infections (chronic suppurative lung disease, subacute bacterial endocarditis).
- Other stigmata of endocarditis (p. 38). Note that nail fold infarcts also occur in vasculitic connective tissue disease.

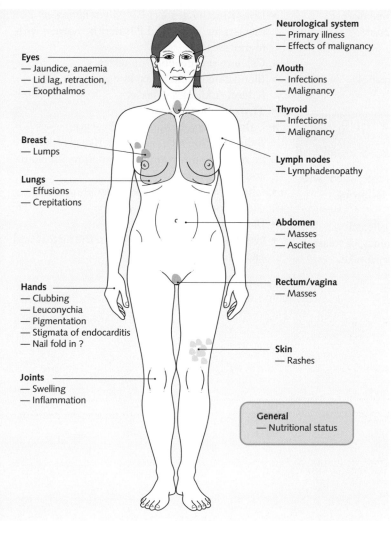

Fig. 10.2 Examining the patient with weight loss.

Neurological system
— Primary illness
— Effects of malignancy

Eyes
— Jaundice, anaemia
— Lid lag, retraction,
— Exopthalmos

Mouth
— Infections
— Malignancy

Thyroid
— Infections
— Malignancy

Breast
— Lumps

Lymph nodes
— Lymphadenopathy

Lungs
— Effusions
— Crepitations

Abdomen
— Masses
— Ascites

Hands
— Clubbing
— Leuconychia
— Pigmentation
— Stigmata of endocarditis
— Nail fold in ?

Rectum/vagina
— Masses

Skin
— Rashes

Joints
— Swelling
— Inflammation

General
— Nutritional status

- Leuconychia and palmar erythema: liver disease (leuconychia reflects hypoalbuminaemia).
- Koilonychia: iron-deficiency anaemia.
- Pigmentation: increased in Addison's disease (particularly in palmar creases) but decreased in anaemia.

Other signs
Other signs include the following:
- Joint swelling and decreased range of movement: connective tissue diseases.
- Tremor, goitre and eye signs: hyperthyroidism (see Fig. 32.14).
- Uraemia: yellow discoloration of the skin.
- Jaundice and other signs of liver failure (e.g. spider naevi) (see Chapter 11).

- Muscle wasting.
- Skin rashes.
- Blood pressure: phaeochromocytoma.
- Mouth: infections and malignancies.
- Lymphadenopathy.

Examination of individual systems
The following individual systems should be examined:
- Respiratory system: infection or malignancy. Do not overlook Horner's syndrome.
- Cardiac system.
- Gastrointestinal system: including careful palpation for abdominal masses, rectal examination, and organomegaly (e.g. liver metastases).

- Neurological system: motor neurone disease, myopathy, paraneoplastic or metastatic manifestations of malignancy.
- Breast lumps.
- Vaginal examination: pelvic malignancy.

Investigating the patient with weight loss

An algorithm for the investigation of the patient with weight loss is given in Fig. 10.3. The following investigations should be carried out:
- Full blood count: anaemia with malignancy, iron deficiency, vitamin B_{12} deficiency, or folate deficiency, with inadequate dietary intake.
- Urea and electrolytes for uraemia.

- Liver function tests (LFTs): liver failure or metastases, although LFTs may be normal with metastases.
- Calcium profile: bone metastases.
- Blood glucose: diabetes, low glucose in liver failure, Addison's disease.
- Thyroid function tests.
- Inflammatory markers (erythrocyte sedimentation rate and C-reactive protein): increased in infection, inflammation, myeloma and other malignancies.
- Chest X-ray: infection or tuberculosis, and malignancy.
- Blood cultures: infection.
- Other investigations depend on the history and examination.

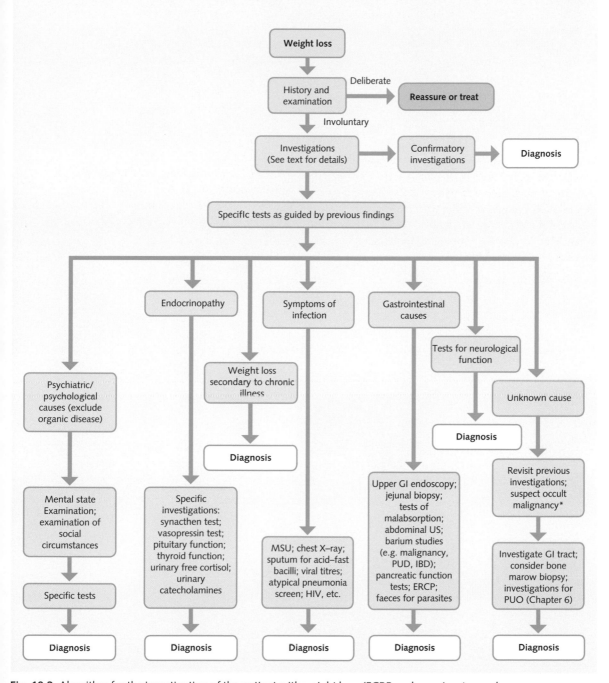

Fig. 10.3 Algorithm for the investigation of the patient with weight loss. (ECRP, endoscopic retrograde cholangiopancreatography; GI, gastrointestinal; HIV, human immunodeficiency virus; IBD, inflammatory bowel disease; MSU, mid-stream urine; PUD, peptic ulcer disease; PUO, pyrexia of unknown origin; US, ultrasound.) *Investigate site under suspicion (e.g. endoscopy for GI tract; look for metastases).

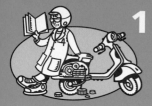

11. Jaundice

Introduction

Jaundice (icterus) is the yellow discoloration of the skin, sclera and mucosae, which is detectable when serum bilirubin concentrations exceed approximately 30 μmol/L. Normal bilirubin metabolism is summarised in Fig. 11.1. Jaundice can arise as a result of increased red blood cell (RBC) breakdown, disordered bilirubin metabolism or reduced bilirubin excretion.

Jaundice is a common examination topic. You need to know the causes and have a logical approach to the patient

Differential diagnosis of jaundice

The causes of jaundice are outlined in Fig. 11.2. 'Prehepatic' jaundice usually results from the excessive production of bilirubin by haemolysis (see Fig. 11.1), but can also result from inherited metabolic defects, the commonest of which is Gilbert's syndrome. 'Hepatic' jaundice results from hepatocyte dysfunction causing disordered bilirubin metabolism. It is important to note that hepatocellular dysfunction usually causes some cholestasis, and may also cause 'pale stools/dark urine' (see below). 'Posthepatic' jaundice is caused by reduced bilirubin excretion due to intra- or extra-hepatic biliary obstruction.

History in the patient with jaundice

The following factors should be assessed when obtaining a history in a patient with jaundice:
- Pruritus, dark urine and pale stools: underlying cholestasis.
- Duration of illness: a short history of malaise, anorexia and myalgia are suggestive of viral hepatitis. If there is a prolonged history of weight loss and anorexia in an elderly patient, carcinoma is more likely.
- Abdominal pain: the episodic, colicky, right hypochondrial pain of biliary colic will commonly

be due to gallstones. A dull, persistent epigastric or central pain radiating to the back may suggest a pancreatic carcinoma.
- Fevers or rigors: cholangitis.
- Full recent drug history: particularly paracetamol, oral contraceptive pill.
- Alcohol consumption: acute alcoholic hepatitis, cirrhosis.
- Infectious contacts: hepatitis A.
- Recent foreign travel to areas of high hepatitis risk.
- Recent surgery: halothane exposure, surgery for known malignancy, biliary stricture due to previous endoscopic retrograde cholangiopancreatography (ERCP).
- Intravenous drug abuse, tattoos, homosexuality: increased risk of hepatitis B and C.
- Occupation: sewage workers are at an increased risk of leptospirosis.
- Family history of recurrent jaundice: inherited haemolytic anaemias and Gilbert's syndrome.

Examining the patient with jaundice

There are three important groups of abnormalities that should be looked for in the jaundiced patient:
- How severe is the jaundice? Is there any evidence of encephalopathy?
- Is this an acute or chronic problem? (Are there any signs of chronic liver disease?)
- Are there any signs of specific disorders?

This approach is summarised in Fig. 11.3.

Is there evidence of encephalopathy?
The following factors suggest the presence of encephalopathy:
- Drowsiness: this will eventually progress through stupor to coma.
- Slurred speech.
- Asterixis: flapping tremor of outstretched hands.
- Seizures.
- Constructional apraxia: test by asking the patient to copy a five-pointed star.
- Hepatic fetor.

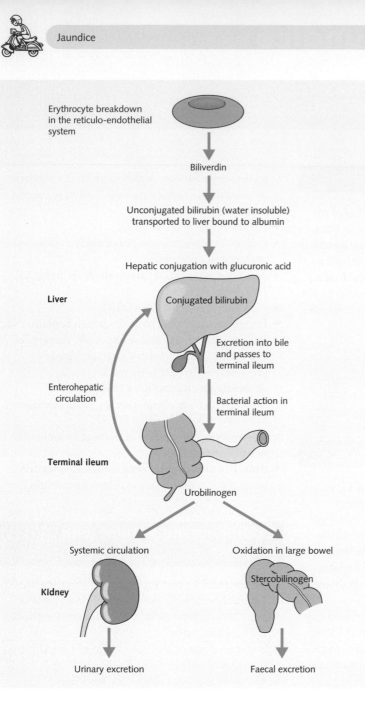

Fig. 11.1 Normal bilirubin metabolism.

Hepatic encephalopathy can arise as a result of fulminating acute liver failure or when chronic disease decompensates. Precipitating factors, grading and management are described in Chapter 29.

Are there any signs of chronic liver disease?

There are few clinical signs specific to acute liver disease. However, the following signs may commonly be found when liver pathology is longstanding:

- Palmar erythema.
- Leuconychia and oedema: hypoalbuminaemia.
- Clubbing.
- Dupuytren's contractures: particularly in alcoholic cirrhosis.
- Spider naevi: greater than five in the distribution of superior vena cava.
- Scratch marks: cholestasis.
- Gynaecomastia, loss of body hair and testicular atrophy: elevated oestrogen.
- Bruising: disordered coagulation.
- Hepatomegaly: not in well-established cirrhosis.
- Splenomegaly, ascites and Caput Medusae: portal hypertension.

The differential diagnosis of jaundice				
Pre-hepatic (see Chapter 34)	**Hepatic** (see Chapter 29)		**Posthepatic** (see Chapter 29)	
	Acute hepatocellular damage	Chronic hepatocellular damage	Extrahepatic obstruction	Intrahepatic obstruction
Haemolysis	Viral infection e.g hepatitis A,B,C,E; EBV; CMV	Inherited defects (e.g. primary haemochromatosis, Wilson's disease, alpha-1-antitrypsin deficiency)	Gallstones	Primary biliary cirrhosis
Inherited metabolic defects (e.g. Gilbert's syndrome)	Non-viral infection (e.g. Leptospira icterohaemorrhagiae)	Alcohol and other drugs (e.g. methotrexate)	Carcinoma-bile duct, head of pancreas, ampulla of Vater	Alcohol
	Drugs (e.g. paracetamol overdose, alcohol)	Chronic infection (e.g. hepatitis B, C)	Sclerosing cholangitis	Viral hepatitis
	Pregnancy	Cryptogenic	Benign stricture (e.g. post ERCP)	Drugs (e.g. OCP)
	Shock	Autoimmune hepatitis	Pancreatitis	Pregnancy
		Metastatic carcinoma Vascular congestion (e.g. Budd–Chiari, right heart failure)	Biliary atresia	

Fig. 11.2 The differential diagnosis of jaundice. (EBV, Epstein–Barr virus; CMV, cytomegalovirus; ERCP, endoscopic retrograde cholangiopancreatography; OCP, oral contraceptive pill.)

Are there any signs of specific diseases?

- Xanthelasmata: primary biliary cirrhosis.
- Kayser–Fleischer rings: Wilson's disease.
- Slate-grey pigmentation: haemochromatosis.
- Hard, irregular hepatomegaly: malignant metastases.
- Palpable gallbladder: carcinoma of head of pancreas (Courvoisier's law).
- Parotid gland enlargement: alcohol.
- Needle marks or tattoos: hepatitis B, C.

Investigating the patient with jaundice

The investigation of jaundiced patients falls into two stages. First, the type of jaundice must be determined (prehepatic, hepatic, posthepatic), then more detailed tests should be performed to determine the specific aetiology. Fig. 11.4 summarises this approach.

Establish the type of jaundice

Quantification of urinary urobilinogen and conjugated bilirubin, along with measurement of serum liver enzymes (alanine aminotransferase, aspartate aminotransferase, alkaline phosphatase, and γ-glutamyltransferase and bilirubin) will give a reasonable indication as to the type of abnormality present (Fig. 11.5). Abdominal ultrasound scan is then essential to exclude biliary obstruction.

The measurement of serum albumin (in the absence of inflammation) and prothrombin time (reflects clotting factor synthesis) help to provide an estimate of hepatic synthetic function.

Tests to determine specific aetiology

The following tests should be used as guided by the above initial investigations.

Haemolysis screen

The haemolysis screen is detailed in Chapter 26.

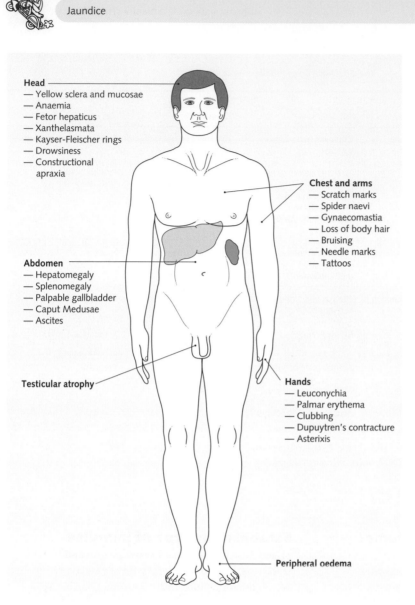

Head
— Yellow sclera and mucosae
— Anaemia
— Fetor hepaticus
— Xanthelasmata
— Kayser–Fleischer rings
— Drowsiness
— Constructional apraxia

Chest and arms
— Scratch marks
— Spider naevi
— Gynaecomastia
— Loss of body hair
— Bruising
— Needle marks
— Tattoos

Abdomen
— Hepatomegaly
— Splenomegaly
— Palpable gallbladder
— Caput Medusae
— Ascites

Testicular atrophy

Hands
— Leuconychia
— Palmar erythema
— Clubbing
— Dupuytren's contracture
— Asterixis

Peripheral oedema

Fig. 11.3 Examining the patient with jaundice.

Hepatocellular screen

- Viral serology: hepatitis A, B, and C; Epstein–Barr virus (EBV), cytomegalovirus (CMV).
- Autoantibody screen: antimitochondrial antibodies, antinuclear antibodies.
- Ferritin: haemochromatosis.
- Serum caeruloplasmin and urinary copper excretion: Wilson's disease.
- α_1-antitrypsin.
- Liver biopsy: definitive diagnostic test for intrinsic liver disease.

Cholestasis screen

- ERCP and percutaneous transhepatic cholangiography: detailed information regarding the biliary tree; also used to perform therapeutic manoeuvres such as stent insertion.

- Computed tomography scan: good images of the pancreas, which is often poorly visualised on an ultrasound scan.
- Magnetic resonance cholangiopancreatography and endoscopic ultrasound: modern techniques for obtaining accurate images of the pancreas and biliary tree.

Liver dysfunction affects the synthesis of clotting factors and therefore the prothrombin time must be checked and corrected (with fresh frozen plasma) before an invasive procedure e.g. liver biopsy

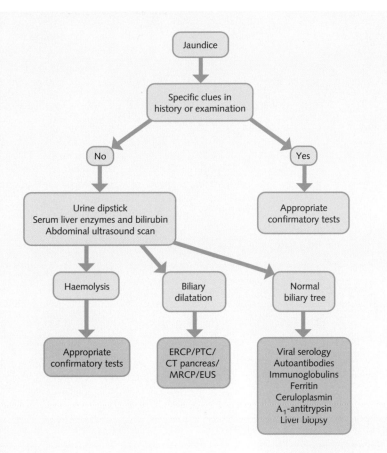

Fig. 11.4 Investigation of the patient with jaundice. (CT, computed tomography; ERCP, endoscopic retrograde cholangiopancreatography; PTC, percutaneous transhepatic cholangiography; MRCP, magnetic resonance cholangiopancreatography; EUS, endoscopic ultrasound.)

Biochemical abnormalities in different types of jaundice				
Specimen	**Test**	**Haemolysis**	**Hepatocellular**	**Cholestasis**
Urine	Urobilinogen	Raised	Normal or raised	Decreased or absent
	Conjugated bilirubin	Absent	Present	Raised
Faeces	Stercobilinogen	Raised	Normal or decreased	Decreased or absent
Serum	Bilirubin	Unconjugated	Unconjugated and conjugated	Conjugated
	Liver enzymes raised	Normal	AST, ALT	alkaline phosphatase, GGT

Fig. 11.5 Biochemical abnormalities in different types of jaundice. (ALT, alanine aminotransferase; AST, aspartate aminotransferase; GGT, γ-glutamyltransferase.)

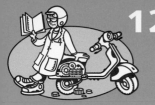

12. Abdominal Pain

Introduction

Abdominal pain is a common cause for consultation (and therefore is often found in examinations). The underlying problem can often be identified by considering which structures normally lie at the site of the pain.

Differential diagnosis of abdominal pain

This is summarised in Fig. 12.1.

History in the patient with abdominal pain

When a patient presents with abdominal pain, the first priority is to determine whether he or she has an 'acute abdomen' requiring urgent admission to hospital. The history should focus on the pain itself and then associated symptoms.

The pain itself

The onset, course, nature, and site of the pain must be accurately assessed.

Sudden onset of sustained severe pain is often due to perforation or rupture of a viscus, such as the bowel, spleen, or abdominal aorta.

Colicky pain is a griping pain that comes and goes. It is due to muscular spasm in a viscus wall, such as the bowel, ureters, and gallbladder. The muscles contract in an attempt to overcome obstruction caused by a stone, tumour, foreign body, strictures, strangulated hernias, or intussusception.

Gradual onset with sustained pain can be seen in inflammatory conditions, such as ulcerative colitis or Crohn's disease, infection including abscess formation, or gastroenteritis and malignancy.

The site and radiation of pain may help to determine the organ involved (as above). Pancreatic and aortic pain may radiate to the back, ureteric pain often radiates from 'loin to groin', and diaphragmatic irritation caused by subphrenic pathology such as an abscess causes referred shoulder tip pain.

Exacerbating and relieving factors may be helpful. Pain from peritoneal irritation is made much worse by movement and relieved by keeping still, whereas patients with colic often curl into a ball and may roll around.

Associated symptoms

The history should now assess other symptoms that may suggest the cause of pain or the consequence of the disease.

Vomiting is common. Haematemesis is seen in upper gastrointestinal bleeding from ulcers or varices, projectile vomiting is seen in pyloric stenosis, and faeculent vomiting results from severe large bowel obstruction.

Rigors suggest sepsis (e.g. abscess, cholangitis, or urinary tract infection). Rigors are particularly common with Gram negative septicaemia.

Change in bowel habit may be an important symptom. Absolute constipation (no faeces or wind passed rectally) indicates complete bowel obstruction, whereas gastroenteritis or diverticulitis often cause diarrhoea. Constipation alternating with diarrhoea is a feature of colonic malignancy but is also seen in irritable bowel syndrome.

Rectal bleeding may indicate malignancy, inflammatory bowel disease, diverticulitis, dysentery, and angiodysplasia. Dark-red bleeding is a feature of bowel infarction.

Dysuria, haematuria, and urinary frequency indicate urinary infection. Renal stones are occasionally passed per urethra.

Vaginal discharge will often be present in pelvic inflammatory disease.

Other factors

The remainder of the history is often relevant and must be obtained (e.g. past surgical history, ? adhesions), past medical history (e.g. under follow up for abdominal aortic aneurysm), details of any similar previous episodes (e.g. recurrent urinary tract infections), family history (e.g. porphyria) and drug history (e.g. opiates causing constipation).

Differential diagnosis of abdominal pain	
Site of pain	Causes
Epigastric	Lower oesophageal: oesophagitis, malignancy, perforation Stomach: peptic ulcer, gastritis Pancreas: pancreatitis, malignancy See Chapter 29
Right hypochondrium	Biliary tree: biliary colic, cholecystitis, cholangitis Liver: hepatitis, malignancy, abscess, right ventricular failure Subphrenic space: abscess See Chapters 29 and 27
Left hypochondrium	Spleen: traumatic rupture, infarction (sickle cell disease) Pancreas: pancreatitis, malignancy Subphrenic space: abscess See Chapter 29
Central abdomen	Pancreas: pancreatitis, malignancy Small/large bowel: obstruction, perforation, intussusception, ischaemia, Crohn's disease, lymphoma, IBS, adhesions, early appendicitis. Lymph nodes: mesenteric adenitis, lymphoma Abdominal aorta: ruptured aortic aneurysm See Chapter 29
Right iliac fossa	Terminal ileum: Crohn's disease, infection (e.g. tuberculosis), Meckel's diverticulum Appendix: appendicitis, tumour (including carcinoid) Caecum/ascending colon: diverticulitis, paracolic abscess, ulcerative colitis, malignancy Ovary/fallopian tubes: malignancy, ectopic pregnancy, pelvic inflammatory disease, cyst (bleeding or torsion) See Crash Course in Obstetrics and Gynaecology and Chapter 29
Left iliac fossa	Sigmoid/descending colon: diverticulitis, paracolic abscess, ulcerative colitis, malignancy Ovary/fallopian tube: malignancy, ectopic pregnancy, pelvic inflammatory disease, cyst (bleeding or torsion) See Crash Course in Obstetrics and Gynaecology and Chapter 29
Loin	Kidneys: malignancy, pyelonephritis, polycystic disease Ureters: colic due to stone or clot See Chapter 30
Suprapubic	Bladder: UTI, acute urinary retention Uterus/adnexae: pelvic inflammatory disease, endometriosis See Crash Course in Obstetrics and Gynaecology and Chapter 30
Other causes of abdominal pain	Anxiety (see Crash Course in Psychiatry) Myocardial infarction (especially inferior causing epigastric discomfort) (see Chapter 27) Lower lobe pneumonia (causing hypochondrial or loin pain) (see Chapter 28) Vasculitis (especially HSP and PAN) (see Chapter 33) Diabetic ketoacidosis (see Chapter 32) Addison's disease (see Chapter 32) Sickle cell crisis (see Chapter 34) VERY RARELY-lead poisoning, porphyria, familial Mediterranean fever

Fig. 12.1 The differential diagnosis of abdominal pain. (IBS, irritable bowel syndrome; UTI, urinary tract infection; HSP, Henoch Schönlein Purpura; PAN, polyarteritis nodosa.)

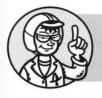

Do not forget constipation as a cause of abdominal pain in the elderly

Examining the patient with abdominal pain

The first question that must be asked is 'Is the patient acutely ill?' Signs of shock and peritonism should be looked for. The examination should then focus on specific signs. Fig. 12.2 summarises the examination approach.

Is the patient acutely ill?
Pulse and blood pressure
Tachycardia and hypotension indicate shock. Other signs include delayed capillary refill (except in sepsis where the peripheries are warm due to vasodilation) and reduced urine output. Consider septicaemia (particularly Gram-negative), severe bleeding (ruptured abdominal aortic aneurysm, spleen), fluid loss (vomiting, diarrhoea, pancreatitis, third spacing in bowel obstruction) and, rarely, acute Addisonian crisis.

Peritonism
The patient often lies still as movement exacerbates the pain. Look for rebound tenderness and guarding (involuntary spasm of the abdominal wall on palpation). When the peritonism becomes generalised, the abdomen will be rigid and bowel signs will be absent due to paralysis of peristalsis. Causes of peritonism are summarised in Fig. 12.3.

What is the underlying cause?
- Pyrexia: high temperature indicates infection; low-grade pyrexia can be found in malignancy, bowel infarction, inflammatory bowel disease and pancreatitis.
- Jaundice: hepatitis or pancreatitis (causing periampullary oedema).
- Dehydration: rapid fluid loss.
- Cachexia: suggests a chronic pathology, particularly malignancy.
- Clubbing: inflammatory bowel disease, small bowel lymphoma or chronic liver disease.
- Lymphadenopathy: lymphoma; or may be due to metastases (remember Virchow's node, see p. 42).
- Cullen's sign (periumbilical or central bruising) and Grey Turner's sign (bruising in the flanks): severe haemorrhagic pancreatitis, rarely leaking abdominal aortic aneurysm.
- Recent surgical scar: may indicate a source of peritoneal sepsis, such as an anastomotic leak.

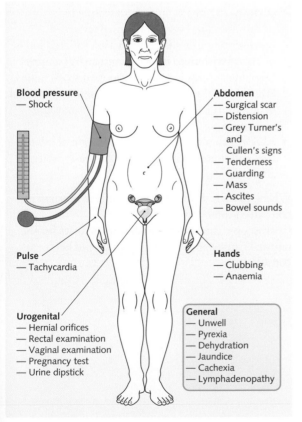

Blood pressure
— Shock

Abdomen
— Surgical scar
— Distension
— Grey Turner's and Cullen's signs
— Tenderness
— Guarding
— Mass
— Ascites
— Bowel sounds

Pulse
— Tachycardia

Hands
— Clubbing
— Anaemia

Urogenital
— Hernial orifices
— Rectal examination
— Vaginal examination
— Pregnancy test
— Urine dipstick

General
— Unwell
— Pyrexia
— Dehydration
— Jaundice
— Cachexia
— Lymphadenopathy

Fig. 12.2 Examining the patient with abdominal pain.

Causes of peritonism	
Cause	Examples
Infection	Spread from paracolic/subphrenic abscess following surgery or paracentesis Bowel perforation
Chemical irritation	Bile Faeces Gastric acid Pancreatic enzymes
Transmural inflammation	Crohn's disease Salpingitis

Fig. 12.3 Causes of peritonism.

65

- Older surgical scar: may indicate presence of adhesions.
- Abdominal distension: if marked, indicates bowel obstruction and is accompanied by a resonant percussion note. Occasionally, visible peristalsis may be present. The abdomen may also be distended in generalised peritonitis.
- Tenderness: it is important to consider what structures lie at the site of tenderness. As discussed, rebound tenderness and guarding indicate peritonism.
- Mass: this can be neoplastic or inflammatory as in Crohn's disease.
- Ascites: malignancy, peritoneal sepsis, pancreatitis, portal hypertension.
- Bowel sounds: high-pitched (tinkling) suggests obstruction; absence indicates an ileus (paralysis of bowel) from whatever cause.
- Hernial orifices (inguinal and femoral): these must be examined, particularly if obstruction is suspected.
- Pelvic and rectal examination: pelvic inflammation, cervical excitation, ectopic pregnancy, rectal mass or bleeding, stool consistency.
- Urine dipstick: should be used to determine the presence of white blood cells (infection), red blood cells (stone, tumour or infection), glucose, and ketones.Cardiorespiratory examination: consider myocardial infarction and basal pneumonia.

Murphy's sign—deep inspiration is arrested by discomfort with two fingers in the right upper quadrant in cholecystitis. Rovsing's sign—a sudden release of pressure in the left iliac fossa causes pain in the right iliac fossa in appendicitis

diagnosis. The diagnostic pathway is outlined in Fig. 12.4:

- Full blood count: leucocytosis is seen in infection and occasionally inflammation and malignancy. Anaemia may be due to acute blood loss or chronic pathology such as malignancy.
- Serum amylase: very high in acute pancreatitis, but may also be raised in perforated peptic ulcer, diabetic ketoacidosis, cholecystitis, abdominal trauma, and myocardial infarction.
- Urea and electrolytes: dehydration, renal failure as a consequence of obstructive uropathy or shock.
- Serum calcium: hypercalcaemia may cause renal stones and pancreatitis; hypocalcaemia may be a consequence of pancreatitis.
- Blood glucose: hypoglycaemia will result from liver failure or Addison's disease; hyperglycaemia will be present in ketoacidosis and may complicate acute pancreatitis.
- Liver function tests: abnormal in acute hepatitis, biliary disease, and shock.
- Microscopy, culture, and sensitivity of mid-stream urine: to exclude infection.
- Abdominal X-ray: erect and supine films should be performed if the following are suspected: perforation (air beneath the diaphragm representing free gas); obstruction (dilated loops of bowel with fluid level); pancreatitis (sentinel loop due to ileus in overlying loop of small bowel); infarction ('thumb printing' representing mucosal oedema); renal stone (90% of such stones are radio-opaque).
- Abdominal ultrasound scan: dilatation of biliary tree and ureters; intra-abdominal mass; ascites; abscess.

Where there is difficulty in making the diagnosis, a computed tomography scan, laparoscopy/laparotomy, or diagnostic tests for the unusual causes of abdominal pain should be considered.

Investigating the patient with abdominal pain

All patients admitted to hospital with abdominal pain should have a full blood count and serum biochemistry performed. The use of radiology and other tests will depend on a focused differential

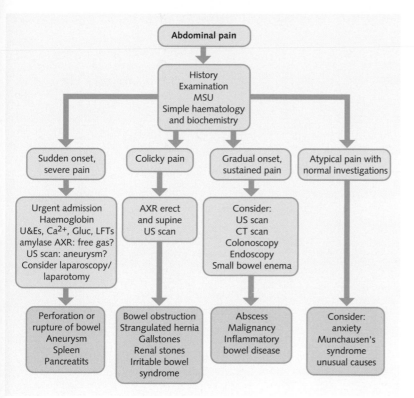

Fig. 12.4 Diagnosis in the patient with abdominal pain. (AXR, abdominal X-ray; CT, computed tomography; CXR, chest X-ray; Gluc, glucose; LFTs, liver function tests; MSU, midstream urine; U&Es, urea and electrolytes; US, ultrasound.)

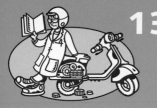

13. Polyuria and Polydipsia

Introduction

Polyuria is the passage of excessive volumes of urine. Urine output depends on fluid intake and body losses, and typically ranges from 1–3.5 L/day. Polydipsia, the ingestion of excessive volumes of fluid, is usually a consequence of polyuria.

Water is normally reabsorbed from the loop of Henle as it passes through the hyperosmolar renal medulla. Fluid in the collecting ducts enters the hyperosmolar renal medulla, with water reabsorption being controlled by antidiuretic hormone (ADH) (Fig. 13.1). The secretion of this is controlled by the hypothalamus in response to osmolality changes in the blood. A rise in osmolality leads to an increase in ADH secretion, and a fall results in a decrease in ADH secretion.

Differential diagnosis of polyuria

 There are many causes of polyuria but those seen most commonly in clinical practice are hyperglycaemia and hypercalcaemia

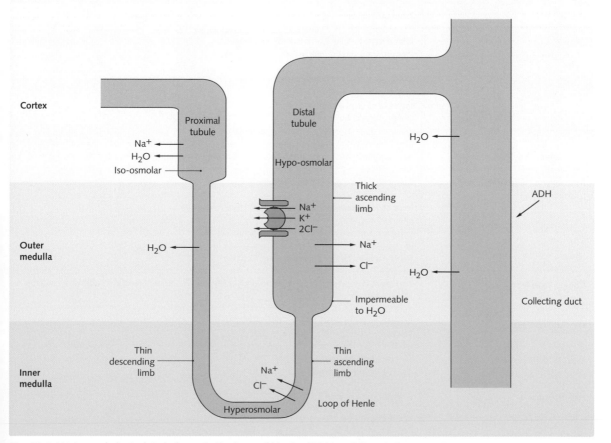

Fig. 13.1 Water and electrolyte balance in the loop of Henle. (ADH, antidiuretic hormone.)

The differential diagnosis of polyuria is summarised in Fig. 13.2.

History in the patient with polyuria or polydipsia

After asking general questions, focus on suspected causes. The following should be ascertained:

- Differentiate between polyuria (an increase in urine production) and frequency (the frequent passage of small amounts of urine).
- Weight loss: think of diabetes; malignancies (especially of the brain – does the patient have headaches?); myeloma leading to renal failure; and bony metastases causing hypercalcaemia.
- Family history: this is relevant in diabetes mellitus and both forms of diabetes insipidus.

- Previous medical history: in particular, consider previous neurosurgery or radiotherapy, head injuries and meningitis.
- Drug history: analgesic abuse may cause renal papillary necrosis; lithium may cause nephrogenic diabetes insipidus; vitamin D or milk-alkali syndrome may lead to hypercalcaemia; nephrotoxic drugs.
- Recurrent infections – may be due to diabetes mellitus.
- Features of hypercalcaemia (see p. 32), hypokalaemia (see p. 32), chronic renal failure (see p. 30) and its common causes—hypertension, diabetes mellitus, polycystic kidneys, urinary tract obstruction, chronic pyelonephritis, glomerulonephritis. Brief psychiatric history: especially if thirst is predominant. These patients may drink surreptitiously, resist investigation,

Differential diagnosis of polyuria	
Causes	**Examples/notes**
Cranial DI (insufficient ADH secretion)	Idiopathic (often familial and commonest form) Post pituitary surgery/irradiation Post head trauma Malignancy (e.g. craniopharyngioma, pinealoma, glioma, metastases) Infections (e.g. meningitis) Infiltrations (e.g. sarcoid and histiocytosis X) Drugs (e.g. alcohol)
Psychogenic polydipsia	Relatively common psychiatric disturbance characterised by excessive water intake (if prolonged can cause temporary 'renal medullary washout' with reduction of kidney's concentrating ability)
Nephrogenic DI (inability of kidney to respond to ADH)	Congenital (primary renal tubular defect) Electrolyte imbalance (hypokalaemia and hypercalcaemia) Lithium toxicity Longstanding pyelonephritis or hydronephrosis Renal papillary necrosis (analgesic nephropathy)
Chronic renal failure	Can result in depressed renal concentrating ability and therefore higher urine volume to excrete a given solute load
Acute renal failure	Diuretic phase of ATN Following relief of obstructive uropathy
Osmotic diuresis	Glucose (diabetes mellitus) Calcium (hypercalcaemia)
ANP release	Arrhythmia (e.g. after SVT)

Fig. 13.2 The differential diagnosis of polyuria. (DI, diabetes insipidus; ADH, anti-diuretic hormone; ATN, acute tubular necrosis; ANP, atrial natriuretic peptide; SVT, supraventricular tachycardia.)

have other neurotic symptoms, and may lack nocturnal symptoms.

Examining the patient with polyuria or polydipsia

The examination approach in the patient with polyuria or polydipsia is summarised in Fig. 13.3.

General appearance
- Wasting/cachexia (malignancy and diabetes mellitus) and hydration status.

- Skin manifestations: diabetes mellitus and malignancy (see p. 38), yellow–brown skin of chronic renal failure.
- Nails: brown arcs in chronic renal failure; clubbing—associated with bronchogenic carcinoma which may produce excess adrenocorticotropic hormone (and therefore hypokalaemia and nephrogenic diabetes insipidus) or parathyroid hormone (and therefore hypercalcaemia).
- Anaemia: malignancy or chronic renal failure.
- Lymphadenopathy: malignancy or infiltrative disorder.
- Optic signs: fundal changes of hypertension or diabetes.

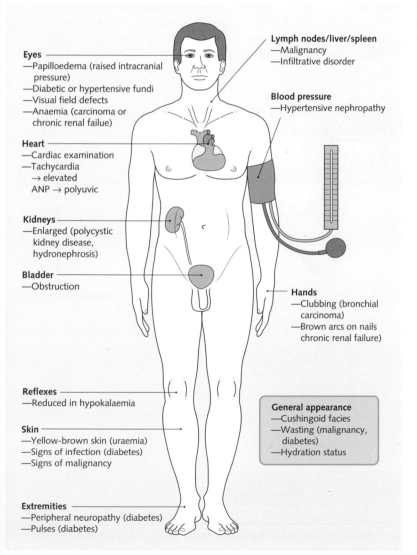

Fig. 13.3 Examining the patient with polyuria or polydipsia (ANP, atrial natriuretic peptide).

Cardiovascular system

Check the heart rhythm (atrial natriuretic peptide production) and the blood pressure for hypertensive nephropathy.

Abdominal examination

Palpate the kidneys as they may be palpable in polycystic kidney disease or hydronephrosis. A large bladder may indicate urinary tract obstruction. The liver and spleen may be enlarged in malignancy and infiltrative disorders.

Neurological examination

The neurological examination should assess the following:

- Diabetic peripheral neuropathy.
- Hypotonia and areflexia with hypokalaemia.
- Wasting in malignancy.
- Paraneoplastic syndromes. Visual fields (classically bitemporal hemianopia with pituitary

pathology) and papilloedema (raised intracranial pressure).

Investigating the patient with polyuria and polydipsia

An algorithm for the investigation of the patient with polyuria and polydipsia is given in Fig. 13.4. The following investigations should be carried out:

- Urinalysis: specific gravity is a measure of the weight of dissolved particles in the urine and osmolality is a measure of their number. (They are closely related unless there is a small number of large particles e.g. myeloma.)
- Biochemistry: renal failure (see p. 30), hypercalcaemia (see p. 32), hypokalaemia (see p. 32) and hyperglycaemia (see p. 32).
- Full blood count: anaemia with chronic renal failure, or malignancy (e.g.leukaemia), and reticuloses.

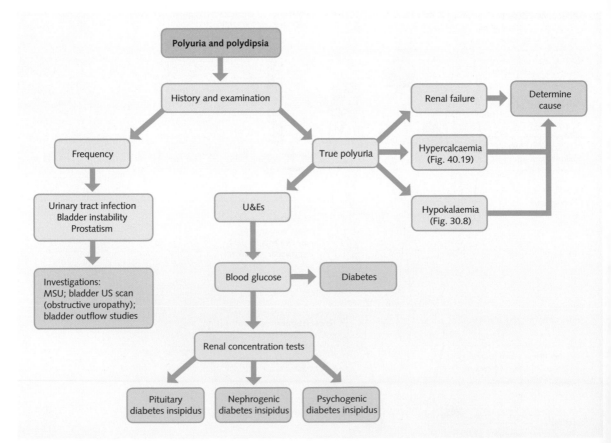

Fig. 13.4 Algorithm for the investigation of the patient with polyuria and polydipsia. (MSU, mid-stream urine; U&Es, urea and electrolytes; US, ultrasound.)

Procedure for testing patients with polyuria and polydipsia
• weigh the patient • Deprive of all fluids the night before the tests • The next morning, weigh the patient every 2 hours (a decrease in weight by >3% indicates dehydration, so stop the test) • Collect urine and blood for osmolality • If the urine osmolality fails to reach 800 mmol/kg give intramuscular DDAVP (DDAVP is synthetic vasopressin which acts in the same way as ADH) • Collect blood and urine for osmolality

Fig. 13.5 Procedure for testing patients with polyuria and polydipsia. (ADH, antidiuretic hormone; DDAVP, desmopressin.)

Interpretation of patient test results

	Fluid deprivation		I.M. DDAVP	
	Plasma osmolality	Urine osmolality	Plasma osmolality	Urine osmolality
Pituitary DI	↑	→	↑	↑
Psychogenic DI	↑	↑*	↑	↑
Nephrogenic DI	↑	→	↑	→

Fig. 13.6 Interpretation of patient test results. (DI, diabetes insipidus; *urine is concentrated, but less than in normal response; ↑, increase in osmolality; →, no significant change in osmolality.)

- Chest X-ray: if any suspicion of sarcoidosis, primary or secondary malignancy.
- Computed tomography or magnetic resonance imaging of brain: to investigate intra-cranial pathology (e.g. if considering a space occupying lesion).
- Renal concentration tests: if either a hypothalamic or pituitary cause or renal tubular dysfunction is suspected. It is mandatory to exclude other potential causes for polyuria, as renal concentration tests may be dangerous.

The patient is told to drink nothing from 16.00 hours the day before attending the outpatient department. If the urine osmolality the next morning is not above 800 mmol/kg, inpatient tests are required (Figs 13.5 and 13.6).

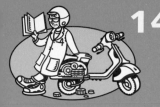

14. Haematuria and Proteinuria

Introduction

Haematuria and proteinuria are common presentations of renal disease, although both may also be due to systemic conditions. They are often incidental findings on urine dipstick testing. Haematuria is abnormal if there are more than two red blood cells per high-power field; proteinuria is defined as more than 150 mg of protein per 24-hour collection of urine. Red-coloured urine may also be due to haemoglobinuria, myoglobinuria, porphyria, drugs (e.g. rifampicin), or even the ingestion of beetroot.

Differential diagnosis of haematuria and proteinuria

Haematuria

This is best classified by the site of pathology.

Systemic conditions

- Clotting disorders and anticoagulants.
- Thrombocytopenia.
- Sickle cell disease.
- Endocarditis.
- Vasculitides.

Kidneys

- Glomerular disease (e.g. immunoglobulin A nephropathy, one of the multiple glomerulonephritides, infective endocarditis).
- Infections (e.g. pyelonephritis, tuberculosis).
- Tumours (e.g. renal cell carcinoma, angioma, adenoma, papilloma).
- Cystic disease (e.g. polycystic kidney disease, medullary sponge kidney).
- Interstitial nephritis: drugs (>75% cases) (e.g. penicillins, sulphonamides and non-steroidal anti-inflammatory drugs).
- Trauma (e.g. both spontaneous and after renal biopsy).
- Papillary necrosis.

Ureters

- Calculi.
- Tumours: transitional cell carcinoma, papilloma.
- Trauma.

Bladder

- Cystitis: infection, chemical-induced cystitis, postradiation cystitis.
- Tumours: transitional cell carcinoma, papilloma.
- Trauma.
- Calculi.
- Infections: tuberculosis and schistosomiasis.

Prostate

- Prostatic carcinoma.
- Tuberculosis.
- Infection: prostatitis.

Urethra

- Calculi.
- Trauma.
- Tumours.
- Foreign bodies (e.g. urinary catheters).

Other sites

Haematuria may result from lesions in adjacent organs (by fistula formation or inflammation) such as:

- Colonic diverticulitis.
- Inflammatory bowel disease.
- Acute appendicitis in a pelvic appendix.
- Acute salpingitis and pelvic inflammatory disease.
- Carcinoma of the colon or genital tract.

Proteinuria

Whilst small amounts of proteinuria can occur in non-renal disease such as urinary tract infection and with vaginal mucus, significant proteinuria >1 g/day usually indicates primary renal pathology (Fig. 14.1).

Benign proteinuria may result from the following:

- Functional proteinuria: pyrexia, strenuous exercise, congestive cardiac failure, acute illnesses, pregnancy.
- Orthostatic proteinuria: common in males aged under 30 years; proteinuria when upright but normal when supine.

Pathological proteinuria can result from all glomerular disease as the basement membrane is damaged and becomes 'leaky'. Differential diagnoses include:

Levels of proteinuria	
	G/day
Normal	0.02
Microalbuminuria	0.02–0.2
Detectable with urinary dipstick	>0.2
Significant	>1.0
Nephrotic range	>3.0
Heavy	>5.0

Fig. 14.1 Levels of proteinuria.

- Diabetes mellitus.
- Glomerulonephritis.
- Other causes of nephrotic syndrome (Fig. 14.2).

In addition to the above, tubular proteinuria, due to tubular or interstitial damage, may occur. Proteinuria results from failure of the tubules to reabsorb some of the plasma proteins that have been filtered by the normal glomerulus. The loss of protein is usually mild and may result from the following:

- Congenital disorders: Fanconi's syndrome, cystinosis, renal tubular acidosis.
- Heavy metal poisoning: lead, cadmium, Wilson's disease.
- Acute tubular necrosis.
- Chronic nephritis and pyelonephritis.
- Renal transplantation.

Finally, overflow proteinuria may occur. This is when abnormal amounts of low molecular weight protein (filtered at the glomerulus) are neither reabsorbed nor catabolised completely by the renal tubular cells (e.g. as in acute pancreatitis; amylase). The following may be responsible:

- Multiple myeloma: Bence-Jones protein.
- Haemolytic anaemia and march haemoglobinuria: haemoglobin.
- Rhabdomyolysis: myoglobin.

Causes of nephrotic syndrome	
Cause	Examples
Renal disease	**Glomerular disorders** -Primary -Secondary to cause Reflux nephropathy
Systemic disease	**Amyloidosis** **Systemic lupus erythematosus** Henoch -Schönlein Purpura
Metabolic disease	**Diabetes mellitus**
Infection	HIV Infective endocarditis Malaria Hepatitis B
Malignancy	Lymphoma Myeloma
Drugs	Gold Penicillamine Heroin Heavy metals
Familial disorders	Alport's syndrome Finnish-type nephrotic syndrome Sickle cell disease
Allergy	Bee stings Pollen

Fig. 14.2 Causes of nephrotic syndrome. Common causes in bold.

History in the patient with haematuria and proteinuria

If haematuria is present in a young woman, ensure that she is not menstruating

Bear the differential diagnoses in mind.

The following factors should be determined when obtaining a history in the patient with haematuria or proteinuria:

- Has there been a history of acute illness especially fever (e.g. with urinary tract infection or post streptococcal glomerulonephritis)?
- Ask about the appearance of the urine. Is there frank blood (malignancy), the frothy urine of heavy proteinuria or foreign matter (e.g. vesicocolic fistula)?
- Ask about the urine volume; oliguria may indicate renal failure, polyuria could be a sign of systemic disease(e.g. diabetes or interstitial renal disease and loss of tubular concentrating ability).
- Ask about associated urinary symptoms, such as frequency (urinary tract infection, bladder calculus, prostatism), hesitancy, strangury (the desire to pass something that will not pass; e.g. a calculus) and dysuria (painful micturition reflecting urethral or bladder inflammation).
- When does it occur in the urinary stream? Is the haematuria worse with exercise? This suggests tumour or calculus.
- Ask about loin pain. This suggests pyelonephritis or renal calculi.
- Ask about colicky pain. This suggests a ureteric calculus.
- Ask specifically about diabetes mellitus, hypertension, previous calculi and recurrent urine infections.
- Is there any evidence of systemic or chronic illness (e.g. arthralgia or rash with vasculitis/connective tissue disease or retinopathy with diabetes mellitus)?
- Are there generalised features of carcinoma (e.g. anorexia and weight loss)?
- Ask about symptoms arising from lesions in adjacent organs.

- Ask about past and current medications (e.g. analgesics (nephropathy) or anticoagulants).
- Is there a history of trauma?
- Has there been recent foreign travel (e.g. schistosomiasis or tuberculosis)?
- Is there a family history? Are there clotting disorders – does the patient bruise easily? Is there a history of renal problems (e.g. polycystic kidney disease, sickle cell disease)?
- Does the patient have a vaginal or penile discharge?
- Are there symptoms of fluid overload or hypoalbuminaemia (e.g. shortness of breath, orthopnoea, ankle swelling)?
- Ask about heavy metal exposure.
- Are there any risk factors for HIV or hepatitis?
- Is the proteinuria only present after vigorous exercise?
- Is the proteinuria absent in early morning specimens (orthostatic proteinuria)?
- Ensure the patient is not pregnant. Whilst usually benign, never forget pre-eclampsia.
- Do not forget to keep the causes of nephrotic syndrome in mind (Fig. 14.2).

Ask about the appearance of the urine:
- If the urine is blood stained at the start of micturition and clear later on, the site of pathology is likely to be the urethra or prostate.
- If the urine is more blood stained towards the end of micturition, the site of pathology is likely to be the bladder.
- If the urine is evenly blood stained throughout micturition, the site of pathology is likely to be the kidney or ureter

Examining the patient with haematuria and proteinuria

The examination approach is summarised in Fig. 14.3.

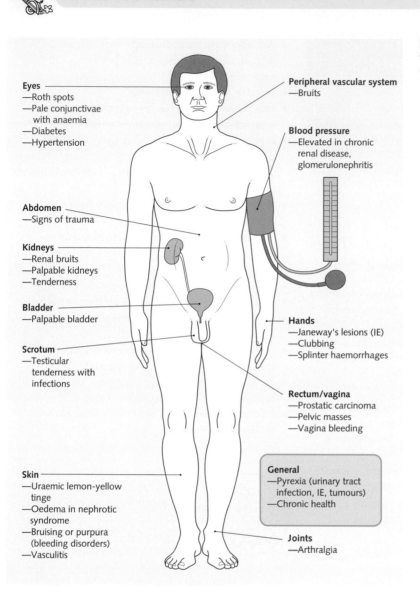

Fig. 14.3 Examining the patient with haematuria and proteinuria. (IE, infective endocarditis.)

Eyes
—Roth spots
—Pale conjunctivae with anaemia
—Diabetes
—Hypertension

Peripheral vascular system
—Bruits

Blood pressure
—Elevated in chronic renal disease, glomerulonephritis

Abdomen
—Signs of trauma

Kidneys
—Renal bruits
—Palpable kidneys
—Tenderness

Bladder
—Palpable bladder

Hands
—Janeway's lesions (IE)
—Clubbing
—Splinter haemorrhages

Scrotum
—Testicular tenderness with infections

Rectum/vagina
—Prostatic carcinoma
—Pelvic masses
—Vagina bleeding

Skin
—Uraemic lemon-yellow tinge
—Oedema in nephrotic syndrome
—Bruising or purpura (bleeding disorders)
—Vasculitis

General
—Pyrexia (urinary tract infection, IE, tumours)
—Chronic health

Joints
—Arthralgia

Investigating the patient with haematuria and proteinuria

An algorithm for the investigation of the patient with haematuria and proteinuria is given in Fig. 14.4. Renal biopsy may provide the best information but is invasive and not without risk. Start with urine, blood and radiological tests.

Urine
The following urinary tests should be performed:

Initial tests
- Gross appearance: frank haematuria should always make the doctor consider malignancy.

- Urinary dipstick: provides initial information about presence or absence and degree of protein and haematuria. Many sticks also test for nitrites/leucocytes/ketones/pH and glucose.
- Microscopy: red blood cells (dysmorphic or normal), white blood cells, casts (red cell casts imply glomerulonephritis), organisms and crystals.
- Culture: infection.
- Early morning urine: acid-fast bacilli if tuberculosis is suspected.
- Cytology: malignancy.

24-hour collection of urine
The level of proteinuria is important as both an indicator of the severity and likely rate of progression

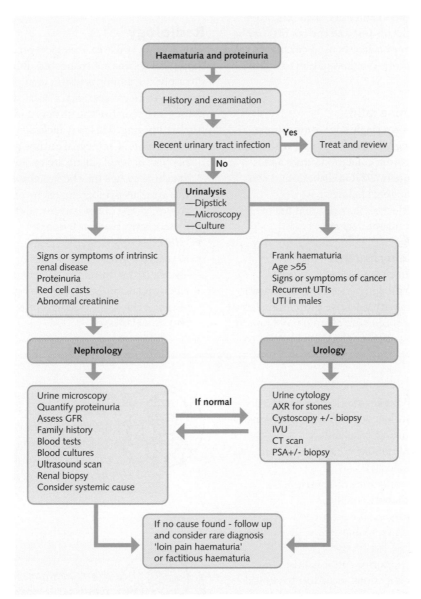

Fig. 14.4 Algorithm for investigation of haematuria and proteinuria. (UTI, urinary tract infection; GFR, glomerular filtration rate; AXR, abdominal X ray; IVU, intravenous urogram; CT, computerised tomography; PSA, prostate specific antigen.)

of renal disease. Reduction of proteinuria correlates with slowing of the loss of renal function. It is usually done on a 24-hour sample of urine. The glomerular filtration rate (GFR) can be assessed from creatinine measurements in blood and urine. Patients often comply poorly with this test and the results may be erroneous. Many nephrologists use a calculated value (e.g. via the Cockcroft–Gault equation to follow GFR).

Protein to creatinine ratio

This is performed on a single spot urine sample (preferably morning). It correlates well with accurate 24-hour urinary protein collection values and is predictive of decline in GFR in diabetic and non-diabetic proteinuric renal failure.

It is easier to collect and process and has been widely adopted by diabetologists.

Differential protein clearance

Differential protein clearance (selectivity) is occasionally performed in patients with nephrotic syndrome. Patients with selective proteinuria (small molecular weight proteins are cleared more rapidly than large proteins) are more likely to respond to steroid therapy.

Blood

The following blood tests should be performed:
- Full blood count: leucocytosis with infections, anaemia with chronic renal failure.
- Erythrocyte sedimentation rate and C-reactive protein (e.g. vasculitis).
- Clotting studies: bleeding diathesis.
- Blood glucose: diabetes mellitus.
- Urea and electrolytes: renal function.
- Creatine kinase: myoglobinuria.
- Urate: gout.
- Blood cultures: infective endocarditis.
- Specialised investigations according to clinical suspicion (e.g. serum complement, anti streptococcal titres and autoantibodies for glomerulonephritis).

- Protein electrophoresis and urinary Bence Jones protein (myeloma).
- HIV and hepatitis serology: potential causes of nephrotic syndrome.

Radiology

This is of most use in urological practice where structural lesions are suspected. Renal tract ultrasound scanning is useful in nephrological practice to assess size and cortical structure of the kidney and visualise the ureters and bladder to guide further imaging. This may include:
- Abdominal X-ray: renal outline and stones. Ninety percent of renal calculi are opaque; urate and xanthine stones may be radiolucent.
- Intravenous pyelogram: excretory function, stones, shape of the calyces, ureters and bladder.
- Cystoscopy: bladder lesions.
- Ureteroscopy: ureter lesions.
- Retrograde pyelogram: stones or obstructive lesions in the ureters are suspected.
- Abdominal computerised tomography scan: to visualise the kidneys, adjacent organs, and other abdominal masses.

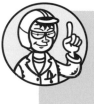

When thinking of causes of haematuria, think of the site of pathology along the renal tract. At each site, tumours, calculi, and infection are possible

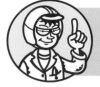

Frank haematuria in the elderly needs urological investigation for malignancy first

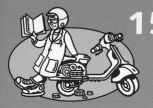

15. Hypertension

Introduction

The level of blood pressure above which someone is 'hypertensive' is controversial and varies between different countries. However, most clinicians and published British guidelines would initiate drug treatment when blood pressure is persistently elevated above 160/100 mmHg and consider it when the blood pressure is above 140/90 mmHg. This is an arbitrary cut-off point and is influenced by age, end-organ damage, and other risk factors. Approximately 95% of all hypertensive patients have 'essential' or 'primary' hypertension and have no underlying disease. Secondary hypertension can be the result of a range of different pathological processes.

Differential diagnosis of hypertension

Essential hypertension
Essential hypertension comprises 95% of cases. There is no specific underlying cause though lifestyle may play a part (e.g. obesity, alcohol, lack of exercise, high salt diet).

Secondary hypertension
Secondary hypertension comprises 5% of cases. Factors leading to secondary hypertension are:
- Renal parenchymal disease (e.g. chronic pyelonephritis, glomerulonephritis, polycystic disease, tumour).
- Renal artery disease (e.g. atherosclerosis, fibromuscular dysplasia, vasculitis).
- Obstructive uropathy (e.g. hydronephrosis due to a stone or tumour).
- Congenital (e.g. coarctation of the aorta).
- Drugs (e.g. combined oral contraceptive pill, non-steroidal anti-inflammatory drugs).
- Endocrine (e.g. phaeochromocytoma, hyperaldosteronism, Cushing's syndrome, acromegaly).
- Raised intracranial pressure. Usually coupled with bradycardia, the 'Cushing reflex'.

95% of patients with hypertension have no underlying disease

History in the patient with hypertension

Hypertension is usually asymptomatic and is often found incidentally. Ideally, all people should have their blood pressure measured every 5 years as a minimum. The history should be approached in three parts.

First, how long has the patient had hypertension and what treatments have been given so far? Second, how severe is the hypertension and has it resulted in complications? Finally, are there any risk factors suggesting that an underlying pathology may be present?

Presentation and history of hypertension
Important questions to address are as follows:
- How was the hypertension discovered? For example, at a routine assessment or with malignant (accelerated) hypertension? Liaison with the patient's general practitioner or other health care professionals is often needed for a full history.
- For how long has the blood pressure been monitored? Unless severe, the diagnosis should not be made until blood pressure is persistently elevated for at least 6 months.
- What treatments, if any, has the patient been given so far? If blood pressure control is poor despite taking correct doses of three antihypertensive agents, the patient is said to have 'resistant hypertension'.

How severe is the hypertension and are there complications?
Mild hypertension is asymptomatic. However, when hypertension is severe or chronic, it can be associated with complications resulting from end organ damage; the following symptoms may occur:

- Headaches.
- Dyspnoea.
- Symptoms of cardiac failure.
- Angina pectoris or myocardial infarction.
- Transient ischaemic attacks or stroke.
- Visual disturbance.

Is the history suggestive of an underlying cause?

Ask about the following:

- Lifestyle history, paying particular attention to alcohol and smoking (atherosclerosis).
- Precise drug history.
- Previous medical history (e.g. recurrent pyelonephritis, nephrectomy).

- Family history may suggest an underlying disease (e.g. adult polycystic kidney disease).
- Symptoms of phaeochromocytoma are rare but include episodic pallor, headache, tremor, palpitations, and nausea.

Examining the patient with hypertension

Patients with uncomplicated mild essential hypertension will have no associated clinical signs. However, when a patient is found to be hypertensive, one should search for evidence of complications or an underlying cause (Fig. 15.1).

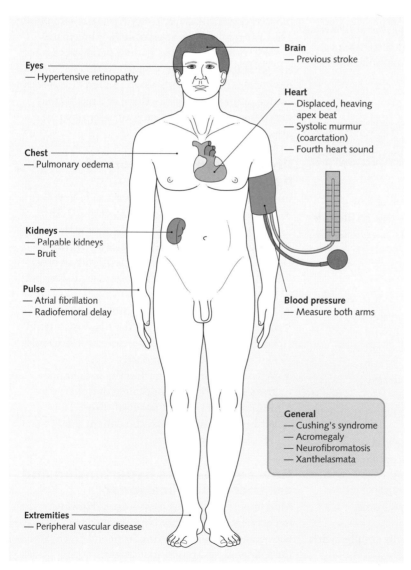

Fig. 15.1 Examining the patient with hypertension.

Eyes
— Hypertensive retinopathy

Brain
— Previous stroke

Heart
— Displaced, heaving apex beat
— Systolic murmur (coarctation)
— Fourth heart sound

Chest
— Pulmonary oedema

Kidneys
— Palpable kidneys
— Bruit

Pulse
— Atrial fibrillation
— Radiofemoral delay

Blood pressure
— Measure both arms

General
— Cushing's syndrome
— Acromegaly
— Neurofibromatosis
— Xanthelasmata

Extremities
— Peripheral vascular disease

Evidence of an underlying cause

- Palpable kidneys: polycystic disease, renal tumour.
- Peripheral vascular disease and xanthelasmata: renal artery stenosis.
- Renal bruits are rarely heard. Other vascular bruits are equally valid indicators of atherosclerosis: renovascular disease.
- Radiofemoral delay: coarctation of the aorta.
- Neurofibromatosis: renal artery stenosis.
- Cushing's disease, acromegaly.

Evidence of complications

- Atrial fibrillation.
- Displaced, thrusting apex beat indicating left ventricular hypertrophy.
- Frank cardiac failure.
- Retinopathy.
- Previous stroke.

Investigating the patient with hypertension

An algorithm for the investigation of the patient with hypertension is given in Fig. 15.2. At presentation all hypertensive patients should have the following tests:

- Urine dipstick for blood and protein: parenchymal disease, urinary tract infection, stone.
- Urea and electrolytes: may indicate renal impairment or suggest a cause (e.g. Conn's syndrome).
- Blood glucose and lipid profile: screen for modifiable cardiovascular risk factors. A quantitative value can be obtained from published risk assessment charts.
- Electrocardiogram: significant hypertension may result in left ventricular hypertrophy.

- Fundoscopy: retinopathy indicating end-organ damage.

The blood pressure should be measured reproducibly (i.e. with the correct cuff size, the patient seated, relaxed and the cuff at the level of the heart). Diastolic pressure is recorded when the audible pulse disappears (Korotkoff V). If an automated monitor is being used, it should one that is validated for the purpose by organisations such as the British Hypertension Society.

Figure 15.3 shows those patients who should then be investigated further, using the following tests:

- 24-hour ambulatory blood pressure measurement (e.g. when blood pressure is abnormally variable, resistant to drug treatment or to exclude 'white coat hypertension').
- 24-hour urinary catecholamine and metanephrine excretion: phaeochromocytoma.
- Radiological investigations: renovascular disease, renal parenchymal disease, obstructive uropathy. This may include abdominal ultrasound scanning, or nuclear medical investigation.
- Renal angiography: renal artery disease; this is a definitive test and should be performed if indicated by the radiological tests or clinical circumstances. Magnetic resonance angiography is now the first-line non-invasive test.

 All hypertensive patients should have urine dipstick, urea and electrolytes, cardiovascular risk stratification and an electrocardiogram. Only a few need any further tests

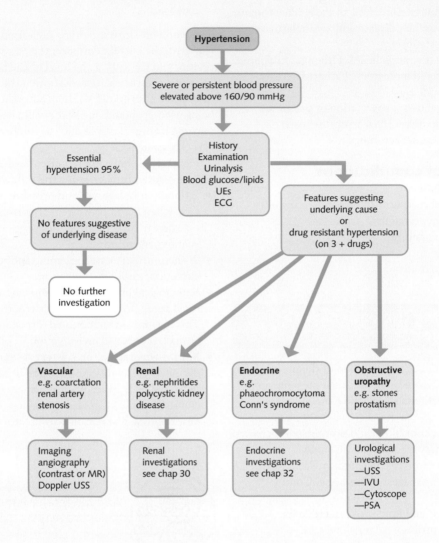

Fig. 15.2 Algorithm for the investigation of the patient with hypertension. (ECG, electrocardiogram; IVU, intravenous urogram; U&Es, urea and electrolytes; USS, ultrasound scan; PSA, prostate specific antigen.)

Indications for detailed investigation of hypertension

- Recent onset or worsening of hypertension
- Malignant (accelerated) hypertension
- Uncontrolled hypertension despite three antihypertensive drugs (beware of and check for non adherence to medication)
- Abdominal bruit
- Proteinuria, haematuria, or abnormal renal function
- Hypokalaemia not otherwise explained, e.g. by diuretic therapy
- Renal failure caused by angiotensin-converting enzyme (ACE) inhibitors
- Young age (<30 years)
- Severe generalized atherosclerosis
- Unexplained ('flash') pulmonary oedema

Fig. 15.3 Indications for detailed investigation of hypertension.

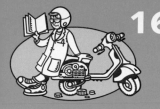

16. Headache and Facial Pain

Introduction

Headache is one of the most common presenting symptoms. There are often few clinical signs and the history is the main diagnostic tool. Many different pathological processes can result in headache and facial pain.

Differential diagnosis of headache and facial pain

The differential diagnosis of headache and facial pain is summarised in Fig. 16.1.

History in the patient with headache and facial pain

This is the key to diagnosis and the onset, nature, and subsequent pattern of pain will usually provide a good shortlist of likely causes. The presence of additional symptoms and risk factors may add further weight to this list.

Solitary acute episode

This pattern is seen in infection, vascular events and trauma. (Note that it may also be the first presentation of the other causes of headache.)

Subarachnoid haemorrhage presents with a sudden onset of severe pain, 'as if someone had hit them on the back of the head'. Nausea, vomiting, neck stiffness, and photophobia result from meningeal irritation. Altered conscious level and focal neurological deficits may also occur depending on the site and size of the bleed.

Fits, focal neurological symptoms, and symptoms of raised intracranial pressure can also result from dural venous sinus thrombosis. This is a rare complication of pregnancy, oral contraceptive pill use, dehydration, paranasal sinus infection, and severe intercurrent illness. Rarely dissection of a carotid or vertebral artery can cause a sudden onset of pain associated with focal neurology.

Patients with infective meningitis present with a short history of headache, symptoms of infection (malaise, fever, and rigors) and symptoms of meningeal irritation (vomiting, photophobia, and neck pain and stiffness). However, tuberculous and carcinomatous meningitis have a more subacute presentation which can be easily missed.

Cerebral abscess causes headaches, fits, symptoms of infection, and symptoms of raised intracranial pressure as the lesion expands (see below). The infection may have spread from a primary focus, such as the lung in bronchiectasis, middle ear, or paranasal sinuses.

Progressive headache

A headache that comes on gradually over days or weeks and increases in severity is often a feature of a tumour, benign intracranial hypertension, or hydrocephalus. In all three the headache results from raised intracranial pressure and has the characteristic features shown in Fig. 16.2. Temporal arteritis also presents gradually, but the nature of the headache is very different.

Cerebral tumours can be primary or secondary. The patient may have a history of malignancy elsewhere. The most common tumours to metastasise to the brain are those of the thyroid, bronchus, and breast, as well as gastric, renal and prostate tumours. In addition to headache, the patient may also develop fits and focal neurological deficits related to the site of the lesion.

Benign intracranial hypertension is most common in young women. Headache, nausea, and visual disturbance are the presenting symptoms. There is an association with obesity, empty sella turcica, and certain drugs. If left untreated, the patient may become blind due to infarction of the optic nerve.

Temporal arteritis predominantly affects the elderly. The patient presents with a superficial headache overlying the temporal arteries. The pain may be exacerbated by brushing or combing the hair. Jaw claudication may arise as a consequence of inflammation of the branches of the external carotid artery. Visual loss may be temporary (amaurosis fugax) or permanent if the ciliary or central retinal

Differential diagnosis of headache and facial pain (see Chapter 31)	
Pattern	Causes
Solitary acute episode	Infection—meningitis, encephalitis, abscess Vascular event—intracranial haemorrhage (especially subarachnoid), venous sinus thrombosis, occasionally infarction (especially if arterial dissection occurred) Trauma
Progressive headache	Raised intracranial pressure (including benign intracranial hypertension) Giant cell arteritis
Episodic headache/facial pain	Migraine Cluster headache (migrainous neuralgia) Trigeminal neuralgia Coital cephalgia
Chronic headache/facial pain	Tension headache/analgesic rebound headache Postherpetic neuralgia Post head injury Paget's disease of the skull
Other causes of facial pain	Dental problems Temporomandibular joint Ears/nose/sinuses Cervical spine Eye Myocardial ischaemia (rarely)

Fig. 16.1 The differential diagnosis of headache and facial pain.

artery are affected. Weight loss, anorexia, fever, and proximal muscle stiffness (but not tenderness) may also occur.

Consider temporal arteritis in any patient aged over 50 years old with a headache

Episodic headache and facial pain

Migraine and cluster headaches present with episodes of pain (often severe) interspersed with long symptom-free periods. Paroxysms of pain are also a feature of trigeminal neuralgia.

Symptoms of raised intracranial pressure
• Headache worse on coughing, sneezing, stooping down • Headache worse in the morning • Visual disturbance due to papilloedema • Nausea and vomiting • Diplopia (false localizing 6th cranial nerve palsy)

Fig. 16.2 Symptoms of raised intracranial pressure.

Classical migraine usually starts with an aura lasting 15–60 minutes, characterised by a sense of ill health and visual abnormalities (fortification spectra, scotomata or teichopsia). Occasionally, the aura may include focal neurological symptoms such as hemiplegia, ophthalmoplegia, ataxia, vertigo, or unilateral facial palsy. A throbbing headache then develops, which tends to be unilateral but can become generalised. This is associated with nausea, vomiting, photophobia, and phonophobia. The attack resolves spontaneously after several hours and is often followed by sleep. Sometimes the aura can occur without an headache or the headache without an aura ('common migraine').

Migraine is more common in women. Provoking factors include menstruation, fatigue, cheese, red wine, and the oral contraceptive pill.

Cluster headache (migrainous neuralgia) is a severe unilateral pain centred around one eye. The pain lasts for around 1 hour and occurs daily (commonly at a predictable time) for several weeks, often waking the patient from sleep. There is ipsilateral nasal congestion and the eye becomes watery. Horner's syndrome can develop and is occasionally permanent. Symptom-free periods of many months occur between attacks. Cluster headaches are more common in men and may be precipitated by alcohol.

Trigeminal neuralgia (tic douloureux) is characterised by paroxysms of lancinating pain in the distribution of the fifth cranial nerve. It is stimulated by touching 'trigger zones' on the face such as the lips, or by eating, or drinking. The pain lasts for up to 1 minute and does not occur during sleep. Spontaneous remissions can last several months.

Chronic headache and facial pain

Persistent pain is a feature of postherpetic neuralgia, post-traumatic headache, Paget's disease of the skull or tension headache.

Following shingles of the trigeminal nerve (usually the ophthalmic division), a persistent burning pain known as postherpetic neuralgia may develop. Facial scarring is usually apparent and the pain may disturb sleep. It is uncommon in the young.

Tension headaches are the commonest cause of headaches presenting to doctors. The feeling is often described as a 'tight band around the head', being most common in the frontal and occipital regions, or as a 'pressure' behind the eyes. It is a constant pain, which tends to be worse towards the end of the day or at times of particular stress. There may be coexistent depression. Persistent headache may occur if analgesics are overused–analgesic rebound headache.

Following head injury, which may not necessarily be severe, a few patients develop persistent headache, similar to a tension headache. It is associated with poor memory and concentration, dizziness, irritability, and symptoms of depression. The patient may be involved in litigation related to the accident responsible.

Examining the patient with headache and facial pain

The diagnosis is often clear from the history. On examination look for evidence of the pathological processes, such as raised intracranial pressure and meningism. Focal neurological deficits, if present, help to determine the site of the lesion. Fig. 16.3 summarises the examination approach.

Signs of raised intracranial pressure
- Papilloedema: commonly, the only sign.

- False localizing sign (ipsilateral then bilateral sixth cranial nerve palsy).
- Altered level of consciousness, bradycardia, hypertension if acute or severe, which can progress to decerebrate posturing and death.

Signs of meningism
- Irritability: with a preference for a quiet, darkened room.
- Neck stiffness.
- Positive Kernig's sign: spasm and pain in hamstrings on knee extension.
- Positive Brudzinski's sign: neck flexion causes leg flexion.
- Delirium, fever, and petechial rash: may also be present in infectious meningitis.

If subarachnoid haemorrhage is suspected, look for subhyaloid (retinal) haemorrhage, bruit of an arteriovenous malformation, and a third cranial nerve palsy caused by direct pressure from a posterior communicating artery aneurysm.

Signs of temporal arteritis
- Temporal artery tenderness.
- Loss of temporal artery pulsation—there may be overlying erythema.
- Optic atrophy.
- Low-grade pyrexia.

Focal neurological deficit

Focal neurological signs will help to determine the site of the lesion (see Chapter 21), and may be found in addition to other signs, such as meningism or raised intracranial pressure.

Investigating the patient with headache and facial pain

An algorithm for the investigation of the patient with headache and facial pain is given in Fig. 16.4. Investigations used in this type of patient include:
- Full blood count: normochromic normocytic anaemia suggests chronic pathology (e.g. temporal arteritis, tuberculous meningitis); leucocytosis will be seen in infection.
- Erythrocyte sedimentation rate: high in temporal arteritis but may also be raised in infection and malignancy.
- Temporal artery biopsy: temporal arteritis. This is a definitive test, but as there is often patchy

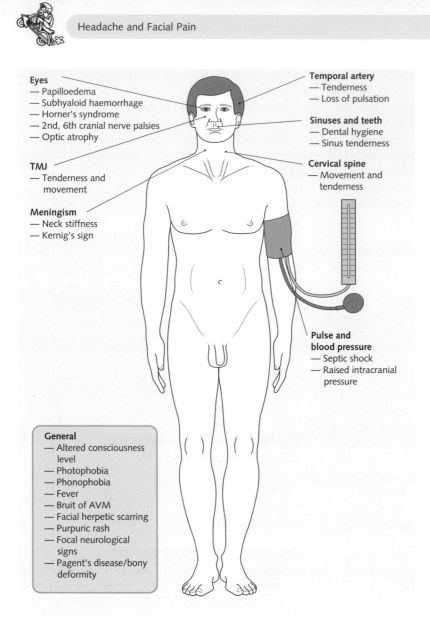

Eyes
— Papilloedema
— Subhyaloid haemorrhage
— Horner's syndrome
— 2nd, 6th cranial nerve palsies
— Optic atrophy

TMJ
— Tenderness and movement

Meningism
— Neck stiffness
— Kernig's sign

Temporal artery
— Tenderness
— Loss of pulsation

Sinuses and teeth
— Dental hygiene
— Sinus tenderness

Cervical spine
— Movement and tenderness

Pulse and blood pressure
— Septic shock
— Raised intracranial pressure

General
— Altered consciousness level
— Photophobia
— Phonophobia
— Fever
— Bruit of AVM
— Facial herpetic scarring
— Purpuric rash
— Focal neurological signs
— Pagent's disease/bony deformity

Fig. 16.3 Examining the patient with headache and facial pain. (AVM, arteriovenous malformation; TMJ, temporomandibular joint.)

vascular involvement, a negative result does not exclude the diagnosis.

- Computed tomography scan or magnetic resonance imaging of the head: presence of blood, space-occupying lesion (tumour, abscess), or hydrocephalus. Contrast enhancement should be used if tumour is suspected.
- Lumbar puncture: this should never be performed when raised intracranial pressure is a possibility, as it causes coning. Cerebrospinal fluid (CSF) examination is invaluable in the diagnosis of meningitis. CSF should be sent to the laboratory for assessment of glucose and protein, microscopy, culture, and cytology (see p. 137).
- Cerebral angiography: should be performed if surgery is considered in subarachnoid haemorrhage. It identifies and localises berry aneurysms and arteriovenous malformations.
- Visual fields: these should be serially measured in patients with benign intracranial hypertension, which carries a serious risk of optic nerve infarction.
- Electroencephalography: herpes simplex encephalitis shows characteristic features.

When meningitis is suspected clinically, treat with antibiotics (after blood cultures if in hospital) and then complete investigations. Patients can die awaiting confirmation of the diagnosis

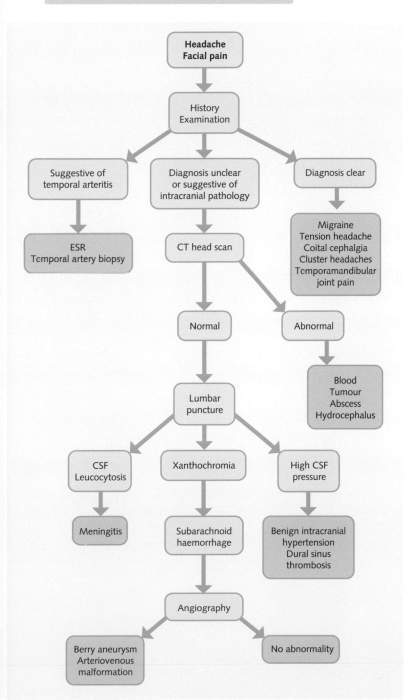

Fig. 16.4 Algorithm for the investigation of the patient with headache and facial pain. (CSF, cerebrospinal fluid; CT, computed tomography; ESR, erythrocyte sedimentation rate.)

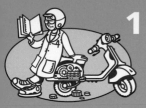

17. Joint Disease

Differential diagnosis of joint disease

Possible causes of joint disease are extensive although in practice the common conditions include the following:

- Rheumatoid arthritis (RA).
- Osteoarthritis (OA).
- Gout.
- Seronegative arthritides: ankylosing spondylitis, Reiter's syndrome, and psoriatic arthritis.
- Septic arthritis.

The causes of a single, hot, red joint is a favourite question. They are as follows:
- Septic arthritis—until proven otherwise.
- Trauma.
- Gout.
- Pseudogout.
- Haemarthrosis.
- Gonococcal arthritis.
- Rheumatoid arthritis.

Arthritis and arthralgia may also be a feature of systemic disease including connective tissue diseases, especially systemic lupus erythematosus (SLE).

Less common causes include the following:
- Enteropathic arthropathies (e.g. inflammatory bowel disease).
- Behçet's syndrome.
- Leukaemia and lymphoma.
- Metastases: bronchial, breast, thyroid, kidney, and prostate carcinomas.
- Hypertrophic pulmonary osteoarthropathy: bronchial carcinoma.
- Viral, bacterial, and fungal infections.
- Endocrine causes: acromegaly, myxoedema and hyperparathyroidism.
- Metabolic diseases: Wilson's disease, haemochromatosis, chondrocalcinosis, ochronosis, pyrophosphate arthropathy.

- Others: familial Mediterranean fever, sarcoidosis, amyloidosis, sickle cell disease, Wegener's granulomatosis.

The differential diagnosis of joint disease is illustrated in Fig. 17.1.

History in the patient with joint disease

The different types of joint disease have many features in common, and examination will provide further additional important clues to the aetiology. Ask about the following:

- Onset: rapid or slowly progressive.
- Persistent or relapsing.
- Early morning stiffness and effect of rest and exercise: classically inflammatory arthritis (e.g. RA is worse first thing in the morning and relieved by exercise). Degenerative arthritis (e.g. OA is worse at the end of the day and relieved by rest, although there is considerable overlap).
- Weakness: with or without wasting of muscles.
- Swelling and deformity.
- Pain: the site, character and exacerbating and relieving factors should be elucidated. Arthralgia is joint pain whereas arthritis indicates an inflammatory process (i.e. swelling, hot and erythema).
- Distribution of the affected joints (see below)— symmetrical or asymmetrical, mono or polyarthritis.
- Patient's age: RA classically affects women aged 25–55 years, and OA usually occurs in the over 40s age group.
- Any history of trauma.
- Recent infection (e.g. viral illness and reactive arthritis or septic arthritis).
- Systemic features associated with different arthropathies: inflammation of the eye (RA and seronegative arthropathies), shortness of breath (fibrosis in RA and ankylosing spondylitis), paraesthesiae (entrapment neuropathies), gastrointestinal symptoms (enteropathic arthropathies).

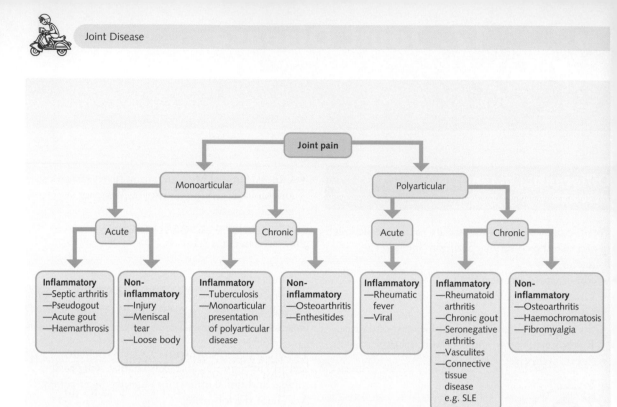

Fig. 17.1 Differential diagnosis algorithm for joint disease.

- In patients with chronic arthritis, it is important to explore the extent of loss of function. How limited are the activities of daily living? This often correlates poorly with the disease activity.
- Chronic arthritis and disability can lead to feelings of helplessness and depression. Assessment of these features is also an important part of the history.

The causes of joint pain can be remembered by the mnemonic SOFTER TISSUE: **s**epsis, **o**steoarthritis, **f**ractures, **t**endon/muscle, **e**piphyseal, **r**eferred, **t**umour, **i**schaemia, **s**eropositive arthritides, **s**eronegative arthritides, **u**rate, **e**xtra-articular rheumatism (e.g. polymyalgia)

Examining the patient with joint disease

Rheumatoid arthritis

RA is a systemic connective tissue disorder, the joints being one of many body parts affected. Look for the following (see Fig. 33.1):
- Symmetrical deforming arthropathy.
- Swelling of the proximal interphalangeal (PIP) and metacarpophalangeal (MCP) joints.
- Wasting of the small muscles of the hand.
- Nodules on the elbows and extensor tendons.
- Ulnar deviation of the fingers: subluxation and dislocation at the MCP joints.
- Swan neck deformity: hyperextension of the PIP joints and flexion of the MCP and terminal interphalangeal (TIP) joints.
- Boutonnière deformity: flexion of the PIP joints and extension of the TIP and MCP joints.
- 'Z'-shaped thumb.
- Trigger finger.
- Iatrogenic Cushing's disease: steroids used in treatment.

- Involvement of other joints.
- Cervical spine disease.
- Anaemia.
- Arteritic lesions: nail-fold infarcts, chronic leg ulceration, and purpuric rash.

You must also carry out a general examination. In particular, look for the following:
- Eye signs: keratoconjunctivitis sicca, keratitis, episcleritis, scleromalacia perforans, cataracts due to steroids.
- Dry mucous membranes: Sjögren's syndrome.
- Chest signs: pleural effusion, fibrosing alveolitis.
- Neurological signs: peripheral neuropathy, mononeuritis multiplex, entrapment neuropathy.
- Vasculitic leg ulceration.
- Felty's syndrome: splenomegaly, neutropenia.
- Cardiac signs: pericarditis, myocarditis, conduction defects, and valvular incompetence.
- Secondary amyloidosis.
- Other autoimmune disorders.

Five causes of anaemia in rheumatoid arthritis:
- Normochromic normocytic anaemia of chronic disease.
- Microcytic anaemia from chronic blood loss secondary to drug treatment.
- Bone marrow suppression from treatment (e.g. gold or penicillamine).
- Megaloblastic anaemia from impaired folate release or pernicious anaemia.
- Felty's syndrome.

Osteoarthritis
In the hands in OA look for the following (see Fig. 33.4):
- Heberden's nodes: swelling of the TIP joints.
- Bouchard's nodes: swelling of the PIP joints.
- Subluxation of the first metacarpal: square hand appearance.
- Crepitus of affected joints.
- Wasting and weakness of the muscle groups involved around the joint.
- Positive Trendelenburg's sign: this is a downward tilting of the pelvis when the patient stands on the affected leg.

- Joint effusions.
- Intermittent locking of the joints due to loose bodies.
- Loss of function.

Gout
Acute gout presents with severe pain, swelling and erythema of the affected joint. Traditionally this is the first metatarsophalangeal joint.

Chronic tophaceous gout follows from recurrent attacks; look for the following:
- Asymmetrical swelling of the small joints of the hands and feet.
- Tophi: look especially on the helix of the ear and tendon sheaths.
- Causes of secondary hyperuricaemia.

Seronegative arthritides
Ankylosing spondylitis
Ask the patient to sit or stand up. Look for the following:
- Loss of lumbar lordosis and a fixed kyphosis and hyperextension of the neck.
- A stooped 'question mark' posture.
- Rigid spine.
- Reduced chest expansion.
- Prominent abdomen.

Also examine for complications and extra-articular manifestations:
- Eyes: iritis.
- Cardiovascular system: aortitis (listen for aortic regurgitation and conduction defects).
- Chest: apical fibrosis.
- Neurological: atlantoaxial dislocation leading to paraplegia or sciatica.
- Secondary amyloidosis: feel for organomegaly.

Reiter's syndrome
This is a triad of urethritis, conjunctivitis, and seronegative arthritis. It follows non-specific urethritis or occasionally dysentery. Look for the following:
- Large joint mono- or oligoarthritis.
- Iritis.
- Keratoderma blenorrhagica (brown, aseptic abscesses on the soles and palms).
- Mouth ulcers.
- Circinate balanitis.
- Enthesopathy (plantar fasciitis or Achilles tendonitis).
- Aortic regurgitation.

Psoriatic arthritis

Look for the following:

- Asymmetrical arthropathy.
- Usually involvement of the TIP joints.
- Pitting of the fingernails and onycholysis.
- Thickened nails.
- Psoriatic plaques: look particularly at the elbows, extensor aspects of limbs, scalp, behind the ears, and the navel.
- Other forms of psoriatic arthropathy: arthritis mutilans, a RA-like picture, asymmetrical mono- or oligoarthropathy, ankylosing spondylitis.

Septic arthritis

This must be recognised and treated promptly because of potential destruction of the joint and widespread infection. It usually presents as a monoarthritis. The affected joint is swollen, painful, hot, and red.

Investigating the patient with joint disease

An algorithm for the investigation of patients with joint disease is provided in Fig. 17.2. The following investigations should be performed:

- Full blood count: anaemia; raised white cell count in infection and occasionally in RA, leucopenia and thrombocytopenia in SLE, neutropenia in Felty's syndrome.
- Erythrocyte sedimentation rate and C reactive protein: non-specific but raised in the presence of inflammation (therefore often high in RA but less so in OA).
- Rheumatoid factor: positive in about 75% of patients with RA. It may also be positive in SLE, mixed connective tissue diseases, scleroderma, and Sjögren's syndrome.

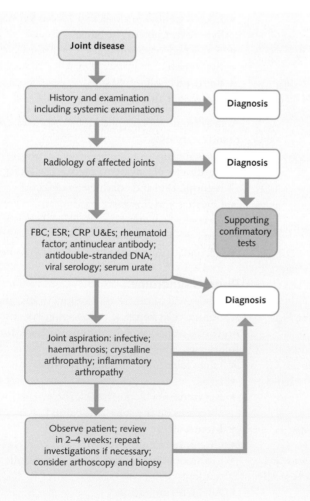

Fig. 17.2 Algorithm for the investigation of the patient with joint disease. (ESR, erythrocyte sedimentation rate; CRP, C-reactive protein; FBC, full blood count; U&Es, urea and electrolytes.)

- Antinuclear antibodies: positive in 30% of patients with RA and in 80% of patients with SLE.
- Antidouble-stranded DNA antibodies: high titres in SLE.
- Other autoantibodies according to clinical suspicion (e.g. anti-Ro and anti-La antibodies in Sjögren's syndrome, and anti-Scl70 antibodies in scleroderma).
- Viral serology: if a viral cause for the arthropathy is suspected (e.g. rubella, mumps, infectious mononucleosis, coxsackie virus and hepatitis B virus).
- Urea and electrolytes: associated renal involvement.
- Liver function tests: liver involvement or drug treatment.
- Creatine kinase: myositis.
- Serum urate: usually high in gout but beware of false positives and false negatives.

Joint aspiration should be performed. Examine the following:
- Appearance: purulence indicates infection, frank blood indicates haemarthrosis or traumatic tap.
- Microscopy for bacteria and crystals: monosodium urate indicates gout, calcium pyrophosphate indicates pseudogout.
- White cell count: high in inflammatory arthropathies.
- Culture: gonococci, tubercle bacillus, or fungi when indicated.

- Rheumatoid nodules or cavities.
- Obliterative bronchiolitis.
- Rheumatoid pneumoconiosis: Caplan's syndrome.

An X-ray of the affected joints may indicate the following:
- RA: soft tissue thickening, juxta-articular osteoporosis, loss of joint space, bony erosions, subluxation.
- OA: loss of joint space, subchondral sclerosis and cysts, marginal osteophytes.
- Gout: soft tissue swelling and punched-out lesions in juxta-articular bone.
- Ankylosing spondylitis: 'bamboo spine' (squaring of the vertebrae and obliteration of sacroiliac joints); also found in Reiter's syndrome and Crohn's disease.

An X-ray of the cervical spine should also be used to look for displacement of the odontoid peg.

Magnetic resonance imaging is now widely used to provide images of soft tissue injury including ligaments, muscle and intervertebral discs. Computerised tomography is very good for assessing bones and joints. Reconstruction of the images using improved software gives three-dimensional pictures of the anatomy of an injury.

Finally, arthroscopy allows direct visualisation inside the joint space, and can be used for biopsy and the removal of foreign bodies.

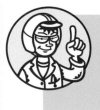

In **p**seudogout, crystals are **p**ositively birefringent in **p**lane-**p**olarised light. Remember this by the 'P's. In gout, the crystals are negatively birefringent

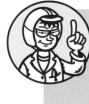

Determine how the joint disease affects the patient's daily activities. Your concerns are not always the same as those of your patient

A chest X-ray should be performed to look for associated diseases or complications of RA:
- Pleural effusion.
- Diffuse fibrosing alveolitis.

18. Skin Diseases

Dermatology is potentially a large subject for the student and junior doctor. Skin disease may be primary or it may be the manifestation of a systemic condition. Students should become familiar with the descriptive terminology used and learn how to manage the most common conditions. For exams a picture book is essential for revision.

Differential diagnosis by appearance

Pigmented lesions
- Freckles (ephelides): flat, brown spots.
- Lentigo: similar to freckles but darker and not affected by sunlight.
- Seborrhoeic keratosis: benign, beige/brown plaques, 3–20 mm in diameter, with a velvety or warty surface.
- Naevus: moles.
- Blue naevus: small, slightly elevated, blue-black lesions.
- Atypical (dysplastic) naevus: over 5 mm across, ill-defined, irregular border, irregularly distributed pigmentation with erythema and accentuated skin markings.
- Melanoma: flat or raised pigmented lesion with possibly a recent change in appearance. It has varying colours and typically irregular borders.

Scaly lesions
- Psoriasis: silvery, scaled, well-demarcated plaques on skin, usually over the extensor surfaces. It can be pustular and involve the nails.
- Dermatitis and eczema: a pruritic, exudative, or lichenified eruption on the face, neck, upper trunk, wrists, and hands, and in the antecubital and popliteal fossae.
- Xerosis: dry skin.
- Lichen simplex chronicus: chronic itching associated with pigmented, lichenified skin lesions. Lichenified lesions exhibit exaggerated skin lines overlying thickened, well-circumscribed, scaly plaques.

- Tinea corporis: ring-shaped lesion with an advancing scaly border and central clearing or scaly patches with a distinct border.
- Tinea versicolor: pale or hyperpigmented macules, or velvety, tan, pink, whitish, or brown macules that scale with scraping.
- Secondary syphilis.
- Pityriasis rosea: oval, fawn-coloured, scaly eruption following the cleavage lines of the trunk. It is commonly preceded by a herald patch.
- Discoid lupus erythematosus: red, asymptomatic, localised plaques, usually on the face and often in a 'butterfly' distribution. There is scaling, follicular plugging, atrophy, and telangiectasia of involved areas.
- Exfoliative dermatitis: scaling and erythema over a large area of the body.
- Actinic keratoses: small, pink patches that feel like bits off sandpaper when the finger is drawn over them. They are premalignant.
- Bowen's disease (intraepidermal squamous cell carcinoma): small, well-demarcated, slightly raised, pink-to-red, scaly plaques.
- Extramammary Paget's disease: this resembles chronic eczema and may involve apocrine areas such as the genitals.
- Intertrigo: fissuring, erythema, and sodden epidermis, with superficial denudation in the body folds.

Vesicular lesions
- Herpes simplex: recurrent, small, grouped vesicles on an erythematous base, especially around the oral and genital areas.
- Herpes zoster: vesicular lesions in a dermatomal distribution.
- Pompholyx: pruritic 'tapioca' vesicles or bullae on the palms, soles, and sides of fingers.
- Dermatophytid (allergy or sensitivity to fungi): pruritic, grouped, vesicular lesions involving the sides and flexor aspects of the fingers and palms.
- Dermatitis herpetiformis: pruritic papulovesicular lesions mainly on the elbows, knees, buttocks, posterior neck, and scalp. It is associated with gluten-sensitive enteropathy.

- Miliaria (heat rash): superficial, aggregated, small vesicles, papules, or pustules on covered areas of the skin.
- Scabies: pruritic vesicles and pustules especially on the sides of the. Red papules or nodules on the penile glans and shaft are pathognomonic.
- Photosensitivity.

Weepy or encrusted lesions

- Impetigo: vesiculopustular lesions with thick, golden-crusted exudate associated with group A β-haemolytic streptococci or coagulase-positive *Staphylococcus aureus*, or bullous lesions associated with *Staphylococcus aureus*.
- Acute-contact allergic dermatitis: erythema and oedema, with pruritus, often followed by vesicles and bullae in an area of contact with a suspected agent. They may later weep, crust, and become infected.
- Any vesicular dermatitis.

Pustular lesions

- Acne vulgaris: the most common skin condition, characterised by open and closed comedones. It varies from purely comedonal to pustular inflammatory acne to cysts to nodules.
- Acne rosacea: erythema and telangiectasia and a tendency to flush easily. May have an acneiform component, or hyperplasia of the soft tissue of the nose (rhinophyma).
- Folliculitis: pustules in the hair follicles.
- Candidiasis: superficial, denuded, beefy-red areas with or without satellite vesicopustules. Whitish, curd-like concretions on the oral and vaginal mucous membranes.
- Miliaria.
- Any vesicular dermatitis.

Figurate erythema

Figurate erythema lesions look like rings or arcs.

- Urticaria: eruptions of evanescent wheals or hives.
- Erythema multiforme: symmetrical erythematous lesions on the extensor surfaces, palms, soles, or mucous membranes, which may be macular, papular, urticarial, bullous, or purpuric. May be target lesions with clear centres and concentric erythematous rings.
- Erythema migrans: a red expansion around an initial papule with an advancing border, which is usually raised, warm, and red. The centre may clear or become indurated, vesicular, or necrotic.

- Cellulitis: a hot, red, diffuse, spreading infection of the skin.
- Erysipelas: oedematous, spreading, circumscribed, hot, erythematous area, with or without vesicle or bulla formation, frequently involving the face.
- Erysipeloid: purplish erythema, most often of a finger or the back of the hand, which gradually extends. Caused by *Erysipelothrix insidiosa*, it is often seen in fishermen and meat handlers.

Bullous lesions

- Impetigo: superficial bacterial infection caused by group A β-haemolytic streptococci or *S. aureus*.
- Pemphigus: relapsing crops of bullae appearing on normal skin, often preceded by mucous membrane bullae, erosions, and ulcerations. There may be superficial detachment of the skin after pressure or trauma (Nikolsky's sign).
- Bullous pemphigoid: tense blisters in flexural areas. They may be preceded by urticarial or oedematous lesions.
- Porphyria cutanea tarda.
- Erythema multiforme: 'target' lesions (i.e. symmetrically distributed, circular lesions, often with a central blister).
- Toxic epidermal necrolysis: usually secondary to drugs (e.g. sulphonamides, penicillins, and anticonvulsants).

Papular lesions

- Hyperkeratotic: warts, corns, seborrhoeic keratoses.
- Purple: lichen planus—pruritic, violaceous, flat-topped papules with fine white streaks and a symmetrical distribution, commonly seen along linear scratch marks on the anterior wrists, sacral region, penis, legs, and mucous membranes; drug eruptions; Kaposi's sarcoma—malignant skin lesions with dark plaques or nodules on cutaneous or mucosal surfaces, common in people with human immunodeficiency virus infection.
- Flesh-coloured and umbilicated: molluscum contagiosum—a viral infection causing single or multiple, rounded, dome-shaped, waxy papules, 2–5 mm in diameter, which are umbilicated and contain a caseous plug.
- Pearly: basal cell carcinoma—most commonly papules or nodules with a central scab or erosion; intradermal naevi.
- Small, red, and inflammatory: acne, miliaria, candidiasis, intertrigo, scabies, folliculitis.
- Nodular, cystic lesions

- Erythema nodosum: painful red nodules without ulceration on the anterior aspects of the legs; they may regress over weeks to resemble contusions.
- Furuncle (boils): painful inflammatory swellings of a hair follicle forming an abscess, caused by *S. aureus*.
- Cystic acne.
- Follicular (epidermal) inclusion cyst.

Photodermatoses

Painful erythema, oedema, and vesiculation on sun-exposed surfaces, usually the face, neck, hands, and V of the chest. Causes include drugs (e.g. amiodarone, phenothiazines, sulphonamides, and related drugs), polymorphic light eruption, and SLE.

Maculopapular lesions

Viral causes, and secondary syphilis.

Erosive lesions

- Any vesicular dermatitis.
- Impetigo.
- Lichen planus.
- Erythema multiforme.
- Oral erosions.

Ulcerated lesions

- Decubiti: bed sores or pressure sores.
- Herpes simplex.
- Skin cancers.
- Parasitic infections.
- Syphilis: chancre.
- Vasculitis.
- Stasis.
- Arterial disease.

History in the patient with skin rashes

The following long list of factors should be assessed when taking a history in the patient with skin rashes:
- Rash: onset, duration.
- Aggravating factors: physical or chemical agents; cold (cold urticaria or cryoglobulinaemia); heat (worsens seborrhoeic conditions and superficial skin conditions).
- Precipitants: stress may lead to alopecia or eczema.
- Site of origin: contact dermatitis and pityriasis rosea (herald patch).

- Rate of progression.
- Timing of change in skin lesions, particularly for moles.
- Character: any alteration or progression in lesions.
- Hair and nails.
- Family history: eczema, psoriasis, inherited skin disorders.
- Infective agents: foreign travel (tropical infections), pets (papular urticaria or animal scabies).
- Farm animals: orf (poxvirus), ringworm.
- Occupation.
- Chemical exposure: at home or work, acting as antigens or direct irritants.
- Drugs taken: over-the-counter drugs; steroids may make the rash better (as in dermatitis) or worse (as in acne). How are the drugs being used?
- Foods: nuts and shellfish.
- Washing powder or soap.
- Contacts: family and friends.
- Light exposure: herpes simplex, systemic lupus erythematosus (SLE), and vitiligo.
- Hobbies: sportsmen are more prone to viral or fungal infections.
- General state of health and past medical history.
- Patient's explanation for rash.

Systemic symptoms should be assessed, and may take the following forms:
- Itching (Fig. 18.1): atopy or urticaria (e.g. scabies which is worse in bed), eczema, dermatitis herpetiformis, lichen planus, flexural psoriasis.
- Pain: inflammatory conditions, skin tumours.

Finally, the mode of spread is significant and may take the form of an annular appearance (e.g. erythema annulare, erythema multiforme, and fungal infections) or irregular spread (e.g. pyoderma gangrenosum or malignancy).

Examining the patient with a skin rash

Always examine the entire skin, but maintain the dignity of the patient, and look in the mouth (e.g. with lichen planus, herpes simplex and zoster, and infective exanthemata). Rashes may change with time and become characteristic or diagnostic of common dermatoses, such as the infectious exanthemata. Look at the distribution of lesions:
- If widespread and symmetrical, suspect systemic disease.

Fig. 18.1 Causes of generalised and localised itching.

Possible causes of generalized and localized itching	
Generalised itching	**Localised itching**
• Uraemia • Cholestasis • Iron–deficiency anaemia • Lymphoma • Hypo- and hyperthyroidism • Pregnancy • Carcinoma • Multiple sclerosis • Syphilis • Intestinal parasites • Morphine ingestion • Allergies, e.g. atopic eczema • Diabetes mellitus	• Scabies and other mite infestations • Contact eczema • Dermatitis herpetiformis (associated with coeliac Disease) • Urticaria ('nettle rash') • Lichen planus • Prickly heat • Winter itch • Aquagenic pruritus • Old age

- If only areas exposed to the sun are involved, suspect light sensitivity.
- Patterns involving a dermatome distribution suggest herpes zoster.
- Dermatitis involving the hands, face, axillae, ears, and eyelids suggests contact dermatitis.
- Dermatitis involving the axillae, groins, scalp, the central chest and back, eyebrows, ears, and beard suggests seborrhoeic dermatitis.
- Dermatitis involving the popliteal and cubital fossae, and the face suggests atopic dermatitis.

Describe the lesion:
- Bizarrely shaped lesions suggest the cause is an external agent (e.g. caustic liquid, a self-induced injury).
- Fungal infections are characterised by slow growth, a smooth outline, an active edge with a healing centre, and asymmetry.

Terms and characteristics of dermatological lesions are given in Fig. 18.2.

Investigating the patient with skin rashes

Drug eruptions may mimic any inflammatory skin condition. They usually start abruptly and are a widespread, symmetrical, erythematous eruption.
Constitutional symptoms such as malaise, arthralgia, headache, and fever may be present

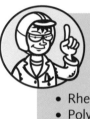

In the patient presenting with subcutaneous nodules, think of the following:
- Rheumatoid nodules.
- Rheumatic fever.
- Polyarteritis.
- Xanthelasmata.
- Tuberous sclerosis.
- Neurofibromatosis.
- Sarcoidosis.

The history and examination may be enough to determine the diagnosis. If the patient is not unwell it may be possible to examine for skin changes over time to allow for the development of possible characteristic lesions. The following investigations should be performed:
- Blood tests: full blood count, urea and electrolytes, bacterial and viral titres with immunological tests for tropical diseases if appropriate, and blood cultures.
- Skin scrapings and nail clippings: fungi.
- Examination of the skin under Wood's light (e.g. fungal infections and tuberous sclerosis).
- Examination of brushings of household pets: mites.
- Culture of fluid-containing lesions.
- Skin biopsy.
- Biopsy of lesions in lymph nodes or other organs.
- Investigations for associated systemic diseases or malignancy.

Term	Characteristics
Terms and characteristics of dermatological lesions	
Alopecia	Hair loss
Atrophy	Loss of skin thickness
Blister or bulla	Vesicle >1 cm diameter
Crust	Dried exudate on skin surface
Cyst	Epithelium-lined cavity containing fluid or semi-solid material
Erythema	Area of reddened skin which blanches with pressure
Fissure	Linear crack in epidermis
Indurated	Hard and thickened
Köebner's phenomenon	Skin lesions at sites of external injury
Lichenification	Thickened skin with exaggerated skin markings
Macule	Circumscribed change in the skin colour up to 1 cm diameter. It is not elevated above the surface
Nodule	Solid skin lesion over 1 cm diameter
Papule	Solid raised palpable area up to 1 cm diameter
Patch	Macule >1 cm across
Petechiae	Pinpoint haemorrhages
Plaque	Palpable plateau-like elevation of skin
Purpura	Area of reddened skin caused by extravasation of blood Which does not blanch with pressure
Pustule	Circumscribed, pus-filled lesion
Scale	Flake of hard skin
Scar	Connective tissue replacement following loss of dermal tissue
Ulcer	Irregularly shaped break in surface continuity of epithelium
Vesicle	Fluid-filled lesion <1 cm diameter
Wheal	Raised, palpable lesion with pale centre

Fig. 18.2 Terms and characteristics of dermatological lesions

Introduction

Loss of consciousness may be transient (syncope) or ongoing (coma). Many patients are admitted to hospital with 'collapse ? cause'. Patients use the word 'collapse' to describe a variety of situations and it is essential to determine whether or not the patient has actually lost consciousness.

Many 'collapse ? cause' patients are erroneously labelled as TIA when there is little evidence of transient ischaemia in the posterior cerebral circulation and alternative diagnoses are more likely

Differential diagnosis of loss of consciousness

Blackouts

Many patients describe transient episodes of blacking out, which are often recurrent. Some of these patients have syncope, which means a transient loss of consciousness and motor tone due to a reduction in cerebral perfusion, and which recovers spontaneously. The causes of blackouts are summarised in Fig.19.1.

Coma

In coma, the patient remains unconscious and is unrousable. The causes of coma are summarised in Fig. 19.2.

History in the patient with loss of consciousness

Always try to obtain a history from a witness, even if the patient has regained consciousness

When a patient presents in coma, relatives or the general practitioner should be contacted to gain information regarding previous medical history, prodromal illness, known alcohol or drug abuse, and whether the events leading to the coma were witnessed by anyone.

In syncope, the history should focus on the following details.

Presyncope

- What was the patient doing at the time?
- Were there any symptoms before the patient lost consciousness?
- In postural hypotension the patient may have stood up suddenly.
- If the patient had just turned his or her head, consider vertebrobasilar insufficiency or carotid sinus hypersensitivity.
- Prior to an epileptic fit, there is often an aura.
- In arrhythmia, the patient can be aware of palpitations, chest pain, or dyspnoea before blacking out.
- In Stokes–Adams attacks, there is usually no warning.
- Exertional syncope is seen in aortic stenosis and hypertrophic cardiomyopathy (HCM).
- Occasionally, cough or micturition may cause syncope.

The attack itself

- What happened during the episode itself? This is where the history of a witness is vitally important.
- Prolonged seizures associated with tongue biting are suggestive of epilepsy. Any cause of cerebral hypoxia may result in brief anoxic seizures, which may be more prolonged if the patient is upright. Urinary incontinence can be a feature of both syncope and epilepsy.
- In Stokes–Adams attacks, the patient is typically seen to go deathly pale with flushing on recovery. The length of time that the patient remained unconscious should be recorded.
- If available, the pulse rate during the episode can help (e.g. Stokes–Adams attack). If the attack occurs in hospital the blood pressure and blood

Differential diagnosis of blackouts		
Causes	**Subgroups**	**Examples and notes**
Syncope (see Chapters 27 and 31)	Postural hypotension	Old age, anti-hypertensive drugs, autonomic neuropathy
	Neurocardiogenic syncope	Vasovagal and carotid sinus hypersensitivity. Characterised by inappropriate vagal outflow in response to stimulus [e.g. prolonged standing, fear, pain (vasovagal) or contact with carotid sinus]
	Situational syncope	Cough, micturition, defecation
	TIA/vertebrobasilar insufficiency	Need transient ischaemia in posterior circulation to cause LOC (i.e. needs to affect reticular activating system in the brainstem, and as this is diffuse TIA's rarely cause LOC alone—other brain stem structures are affected)
	Cardiogenic syncope	Arrhythmia (Stokes–Adams attack) or structural heart disease (e.g. AS, HCM)
Epilepsy (see Chapter 31)	Complex partial seizure	Focal epileptic activity with altered consciousness (e.g. temporal lobe epilepsy)
	Generalised seizure	Generalised epileptic activity
	Pseudoseizure	Behaviour mimicking a seizure but no epileptic activity in brain
Hypoglycaemia (see Chapter 32)	Fasting	See list in Chapter 32
	Post-prandial	Dumping syndrome

Fig. 19.1 The differential diagnosis of blackouts. (TIA, transient ischaemic attack; LOC, loss of consciousness; AS, aortic stenosis; HCM, hypertrophic cardiomyopathy.)

Differential diagnosis of coma	
Causes	**Examples**
Neurological (see Chapter 31)	Trauma-especially closed head injury
	Cerebrovascular event - intracranial haemorrhage or infarction
	Epilepsy (post ictal or non-convulsive status epilepticus)
	Meningitis, encephalitis, overwhelming septicaemia
	Space occupying lesion
Metabolic	Hypo- or hyperglycaemia
	Myxoedema or Addisonian crisis (see Chapter 32)
	Hypothermia (see Chapter 32)
	Hypoxia or CO_2 narcosis (see Chapter 28)
	Electrolyte disturbance (see Chapter 32)
	Uraemic encephalopathy
	Hepatic encephalopathy (see Chapter 29)
	Drugs and toxins (see Chapter 36)

Fig. 19.2 The differential diagnosis of coma.

glucose should have been recorded during the episode.

Postsyncope

- How quickly did the patient recover? Syncope is generally followed by rapid recovery. However, in epilepsy, there is usually postictal sleepiness.
- Was there any focal neurological impairment after recovery of consciousness—may suggest transient ischaemic attack (TIA) or Todd's paresis following focal seizure (see p. 275).
- It is also very important to ask whether patients hurt themselves during the episode. If there is significant injury consider cardiac syncope (lack of warning).

Risk factors

- Is there a previous history of similar episodes or of epilepsy, cardiac disease, cerebrovascular disease, or obstructive airways disease?

- Does the patient have cardiovascular risk factors or a relevant family history (e.g. Hypertrophic cardiomyopathy).
- Is the patient a diabetic on insulin or a health care worker with access to insulin?
- Is there a history of drug abuse or depression?
- Has there been any trauma to the head?

Examining the patient with loss of consciousness

Fig. 19.3 summarises the examination approach. The emphasis of the examination differs between the sick comatose patient and one with recurrent blackouts. These approaches are outlined below:

Coma patient

- Always start with ABC: Airway, Breathing, Circulation, Disability (i.e. Glasgow coma scale— see Fig. 19.4), Exposure.

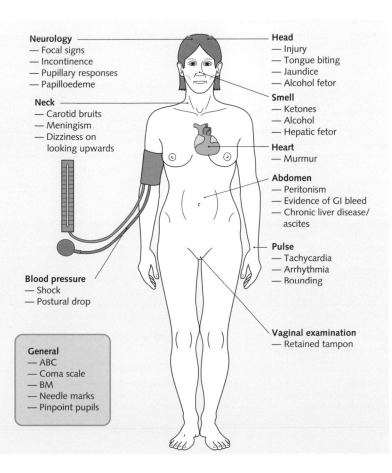

Fig. 19.3 Examining the patient with loss of consciousness. (ABC, the Airway-Breathing-Circulation first-aid mnemonic; BM, stick test for blood sugar.)

Neurology
— Focal signs
— Incontinence
— Pupillary responses
— Papilloedeme

Neck
— Carotid bruits
— Meningism
— Dizziness on looking upwards

Blood pressure
— Shock
— Postural drop

General
— ABC
— Coma scale
— BM
— Needle marks
— Pinpoint pupils

Head
— Injury
— Tongue biting
— Jaundice
— Alcohol fetor

Smell
— Ketones
— Alcohol
— Hepatic fetor

Heart
— Murmur

Abdomen
— Peritonism
— Evidence of GI bleed
— Chronic liver disease/ ascites

Pulse
— Tachycardia
— Arrhythmia
— Bounding

Vaginal examination
— Retained tampon

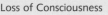

The Glasgow coma scale		
Category	**Response**	**Score**
Best verbal response	Orientated	5
	Confused conversation	4
	Inappropriate speech	3
	Incomprehensible words	2
	No speech	1
Best motor response	Obeys commands	6
(i.e. best response	Localises to pain	5
of any limb)	Withdraws to pain	4
	Flexes to pain	3
	Extends to pain	2
	No response	1
Eye opening	Spontaneous	4
	To speech	3
	To pain	2
	No eye opening	1

Fig. 19.4 The Glasgow coma scale, used for assessing loss of consciousness in a patient.

- Urgent checks: pulse, blood pressure, oxygen saturation, blood sugar estimation and arterial blood gas.
- Survey for injuries—especially closed head injury, and evidence of skull fracture, blood or cerebrospinal fluid in ears.

- Check for known liver disease, diabetes mellitus, intravenous drug use or any clues (e.g. signs of chronic liver disease or injection sites)—consider hepatic encephalopathy, diabetic coma, opiate or other overdose.
- Is there a characteristic smell—alcohol, ketones, hepatic fetor?
- Always think of meningism (meningitis or subarachnoid haemorrhage) and rash (meningococcal meningitis classically gives petechial or purpuric rash).
- Eyes (see Fig. 19.5).
- Cardiovascular examination—?rhythm (atrial fibrillation predisposes to stroke) ?murmur or other evidence of bacterial endocarditis.
- Respiratory—?focal consolidation or collapse.
- Abdomen—?gastrointestinal bleed ?ascites (which may be infected) ? organomegaly ? peritonism.
- Neurological examination -focal neurology suggests intracranial cause.

Patient with blackouts
- Check for a history of injuries.
- Lying and standing blood pressure.
- Full cardiovascular and neurological examination.

Examination of the eyes in the coma patient		
Test	**Findings**	**Interpretation**
Visual fields (by visual threat—normal response is to blink)	Hemianopia	Suggests contralateral hemisphere lesion
Pupil reactions	Normal direct and consensual	Intact midbrain
	Midposition, non-reactive ± irregular	Midbrain lesion
	Unilateral, fixed, dilated	Third nerve compression (e.g. due to tentorial herniation)
	Small, reactive	Pontine lesion
		Opiate overdose
	Horner's syndrome	Ipsilateral lateral medullary or hypothalamic lesion
Doll's head manoeuvre to test vestibulo-ocular reflex (ONLY IF CERVICAL SPINE CLEARED)	Normal if pupils fixed on same point in space when head moved quickly	Brainstem from third to seventh nerve nucleus intact
Fundoscopy	Papilloedema	Raised intracranial pressure (CO$_2$ narcosis)
	Subhyaloid haemorrhage	Subarachnoid haemorrhage
	Hypertensive retinopathy	? Hypertensive encephalopathy

Fig. 19.5 Examination of the eyes in the coma patient.

Investigating the patient with loss of consciousness

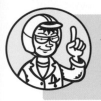

A blood sugar test should be performed urgently in all unconscious patients to exclude hypoglycaemia

Investigation will be guided by findings in the history and clinical examination. The following investigations are useful in the different clinical scenarios (Figs 19.3 and 19.4):

- Full blood count: anaemia in severe haemorrhage or haemolysis (malaria); leucocytosis in sepsis.
- Urea and electrolytes: hypo- or hypernatraemia.
- Calcium: hypocalcaemia.
- Glucose: hypoglycaemia/hyperglycaemia.
- Liver function tests: liver failure.
- Thyroid function tests: hypothyroidism.
- Electrocardiogram: arrhythmia, left ventricular hypertrophy in aortic stenosis and HCM.
- Arterial blood gases: hypercapnia.
- Chest X-ray: pulmonary disease, aspiration pneumonia.
- Drugs screen: urine and blood.
- Electroencephalogram: epilepsy (including non-convulsive status epilepticus), herpes simplex encephalitis.
- Computed tomography head scan: intracranial pathology.
- Carotid dopplers: carotid atheroma.
- 24-hour tape: arrhythmia.

- Electrocardiogram: heart rhythm, source of emboli, aortic stenosis, HCM.
- Lumbar puncture: meningitis, subarachnoid haemorrhage.
- Septic screen, including blood cultures and mid-stream urine.
- Tilt table testing: patients are moved from a recumbent to an upright position with monitoring of their pulse, blood pressure, electrocardiogram and symptoms. Those with orthostatic (postural) hypotension show an early drop in blood pressure (within 2–3 minutes) whereas those with vasovagal syndrome show a delayed response (up to 45 minutes) in which the blood pressure alone may drop (vasodepressor response), a bradycardia causes hypotension (cardio-inhibitory response), or a mixture of the two. In some centres, carotid sinus massage is performed in combination with tilt-table testing to increase its sensitivity at diagnosing carotid sinus hypersensitivity (which may also manifest with a vasodepressor response, cardio-inhibitory response, or a mixture of the two).

Carotid dopplers should only be requested for clinical syndromes suggesting unilateral anterior cerebral circulation infarction where surgery would be considered

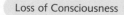

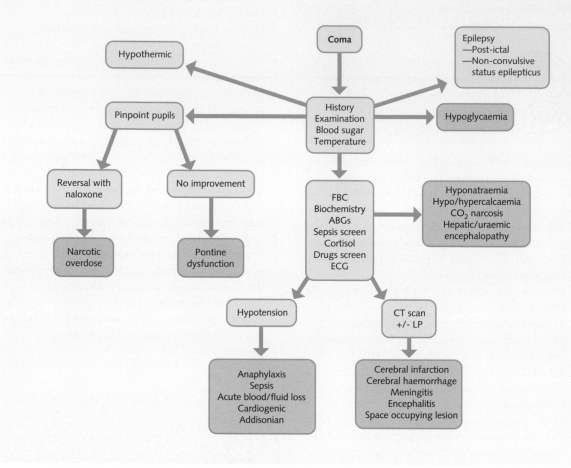

Fig. 19.6 Diagnosis in the patient with coma. (ABGs, arterial blood gases; CT, computed tomography; ECG, electrocardiogram; FBC, full blood count; LP, lumbar puncture.)

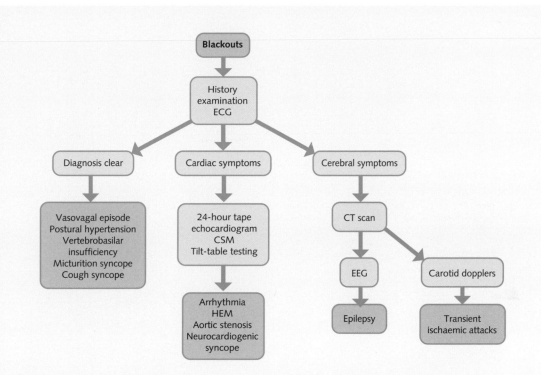

Fig. 19.7 Diagnosis in the patient with blackouts. (CT, computed tomography; ECG, electrocardiogram; EEG, electroencephalogram; CSM, carotid sinus massage; HCM, hypertrophic obstructive cardiomyopathy.)

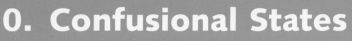

20. Confusional States

Introduction

Confusion can be acute or subacute (delirium), or chronic and progressive (dementia). Any cause of delirium can precipitate an acute exacerbation of dementia—'acute on chronic confusion'. Confusion is very common, particularly in the elderly and is often worsened by admission to hospital.

When a patient presents with confusion, try to establish whether it is a longstanding problem which is getting worse or whether it has arisen 'out of the blue' by talking to the family or carers

Differential diagnosis of confusion

Delirium

Almost anything can present as delirium in the elderly patient and the common causes are summarised in Fig. 20.1.

Dementia

The causes of dementia are summarised in Fig. 20.2.

It is important to remember that deaf people are not necessarily confused and that depression can sometimes mimic dementia ('pseudodementia')

History in the confused patient

The first step is to establish whether the patient has delirium or dementia. A good account from relatives, carers, or close friends is almost always the only way of getting a true picture of the pattern of disease. The previous hospital notes can be an invaluable source of information, and a thorough social history is essential

Differential diagnosis of delirium	
Causes	**Examples**
Infection	Any—commonly urinary tract, pneumonia, cellulitis, meningitis, encephalitis.
Drug intoxication	Opiates, anxiolytics, steroids, tricyclics, anticonvulsants, drugs of abuse (See Chapter 36)
Drug withdrawal	Alcohol, benzodiazepines
Metabolic	Liver, kidney, cardio-respiratory failure (hypoxia and hypercapnia), hyper- or hyponatraemia, hypoglycaemia, hypercalcaemia.
Vitamin deficiency	Wernicke–Korsakoff syndrome (thiamine deficiency) (see *Crash Course in Psychiatry*)
Cerebral pathology	Abscess, tumour, haemorrhage, infarction, trauma, epilepsy/post-ictal (see Chapter 31)
Pain	Any cause
New surroundings	Hospital ward, possibly without hearing (hearing aid?) or vision (spectacles?)

Fig. 20.1 The differential diagnosis of delirium.

Differential diagnosis of dementia (See *Crash Course In Psychiatry*)	
Categories	**Causes**
Common causes	Alzheimer's disease, vascular dementia, Lewy body dementia, fronto-temporal dementia
Rarer causes	Chronic alcohol abuse, Huntington's chorea, Creutzfeldt-Jakob disease, Parkinson's disease, Pick's disease, HIV, pellagra, subacute sclerosing panencephalitis, progressive multiple leukencephalopathy, pellagra (niacin deficiency)
Treatable causes (which MUST therefore be excluded)	B_{12}/folate deficiency, hypothyroidism, thiamine deficiency, subdural haematoma, normal pressure hydrocephalus, neurosyphilis, resectable tumour, depression (pseudodementia)

Fig. 20.2 The differential diagnosis of dementia.

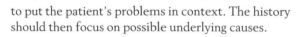

to put the patient's problems in context. The history should then focus on possible underlying causes.

Pattern of confusion

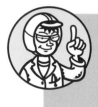

If delirium develops at around 2 days following hospital admission, consider delirium tremens due to alcohol withdrawal

Delirium develops over hours or days. It is characterised by clouding of consciousness, which fluctuates in severity, being worse at night with lucid periods in the day. It can be accompanied by poor recent memory, disorientation, and hallucinations. As a result, the patient may be agitated, uncooperative, and sometimes paranoid.

Dementia usually has a gradual onset over months or years. It is characterised by a global deterioration in higher cerebral functions with no change in level of consciousness, tends to be progressive, and is often exacerbated when the patient is removed from familiar surroundings, such as by admission to hospital. Multi-infarct dementia characteristically progresses in a stepwise fashion.

A more rapid onset is seen in Creutzfeldt–Jakob disease (CJD), hydrocephalus and depression. The depressed patient often complains of memory loss (unlike patients with early dementia who may not be aware of the problem), makes poor effort at testing and may have a personal or family history of depression.

Possible underlying causes

The following should be assessed, as they may reveal an underlying cause:

- Age: dementia becomes increasingly common after the age of 60 years. In younger patients, a thorough search for a treatable underlying cause should be made.
- Symptoms of focal infection (see Chapter 6).
- Symptoms of raised intracranial pressure (see Chapter 16).
- Risk factors for, or known, vascular disease (see Chapter 23).
- Dietary history: vitamin deficiency.
- Alcohol history: whilst chronic alcohol abuse can cause dementia in its own right, it may also be associated with folate and thiamine deficiency.

- Previous head injury: subdural haematoma.
- Drug history: particular attention should be given to sedatives, anticonvulsants, and steroids.
- Other neurological symptoms: cerebrovascular disease, multiple sclerosis, cerebral tumour or abscess.
- Previous medical history of any disease may be relevant: longstanding renal disease (uraemia), malignancy (cerebral metastases, hypercalcaemia or paraneoplastic) or diabetes (insulin overdose).
- Family history: Wilson's disease (autosomal recessive); Huntington's chorea (autosomal dominant); depression.
- Brief psychiatric history—notably for features of depression.

Examining the confused patient

Since the causes of confusion are so varied, a thorough clinical examination is mandatory. This approach is summarised in Fig. 20.3. Particular attention should be given to the following:

- Consciousness: the level of consciousness should be recorded using the Glasgow coma scale (Fig. 19.4).
- Blood pressure: hypotension may be due to overwhelming infection or cardiac failure. Hypertension is a risk factor for cerebrovascular events and can also be caused by raised intracranial pressure.
- Cyanosis: hypoxia is a common cause of confusion in patients in hospital. The oxygen saturation should be measured.
- BM sticks: hypoglycaemia.
- Evidence of head injury: subdural haematoma.
- Signs of infection: measure temperature, look for neck stiffness, consolidation in the chest, signs of endocarditis, abdominal tenderness, otitis media on otoscopy, pressure areas and skin for evidence of cellulitis. (see Chapter 6).
- Mental state: The 10-point abbreviated mental test score (Fig. 20.4) is useful for confirming confusion and may be used serially to monitor progress. The 30 point MMSE (mini-mental state examination) is mandatory if querying a new diagnosis of dementia—to document cognitive function and provide a baseline for future assessment.
- Focal neurological deficit and the pattern of signs may give important clues as to the diagnosis (see Chapters 21 and 23): fundoscopy should be performed looking for papilloedema (raised

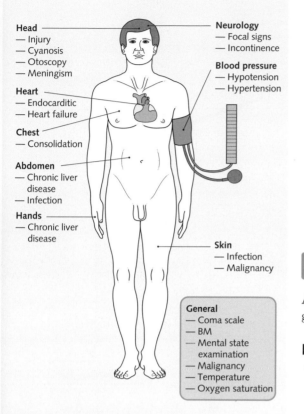

Fig. 20.3 Examining the confused patient. (BM, stick examination for blood sugar.)

	The abbreviated mental test score
1	Age
2	Time (to nearest hour)
3	Address for recall at end of test—to be repeated by patient to ensure it has been heard correctly: 42 West Street
4	Year
5	Name of this place
6	Recognition of two people (e.g. nurse and doctor)
7	Date of birth
8	Year of First World War
9	Name of Monarch
10	Count backwards from 20 to 1

Fig. 20.4 The abbreviated mental test score. One point is awarded for each correct answer. A score of less than 7/10 strongly suggests confusion.

intracranial pressure), optic atrophy (demyelination), or subhyaloid haemorrhages (subarachnoid haemorrhage). Parkinsonism may be present in Parkinson's disease and multisystem atrophy. Myoclonus, extrapyramidal signs and aphasia are features of CJD.

- Signs of chronic liver disease: hepatic encephalopathy can cause confusion. Chronic liver disease may also indicate chronic alcohol abuse or rare disorders such as Wilson's disease.
- Malignancy: examine thoroughly—breasts, digital rectal examination for prostate and bowel pathology, lymph nodes and skin for dermatological malignancy and cutaneous manifestations of malignancy.

Investigating the confused patient

An algorithm for diagnosing the confused patient is given in Fig. 20.5.

Blood

- Full blood count: reactive blood picture in malignancy, infection, or inflammation; anaemia with raised mean corpuscular volume in vitamin B_{12} or folate deficiency.
- Erythrocyte sedimentation rate: raised in malignancy, infection, inflammation.
- Urea and electrolytes: hypo- or hypernatraemia and renal failure.
- Liver function tests: abnormal in liver disease, raised γ-glutamyl transferase in excess alcohol consumption.
- Thyroid function tests: low T_4 in hypothyroidism.
- Serum calcium: hyper- or hypocalcaemia.
- Serum glucose: hypoglycaemia.
- Serum vitamin B_{12} and red blood cell folate: deficiency.
- Syphilis serology.
- Arterial blood gases for hypoxia.
- Blood cultures if considering infection.

Urine

Midstream urine should be obtained for microscopy, culture and sensitivity in urinary tract infection.

Radiology

Chest X-ray may show pneumonia, cardiac failure, or malignancy. Computed tomography scan or magnetic resonance imaging of the head should be performed

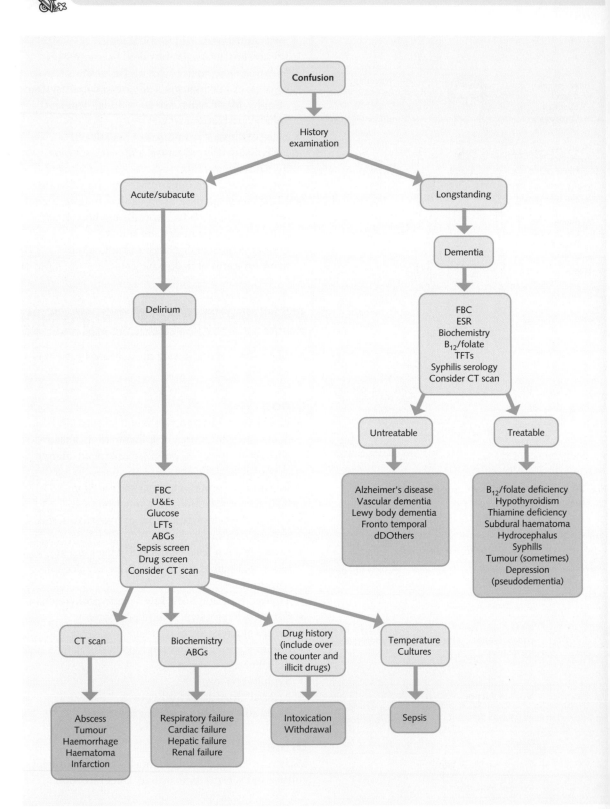

Fig. 20.5 Algorithm for diagnosing the confused patient. (ABGs, arterial blood gases; CT, computed tomography; ESR, erythrocyte sedimentation rate; FBC, full blood count; LFTs, liver function tests; TFTs, thyroid function tests; U&Es, urea and electrolytes.)

to diagnose tumour, infarction, haematoma, hydrocephalus, and abscess.

Other tests

Consider the following when clinically indicated:

- Thick and thin films: malaria.
- HIV serology.
- Urine: toxicology screen.
- Red cell transketolase for thiamine deficiency.
- Serum copper and caeruloplasmin (reduced) and 24-hour urinary copper excretion (increased): Wilson's disease.
- Electroencephalogram: typical changes of herpes simplex encephalitis.
- Lumbar puncture and cerebrospinal fluid examination: protein, glucose, microscopy, culture, and oligoclonal bands.

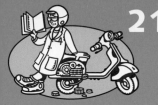

21. Acute Neurological Deficit

Introduction

A stroke is a neurological deficit due to vascular disturbance which develops over minutes (sometimes hours) and persists for at least 24 hours. Identical deficits lasting less than 24 hours are termed transient ischaemic attacks (TIAs). Cerebral infarction (embolism or thrombosis) accounts for 80% of strokes; 20% of strokes are caused by intracerebral haemorrhage. Fig. 21.1 outlines the principal types of stroke.

Differential diagnosis of stroke

The diagnosis is often clear from the history and examination, but the following pathologies can also produce a clinical picture that is identical to stroke and should be considered in atypical presentations:

- Subdural haematoma: elderly, alcoholics.
- Cerebral abscess: consider if patient has bronchiectasis or murmur (infective endocarditis).
- Space occupying lesion (e.g. tumour).
- Epilepsy: Todd's paresis following Jacksonian seizure.
- Hemiplegic migraine: typical features of migraine also present, resolving within 24 hours.
- Demyelination e.g. multiple sclerosis: rare.
- Drugs (e.g. overdose with tricyclic antidepressants: history of depression, younger patients).
- Hypoglycaemia.

Fig. 21.1 Causes of stroke. (PAN, polyarteritis nodosa; SLE, systemic lupus erythematosus.)

Types of stroke	
Cause	**Aetiology**
Haemorrhagic	Hypertension Aneurysm (particularly Charcot–Bouchard microaneurysms; also Berry and mycotic aneurysms) Arteriovenous malformation Tumours Bleeding tendency (thrombocytopenia, coagulation defects, Anticoagulants) Drugs (amphetamines, ecstasy)
Infarction	Hypertension Intracranial arterial atheroma Inflammatory vasculopathy (temporal arteritis, SLE, PAN, Neurosyphilis) Prolonged hypotension (cardiac arrest) Prothrombotic haematological disorders (hyperviscosity, Antiphospholipid syndrome) Drugs (amphetamines, ecstasy) Embolism
Embolic	Carotid or vertebral atheroma Cardiac: • Atrial fibrillation with left atrial thrombosis • Endocarditis • Ventricular thrombus due to myocardial infarction or ventricular aneurysm • Atrial myxoma Paradoxical: • Venous thrombus can reach the cerebral circulation via a patent foramen ovale or an atrial septal defect (rare)

History in the stroke patient

The history should focus on three distinct areas. First, does the story fit with the diagnosis of stroke? Second, where is the anatomical site of the lesion? Finally, are any risk factors present? The assessment for acute stroke treatment will become more common in years to come.

How has the deficit developed?

The key feature in stroke is that the symptoms develop rapidly over a few minutes or, less commonly, hours, but once the deficit is complete it remains stable and usually improves. If there has been gradual neurological deterioration, consider one of the differential diagnoses or hydrocephalus secondary to the stroke (oedema or blood preventing free drainage of cerebrospinal fluid). Improvement can be complete but there is often some residual deficit.

Where is the lesion?

Any intracranial artery can be involved in stroke. The symptoms and signs will reflect which artery and therefore which part of the brain has been involved. This is summarised in Fig. 21.2.

Are there any risk factors for stroke?

Fig. 21.3 shows the main risk factors for stroke and they are the same as for all vascular disease (see Chapter 1).

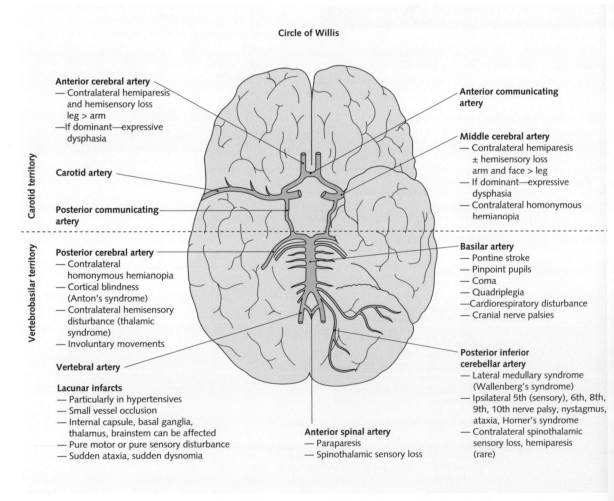

Fig. 21.2 Symptoms and signs associated with different strokes. Note that haemorrhagic strokes have symptoms and signs determined by the site of the bleed. Patients may also develop headache, loss of consciousness and vomiting as a result of raised intracranial pressure.

Risk factors for stroke

- Atrial fibrillation
- Hypertension
- Diabetes mellitus
- Hypercholesterolaemia
- Obesity
- Alcohol
- Oral contraceptive pill
- Established vascular disease (carotid bruit, peripheral vascular disease)
- Previous stroke or transient ischaemic attack
- Smoking
- Thrombophilia
- Family history

Fig. 21.3 Risk factors for stroke.

Examining the stroke patient

Clinical examination gives information regarding four important areas in the stroke patient.

(i) What are the neurological abnormalities and do they fit with the diagnosis of stroke?

(ii) Is there any evidence of an underlying cause?

(iii) Have any complications arisen as a result of the stroke?

(iv) What acute treatment is needed?

Fig. 21.4 summarises this examination approach.

Has the patient had a stroke?

A thorough neurological examination should be performed, including a coma scale. Does the pattern

Fig. 21.4 Examining the stroke patient. (BM, stick blood sugar test.)

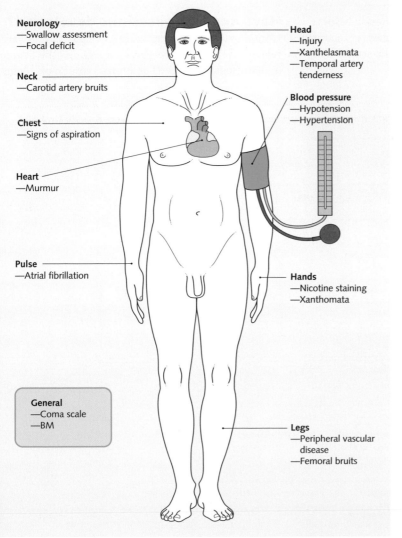

Neurology
—Swallow assessment
—Focal deficit

Neck
—Carotid artery bruits

Chest
—Signs of aspiration

Heart
—Murmur

Pulse
—Atrial fibrillation

General
—Coma scale
—BM

Head
—Injury
—Xanthelasmata
—Temporal artery tenderness

Blood pressure
—Hypotension
—Hypertension

Hands
—Nicotine staining
—Xanthomata

Legs
—Peripheral vascular disease
—Femoral bruits

of neurological deficit fit with disruption of the cerebral vascular supply (Fig. 21.2)? Remember that the Glasgow Coma Scale is imperfect in stroke as an aphasic person will score a maximum of eleven, as their verbal score can only ever be one. Pay particular attention to the pattern of upper motor neurone weakness, hemianopia, dysphasia and sensory/visual inattention. This enables you to place the patient in the Bamford classification which has important prognostic implications (Fig. 21.5).

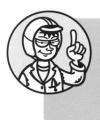 Glasgow Coma Scale is not ideal in stroke as an aphasic person will only ever score one point for the verbal component (i.e. best possible GCS = 11)

Determining the likely site of the lesion helps to focus the search for an underlying cause (e.g. carotid bruits in an anterior or middle cerebral artery stroke).

Is there any evidence of an underlying cause?

There are many causes and risk factors for stroke. However, pay particular attention to the following:
- Carotid bruits: carotid atheroma.
- Murmurs: endocarditis, valvular disease, atrial septal defect.
- Pulse: atrial fibrillation.
- Blood pressure: hypertension can be the cause or result of stroke; prolonged hypotension can also cause stroke.
- Diminished peripheral pulses and femoral bruits: peripheral vascular disease.
- Xanthelasmata, xanthomata: underlying hyperlipidaemia.
- Temporal artery tenderness: giant cell arteritis.
- Tar-stained fingers from smoking.

Have any complications developed?

Complications are common following stroke and are related to the size of cerebral damage and the degree of neurological deficit. The more common problems

Fig. 21.5 The Bamford classification of acute stroke.

The Bamford classification of stroke				
Category	Percentage of overall strokes	Clinical findings	Percentage at one year	
			Dead	Living independently
TACS Total Anterior Circulation Stroke	20	All three of a) Weakness of two or more of face, arm and leg. b) Homonymous hemianopia. c) Disturbance of higher cerebral function e.g. dysphasia, dyspraxia, inattention. If the patient is drowsy then b) and c) are assumed.	60	5
PACS Partial Anterior Circulation Stroke	35	Two of the components of TACS.	15	55
LACS LACunar Stroke	20	Pure motor/sensory stroke. Ataxic hemiparesis. NO disturbance of higher function.	10	60
POCS POsterior Circulation Stroke	25	a) Brainstem and/or cerebellar deficits. b) Isolated homonymous hemianopia.	20	60

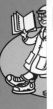

Fig. 21.6 Complications of stroke and measures to prevent them.

Complications of stroke and measures to prevent them

Complications	Prophylactic measures
Cerebral oedema	Particularly in haemorrhagic stroke and usually non-preventable (avoid overenthusiastic rehydration)
Pressure sores	Careful nursing with regular turning
Pneumonia	Patient should be kept nil by mouth until they have a safe swallow
Contractures and spasticity	Regular skilled physiotherapy
Malnutrition	Feeding via nasogastric tube or later, gastrostomy
Depression	Provision of adequate social and practical support
Epilepsy	None
Deep vein thrombosis	Physiotherapy, antiembolism stockings Heparin not used routinely

along with prophylactic measures to avoid them are outlined in Fig. 21.6.

What acute intervention is needed?

There is strong evidence that the acute management of stroke influences outcome. At present this involves the use of aspirin, good fluid balance, glycaemic control, normothermia and correction of hypoxia. Acute thrombolysis is not widely used in the UK though guidelines suggest overall benefit in patients despite the increased risk of haemorrhage if started within 3 hours of symptom onset. This is after exclusion of intracerebral haemorrhage by computerised tomography (CT) scanning and done in centres with expertise and experience in the treatment. Exclusion criteria are wide and include mild or rapidly improving neurological deficits, risk of bleeding, early evidence of infarction on CT and severely uncontrolled hypertension.

Investigating the stroke patient

The diagnosis of stroke remains a clinical one. The purpose of acute investigations is to exclude treatable causes and offer the best supportive care. In the future it may involve the assessment for thrombolysis.

An algorithm for investigating the patient with stroke is given in Fig. 21.7.

The following tests should be performed for all acute stroke patients:

- Full blood count: polycythaemia may cause a stroke; a reactive picture may indicate inflammation (e.g. temporal arteritis).

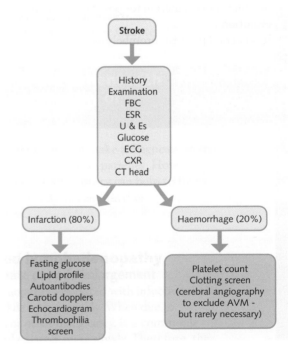

Fig. 21.7 Algorithm for the investigation of the stroke patient. Note that performing a lumbar puncture in patients with haemorrhagic stroke can precipitate coning. (AVM, arteriovenous malformation; CT, computed tomography; CXR, chest X-ray; ECG, electrocardiogram; ESR, erythrocyte sedimentation rate; FBC, full blood count; glucose; U&Es, urea and electrolytes.)

123

Symptoms in local structures

Has the patient noticed pain, erythema or a mass in any of the structures draining into the affected node, e.g. cellulitis in inguinal lymphadenopathy or a breast mass in axillary lymphadenopathy? Neurological signs may be due to a mass pressing on a nerve or plexus distant from the deficit.

Systemic symptoms

In lymphoma the patient may experience pruritus or the so called 'B symptoms' (fever above 38°C, drenching night sweats, weight loss). B symptoms indicate more extensive disease and a worse prognosis (see Chapter 34).

Generalised lymphadenopathy

Infection and underlying malignancy—be it lymphoma or metastatic—are the two top diagnoses here and questions are asked with this in mind. A full systemic enquiry is essential in these patients as most of the causes of generalised lymphadenopathy can affect multiple systems and a distant primary malignancy may require careful pursuit. Special attention should be paid to the following:

- Malaise, anorexia and general debility: common but non-specific.
- 'B symptoms': haematological malignancy.
- Skin rash: rubella, SLE and sarcoidosis.
- Arthralgia and arthropathy: SLE, rheumatoid arthritis, syphilis (Charcot's joints).
- Infectious contacts: rubella, TB and EBV.
- Risk factors for HIV infection, so called persistent generalised lymphadenopathy (see Chapter 35).
- Drug history: phenytoin.

Splenomegaly
Previous medical history

Is the patient known to have a pre-existing illness that can cause splenomegaly [e.g. chronic liver disease resulting in portal hypertension, connective tissue disease, thalassaemia (haemolysis), Gaucher's disease, or damaged cardiac valves (rheumatic fever or prosthetic valve) with infective endocarditis]?

Recent travel abroad or infectious contacts

Consider infectious mononucleosis, TB, schistosomiasis, kala-azar and malaria.

Systemic symptoms

Systemic symptoms suggestive of an underlying cause include arthralgia, rash, and 'B symptoms' (as above).

Symptoms of haematological disturbance

Hypersplenism can affect all three cell lines. It can cause malaise, breathlessness and lethargy if anaemia is present. Recurrent infection may be a symptom of leucopenia and increased or new mucosal and petechial bleeding may indicate thrombocytopenia.

Examining the patient with lymphadenopathy and splenomegaly

When lymphadenopathy or splenomegaly is present, a full clinical examination of the lymphatic system should be made. The examination should then focus on possible underlying causes. Fig. 22.1 summarises this examination approach.

Which lymph nodes are affected? Is there splenomegaly?

First, the extent, sites, size, consistency, tenderness, and fixation of enlarged lymph nodes should be documented. Normal reactive nodes are generally

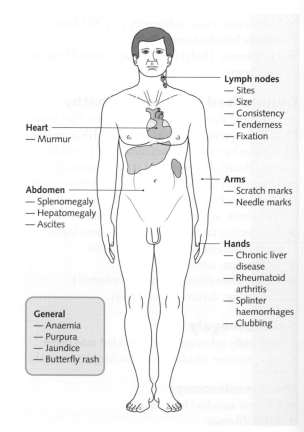

Fig. 22.1 Examining the patient with lymphadenopathy and splenomegaly.

Fig. 22.2 Characteristic clinical features which distinguish between the spleen and left kidney.

Characteristic clinical features which distinguish between the spleen and left kidney	
Spleen	**Left kidney**
No palpable upper border	Palpable upper border
Not bimanually palpable (not ballottable)	Bimanually palpable (ballottable)
Notch on medial border	No notch
Moves inferomedially on inspiration	Moves inferiorly on inspiration
Dull to percussion	Resonant to percussion (overlying bowel)

less than 1 cm in diameter, feel soft, are not fixed, and can be tender. Lymphomatous nodes are often larger and feel rubbery, but are not fixed. Lymph nodes infiltrated by carcinoma feel hard and may be fixed to surrounding tissue. Cervical, occipital, supraclavicular, axillary, and inguinal areas should be palpated carefully.

If splenomegaly is present, the size from the left costal margin must be recorded.

It is important to distinguish the left kidney from the spleen when palpating a mass in the left hypochondrium and the differences between the two are commonly asked for in examinations (Fig. 22.2). The presence or absence of hepatomegaly is important in clinical practice but is more so in examinations; remember hepatosplenomegaly is a common scenario.

Is there evidence of an underlying cause?

Anaemia and petechial bleeds/purpura may be present as described above. Jaundice may result from chronic liver disease, haemolysis, or infective hepatitis. Cachexia heralds underlying malignancy.

Figure 22.3 summarises clinical findings that may point to particular diagnoses. Evidence of chronic liver disease, rheumatoid arthritis, and SLE should also be looked for as described in Chapters 11 and 17. Needle marks may indicate previous exposure to HIV and hepatitis B or C, or provide a source of bacteria in infective endocarditis.

Localised lymphadenopathy

Examine those structures with lymphatic drainage to the affected nodes. Erythema, increased temperature, and tenderness suggest infection, whilst a hard, non-tender mass may indicate malignancy. When there is isolated cervical lymphadenopathy, a formal ear, nose, and throat examination should also be performed since oropharyngeal malignancies commonly metastasise to these nodes.

Splenomegaly and generalised lymphadenopathy

Where there is both splenomegaly and generalised lymphadenopathy consider lymphoproliferative disorders, infection, connective tissue disease, and sarcoidosis.

Additional clinical features of some conditions presenting with splenomegaly	
Disease	**Clinical features**
Portal hypertension	Caput Medusae, venous hum, ascites
Infectious mononucleosis	Palatal petechiae, tonsillar enlargement, jaundice, tender hepatomegaly, rash
Bacterial endocarditis	Clubbing, splinter haemorrhages, Osler's nodes, Janeway's lesions, Roth's spots, changing murmurs, haematuria, pyrexia
AA amyloid	Hepatomegaly, renal involvement causing nephrotic syndrome (see Chapter 13), macroglossia
Gaucher's disease	Adult type: hepatomegaly, pathological fractures, pigmentation Childhood type: mental retardation, spasticity

Fig. 22.3 Additional clinical features of some conditions presenting with splenomegaly.

Investigating the patient with lymphadenopathy and splenomegaly

An algorithm for diagnosis of the patient with lymphadenopathy and splenomegaly is given in Fig. 22.4.

Haematology

- A full blood count may show anaemia, leucopenia, thrombocytopenia, or a combination of these.
- Blood film can provide diagnostic information (Fig. 22.5).
- Erythrocyte sedimentation rate and C-reactive protein will be elevated in infection, malignancy, and inflammation.
- Bone marrow examination includes aspiration, trephine, and cytogenetic analysis. It is indicated if the blood count or film suggest haematological abnormalities, and it is useful in the diagnosis of leukaemias, myeloproliferative disorders, immune thrombocytopenias, and pancytopenia. Occasionally, it is helpful in storage diseases, lymphoma, and carcinoma, where there is marrow infiltration.

Biochemistry

- Liver function tests: transaminases will be abnormal in infective hepatitis and sometimes in EBV and CMV; elevation in alkaline phosphatase and γ-glutamyl transpeptidase will occur when the porta hepatis is obstructed by enlarged lymph nodes; unconjugated hyperbilirubinaemia will be present in haemolysis.
- Lactate dehydrogenase: is a useful prognostic marker in lymphoma.
- Serum calcium: raised in malignancy, sarcoidosis, and sometimes lymphoma.
- Serum uric acid: raised when there is rapid cell turnover such as in malignancy.
- Thyroid function tests: thyrotoxicosis.

Infection screen

- Monospot test: EBV.
- Serology: EBV, CMV, HIV, rubella, viral hepatitis, toxoplasmosis, and brucellosis.
- Blood cultures: repeated if infective endocarditis is suspected.
- Sputum culture: TB.

Autoantibody screen

This is useful in the detection of connective tissue disorders (see Chapter 17).

Imaging

- Chest X-ray: bilateral hilar lymphadenopathy (caused by lymphoma, sarcoidosis, and TB).
- Abdominal ultrasound scan: will confirm the presence of splenomegaly. It is poor at imaging the retroperitoneal lymph node chains.
- Computed tomography scan of the chest, abdomen, and pelvis: gives clear staging information in malignancy and particularly lymphoma where retroperitoneal lymphadenopathy may often be missed by ultrasound scan.

A palpable spleen is at least twice its normal size

A common examination question is to palpate a mass in the left hypochondrium. Make sure you can distinguish the left kidney from the enlarged spleen

Histology

The definitive diagnosis of lymphadenopathy and its classification is often made on excision biopsy of an enlarged node.

Rarely, a lumbar puncture and cytology may be needed to assess intracerebral involvement with malignancy.

Alcohol can produce dramatic pain in the lymphadenopathy associated with Hodgkin's Disease

Remember massive splenomegaly crosses the patient's midline into the right iliac fossa

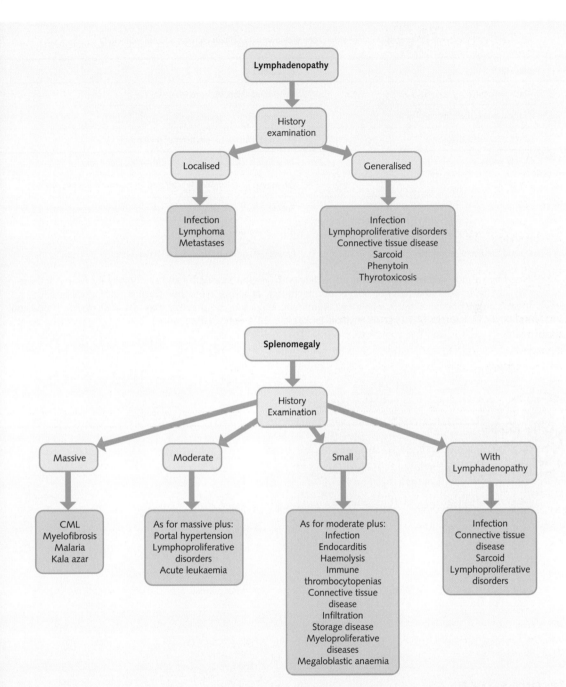

Fig. 22.4 Algorithm for diagnosis in the patient with lymphadenopathy and splenomegaly. (CML, chronic myeloid leukaemia.)

Blood film abnormalities in conditions presenting with lymphadenopathy and splenomegaly	
Disease	Blood film
Acute leukaemia	Circulating blasts (Auer rods in AML)
Chronic lymphocytic leukaemia	Lymphocytosis, smear cells
Chronic myeloid leukaemia	Leucocytosis due to spectrum of myeloid cells
Myelofibrosis	Tear drop poikilocytes, leucoerythroblastic blood film
Lymphoma	Often normal (occasionally mild eosinophilia in Hodgkin's disease)
Haemolysis	Reticulocytosis (polychromasia), microspherocytosis, erythroblasts
EBV, infectious hepatitis, toxoplasmosis	Atypical lymphocytes
Malaria (thick and thin films)	Parasitaemia, thrombocytopenia, haemolysis

Fig. 22.5 Blood film abnormalities in conditions presenting with lymphadenopathy and splenomegaly. Many of these disorders may also be associated with a normocytic normochromic anaemia. A leucoerythroblastic film will be seen wherever there is heavy bone marrow involvement. Autoimmune haemolytic anaemia may also arise in lymphoma and chronic lymphocytic leukaemia. (AML, acute myeloid leukaemia; EBV, Epstein–Barr virus.)

To enhance chances of palpating the spleen have the patient lie on their right side and fix the lower ribs with the left hand, gently pulling against the examining right hand in inspiration

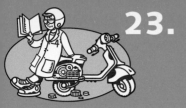

23. Sensory and Motor Neurological Deficits

Introduction

Muscle weakness or abnormal sensation can result from disease occurring anywhere along the pathway from the skin or muscle to the brain and back. Such pathological processes are outlined below.

Differential diagnosis of sensory and/or motor neurological deficits

The differential diagnosis is approached logically according to the neuromuscular pathway (Fig. 23.1).

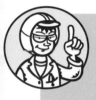

Psychological problems may manifest themselves as neurological (and other physical) symptoms, which may be bizarre—'somatisation'

History in the patient with sensory and/or motor neurological deficits

It is often a daunting prospect to be faced with a patient with neurological symptoms or signs. However, despite the vast number of potential underlying pathologies, a lesion at a particular point in the pathway between brain and muscle or skin will always produce the same clinical signs regardless of the cause. There are five important aspects to consider in the history.

Onset
Sudden onset usually indicates a vascular problem such as infarction, haemorrhage or haematoma. Lesions due to trauma, multiple sclerosis (MS), abscess, acute prolapsed disc, and myelitis can also develop rapidly. An insidious onset is more typical of cervical spondylosis, motor neurone disease, neoplasm, myopathy, and syringomyelia.

Precipitants
Trauma may result in muscular and neurological deficits. Acute myasthenia can be precipitated by intercurrent illness (particularly infection), or drugs (aminoglycosides or penicillamine). MS may relapse during the puerperium and symptoms may be exacerbated by exertion, hot weather, or after a hot bath.

Development
Many lesions cause gradually progressive, unremitting disease, including tumour, motor neurone disease, hereditary ataxias, and degenerative brain diseases. Intermittent deficits can be due to transient ischaemic attacks, epilepsy, migraine, and myasthenia gravis. MS is characterised by the development of different lesions which are dissociated in time and site. Symptoms and signs due to trauma or vascular events may slowly improve with time or remain static following the initial event.

Pattern of deficit
Figure 23.2 summarises characteristic symptoms and signs which arise as a consequence of a lesion at a specific site. If the neurological abnormalities do not fit with a single localised lesion, consider MS, motor neurone disease, paraneoplastic neuropathy or a functional disorder.

Evidence of cause
The following factors provide evidence of cause:
- Family history: hereditary ataxias, phenylketonuria, neurofibromatosis.
- Drug history: e.g. phenytoin (cerebellar signs), vincristine (peripheral neuropathy), penicillamine (myasthenia).
- Dietary history: intake of vitamins B_1, B_6 and B_{12}.
- Alcohol history.
- Pre-existing illness: e.g. diabetes, hypertension (cerebrovascular disease), rheumatoid arthritis, tuberculosis or malignancy.
- History of trauma. Associated features: e.g. swinging pyrexia and rigors (abscess), vasculitic symptoms (connective tissue disease), anorexia and weight loss (malignancy), symptoms of hypo- or hyperthyroidism.

131

Differential diagnosis of sensory and motor deficits	
Site of lesion	Examples
Muscle (see Chapters 31, 32 and 33)	**Congenital**
	Dystrophy: Duchenne, Becker's, limb girdle, facioscapulohumeral.
	Myotonia: myotonic dystrophy, myotonia congenita (Thomsen's disease)
	Acquired
	Drugs: steroids, penicillamine, procainamide, cholesterol lowering drugs (statins and fibrates) Endocrine: Cushing's syndrome, thyrotoxicosis, myxoedema, and hyperparathyroidism
	Infection: bacterial (*Clostridium welchii*), viral (influenza) and parasitic (trichinosis)
	Inflammation: polymyositis, dermatomyositis and sarcoidosis
	Metabolic: periodic paralyses, McArdle's disease and mitochondrial myopathy
	Toxin: alcohol
	Tumour: sarcoma and paraneoplastic syndrome
Neuromuscular junction (see Chapter 31)	Myasthenia gravis
	Lambert-Eaton syndrome
	Clostridium botulinum infection
Peripheral nerves (see Chapters 31, 32, 33, and 35)	**Mononeuropathy** (only one nerve involved)
	Trauma
	Entrapment: carpal tunnel syndrome (median nerve) and meralgia paraesthetica (lateral cutaneous nerve of thigh)
	Stretching: ulnar nerve with increased elbow carrying angle
	Tumour: neurofibromatosis
	Mononeuritis multiplex (two or more nerves involved)
	Connective tissue disease: PAN, SLE, RA
	Infection: leprosy, herpes zoster, HIV
	Inflammation: sarcoid
	Metabolic: DM and amyloid

Differential diagnosis of sensory and motor deficits	
Site of lesion	Examples
	Tumour: infiltration, paraneoplastic syndrome, neurofibromatosis
	Peripheral neuropathy (polyneuropathy with symmetrical deficit most marked distally)
	Congenital
	Charcot–Marie–Tooth disease
	Refsum's disease
	Friedrich's ataxia
	Acquired
	Connective tissue disease: PAN, SLE, RA
	Drugs: nitrofurantoin, metronidazole, vincristine
	Inflammation: AIDP (Guillain-Barré) and CIDP
	Metabolic: DM, renal failure, porphyria, amyloid
	Toxins: alcohol and lead
	Tumour: paraneoplastic syndrome and paraproteinaemias
	Vitamin deficiency: thiamine (B_1), niacin (B_6), B_{12}
Brachial or lumbar plexus	Compression: cervical rib
	Idiopathic: neuralgic amyotrophy
	Metabolic: DM Trauma: birth injury (Erb's and Klumpke's palsies) and motorbike accidents
	Tumour: malignant infiltration
Spinal nerve root	Infection (e.g. pyogenic meningitis and syphilis)
	Prolapsed intervertebral disc
	Spinal stenosis
	Spondylosis
	Tumour
	Vertebral fracture dislocation
Anterior horn cell (see Chapter 31)	Motor neurone disease
	Poliomyelitis

Differential diagnosis of sensory and motor deficits	
Site of lesion	Examples
Spinal cord (see Chapter 31)	
	Degeneration: osteoarthritis
	Infection: abscess, HIV, TB (Pott's disease) Inflammation; MS, sarcoidosis, RA (atlanto-axial subluxation)
	Metabolic: Paget's disease
	Trauma: also prolapsed intervertebral disc and radiotherapy Tumour: metastases, neurofibroma, meningioma, glioma, ependymoma
	Vascular: anterior spinal artery occlusion, dissecting aortic aneurysm, arteriovenous malformation, vasculitis Vitamin deficiency: subacute combined degeneration of the cord (vitamin B_{12})
	Others: syringomyelia, spina bifida, motor neurone disease
Cerebellum (see Chapter 31)	**Congenital**
	Friedrich's ataxia
	Ataxia telangiectasia
	Acquired
	Endocrine: hypothyroidism
	Infection: abscess and postencephalitis
	Inflammation: MS
	Toxins: alcohol, lead, anticonvulsants
	Trauma: 'punch-drunk' syndrome
	Tumour: metastases, acoustic neuroma, haemangioblastoma (von Hippel-Lindau disease), paraneoplastic degeneration.
	Vascular: infarction, haematoma, arteriovenous malformation

Differential diagnosis of sensory and motor deficits	
Site of lesion	Examples
Cerebral hemispheres (see Chapter 31)	Degenerative disease
	Hydrocephalus: primary or secondary
	Infection: abscess, meningitis, encephalitis, HIV, malaria, rabies, tuberculosis, syphilis
	Inflammation: sarcoid, SLE, MS
	Metabolic: phenylketonuria and Wilson's disease (basal ganglia)
	Toxic: alcohol
	Trauma
	Tumour: primary or secondary
	Vascular: infarction, haemorrhage, arteriovenous malformation, aneurysm
	Vitamin deficiency: thiamine, niacin, B_{12}

Fig. 23.1 The differential diagnosis of sensory and/or motor neurological deficits. (PAN, polyarteritis nodosa; SLE, systemic lupus erythematosus; RA, rheumatoid arthritis; HIV, human immunodeficiency virus; DM, diabetes mellitus; AIDP, acute inflammatory demyelinating polyneuropathy; CIDP, chronic inflammatory demyelinating polyneuropathy; TB, tuberculosis; MS, multiple sclerosis.)

Examining the patient with sensory and/or motor neurological deficits

When assessing a patient in clinic or hospital, a full neurological examination should be performed (see Chapter 38). However, in medical school examinations you will only be expected to assess a specific part of the system, such as the eyes, face, legs, arms, or gait. The most common neurological short cases are peripheral neuropathy [usually due to diabetes mellitus (DM), Parkinson's disease, stroke, and MS], but be prepared for anything!

It is important to remember that, in sensory problems, subjective sensation is usually more sensitive than physical examination which should be used to elicit the pattern and delineate and clarify the problem.

The clinical examination should aim to answer three questions. First, where is the anatomical site of the lesion or lesions? Second, is there anything to suggest the underlying pathological process? Finally, what disability does the patient have as a consequence of their neurological deficit?

Where is the lesion?

From the moment you meet the patient, watch like a hawk. How does the patient shake your hand? Can they lift their arm up? Can they let go of your hand (myotonia)? Watch how they undress or get on to the bed. Any severe deficit will often become apparent before you even lay hands on the patient. Examine the area of interest very carefully.

Figure 23.2 should help you identify where the anatomical lesion is likely to be on the basis of those neurological abnormalities present.

What is the underlying cause?

Once the site of the lesion is identified, think of the differential diagnosis as outlined at the beginning of this chapter. Are there any clues around the patient? Look for diabetic drinks (for peripheral neuropathy or amyotrophy).

If the patient is young, looks well, and is sitting in a wheelchair, MS is the most likely diagnosis. An elderly patient with a hemiparesis is most likely to have had a stroke. Is there a blood pressure chart? Is the patient in atrial fibrillation?

Look at the patient's face for myotonic facies (myotonia dystrophica), Cushing's syndrome (proximal myopathy), or hypothyroidism (myopathy or cerebellar dysfunction). Does the patient have neurofibromatosis (spinal cord or peripheral nerve lesions) or connective tissue disease, such as rheumatoid arthritis (entrapment mononeuropathy, mononeuritis multiplex, or peripheral neuropathy)? Is there a cervical rib?

What disability does the neurological deficit cause?

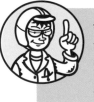

The most important thing for the patient is not locating the anatomical site of the lesion but what that lesion prevents them from doing

It is important to distinguish three related concepts: *impairment* refers to the affected body part (e.g. right arm following stroke), *disability* refers to a

Symptoms and signs associated with different anatomical lesions					
Site of anatomical lesion	Symptoms	Specific signs	Muscle	Reflexes	Sensation
Muscle	Weakness (particularly climbing stairs, getting out of chair) Pain (inflammation)	Myotonia in myotonia dystrophica Calf pseudohypertrophy and Gowers' sign in Duchenne muscular dystrophy	Wasting (usually proximal) Tone normal or reduced Power reduced	Normal Reduced or absent in severe muscle disease only Plantars downgoing	Normal
Neuromuscular junction	Diplopia Choking on food Altered voice Proximal limb weakness	Fatiguable weakness with repetition in myasthenia gravis eg. counting to 10 increasing strength with repetition in Lambert-Eaton syndrome	Wasting only if severe Tone normal Power alters with repetition	Normal	Normal
Peripheral nerve	Muscle weakness Sensory disturbance can be purely sensory, purely motor, or mixed	Mononeuropathy and mononeuritis multiplex –signs in distribution of affected nerves polyneuropathy–signs symmetrical and distal (glove and stocking)	Wasting Fasciculation Reduced tone Reduced power	Reduced or absent	Deficit of all modalities (glove and stocking distribution)

Symptoms and signs associated with different anatomical lesions [cont.]					
Site of anatomical lesion	Symptoms	Specific signs	Muscle	Reflexes	Sensation
Brachial or Lumbar plexus	Muscle weakness Sensory disturbance		Wasting Fasciculation Reduced tone Reduced power In distribution affected nerves	Reduced or absent	Deficit in distribution affected nerves
Anterior spinal root	Muscle weakness		Wasting Fasciculation Reduced tone Reduced power In distribution affected root	Reduced or absent	Normal
Posterior spinal root	Pain in skin and muscle supplied by that root		Normal	Reduced or absent	Deficit in distribution affected root
Anterior horn cell	Muscle weakness		Wasting Fasciculation Reduced tone Reduced power In distribution affected nerve	Reduced or absent	Normal
Spinal cord	Pain at site of lesion worse on coughing, sneezing, at night Urinary/bowel disturbance Leg weakness Sensory disturbance		At level of lesion: Wasting, Fasciculation, Reduced tone, Reduced power Below lesion: Spasticity, Increased tone, Reduced power	At level of lesion: reduced or absent Below lesion: increased, upgoing plantars	Below lesion Ipsilateral posterior column loss (proprioception, vibration sense) Contralateral spinothalamic loss (pain and temperature)
Cerebellum	Unsteadiness Tremor Altered speech Falls Poor coordination	Wide-based gait Fall to side of lesion Intention tremor Past-pointing Dysdiadochokinesis Nystagmus Staccato speech	Reduced tone No wasting Normal power	Pendular	Normal
Cerebral hemispheres	Determined by site of lesion (see Chapters 15, 19, and 20) Limb weakness Seizure Altered speech Disturbed higher functions	Parietal drift Dysphasia Dysarthria Visual disturbance	Increased tone Clasp-knife rigidity Wasting only if disuse Reduced power in pyramidal distribution (flexors stronger than extensors in arms, extensors stronger than flexors in legs)	Brisk Plantars upgoing	Deficit determined by site of lesion

Fig. 23.2 Symptoms and signs associated with different anatomical lesions.

particular activity (e.g. cannot write) and *handicap* refers to social function (e.g. cannot work).

Think what tasks the affected part of the body normally performs, and ask the patient to show you how they manage, such as doing up buttons (for peripheral neuropathy), brushing hair, or standing out of a chair (for proximal myopathy). Watching the patient walk can give useful information (Fig. 23.3).

Investigating the patient with sensory and/or motor neurological deficits

The pathway of investigation is very much determined by findings on the history and clinical examination. The following tests may be useful but each patient will require only those relevant to their presentation:

- Full blood count and erythrocyte sedimentation rate: reactive picture in inflammation, infection, and neoplasm, and raised mean corpuscular volume in vitamin B_{12} deficiency and alcohol abuse.
- Urea and electrolytes: raised urea and creatinine in renal failure, potassium high or low in periodic paralyses.
- Serum calcium: raised in hyperparathyroidism.
- Serum glucose: raised in DM.

- Liver function tests: raised γ-glutamyltransferase in alcohol abuse, raised alkaline phosphatase in Paget's disease, and deranged transamines in metastases, infection, and Wilson's disease.
- Thyroid function tests: hyper- or hypothyroidism.
- Creatine kinase: markedly raised in muscle inflammation and muscular dystrophies.
- Autoantibodies: rheumatoid arthritis, systemic lupus erythematosus, and polyarteritis nodosa.
- Serology: HIV, herpes, and syphilis where appropriate.
- Immunoglobulins: paraproteinaemias.
- Lumbar puncture: the cerebrospinal fluid should be analysed and interpreted as in Fig. 23.4.
- Electroencephalogram: may indicate structural cerebral pathology and is characteristic in herpes simplex encephalitis.
- Electromyogram: primary muscle disease (typical changes in myotonia and myasthenia); it also shows denervation but not its cause.
- Nerve conduction studies demonstrate peripheral neuropathies and the site and type of individual nerve lesions.
- Radiology: plain radiographs may demonstrate degenerative and destructive bone lesions and fractures; computed tomography (CT) scanning and magnetic resonance imaging (MRI) of the brain and spine are extremely useful in diagnosing and localizing central lesions; myelography can be

Fig. 23.3 Abnormalities of gait.

Abnormalities of gait	
Lesion	**Gait**
Hemiplegia	Foot is plantar flexed; leg is stiff and dragged through a semicircle
Spastic paraplegia	Legs stiff; walk in 'scissor fashion', like 'walking through mud'
Proximal myopathy	Waddling gait; trunk moves to swing legs forward; difficulty in climbing stairs or standing out of a chair
Parkinsonism	Stooped posture, hesitation in starting, shuffling, festinant, difficulty in turning, poor arm swing and may freeze
Cerebellar dysfunction	Broad based, ataxic with a tendency to fall to the side of the lesion; unable to walk heel to toe
Dorsal column disease	Stamping; wide based with patient looking at the ground as unable to sense where foot is; clumsy and slaps feet to ground
Foot drop	Stepping; legs lifted high off the ground as no dorsiflexion of the foot
Musculoskeletal disease	Limping; patient avoids weightbearing on affected side due to pain

CSF analysis and interpretation	
Test	**Interpretation**
Microscopy	?Infection ?malignancy
Culture and sensitivity	?Infection
Low glucose (<2/3 blood glucose)	Bacterial/TB/fungal/carcinomatous meningitis
Very high protein (>2 g/L)	GBS, *Froin's syndrome, TB/fungal meningitis, acoustic neuroma, Behcet's syndrome
High protein (0.4-2 g/L)	Bacterial meningitis, viral encephalitis, cerebral abscess, cerebral malignancy
Oligoclonal bands	Multiple sclerosis, SLE, neurosyphilis, neurosarcoidosis, Behçet's syndrome, SSPE
Neutrophils	Bacterial meningitis
Lymphocytes	Partially treated bacterial meningitis, viral encephalitis/meningitis, TB meningitis, CNS vasculitis, Behçet's syndrome, HIV associated, lymphoma/leukaemia, SLE
Xanthochromia (yellow CSF due to haemoglobin breakdown products)	Subarachnoid haemorrhage (xanthochromia from 12 hours after event)

Fig. 23.4 Cerebrospinal fluid (CSF) analysis and interpretation. (*Froin's syndrome—raised CSF protein and xanthochromia, but normal cell count, seen below a block in spinal cord compression; GBS, Guillain–Barré syndrome; TB, tuberculosis; CNS, central nervous system; HIV, human immunodeficiency virus; SLE, systemic lupus erythematosus; SSPE, subacute sclerosing panencephalitis.)

useful in demonstrating compressive cord lesions but this technique has been largely superseded by CT scans and MRI.

- Visual evoked potentials: demonstrate previous retrobulbar neuritis in MS. Auditory and somatosensory evoked potentials may also be performed to look for lesions in these pathways.
- Biopsy: if the diagnosis is in doubt, despite history, examination, and non-invasive procedures. Muscle, nerve, and brain biopsies can be performed to give a definitive histological diagnosis.

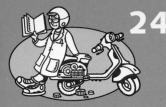

24. Bruising and Bleeding

Introduction

Bruising and bleeding arise when there is abnormal haemostasis. Haemostasis is dependent on normal platelet number and function, an intact coagulation pathway, and normal vessel walls. This chapter is intended to help with stable patients who have a documented increased tendency to bleed. It is not about resuscitating the shocked patient.

Differential diagnosis of bruising and bleeding

Platelet abnormalities

Platelets may be reduced in number or function.

Thrombocytopenia

- Reduced production: bone marrow failure, drugs (commonly cytotoxics, quinine, and cotrimoxazole), postchemotherapy or postradiotherapy, viral infections.
- Increased consumption: immune thrombocytopenic purpura, disseminated intravascular coagulation, thrombotic thrombocytopenic purpura, autoimmune disease, systematic lupus erythematosus and hypersplenism.
- Abnormal distribution: splenic pooling in splenomegaly.
- Dilutional: massive transfusion.
- Factitious: isolated thrombocytopenia may be related to aggregation caused by EDTA used in full blood count bottles.

Heparin is now the most common drug related cause of thrombocytopenia in hospitalised patients. It is usually caused by aggregation and not the heparin induced thrombocytopenia syndrome. It usually resolves and does not need withdrawal or future withholding of heparin.

Remember heparin induced thrombocytopenia (HIT) is a PRO-coagulant state

Platelet dysfunction

- Hereditary: Glanzmann's thrombasthenia (deficiency of glycoprotein IIb/IIIa receptor on platelet surface).
- Acquired: aspirin, heparin, uraemia.

Coagulation abnormalities

Coagulopathies may be due to vitamin K deficiency or specific factor deficiency.

Factor deficiency

- Hereditary: haemophilia A (factor VIII), haemophilia B (factor IX), von Willebrand's factor.
- Acquired: liver disease, decreased production of clotting factors as synthetic function fails.

Vitamin K deficiency

Factors II, VII, IX and X are dependent on vitamin K. Deficiency may be caused by:
- Malabsorption: bowel pathology such as coeliac disease or biliary obstruction (vitamin K is fat soluble).
- Antagonist drugs: coumarins (warfarin).

Vessel wall abnormalities

Vessel wall abnormalities may be inherited or acquired.

Hereditary

- Hereditary haemorrhagic telangiectasia (Osler–Weber–Rendu syndrome).

Acquired

- Trauma.
- Physiological: senile purpura.
- Drugs: corticosteroids.
- Infections: meningococcal septicaemia.
- Vitamin deficiency: scurvy (vitamin C).

- Connective tissue disease: pseudoxanthoma elasticum, Ehlers–Danlos syndrome.
- Endocrine: Cushing's syndrome.

History in the patient with bruising and bleeding

The history should focus on three areas. First, what is the pattern and extent of the bleeding and bruising? Second, are there any clues as to the possible underlying cause? Finally, have complications occurred?

What is the pattern and extent of bleeding and bruising?

As a general rule:

- Platelet abnormalities (low number or dysfunction) cause skin or mucosal purpura and haemorrhage, with prolonged bleeding following trauma or often minor surgery.
- Vessel wall abnormalities cause petechiae and ecchymoses due to bleeding from small vessels, mostly in the skin, but occasionally in mucous membranes.
- Coagulopathies cause haemarthroses, muscle haematomas, post-operative or traumatic bleeding, and mucosal bleeding (von Willebrand's disease).

What is the underlying cause?

- Bleeding and bruising: 'normal' and related to recent trauma, or due to an underlying haemostatic abnormality.
- Age: senile purpura seen mostly on the upper limbs.
- Liver disease: intrinsic liver disease or biliary tree obstruction.
- Drug history: aspirin, clopidogrel, heparin, warfarin, steroids, previous chemotherapy.
- Family history (e.g. haemophilia, hereditary haemorrhagic telangiectasia).
- Symptoms of underlying bone marrow failure (e.g. recurrent infection).
- Hyperextensibility of the skin or joints: Ehlers–Danlos syndrome, pseudoxanthoma elasticum.
- Poor diet: scurvy (ecchymoses predominantly on the lower limbs).
- Known acquired immune deficiency syndrome or risk factors for HIV infection.

Have complications occurred?

- Symptoms of anaemia (see Chapter 26).
- How severe was the bleeding: life threatening or minor irritant?
- Muscle pain or mass.
- Joint pain or deformity.

Examining the patient with bruising and bleeding

The examination should be approached in a similar manner to the history. Fig. 24.1 summarises the examination approach.

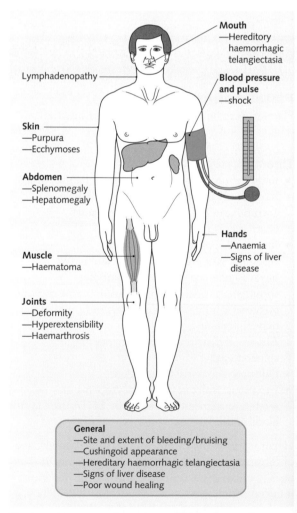

Fig. 24.1 Examining the patient with bleeding and bruising.

What is the pattern and extent of bleeding and bruising?

The sites and types of lesions should be documented (see above). 'Purpura' includes petechiae (small pinpoint bleeds into the skin) and ecchymoses (small bruises).

How severe has the bleeding been?

Anaemia may represent chronic bleeding or a primary haematologic defect (see Chapter 26). Finally, look for joint deformities or a mass in muscle.

Are there signs suggestive of specific diseases?

- Signs of liver disease (see Chapter 11).
- Splenomegaly (whatever cause): platelet pooling.
- Cushingoid appearance: steroid therapy, endocrinopathy.
- Hereditary haemorrhagic telangiectasia: characteristic petechiae on the tongue and lips.
- Scurvy: corkscrew hairs with hyperkeratosis of the follicles, perifollicular haemorrhages, gum hypertrophy, poor wound healing.
- Ehlers–Danlos syndrome: hyperextensible skin and joints, 'fish-mouth' wounds, pseudotumours over the elbows and knees.

- Pseudoxanthoma elasticum: loose skin in neck, axillae, anticubital fossae and groins, 'chicken skin', blue sclera, angioid streaks in the retina, hyperextensible joints.

Investigating the patient with bleeding and bruising

When an abnormality of haemostasis is suspected, a platelet count and simple coagulation assays should be performed. More specific tests to diagnose the underlying cause can then be considered. Fig. 24.2 summarises the normal coagulation pathway.

An algorithm for investigating the patient with bleeding and bruising is given in Fig. 24.3.

Platelet count

If thrombocytopenia is present, request a blood film (exclude artefactual result due to platelet clumping, look for primary haematological cause) and bone marrow aspirate (increased megakaryocytes in consumptive thrombocytopenia; e.g. idiopathic thrombocytopenic purpura or reduced megakaryocytes in bone marrow failure).

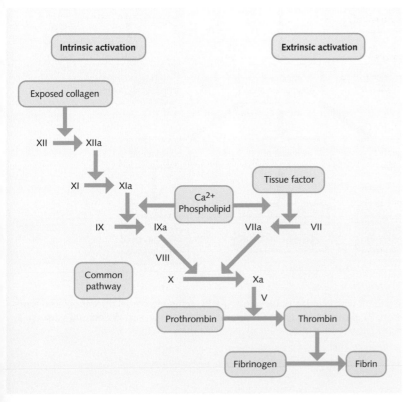

Fig. 24.2 The normal coagulation pathway. (INR measures extrinsic pathway. APTT measures intrinsic pathway.)

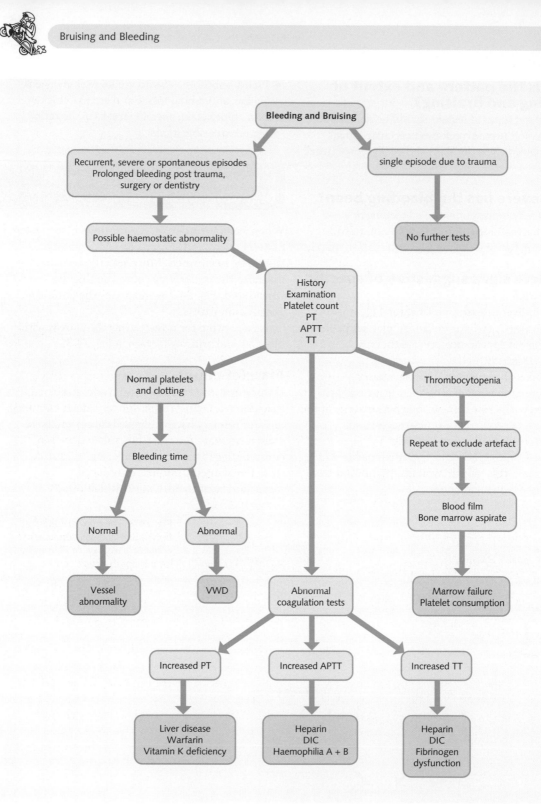

Fig. 24.3 Algorithm for investigating the patient with bruising or bleeding. (APTT, activated partial thromboplastin time; DIC, disseminated intravascular coagulation; PT, prothrombin time; TT, thrombin time; vWD, von Willebrand's disease.)

Summary of common tests of clotting						
	Platelet dysfunction including aspirin	Haemophilia	Vit K deficiency/ Warfarin	Intrinsic liver disease	vWD	Heparin
Platelet count	N	N	N	N	N	N/−
INR	N	N	+	+	N	N/+
APTT	N	+	N/+	N/+	+	+
Bleeding time	+	N	N	N/+	+	N
TT	N	N	N	N/+	N	+

Fig. 24.4 Summary of the common clotting tests. (INR, international normalised ratio; APTT, activated partial thromboplastin time; TT, thrombin time; vWD, von Willebrands disease; N, normal.)

Prothrombin time

Prothrombin time measures the extrinsic system (VII) and common pathway (X, V, prothrombin, and fibrinogen). It is prolonged in liver disease and warfarin therapy, and is generally expressed as international normalised ratio.

Activated partial thromboplastin time

This measures the intrinsic system (XII, XI, IX, and VIII) and common pathway (X, V, prothrombin, and fibrinogen). It is prolonged in unfractionated heparin therapy (not newer low molecular weight heparins), factor deficiency such as factor VIII (haemophilia A) and factor IX (haemophilia B, Christmas disease) and acquired (autoimmune) haemophilia.

Thrombin time

Thrombin time measures the activity of thrombin and fibrinogen in the common pathway. It is prolonged in fibrinogen deficiency (disseminated intravascular coagulation) or fibrinogen dysfunction. Prolonged thrombin time may also result from heparin therapy (inhibition of thrombin activity).

Bleeding time

Bleeding time measures platelet function. It is rarely performed and only if platelet count, coagulation screening tests (as above), blood film, and bone marrow are normal. It is prolonged in aspirin therapy, uraemia, and von Willebrand's disease.

Fibrin degradation products and D-dimers

Fibrin degradation products and D-dimers will be elevated in disseminated intravascular coagulation.

Other tests

Tests for other diseases given in the differential diagnosis list should be performed as indicated from the history, examination, and basic laboratory tests.

Normal range results to the above tests do not exclude a bleeding disorder. There are increasing numbers of sophisticated tests of platelet function and coagulation that are beyond the scope of this book. Referral to a haemotologist specialising in haemostasis is recommended.

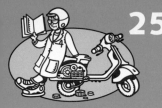

25. Vertigo and Dizziness

Introduction

True vertigo is the false perception (illusion) of movement, usually rotational, of a patient or of his or her surroundings. This is often accompanied by vomiting, sweating, and pallor. It results from either disease in the labyrinth (most common cause), the eighth cranial nerve, or its connections in the brainstem.

Dizziness or unsteadiness without vertigo can result from a variety of unrelated disorders. These are discussed in more detail in their appropriate chapters.

When a patient presents with 'vertigo' or 'dizziness', it is vital to establish whether true vertigo is present or not, as these symptoms result from different pathologies

Differential diagnosis in the patient with vertigo or dizziness

Vertigo
The differential diagnosis in the patient with vertigo includes labyrinth disorders, eighth cranial nerve disease, or brainstem lesions and is summarised in Fig. 25.1. Rarely vertigo can be a feature of temporal lobe pathology (e.g. temporal lobe epilepsy).

Dizziness
The differential diagnosis of dizziness is summarised in Fig. 25.2.

History in the patient with vertigo

The diagnosis in patients with vertigo is largely made on the history. It is important to elicit the time course of the vertigo and the likely site of the lesion by asking about other auditory and neurological symptoms. Typical features of specific diseases are shown in Fig. 25.3.

Differential diagnosis of vertigo (See Chapter 31)	
Location of lesion	**Examples**
Labyrinth	Middle ear disease (e.g. otitis media)
	Ménière's disease
	Benign positional vertigo
	Labyrinthitis
	Traumatic vertigo
	Perilymphatic fistula
	Syphilitic labyrinthitis
Eighth cranial nerve	Vestibular neuronitis
	Acoustic neuroma
	Ramsay Hunt syndrome: herpes zoster of the geniculate ganglion
	Ototoxic drugs: aminoglycosides such as gentamicin
	Petrous temporal bone pathology (e.g. Paget's disease)
Brainstem	Multiple sclerosis: demyelination
	Vertebrobasilar ischaemia: transient ischaemic attack
	Stroke: lateral medullary syndrome (infarction of posterior inferior cerebellar artery)
	Vertebrobasilar insufficiency
	Migraine
	Encephalitis
	Tumour
	Syringobulbia
	Alcohol abuse

Fig. 25.1 The differential diagnosis of vertigo.

Pattern of vertigo
The following should be established:
- Onset: peripheral lesions generally cause acute severe symptoms; central lesions tend to cause a gradual onset with less severe vertigo.

Differential diagnosis of dizziness	
Causes	**Further information**
Low cardiac output	Chapter 27
Hyperventilation, anxiety	*See Crash Course in Psychiatry*
Anaemia	Chapter 34
Hypoglycaemia	Chapter 32
Phaeochromocytoma	Chapter 32
Postural hypotension	Chapter 27
Visual disturbance	*See Crash Course in Neurology*
Cerebrovascular disease	Chapter 31
Pyrexia	Chapter 35

Fig. 25.2 The differential diagnosis of dizziness.

- Duration of vertigo.
- Recurrent episodes or a single attack?
- Relation to head position.

Aural symptoms

The presence of aural symptoms suggests that the lesion is peripheral, involving the labyrinth or eighth cranial nerve:

- Ear pain.
- Ear discharge.
- Deafness (fluctuating or progressive).
- Tinnitus.

Neurological symptoms

The following symptoms suggest central pathology or acoustic neuroma.

- Facial weakness.
- Dysarthria.
- Dysphagia.

Characteristic features of diseases causing vertigo					
Disease	**Cause**	**Length of vertigo**	**Aural symptoms**	**Neurological symptoms**	**Natural history**
Ménière's disease	Excess endolymphatic fluid (hydrops)	1–8 hours often preceded by sensation of ullness in the ear	Fluctuating but progressive deafness Tinnitus	None	Episodic attacks Unilateral at first becomes bilateral in 25% Ceases when deafness complete
Vestibular neuronitis	Possibly viral	Days to weeks explosive onset	None	None	Spontaneously resolves in weeks
Benign positional vertigo	Degeneration of utricular neuroendothelium can follow head injury and vestibular neuronitis	Seconds Precipitated by changes in head position	None	None	Episodic attacks Spontaneous resolution over weeks to months
Perilymphatic fistula	Rupture of round window membrane often due to barotrauma can be spontaneous	Months to years	Deafness and tinnitus	None	Often resolves with bed rest can be surgically repaired
Vertebrobasilar insufficiency	'Nipping' of vertebral arteries by osteophytic cervical vertebrae	Seconds Precipitated by neck extension or rotation	None	Dysarthria Diplopia Visual loss Syncope	Episodic attacks
Acoustic neuroma	Schwannoma of vestibular nerve	Gradual onset progressive	Unilateral deafness and tinnitus	5th and 7th cranial nerve palsies Ipsilateral cerebellar signs	Symptoms progress until surgical removal
Central lesions	Tumour Demyelination Vascular Migraine	Develops gradually Unremitting	Often spared	Usually present and dependent on site of lesion	Symptoms progress until underlying cause treated

Fig. 25.3 Characteristic features of diseases causing vertigo.

- Diplopia.
- Loss of consciousness.
- Seizures.
- Weakness, altered sensation, poor limb coordination.

History suggestive of an underlying cause

- Recent viral illness causes vestibular neuronitis.
- Previous head injury may lead to labyrinth concussion, benign positional vertigo.
- Previous otological surgery.
- Drug history (e.g. aminoglycosides).
- Risk factors for vascular disease: hypertension, high cholesterol, smoking, family history.
- Recent flying or diving (e.g. barotrauma–perilymphatic fistula). Recurrent episodes with subsequent headache (? migraine)

Examining the patient with vertigo

The clinical examination is often normal. The following specific abnormalities should be looked for carefully:

- Nystagmus: horizontal and away (fast phase) from the side of the lesion. Occasionally, brainstem lesions may also cause vertical nystagmus. (see p.397)
- Hallpike's manoeuvre: the patient is asked to lie down quickly with their head tilted to one side; in benign positional vertigo there will be a latent period of a few seconds followed by nystagmus.
- Focal neurological signs: if present, these suggest a central lesion, acoustic neuroma, or Ramsay Hunt syndrome. Pay particular attention to assessment of the eighth cranial nerve, gait, and cerebellar signs.
- Eyes: papilloedema (tumour with raised intracranial pressure), optic atrophy (demyelination), and ophthalmoplegia (cranial nerve defect, demyelination).
- Ears: otoscopy may reveal otitis media or a herpetic rash. Herpetic lesions may also be found on careful examination of the surrounding skin.
- Lying and standing blood pressures: postural hypotension.
- Neck movements—are they limited and/or do they provoke the symptoms (vertebrobasilar insufficiency)?

Figure 25.4 summarises the examination approach.

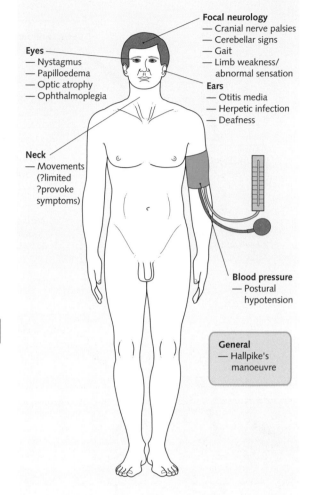

Fig. 25.4 Examining the patient with vertigo.

Investigating the patient with vertigo

- Audiometry: to distinguish between conductive and sensorineural deafness.
- Caloric tests: normally, running cold and then warm water into the external auditory meatus causes contralateral and then ipsilateral nystagmus, respectively; where there is pathology in the ipsilateral labyrinth, eighth cranial nerve, or brainstem, this normal response will be reduced or absent.
- Electronystagmography: a more accurate assessment of the presence and type of nystagmus.

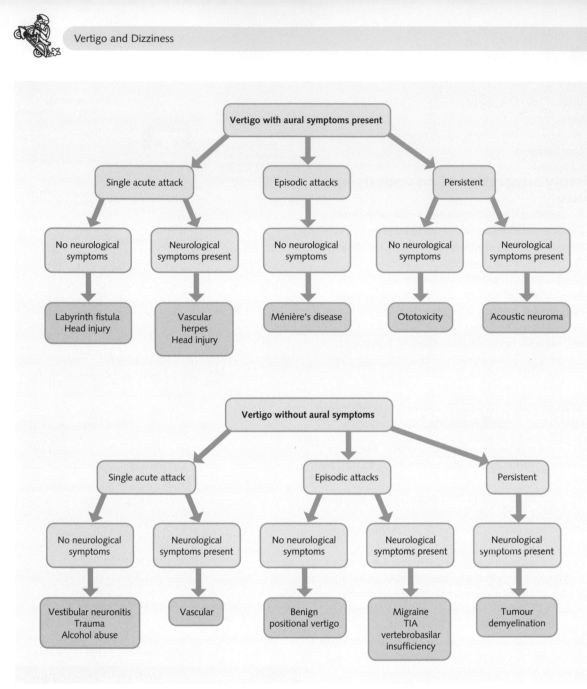

Fig. 25.5 Algorithm for the diagnosis of a patient with vertigo. (TIA, transient ischaemic attack.)

- Imaging: high-resolution computed tomography scanning and magnetic resonance imaging are useful tools when a central lesion or acoustic neuroma are suspected.

An algorithm for approaching the diagnosis in the patient with vertigo is given in Fig. 25.5.

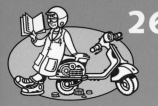

26. Anaemia

Introduction

Anaemia is not a diagnosis. It is a consequence of an underlying problem. A patient is anaemic when the haemoglobin concentration in the blood is less than 13.5 g/dL in men and 11.5 g/dL in women. It is common up to 10% of women in the UK are iron deficient due to menorrhagia.

Differential diagnosis of anaemia

The mean corpuscular volume (MCV) of the red blood cells gives important clues as to the likely underlying abnormality.

Microcytic red blood cells

Microcytic red blood cells (RBCs) have a MCV of less than 80 fL; where fL stands for femtolitre (-10^{-15} L). Causes include:

- Iron-deficiency anaemia (Fig. 26.1).
- Thalassaemia.
- Anaemia of chronic disease (Fig. 26.2).
- Sideroblastic anaemia.
- Lead poisoning.

Normocytic red blood cells

Normocytic RBCs have a MCV of 80–95 fL. Causes include:

- Anaemia of chronic disease (Fig. 26.2).
- Haemolysis (Fig. 26.3).
- Acute blood loss.
- Bone marrow hypoplasia.

Causes of iron-deficiency anaemia	
Mechanism	Examples
Reduced iron intake	Poor diet Malabsorption (gastrectomy, coeliac disease)
Increased iron utilization	Infancy, adolescence, pregnancy
Abnormal iron loss	Chronic bleeding from gastrointestinal tract, uterus, urinary tract

Fig. 26.1 Causes of iron-deficiency anaemia.

Causes of anaemia of chronic disease	
Mechanism	Examples
Malignancy	Breast, prostate, lung
Inflammation	Rheumatoid arthritis, temporal arteritis
Chronic infection	Tuberculosis, subacute bacterial endocarditis

Fig. 26.2 Causes of anaemia of chronic disease.

Macrocytic red blood cells

Macrocytic RBCs have a MCV of more than 95 fL. Causes include:

- Megaloblastic anaemia: folate deficiency (Fig. 26.4), vitamin B_{12} deficiency (Fig. 26.5).

Causes of haemolytic anaemia		
Mechanism		Examples
Intrinsic	Red blood cell membrane defects	Hereditary spherocytosis Hereditary elliptocytosis
	Enzyme deficiencies	Glucose-6-phosphate Dehydrogenase deficiency Pyruvate kinase deficiency
	Abnormal haemoglobin	Thalassaemia Sickle cell disease
Extrinsic	Immune	ABO incompatibility (blood transfusion) haemolytic disease of the newborn Autoimmune (warm): idiopathic, lymphoma, CLL, SLE, methyldopa Autoimmune (cold): idiopathic, lymphoma, mycoplasma, Epstein – Barr virus Drugs
	Non-immune	Mechanical heart valves Burns Malaria Microangiopathic (DIC, TTP, pre-eclampsia) Paroxysmal nocturnal haemoglobinuria Hepatic or renal disease

Fig. 26.3 Causes of haemolytic anaemia. (CLL, chronic lymphocytic leukaemia; DIC, disseminated intravascular coagulation; SLE, systemic lupus erythematosus; TTP, thrombotic thrombocytopenic purpura.)

Causes of folate deficiency

Mechanism	Examples
Reduced intake	Poor diet, e.g. old age, poverty, alcoholics
Reduced absorption	Coeliac disease, extensive Crohn's disease, tropical sprue, gastrectomy
Increased utilization	Physiological, e.g. pregnancy, lactation, prematurity Increased cell turnover, e.g. malignancy, chronic inflammation, haemolysis, dialysis
Drugs	Trimethoprim, sulphasalazine, anticonvulsants, methotrexate

Fig. 26.4 Causes of folate deficiency.

- Normoblastic anaemia: alcohol, liver disease, hypothyroidism, pregnancy, reticulocytosis.

History in the anaemic patient

It is important to establish first how symptomatic the patient is because of their anaemia. The history should then focus on whether any complications of anaemia are present and whether there are any clues as to the likely underlying diagnosis.

Symptoms of anaemia

When anaemia develops over a long time, the haemoglobin can be very low before symptoms

Causes of vitamin B$_{12}$ deficiency

Mechanism	Examples
Reduced intake	Vegans
Reduced absorption	Stomach, e.g. gastrectomy, pernicious anaemia Small intestine, e.g. Crohn's disease, ileal resection, ileal TB or UC
Increased utilization	Blind loop syndrome (bacterial overgrowth), fish tapeworm (*Diphyllobothrium latum*)
Abnormal metabolism	Transcobalamin II deficiency (autosomal recessive)
Drugs	Nitrous oxide, metformin

Fig. 26.5 Causes of vitamin B$_{12}$ deficiency. (TB, tuberculosis; UC, ulcerative colitis)

occur. Anaemia is tolerated less well in the elderly. The following symptoms may present:
- Lethargy.
- Shortness of breath: most marked on exertion.
- Lightheadedness.
- Palpitations.

Symptoms of complications
- Symptoms of cardiac failure (see Chapters 1 and 2).
- Angina.
- Ischaemic claudication.

Evidence to suggest underlying cause
- Specific symptoms: menorrhagia, change in bowel habit, dyspepsia, weight loss, headache.
- Pre-existing illness: rheumatoid arthritis, previous abdominal surgery, chronic renal failure.
- Family history: haemolytic anaemia.
- Drug history: non-steroidal anti-inflammatory drugs (iron deficiency), anticonvulsants (folate deficiency).
- Diet: vegans (vitamin B$_{12}$ deficiency), alcoholics (folate deficiency).
- Pica (craving for specific and often bizarre foods): iron deficiency.
- Pregnancy: folate deficiency.

Dysphagia plus iron-deficiency anaemia: think of Plummer–Vinson or Paterson–Brown–Kelly syndrome (postcricoid oesophageal web)

Examining the anaemic patient

Signs of anaemia and its consequences

Figure 26.6 summarises the examination approach. The following signs of anaemia should be noted:
- Pallor: mucous membranes (mouth and conjunctivae), nails, skin creases.
- Hyperdynamic circulation: tachycardia, collapsing pulse, systolic flow murmur.
- Cardiac failure.

Fig. 26.6 Examining the anaemic patient. (SACDC, subacute combined degeneration of the cord.)

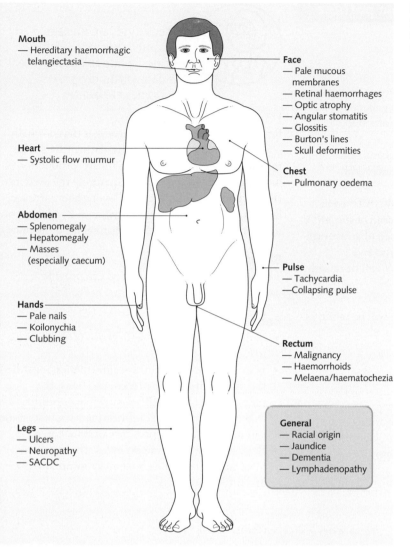

Mouth
— Hereditary haemorrhagic telangiectasia

Face
— Pale mucous membranes
— Retinal haemorrhages
— Optic atrophy
— Angular stomatitis
— Glossitis
— Burton's lines
— Skull deformities

Chest
— Pulmonary oedema

Heart
— Systolic flow murmur

Abdomen
— Splenomegaly
— Hepatomegaly
— Masses (especially caecum)

Pulse
— Tachycardia
— Collapsing pulse

Hands
— Pale nails
— Koilonychia
— Clubbing

Rectum
— Malignancy
— Haemorrhoids
— Melaena/haematochezia

Legs
— Ulcers
— Neuropathy
— SACDC

General
— Racial origin
— Jaundice
— Dementia
— Lymphadenopathy

Signs of underlying disease

A full general examination should always be performed, including breast examination and rectal examination in iron deficiency. Specific abnormalities include the following:

- Glossitis: megaloblastic anaemia, iron deficiency.
- Angular stomatitis and koilonychia: iron deficiency.
- Jaundice: haemolysis, megaloblastic anaemia (mild).
- Splenomegaly: haemolysis, megaloblastic anaemia (see Chapter 22).
- Leg ulcers: rheumatoid arthritis, sickle cell disease.
- Bone deformities: thalassaemia.
- Peripheral neuropathy, optic atrophy, subacute combined degeneration of the cord, dementia are all neurological sequelae of vitamin B_{12} deficiency.
- Blue line on the gums (Burton's line), peripheral motor neuropathy, encephalopathy are seen in lead poisoning.

Note the racial origin of the patient as thalassaemia is more common in people from the Mediterranean to South-East Asia, while sickle cell anaemia is more common among people of Black African origin.

Investigating the anaemic patient

General investigations
Full blood count
- Haemoglobin: anaemia.
- Mean corpuscular volume: underlying pathologies.
- White cell count: if low, consider general bone marrow failure; if high, consider infection, inflammation or malignancy.
- Platelet count: if low, consider general bone marrow failure; if high, consider infection, inflammation or malignancy.
- Red cell distribution width (RDW): offered in many labs, is a measure of the spread of the MCV. A 'normal' MCV may be composed of an average of a mixed population of microcytic and macrocytic red cells but the RDW will be raised.

Erythrocyte sedimentation rate
The erythrocyte sedimentation rate will be raised in infection, inflammation, or malignancy.

Reticulocyte count

 Iron deficiency anaemia is a sinister finding in older adults and needs thorough investigation

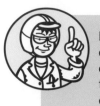 Reticulocytes are nucleated cells and can lead to a falsely elevated white cell count when the count is done on an electronic cell counter

Reticulocytes are young erythrocytes that normally constitute only 0.5–2.0% of circulating RBCs. The reticulocyte count is increased if RBC production is increased and red cells are prematurely released into the circulation. This occurs following haemorrhage, in chronic haemolysis, or with vitamin B_{12}, folate, or iron replacement, when there has been a deficiency.

Blood film
The blood film is mandatory and can provide diagnostic information, as shown in Fig. 26.7.

Bone marrow
- Not necessary when the diagnosis is obvious (e.g. iron deficiency).
- Bone marrow aspirate gives information regarding the development of different cell lines, the proportion of these different cell lines, infiltration by abnormal cells (e.g. infiltration with metastatic carcinoma), and the presence of iron stores.
- Bone marrow trephine provides structural information regarding bone marrow architecture and infiltration.

Abnormalities on the blood film in anaemia	
Abnormality	**Changes on blood film**
Iron deficiency	Hypochromic, microcytic RBCs, target cells, pencil cells, poikilocytosis (variation in RBC shape), anisocytosis (variation in RBC size), often thrombocytosis
Vitamin B_{12}/folate deficiency	Oval-shaped macrocytosis, neutrophil nuclei hypersegmented (greater than six lobes), poikilocytosis; white blood cell and platelet count may be low
Haemolysis	Reticulocytosis, microspherocytes, erythroblasts Many spherocytes in hereditary spherocytosis Elliptocytes in hereditary elliptocytosis
Thalassaemia	Hypochromic, microcytic RBCs, basophilic stippling, target cells, reticulocytosis
Sickle cell disease	Sickle cells, target cells Features of hyposplenism in adults (Howell–Jolly bodies, Pappenheimer bodies, target cells)
Anaemia of chronic disease	Normochromic, normocytic RBCs Neutrophilia and thrombocytosis may be present
Liver disease	Macrocytic RBCs, target cells Features of iron deficiency and folate deficiency may also be present

Fig. 26.7 Abnormalities on the blood film in anaemia. (RBCs, red blood cells)

Specific investigations

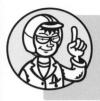

Ferritin is an acute phase protein, so false elevated or normal range results are possible with inflammation

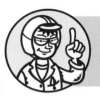

B_{12} deficiency can cause a profound pancytopenia in addition to anaemia

All patients with anaemia should have measurement 'haematinics' [i.e. serum ferritin (storage form of iron and the best non invasive assessment of iron stores)] (Fig. 26.8), vitamin B_{12}, and RBC folate because more than one deficiency can occur at the same time. An algorithm is presented in Fig. 26.9 for the diagnosis of anaemia.

Iron deficiency

- Serum ferritin: low in iron deficiency but raised in iron overload, haemochromatosis and anaemia of chronic disease (occasionally).
- Serum iron: low.
- Total iron-binding capacity: increased.
- Menorrhagia or pregnancy: no further investigations are necessary.
- If no menorrhagia or pregnancy: consider upper gastrointestinal endoscopy, rectal examination,

and sigmoidoscopy with colonoscopy or barium enema. Coeliac disease is a common cause of iron deficiency. Always consider duodenal biopsy at gastroscopy.
- No obvious cause: consider mesenteric angiogram for angiodysplasia.

Vitamin B_{12} deficiency

- Serum vitamin B_{12}: low.
- Bilirubin: mildly raised-intramedullary destruction of abnormal RBCs.
- Lactate dehydrogenase (LDH): elevated-intramedullary destruction of abnormal RBCs.
- Gastric parietal antibodies: positive in 90% of patients with pernicious anaemia.
- Intrinsic factor antibodies: positive in approximately 50% of patients with pernicious anaemia.
- Schilling test (now rare): the patient is given a loading dose of 1000 mg vitamin B_{12} intramuscularly, followed by a small oral dose of radioactive vitamin B_{12}, and excretion is then measured in the urine; vitamin B_{12} malabsorption is corrected by giving intrinsic factor with labelled vitamin in pernicious anaemia, but persists despite the use of intrinsic factor in intestinal disease.
- Endoscopy or barium meal and follow through: may be necessary in underlying intestinal disease.

Folate deficiency

- RBC folate: more reliable than serum folate.
- Bilirubin: mildly raised intramedullary destruction of abnormal RBCs.

Interpretation of iron storage results				
	Ferritin	Serum iron	% Of transferrin saturation	Total iron binding capacity
Iron Deficiency Anaemia	−	−	−	+
Anaemia of Chronic Disease	N/+	−	−	−
Thalassaemia	N/+	N/+	N/+	N
Sideroblastic Anaemia	+	+	+	N
Haemochromatosis	+	+	+	−

Fig. 26.8 Interpretation of iron storage results. (N, normal; −, reduced; + increased.)

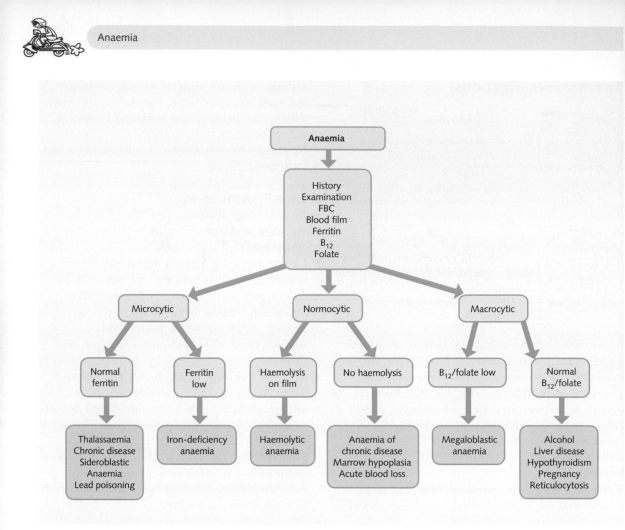

Fig. 26.9 Algorithm for the diagnosis of anaemia. (FBC, full blood count.)

- LDH: elevated intramedullary destruction of abnormal RBCs.
- Tests for intestinal malabsorption: including jejunal biopsy, may be necessary when the diagnosis is not clear.

Haemolysis

- Serum bilirubin: raised and unconjugated.
- Serum haptoglobins: reduced or absent.
- LDH: raised.
- Faecal stercobilinogen: raised.
- Urinary urobilinogen: raised.
- Reticulocyte count: raised.
- Haemoglobin electrophoresis: abnormal in thalassaemia and sickle cell disease.
- Coombs' test/direct antigen test: positive in autoimmune haemolytic anaemias.
- Osmotic fragility: increased if spherocytes are present.

- Enzyme assays: available in specialist centres only for glucose-6-phosphate dehydrogenase and pyruvate kinase deficiencies.
- Ham's test: positive in paroxysmal nocturnal haemoglobinuria. Ham's test is an examination favourite but increasingly rare in clinical practice.

Anaemia of chronic disease

- Ferritin: high (ferritin is an acute phase protein).
- Serum iron: low.
- Total iron-binding capacity: low.
- Serum vitamin B_{12}: normal.
- RBC folate: normal.

The clinical scenario should direct other investigations. Consider erythrocyte sedimentation rate, C-reactive protein, autoantibody screen, sepsis screen, and search for occult malignancy.

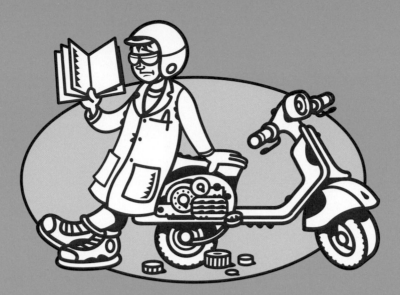

DISEASES AND DISORDERS

27. **Cardiovascular system**   157

28. **Respiratory Disease**   195

29. **Gastrointestinal and Liver Disease**   221

30. **Genitourinary System**   245

31. **Central Nervous System**   261

32. **Metabolic and Endocrine Disorders**   283

33. **Musculoskeletal and Skin Disorders**   315

34. **Haematological Disorders**   333

35. **Infectious Diseases**   355

36. **Drug Overdose**   363

27. Cardiovascular System

Ischaemic heart disease

Ischaemic heart disease (IHD) is the result of an imbalance between myocardial oxygen supply and demand. The term covers a group of clinical syndromes, including chronic angina pectoris; the acute coronary syndromes: both non-ST segment elevation myocardial infarction (NSTEMI) and ST segment elevation myocardial infarction (STEMI); and sudden death. The commonest underlying pathology is atherosclerosis of the coronary arteries. More rarely, IHD can result from coronary artery spasm, emboli, coronary ostial stenosis, aortic stenosis, hypertrophic obstructive cardiomyopathy, arrhythmias causing decreased coronary perfusion pressures, and anaemia.

Ischaemia also occurring with normal coronary arteries is termed syndrome X. It is thought to be due to abnormalities of small coronary vessels resulting in a reduction of coronary flow reserve.

The incidence of IHD shows large geographical variations, ranging from a mortality rate below 100 in 100 000 in Japan to 600 in 100 000 in Finland and Northern Ireland. The incidence is declining in Western Europe. In England and Wales, 1 in 6 men aged 40–44 years have some evidence of IHD; at 55–59 years, this rises to 1 in 3, showing the increase in prevalence with age.

Risk factors for ischaemic heart disease

A number of predictors have been found to be associated with an increased likelihood of developing IHD, and are called risk factors (Fig. 27.1).

The complete list of possible risk factors for IHD is extremely long and includes environmental factors as well as personal characteristics. Not all these factors will ultimately be shown to be truly causal. For example, obesity may act as a risk factor because it is associated with raised serum cholesterol, hypertension, and decreased glucose tolerance.

Age

Mortality from IHD rises steeply with increasing age. This may be due to the cumulative effects of raised serum cholesterol, hypertension, cigarette smoking, and other factors over time.

Major risk factors for coronary artery disease	
Type	**Risk factors**
Fixed	Age Male sex Positive family history Race
Modifiable	Cigarette smoking Hyperlipidaemia Hypertension Diabetes mellitus Left ventricular hypertrophy

Fig. 27.1 Major risk factors for coronary artery disease.

Sex

The rate in young men is about six times higher than in women of the same age, although this difference diminishes with increasing age. Premenopausal women are thought to be protected by their hormonal status, and this protection diminishes progressively during and after the menopause such that the ratio of IHD in men and women aged 70 years is equal.

Family history

The effect of family history appears to be independent of other major risk factors if first-degree relatives below the age of 50 years are affected. Although high levels of serum total cholesterol may cluster in families, only a very small proportion of these are associated with the genetic condition 'familial hypercholesterolaemia'.

Cigarette smoking

The risk of developing coronary artery disease is directly proportional to the number of cigarettes smoked. The rate of IHD in current smokers is about three times that of those who have never smoked. Giving up smoking leads to an initial rapid decrease in the risk of developing IHD followed by a more gradual decline in risk, so that the risk of IHD is almost the same as a non-smoker after approximately 10 years.

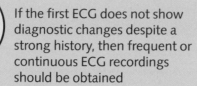

If the first ECG does not show diagnostic changes despite a strong history, then frequent or continuous ECG recordings should be obtained

Blood lipids

The risk of IHD increases as serum total cholesterol and low density lipoprotein (LDL) cholesterol increases. High density lipoprotein (HDL) cholesterol is 'protective' for IHD, and the risk of IHD decreases as HDL increases. Triglycerides are also positively related to IHD risk, although, when the relationship of IHD to other blood lipids is taken into account, the independent contribution of triglycerides to IHD may be small.

Hypertension

Both systolic and diastolic hypertension is associated with the risk of developing IHD, as well as hypertensive heart disease, stroke, and renal failure. Treatment of hypertension with drugs reduces the incidence of cardiac events by approximately 16% overall, with a greater benefit obtained in the elderly.

Diabetes mellitus

In countries where IHD is prevalent, diabetes mellitus (DM) is associated with an approximately two-fold increase in the risk of a major IHD event.

Race

The prevalence of IHD in British Asians is high compared with their family members remaining in the Indian subcontinent. The explanation is only partly accounted for by a low HDL cholesterol and a higher prevalence of DM and glucose intolerance.

Weight

Overweight individuals have twice the risk of a major IHD event. This is probably mediated through increased blood pressure levels, total cholesterol, insulin resistance, and with decreased HDL and physical activity.

Obstructive sleep apnoea

Although associated with obesity and hypertension, obstructive sleep apnoea appears to have an independent association with cardiovascular and cerebrovascular disease.

Novel risk factors

In recent years, newer risk factors have been suggested, these include elevated C-reactive protein (CRP) and hyperfibrinogenaemia plus hyperhomocysteinaemia. Whether these are truly independent risk factors or markers of underlying inflammation should become clear from further studies.

Psychosocial factors

Although stress and other strong emotional responses can precipitate major IHD events in individuals with severe atherosclerosis, it remains to be shown whether stress plays a role in the pathogenesis of coronary artery disease in the absence of other standard risk factors.

Combining risk factors is a more accurate way of predicting those at risk from IHD than relying on any one individual risk factor. Many models and scoring systems have been devised incorporating the different risk factors so that those at high risk may be targeted for preventative treatment. The commonly used Sheffield risk tables can be found at the back of the British National Formulary (See Fig. 32.4). This should be accompanied by population-based measures to reduce the risk of IHD.

Pathology

Atherosclerosis is a slowly progressive focal proliferation of connective tissue within the arterial intima, which begins early in life. It is linked to high lipid level. LDL is the main atherogenic lipid, although the principal constituent of atherosclerotic plaques is collagen synthesised by smooth muscle cells.

The initial process consists of endothelial dysfunction in association with a high circulating cholesterol, inflammation and shear forces. Macrophages enter the arterial wall between endothelial cells, taking up lipids and forming 'foam cells'. The accumulation of lipid-laden macrophages in the subendothelial zone leads to the formation of fatty streaks. Toxic products released from the macrophages lead to the adhesion of platelets and result in smooth muscle cell proliferation and thrombus formation. This then becomes organised, leading to the development of an atherosclerotic plaque surrounded by a fibrotic cap. Progressive enlargement of these lesions leads to segmental narrowing of the lumen, which, when sufficient to be flow-limiting on exercise, causes stable exertion-associated angina. Atherosclerotic plaques are liable to rupture resulting in sudden thrombosis, which is responsible for acute coronary syndromes. Factors associated with plaque disruption and consequent thrombosis include a large lipid core, a high monocyte density, and low smooth muscle cell density.

The association of high levels of CRP and other inflammatory markers with IHD has led many to suggest that atherosclerosis may be an inflammatory process. Various pathogens have been advanced including *Helicobacter pylori* and *Chlamydia pneumoniae* though this remains speculative.

Investigations

Electrocardiogram

A normal electrocardiogram (ECG) does not exclude a diagnosis of angina. During attacks, there may be ST segment depression or symmetrical T wave inversion. T wave inversion in leads V_{1-3} often indicates left anterior descending coronary artery stenosis. The ECG may show signs of an old MI or left ventricular hypertrophy.

Exercise electrocardiogram

In ischaemic heart disease the exercise ECG is an indicator of exercise performance and is an independent indicator of prognosis. It is contraindicated in acute coronary syndromes, severe aortic stenosis, severe pulmonary hypertension, and significant rhythm disturbances. The test is usually regarded as positive if there is more than 1 mm of downsloping ST segment depression after the J point (the junction of the ST segment and the T wave). If the pretest probability of angina is high, the number of false positives is low. Causes of false positive tests include hyperventilation, digoxin, hypokalaemia, hypertension, valvular heart disease, left ventricular hypertrophy and pre-excitation syndromes. The test should be terminated if there is more than 3 mm of ST depression, a fall in blood pressure, ventricular tachycardia, pallor, indicating peripheral circulatory collapse or if the end point is reached.

Echocardiography

This can be used to assess ventricular function and localise areas of ventricular wall involvement. In patients with angina but no evidence of infarction, the echocardiogram may be normal. With diffuse ischaemic changes, left ventricular function may be globally impaired. Exercise or pharmacological stress echocardiography may be used to detect areas of 'hibernating' myocardium. These are areas that show reduced function with exercise, due to decreased blood flow secondary to decreased coronary flow reserve, but which show improved function at rest. They indicate areas that may improve with revascularisation procedures.

Nuclear imaging

This technique may be used to assess myocardial structure and function. A radioactive isotope (e.g. thallium) is injected during exercise and an image is taken soon after. The isotope is taken up by healthy myocardium whereas areas of infarction show up as 'cold spots'. If exercise is not feasible, pharmacological stress can be induced with agents such as adenosine.

Repeat images are taken at rest to obtain a redistribution image. The disappearance of the cold spot implies ischaemia provoked by exertion and reversed by rest; a fixed cold spot indicates infarction. It is a useful technique when the exercise test is equivocal or contraindicated, or to indicate the clinical significance of angiographically equivocal stenoses.

Coronary angiography

This is a technique for visualising the coronary arteries radiographically, measuring intracardiac pressures, blood oxygen saturation in different cardiac chambers, and cardiac output. The test is usually used to determine the exact coronary anatomy and is used to decide on further management (i.e. medical therapy, coronary angioplasty, or coronary artery bypass surgery). In stable angina, it is usually reserved for patients with:

- Angina resistant to optimal medical treatment.
- Strongly positive exercise tests indicating a poor prognosis.
- Evidence of reversible ischaemia on stress testing with reduced left venticular function.
- After confirmed troponin positive acute coronary events especially if pain continues.

More rarely, coronary angiography is used as a diagnostic test when other non-invasive tests have not been helpful and symptoms persist.

The mortality from the procedure is approximately 1 in 1000. Complications include:
- Haemorrhage and haematoma at the site of arterial puncture.
- Emboli into arteries resulting in coronary or peripheral ischaemia.
- Stroke.
- Arrhythmias.
- Coronary artery dissection.

Treatment of ischaemic heart disease

Chronic stable angina provides considerable morbidity for patients and a high workload for health services. Similar to all chronic disease, the optimal management comprises patient education, lifestyle change and medication. Non-coronary causes for angina should be sought and treated (e.g. valvular heart disease and anaemia).

General measures

Risk factors should be sought and addressed. Weight loss, smoking cessation, exercise within the capacity of the patient and healthy diet should all be encouraged. Exercise may improve the collateral circulation in the heart in the same way as in peripheral vascular disease. Factors precipitating angina (e.g. cold weather or extremes of emotion) should be avoided. All patients should be provided with a sublingual nitrate, either spray or tablet, for relief of acute attacks or prophylactic use before exercise.

Drugs

Antiplatelet drugs

All patients should be prescribed aspirin 75 mg daily as this lowers the incidence of subsequent MI and death. There is a risk of gastrointestinal bleeding so patients should be given advice to take the aspirin with food and made aware of warning signs such as melaena; if a history of previous bleeding is present, a proton pump inhibitor can be added. If aspirin is contraindicated then clopidogrel, an inhibitor of platelet aggregation, is an alternative, although its proven use is in NSTEMI and post-angioplasty.

β-Blockers

These act by reducing sympathetic tone, depressing myocardial contractility (negatively inotropic), and reducing the heart rate (negatively chronotropic). In addition to these effects (which reduce the oxygen demand), β-blockers may also increase the perfusion of the ischaemic area because the decrease in heart rate increases the duration of diastole and hence the time available for coronary blood flow.

Typical β-blockers include atenolol, bisoprolol and metoprolol. Relative contraindications include asthma, peripheral vascular disease with skin ulceration. They are contraindicated in second and third degree heart block.

Of all antianginal drugs, β-blockers improve survival post myocardial infarction and so should be first line. It was formerly taught that β-blockers were contraindicated in heart failure. It remains true that they are not appropriate in acute or overt heart failure but they have proven beneficial in chronic heart failure adding further importance to their use.

Nitrates

Nitrates cause peripheral vasodilatation, especially in the veins. This reduces venous return and ventricular preload is decreased. Reduction in the distension of the heart wall decreases oxygen demand resulting in relief of angina. Nitrates work by conversion to nitric oxide, which results in an increase in intracellular cyclic GMP in smooth muscle. This stimulates calcium binding processes and the free calcium available to trigger muscle contraction is reduced.

Short-acting nitrates are the mainstay of relief of acute angina and, when combined with rest, they relieve the pain in minutes. If it continues, then this should be a warning sign to patients. Longer-acting nitrates are more stable and can be effective for several hours. Isosorbide dinitrate (ISDN) is rapidly metabolised by the liver to mononitrate, which is the main active metabolite. Isosorbide mononitrate (ISMN) may avoid the variable absorption and unpredictable first-pass metabolism of the dinitrate.

Adverse effects are normally due to arterial dilatation and include headaches, flushing, hypotension, and rarely fainting. Patients may become tolerant to nitrates, reducing their effectiveness. Nitrate 'holidays' are the traditional way of minimising the problem although newer once-daily preparations reduce this effect.

Calcium channel blockers

Calcium antagonists inhibit the influx of calcium into the myocyte during the action potential and relax peripheral vascular smooth muscle. They reduce angina by a combination of reduced afterload and hence myocardial oxygen demand plus reduced heart rate and increased coronary vasodilation. They are especially useful if there is a degree of coronary artery spasm. Dihydropyridines such as nifedipine can cause reflex tachycardia secondary to peripheral vasodilatation and therefore may be combined with a β-blocker. Diltiazem has slight negative inotropic and chronotropic effects, and the patient should be monitored if on β-blockers for the development of bradycardias. Verapamil is the drug of choice for supraventricular tachycardias if β-blockers are contraindicated. All calcium channel blocking drugs are negatively inotropic to some degree and, although amlodipine has demonstrated its safety in heart failure, extreme care should be taken with prescribing any of them to patients with impaired left ventricular function.

Side effects include headache, flushing, dizziness, constipation and gravitational oedema.

Potassium channel activators

This is a new class of drug with arterial and venous vasodilating properties. It may be useful in patients refractory to treatment with other antianginal agents. The only licensed drug at present is nicorandil.

Statins

Statins (HMG CoA reductase inhibitors) are the mainstay of lipid lowering therapy. The current maxim is the 'lower the better'. Statins may also help to stabilise atherosclerotic plaques and reduce the frequency of acute cardiac events and as such most patients with IHD should be on a statin even if their cholesterol is within the normal range.

Angioplasty and stenting

Coronary artery stenoses can be dilated using a balloon after plaque visualisation at angiography. This improves blood flow. The best results in terms of patency and flow are achieved with stent insertion. It is a very safe procedure and is now preferred to surgery in most cases. Use of clopidogrel and IIb/IIIa receptor antagonists has further reduced stent restenosis. Drug eluting stents (e.g. with sirolimus) may further enhance this. Patients need only stay in hospital overnight and return to activity quickly compared to surgery.

Surgical management

Coronary artery bypass graft (CABG) surgery should be considered in patients who have angina despite optimal medical therapy and are not suitable for or have failed angioplasty. It has a low mortality in otherwise well patients (2%). Bypass using one or both of the internal mammary arteries is preferred to the traditional vein graft. They result in better patency, flow and graft survival. Certain patient groups are better served by surgery rather than stents (Fig. 27.2). Post-operatively the number and dose of antianginal drugs can be reduced.

Acute coronary syndromes

The terminology used to classify acute cardiac ischaemic events has changed in the last few years. Subendocardial and non Q wave myocardial infarctions are now termed non ST segment elevation myocardial infarction (NSTEMI). Acute myocardial infarction with ST elevation is hence a

Patient factors associated with reduction in mortality with surgery
• Left main stem stenosis
• Triple vessel coronary artery disease
• Two vessel disease with proximal LAD disease
• Benefit is greater in those with left ventricular impairment

Fig. 27.2 Factors associated with reduction in mortality with coronary artery bypass surgery compared to medical management of patients with coronary artery disease. (LAD, left anterior descending coronary artery.)

STEMI. This reflects that the key to appropriate treatment is the presence or absence of ST elevation because there are good evidence-based guidelines for their different management. When combined with unstable angina, all three are the 'acute coronary syndromes'.

Non ST segment elevation myocardial infarction

Symptoms

The patient may have characteristic central ischaemic chest pain (see Chapter 1) or more non specific symptoms. Patients with chronic stable angina may note that their pain is no longer relieved fully by GTN, that it is increasing in intensity or that it is occurring at rest. These are all symptoms requiring urgent assessment. As approximately one-third of referrals to general medicine are for chest pain, many hospitals in the UK are now developing chest pain assessment units allowing more rapid and effective assessment, monitoring and discharge.

Diagnosis

As well as symptoms, the other important assessment is the ECG. It may show ST segment depression, T wave flattening, biphasic changes or inversion. The deeper the changes, the more worrying. The initial ECG may be normal and serial ones are needed, preferably when pain occurs, to demonstrate the dynamic ischaemia.

Management
Emergency

Adequate analgesia and oxygen are vital. They alleviate the patient's distress and help reduce stress on the heart. Nitrates either sublingually or as an infusion relieve pain and offload the heart and should be started unless a low blood pressure prevents this.

Opiates may be needed if nitrates are not fully effective.

Drugs

Aspirin   Aspirin (300 mg) should be given straight away and is often administered by paramedics. It should be continued daily at 75 mg.

Clopidogrel   This is a novel antiplatelet agent that has demonstrated significant improved outcomes in combination with aspirin in patients with NSTEMI. It should also be used if aspirin is contraindicated. The first dose is 300 mg and subsequently 75 mg daily.

Heparin   Heparin should be given until pain free for 48 hours. It can be as a continuous i.v. infusion of unfractionated heparin or twice daily low molecular weight heparin (LMWH) for easier administration. Most hospitals use enoxaparin as it may be beneficial over conventional heparin. However, this is still the subject of debate.

These three medications are aimed at moderating thrombosis and preventing occlusion of the artery and subsequent STEMI. They have proven very effective. They are associated with an increased risk of bleeding.

β-Blockers   Unless contraindicated (e.g. overt heart failure or known marked LV dysfunction), β-blockers should be started. They have immediate antianginal effects and reduce the progression to acute STEMI, reduce arrhythmias and improve survival. Examples include metoprolol, atenolol and carvedilol.

Diltiazem   This is an anti-anginal drug which has negatively chronotropic effects. If β-blockers are contraindicated, then it is an alternative agent.

Statins   Statins should be started on admission regardless of cholesterol levels as they may improve outcomes by anti-inflammatory plaque stabilising effects.

Angiotensin-converting enzyme (ACE) inhibitors ACE inhibition should start early in patients with NSTEMI. It is reasonable to start at a low dose and wait 12 hours until the acute event has settled as hypotension is a risk.

Glycoprotein IIb/IIIa receptor antagonists These are potent antiplatelet agents which block the binding of fibrinogen to the IIb/IIIa receptor on the platelet surface. They are started if the pain continues or ECG changes progress. They may settle the acute events on their own but are usually part of a strategy including cardiac catheterisation. The most common are tirofiban or eptifibatide. They have a significant risk of causing bleeding which should be assessed.

Over 90% of patients with NSTEMI will become pain free and respond well to the above treatments. If pain continues, complications such as cardiogenic shock and/or the ECG changes progress then additional therapy is needed and the patient should be transferred to a centre with interventional cardiology support.

Place of thrombolysis or angioplasty

Thrombolysis is not indicated in patients without STEMI or new left bundle branch block because it has no demonstrated benefit. Angiography and angioplasty is the best option in ongoing NSTEMI. In patients who have responded well to therapy and undergone confirmed NSTEMI, the place of early or more conservative interventional strategies is debated by cardiologists.

Troponin

The measurement of troponin I or T concentrations at 8–12 hours after the onset of pain is crucial. As well as being a highly specific marker of myocardial damage, it has shown prognostic value. Therefore, patients with non-evolving ECGs, who are pain free and with a negative troponin result can be safely discharged and have an exercise test and cardiovascular risk stratification as an outpatient. Patients with positive troponin NSTEMI events are at high risk for further events and they should be evaluated for revascularisation procedures as an inpatient.

Prevention

In patients with proven NSTEMI the mortality at 1 year is up to 20%. All patients should have their cardiovascular risks assessed and modified. Long term antiplatelet medications, statins, beta-blockers and ACE inhibitors should be prescribed unless contraindicated. The need for angioplasty or bypass surgery should be considered with stress testing or angiography.

Acute myocardial infarction (STEMI)

Myocardial infarction affects 5 in 1000 of the general population per year in the UK and is the most common cause of mortality in the Western world. Ninety per cent of transmural MIs are caused by an

Fig. 27.3 Changes induced by acute myocardial infarction.

Changes induced by acute myocardial infarction		
Time after onset of symptoms	**Macroscopic changes**	**Microscopic changes**
Up to 18 hours	None	None
24–48 hours	Pale oedematous muscle	Oedema, acute inflammatory cell infiltration, necrosis of myocytes
3–4 days	Yellow rubbery centre with haemorrhagic border	Obvious necrosis and inflammation, early granulation tissue
3–6 weeks	Silvery scar becoming rough and white	Dense fibrosis

occlusive intracoronary thrombus overlying an ulcerated or fissured stenotic plaque. Underlying most cases, there is a dynamic interaction between severe coronary atherosclerosis, an acute atheromatous plaque change, superimposed thrombosis, platelet activation, and vasospasm. The microscopic changes of acute MI follow a predictable sequence (Fig. 27.3).

The overall fatality from acute MI has improved markedly in the last 20 years with better medical care, the development of coronary care units and the recognition of the importance of opening the occluded artery to reperfuse the damaged myocardium and limit infarct size. This is so important that the 'door to needle' time is used to assess quality of acute cardiac care.

Adverse risk factors in patients admitted to hospital with acute MI are:
- Older age.
- Previous medical history (diabetes, previous MI).
- Indicators of a large infarct size, including the site of infarction (anterior versus inferior).
- Low initial blood pressure.
- The presence of pulmonary congestion.
- The extent of ischaemia as expressed by ST elevation with or without depression on the ECG.

Diagnosis

The diagnosis of acute MI is based on two or three out of: the history (see p. 3), ECG changes, and enzyme changes.

Cardiac enzymes

Cardiac enzymes are intracellular enzymes which leak out of infarcted myocardium into the bloodstream (Fig. 27.4):

- Creatine kinase (CK) peaks within 24 hours. It is a cardiac enzyme that is also produced by skeletal muscle and brain. In cases of doubt, the myocardial-bound isoenzyme fraction of CK (i.e. CKMB) can be requested, which is specific for heart muscle damage. The site of the infarct is related to the serum level of enzyme.

Aspartate aminotransferase and lactate dehydrogenase were formerly used to assess MI as they remain elevated for several days after CK has settled. They are now largely obsolete.

- Elevated troponin I or T concentrations in the blood are highly reliable markers of myocardial damage. They are not 'enzymes' but proteins involved in myocyte contraction. They are most

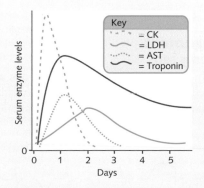

Fig. 27.4 The pattern of serum enzymes after acute myocardial infarction. (AST, aspartate aminotransferase; CK, creatinine kinase; LDH, lactate dehydrogenase.)

163

reliable 8–12 hours post event and remain elevated for several weeks. CK is therefore still used to assess reinfarction in patients whose troponin is elevated from a previous MI.

Electrocardiogram

The earliest ECG changes or 'hyperacute' changes consist of tall, pointed T waves, followed by elevation of the ST segment. This is followed by T wave inversion, the R wave voltage decreases, and Q waves develop. After weeks or months, the T wave may become upright again but the Q waves remain (Fig. 27.5).

The site of the infarction may also be deduced from the affected leads on the ECG.

- Inferior MI involves leads II, III, and aVF.
- Anterior MI: affects the precordial leads.
- Anteroseptal MI: affects leads V_{1-3}.
- Lateral MI: affects leads I and aVL and V_{4-6}.
- Posterior MI; there is a tall R wave in leads V_1 and V_2 with ST segment depression and upright T waves.

There may also be 'reciprocal' ECG changes with ST segment depression in leads opposite to the site of infarction.

The development of new onset left bundle branch block is an indicator of acute MI and if coupled with pain is an indication for thrombolysis. However, it is a common abnormality and old ECGs are invaluable.

Other investigations to help with management include:

- A full blood count (FBC): anaemia.
- Urea and electrolytes (U&Es): renal and electrolyte abnormalities.
- Chest X-ray (CXR): aortic dissection, signs of heart failure and to assess cardiac size.
- Blood glucose.

Management
Emergency care

The main aims are to prevent or treat cardiac arrest, and to relieve pain–the patient should ideally be managed on a coronary care unit with continuous

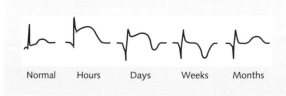

Normal   Hours   Days   Weeks   Months

Fig. 27.5 Progressive electrocardiogram changes in myocardial infarction.

cardiac monitoring and an intravenous cannula should be inserted for emergency medicines. Sublingual nitrates, intravenous nitrate and opiates such as diamorphine are given for pain relief. This relieves pain not only for humane reasons, but also alleviates sympathetic activation associated with the pain which causes vasoconstriction and increases the work of the heart.

Side effects include nausea and vomiting, hypotension with bradycardia, and respiratory depression. Antiemetics should be administered with opiates. If respiratory depression occurs, intravenous naloxone, which is a specific opioid antagonist, is given. High-dose oxygen should be given via a face-mask or nasal cannula, especially to those who are breathless or who have any features of heart failure or shock.

Anxiety is a natural response to the pain and to the circumstances surrounding a heart attack. Reassurance of patients and those closely associated with them is therefore of great importance.

Early care

The aims are to initiate reperfusion therapy, limit infarct size, prevent infarct extension, and to treat life-threatening arrhythmias.

Thrombolytic treatment

Within 12 hours of the onset of pain, treatment with thrombolysis should be given for patients with ST elevation or new left bundle branch block. This prevents death and the earlier it is given the greater the benefit. Administration within 30 minutes of arrival in hospital should be possible in most patients with clear MI. The improvement from aspirin is additive so that more lives are saved than either therapy alone.

The largest benefit is seen for those at highest risk; these include:

- The elderly.
- Those with presenting systolic blood pressure of below 100 mmHg.
- Those with anterior infarction.
- Those treated soonest after the onset symptoms.

Contraindications to thrombolytic therapy are given in Fig. 27.6. Major bleeding complications are seen in approximately 1–3% of patients.

The two main thrombolytics are streptokinase and recombinant tissue plasminogen activator (tPA). Streptokinase induces an antibody response which reduces the effectiveness of a repeat dose and

Contraindications to thrombolytic therapy	
Contraindications	Stroke
	Major surgery, trauma, or head injury within 3 weeks
	Gastrointestinal bleed within the last week
	Known bleeding disorder
	Dissecting aneurysm
Relative contraindications	Transient ischaemic attack in the preceding 6 months
	Warfarin therapy
	Pregnancy
	Non-compressible punctures
	Traumatic resuscitation
	Refractory hypertension (SBP >180 mmHg)
	Recent retinal laser treatment

Fig. 27.6 Contraindications to thrombolytic therapy. (SBP, systolic blood pressure.)

increases the risk of an anaphylactic reaction. It should therefore not be readministered in the period between 5 days and a minimum of 2 years following initial treatment. tPA may have benefits in patients with anterior MI or those with hypotension. It is also used when streptokinase is contraindicated. Frequently used thrombolytic regimens are given in Fig. 27.7.

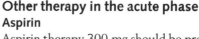

Remember the causes of pericarditis by the mnemonic CARDIAC RIND: **C**ollagen vascular disease, **A**ortic aneurysm, **R**adiation, **D**rugs, **I**nfections, **A**cute renal failure, **C**ardiac infarction, **R**heumatic fever, **I**njury, **N**eoplasms, and **D**ressler's syndrome

Primary angioplasty

If facilities exist and can be accessed rapidly then it is thought that immediate primary angioplasty and stenting leads to better immediate and long-term outcomes in acute STEMI than thrombolysis. This is not possible in many parts of the UK and thrombolysis is used. It is also appropriate if contraindications to thrombolysis are present.

Other therapy in the acute phase
Aspirin

Aspirin therapy 300 mg should be prescribed early. This leads to a 30% reduction in deaths or 24 lives saved in 1000 treated. If aspirin sensitivity is present then clopidogrel should be used.

β-Blockers

The intravenous administration of β-blockers in the acute phase potentially limits infarct size, reduces the risk of fatal arrhythmias, and relieves pain. There is a 15% reduction in mortality at 1 week. It is

Frequently used thrombolytic drugs	
Drug	**Comment**
Streptokinase	Cheapest. Often first line in inferior MI. Can result in hypotension and allergic reaction. Usually only given once
Alteplase (tPA)	Less hypotension. Better than streptokinase for anterior MI. Requires heparin infusion for 48 hours post administration
Tenecteplase	Given as a bolus injection so can reduce 'door to needle' times

Fig. 27.7 Frequently used thrombolytic regimens.

particularly appropriate when the patient has a tachycardia (in the absence of heart failure), relative hypertension, or pain unresponsive to opioids. If the intravenous formulation is not available, start oral therapy.

Angiotensin-converting enzyme inhibitors

All patients should be commenced on ACE inhibitors if tolerated as they produce survival benefit. ACE inhibitors are of most value in patients with clinical symptoms or signs of heart failure, or impaired left ventricular function echocardiographically. Opinions differ as to the best time to initiate treatment – whether acutely or after a few days. The benefits appear to be a class effect, and doses should be titrated to the target dose.

Statins

Statin therapy should be started immediately as per management of NSTEMI.

Heparin

Heparin forms part of most thrombolytic regimes. Once these are completed, then heparin prophylaxis until mobile should be given.

Control of blood glucose

Improved outcome after MI has been shown if the blood glucose is tightly controlled using an insulin sliding scale. This should be commenced even if the patient is not a known diabetic as blood glucose is often raised with a variety of physical stressors.

Complications of myocardial infarction

A summary of the complications that may occur in MI is given in Fig. 27.8.

Cardiac failure and shock

Left ventricular failure (LVF) during the acute phase of MI is associated with a poor prognosis. Repeated examination of the heart and lungs for signs of incipient heart failure should be performed on all patients (Fig. 27.9).

Chest X-rays and echocardiography for assessing ventricular function, mitral regurgitation, and ventricular septal defects may be of help.

The management of heart failure is described on pp 176. Cardiogenic shock is defined as a systolic blood pressure less than 90 mmHg in association

Complications of myocardial infarction		
Complication	**Interval**	**Mechanism**
Sudden death	Usually within hours	Often ventricular fibrillation
Arrhythmias	First few days	–
Persistent pain	12 hours to a few days	Progressive myocardial necrosis (extension of MI)
Angina	Immediate or delayed (weeks)	Ischaemia of non-infarcted muscle
Cardiac failure	Variable	Ventricular dysfunction following muscle necrosis; arrhythmias
Mitral incompetence	First few days	Papillary muscle dysfunction, necrosis or rupture
Pericarditis	2–4 days	Transmural infarct with inflammation of the pericardium
Cardiac rupture and ventricular septal defects	3–5 days	Weakening of wall following muscle necrosis and acute inflammation
Mural thrombus	One week or more	Abnormal endothelial surface following infarction
Ventricular aneurysm	4 weeks or more	Stretching of newly formed collagenous scar tissue
Dressler's syndrome	Weeks to months	Autoimmune
Pulmonary emboli	1 week or more	Deep venous thrombosis in lower limbs
Late ventricular arrhythmias	–	–

Fig. 27.8 Complications of myocardial infarction.

The Killip classification	
Class	Features
1	No crepitations or third heart sound
2	Crepitations over less than 50% of lung fields or third heart sound
3	Crepitations over 50% of the lung fields
4	Shock

Fig. 27.9 The Killip classification for the assessment of heart failure.

with signs of circulatory deterioration expressed as peripheral vasoconstriction, low urinary output (<0.5 ml/kg/hour), and mental confusion.

Other causes of hypotension should be excluded such as hypovolaemia, vasovagal reactions, electrolyte disturbance, drugs, or arrhythmias. Ventricular and valvular function should be evaluated by echocardiography, and a pulmonary artery catheter may be used though their value is much debated in critical care. Inotropic agents are of value, dobutamine (5–20 μg/kg/min) is first line. Correction of acidosis is important for myocardial function though usually improves if cardiac output improves as it is usually a lactic acidosis.

Emergency angiography and angioplasty or surgery should be considered.

Cardiac rupture and mitral regurgitation
Free wall rupture, if acute, is usually fatal within minutes. If subacute, there is haemodynamic deterioration with hypotension and signs of cardiac tamponade. Immediate surgery is needed.

Ventricular septal defect (VSD) occurs in 1% of all infarctions, appearing early after MI. Without surgery, the mortality is 50% within the first week and 90% within the first year. It should be suspected if there is clinical deterioration and a loud pansystolic murmur at the left sternal edge. Treatment is by surgical closure of the defect and bypass grafts as necessary.

Mitral regurgitation
The incidence of moderately severe or severe mitral regurgitation is approximately 4% and the mortality without surgery is high at approximately 20%. Valve replacement is the procedure of choice in papillary muscle dysfunction and rupture.

Arrhythmias and conduction disturbances
These are extremely common in the early period following MI. Often, the arrhythmias are not hazardous in themselves but are a manifestation of a serious underlying disorder such as continuing ischaemia, vagal overactivity, or electrolyte disturbance that requires attention. Arrhythmias are also discussed on pp. 169.

Ventricular arrhythmias
Ventricular arrhythmias may present as ventricular ectopics, ventricular tachycardia (VT), or ventricular fibrillation.

Ventricular ectopics are almost universal on the first day and require no treatment if the patient is asymptomatic.

Short episodes of VT may be well tolerated and require no treatment. More prolonged episodes may cause hypotension and heart failure. Amiodarone or lidocaine are the drugs of choice. Direct current (DC) cardioversion may be required if haemodynamically significant VT persists.

If ventricular fibrillation occurs, immediate defibrillation should be performed.

Supraventricular arrhythmias
Atrial fibrillation complicates 15–20% of MIs and is often associated with severe left ventricular damage and heart failure; it is usually self-limiting. If the heart rate is fast, digoxin is effective in slowing the rate, but amiodarone may be more efficacious in terminating the arrhythmia.

Other supraventricular arrhythmias are rare but are also usually self-limiting. They may respond to carotid sinus massage. β-Blockers may be effective and DC shock should be employed if the arrhythmia is poorly tolerated.

Sinus bradycardia and heart block
Sinus bradycardia is common early on, especially in inferior MI, and emergently responds to atropine in boluses titrated against response. The administration of unnecessarily large doses of atropine should be avoided.

Atrioventricular (AV) block is common in inferior MI as the right coronary artery supplies the AV node and may respond to atropine, though many patients will need a permanent pacemaker. However, it may take up to 14 days before normal conduction is restored.

Heart block with anterior MI is ominous because it indicates a large infarct. The development of left bundle branch block or bifasicular block may presage complete heart block and is an indication for temporary pacemaker insertion. If complete heart block does occur and persists, a permanent pacemaker will be needed.

Subsequent inpatient management
General
Patients should be on bed rest for the first 24 hours. If uncomplicated, the patient can then sit out of bed, use a commode, and undertake self-care and self-feeding. Ambulation can be started the next day and the exercise is gradually built up to climbing stairs within a few days.

Deep venous thrombosis and pulmonary embolism
Deep venous thrombosis (DVT) and pulmonary embolism may be prevented by subcutaneous heparin when in bed. If they do occur, the patient should be treated initially with heparin, followed by oral anticoagulation. Patients are usually started on subcutaneous heparin or a low molecular weight heparin after admission to the coronary care unit.

Intraventricular thrombus and systemic emboli
This may be confirmed on echocardiography and treated with intravenous heparin followed by oral anticoagulation.

Pericarditis
This can occur within the first few days, causing pain that is sharp in nature and varies with posture and respiration. The diagnosis can be confirmed by a pericardial rub. If troublesome, it may be treated with high-dose aspirin, non-steroidal anti-inflammatory drugs (NSAIDs), or steroids. Dresslers's syndrome is fever, leucocytosis, pericarditis and serositis occurring up to 3 months after MI due to an autoimmune response to the damaged myocardium. Treatment is as for pericarditis.

Late ventricular arrhythmias
When arrhythmias occur late in the course of MI, they are liable to recur and are associated with a high risk of death. If it is probable that the arrhythmia is induced by ischaemia, revascularisation should be considered. If this is unlikely, anti-arrhythmic agents (e.g. β-blockers and amiodarone) and electrophysiologically-guided treatment may be given. In some cases, an implantable defibrillator is indicated.

Rehabilitation
Rehabilitation is aimed at restoring the patient to as full a life as possible, and must take into account physical, physiological, and socio-economic factors. The process should start as soon as possible after hospital admission and should be continued in the succeeding weeks and months. Depression and denial are common. Lifestyle advice should be individualised and include advice on diet, exercise, and smoking cessation.

Secondary prevention
Risk stratification
All patients post MI should undergo echocardiography to assess valve and systolic function. Most patients can safely undergo a limited exercise test after being pain free for 5–7 days. If normal, then they can be followed up in clinic with no further testing. Increased risk of further events and death include:
- Continuing angina.
- Heart failure.
- Positive exercise or pharmacological stress test.

These patients should then have angiography prior to discharge.

Smoking
Observational studies show that those who stop smoking have a mortality in the succeeding years of less than half that of those who continue to smoke. It is potentially the most effective of all the secondary prevention measures. All smokers should be counselled to stop smoking. Nicotine replacement therapy may be of value.

Diet
Weight reduction should be encouraged if overweight. Eating fatty fish rich in omega-3 fatty acids at least twice a week may reduce the risk of reinfarction and death.

Hypertension
The blood pressure should be controlled to 130/85 mmHg if possible.

Fasting glucose and lipids
Assessment for diabetes before discharge is essential as it indicates a worse prognosis. Immediately after MI lipid levels are unreliable and all patients should be on statin therapy. Fasting lipid levels should be part of routine follow up in clinic over subsequent years.

All patients should be discharged on 'the big four' drugs unless contraindicated because all show benefit in secondary prevention.

Antiplatelet treatment

Aspirin 75 mg daily reduces the risk of reinfarction and death by 25%. There is no clear benefit of oral anticoagulation over antiplatelet therapy, although it may be considered for patients with left ventricular aneurysm, atrial fibrillation, or echocardiographically proven left ventricular thrombus.

β-Blockers

β-Blockers reduce the risk of mortality and reinfarction by 20–25%. Approximately 25% of patients have relative contraindications to β-blockers because of uncontrolled heart failure, respiratory disease, or other conditions. Calcium channel blockers such as diltiazem and verapamil may be used if β-blockers are contraindicated.

Angiotensin-converting enzyme inhibitors

Provided there are no contraindications, ACE inhibitors are of benefit to all after MI. However, patients at low risk gain only marginal benefit, and they are often reserved for people with clinical signs of heart failure, low ejection fraction on echocardiography or anterior MI.

Lipid-lowering agents

There are clear benefits from treatment with statins. The risk of subsequent major coronary heart disease events is lowered. All subgroups of patients appear to benefit from treatment.

Arrhythmias

Arrhythmias are usually secondary to IHD, particularly after MI. Ventricular ectopic beats are extremely common in the first 24 hours following an MI, but any arrhythmia including conduction disturbances may occur.

Other causes include drugs, cardiomyopathy, myocarditis, thyroid dysfunction, and electrolyte disturbances.

Clinical features

Arrhythmias may present with palpitations (see Chapter 3), dizziness, angina, shortness of breath (see Chapter 2), syncope, cardiac arrest, or sudden death; they may also be symptomless. The history should focus on symptoms and possible underlying aetiologies.

Investigations

An ECG with a long rhythm strip will allow diagnosis of the arrhythmia, if present at the time of the test. For infrequent symptoms, 24-hour Holter monitoring (with a diary of events) may record the rhythm disturbance. Other routine investigations should include FBC, U&Es, calcium, magnesium, thyroid function tests (TFTs), and a chest radiograph. An echocardiogram should be considered to look for structural cardiac disease.

Finally, electrophysiological studies may reveal an arrhythmogenic focus; radiofrequency ablation can destroy this focus and response to treatment may be assessed, but this is only available in specialised centres.

Supraventricular arrhythmias

Sinus tachycardia

There is usually an underlying cause, which should be treated as required (see also p. 16).

Atrial fibrillation

This is an irregular, chaotic atrial rhythm at a rate of 300–600 b.p.m. It is transmitted to the ventricles via the AV node at different intervals leading to an irregular heart rate, dependent on the speed of conduction and refractoriness down the AV node. The incidence rises with age and is over 10% in the elderly. It may be idiopathic, secondary to chronic heart disease or a response to acute illness. Causes include:

- IHD.
- Mitral valve disease.
- Hyperthyroidism.
- Hypertension.
- Cardiomyopathy.
- Pericarditis.
- Pneumonia.
- Atrial myxoma.
- Endocarditis.
- Infiltrative diseases of the heart (e.g. sarcoidosis).

Clinically, there is an irregularly irregular pulse and the apical rate can be greater than the rate at the radial artery. The first heart sound is of variable intensity.

The ECG shows absent P waves and irregular narrow complex QRS complexes (unless there is associated bundle branch block) (Fig. 27.10).

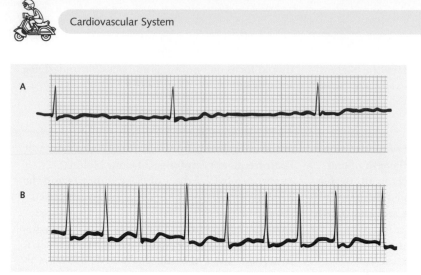

Fig. 27.10 Electrocardiogram of atrial fibrillation with a slow ventricular rate (A), and fast ventricular rate (B).

Treatment

In longstanding AF there is debate as to whether conversion back to sinus rhythm or simple rate control is best. The ventricular rate can usually be controlled with digoxin or a β-blocker. If not, verapamil can be added if left ventricular function is good. Other classes of drugs may sometimes be required. Patients should be anticoagulated to reduce the risk of systemic emboli, especially stroke. If the patient has contraindications to warfarin, aspirin should be used.

If the atrial fibrillation is of recent onset, DC cardioversion or intravenous flecainide to restore sinus rhythm may be attempted. If after more than 2 days, the patient should be 'warfarinised' for at least 1 month before cardioversion. If this is unsuccessful, the aim is control of the ventricular rate.

If the atrial fibrillation is paroxysmal, amiodarone or sotalol may maintain the patient in sinus rhythm.

Atrial flutter

This is due to a regular circus movement of continuous atrial depolarisation. As the AV node cannot conduct that fast, it is usually transmitted with a degree of block.

The causes and treatment are similar to those for atrial fibrillation.

The ECG shows a 'sawtooth' appearance to the baseline at 300 b.p.m. due to flutter or F waves (Fig. 27.11). The ventricular rate is usually divisible into this (e.g. 150 b.p.m. in 2 : 1 block, or 100 b.p.m. in 3 : 1 block).

Paroxysmal supraventricular tachycardias

This is normally due to the presence of a second pathway between the atria and ventricles. An impulse is conducted normally through one AV connection and is then conducted retrogradely up the other, causing a premature atrial contraction. This is then conducted down the first AV connection. On each occasion, the ventricle also depolarises, giving rise to a fast

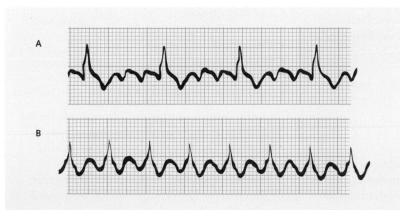

Fig. 27.11 Electrocardiogram of atrial flutter. (A) Atrial flutter with 4:1 block. (B) Atrial flutter with 2:1 block.

ventricular rate. The refractory period for an accessory pathway may be shorter than the AV node, leading to ventricular rates exceeding 200 b.p.m.

Management
Initially, try vagal stimulation, which can be achieved in the following ways:
- Valsalva manoeuvre: ask the patient to blow against resistance (the closed glottis) for approximately 15 seconds, as if straining at stool. The tachycardia usually terminates in the relaxation (parasympathetic) phase.
- Carotid sinus massage: massage of the carotid artery at the level of the thyroid cartilage.
- Diving reflex: the patient holds his breath while the face is wetted with cold water.
- Eye pressure: this should not now be done as it may cause retinal detachment.

 If the heart rate is 150 b.p.m., always consider atrial flutter with 2 : 1 block as the diagnosis

Drug treatment
Intravenous adenosine is the treatment of choice. Digoxin or intravenous β-blockers may also be effective. Intravenous verapamil can be useful for patients without MI or valvular disease. If the arrhythmia is poorly tolerated, synchronised DC shock usually provides rapid relief.

Potassium and magnesium levels should be checked and corrected.

If the patient is already on digoxin, the levels should be checked to exclude toxicity.

Ventricular tachycardia
This is defined as three or more consecutive ventricular extrasystoles with a rate greater than 120 b.p.m. (Fig. 27.12).

Treatment
If there is no pulse or circulatory collapse, then treat with DC shock as per advanced life support algorithms or synchronised DC cardioversion respectively. If conscious, the patient will require an anaesthetic. Electrolyte abnormalities should be corrected. If the patient has a stable blood pressure then response to amiodarone can be assessed in a monitored environment.

Drug treatment is also used for prophylaxis of recurrent attacks. The most common setting is after MI; amiodarone is the preferred therapy for emergency use. Other options include lidocaine or procainamide.

Torsade de pointes ('twisting of the points')
This is a special form of so called 'polymorphic' VT, which tends to occur in the presence of a long QT interval. It may progress to ventricular fibrillation and is often refractory to treatment, which is with intravenous magnesium sulphate. Anti-arrhythmics may further prolong the QT interval and worsen the condition. Overdrive pacing may be effective.

Ventricular fibrillation
This is an emergency and requires immediate advanced life support, DC shock with cardiopulmonary resuscitation (Fig. 27.13).

 Before carotid sinus massage:
- Always check that there are two carotid pulses.
- Never massage both carotids at the same time.
Listen for carotid bruits first—do not massage if one is present because it may cause a cerebral embolus

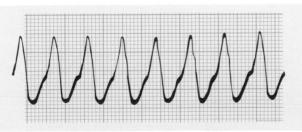

Fig. 27.12 Electrocardiogram of ventricular tachycardia.

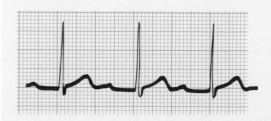

Fig. 27.13 Electrocardiogram of ventricular fibrillation. Coordinated activity of the ventricles ceases. The electrocardiogram shows irregular waves of no defined shape. In this trace there are short periods suggestive of ventricular flutter.

A favourite examination question is how to distinguish VT from SVT with aberrant conduction. The following features suggest VT:
- Fusion or capture beats (these are pathognomonic).
- Different QRS morphology to that in sinus rhythm.
- QRS duration 0.14 seconds with RBBB configuration or 0.16 seconds with LBBB configuration.
- QRS axis: left axis deviation with RBBB morphology, or extreme left axis deviation (northwest axis) with LBBB morphology.
- Concordance in the chest leads (all complexes have similar polarities).

Bradycardias
Sinus bradycardia
For notes on sinus bradycardia, see p. 17.

Sick sinus syndrome
This is due to dysfunction of the sinus node and can lead to periods of sinus bradycardia with periods of asystole, and tachycardia. Dual chamber pacemakers are now fitted as standard though they will only function as an atrial pacemaker if there is no AV conduction defect.

Heart block
This refers to aberrant conduction through the heart and has three forms termed first, second and third degree block. As the 'degree of block' increases so does the seriousness of the problem (i.e. first degree block is usually unimportant whilst third degree block is an emergency).

First degree heart block
The ECG shows a prolonged PR interval (more than 0.2 seconds) (Fig. 27.14). All impulses are conducted to the ventricles.

Second degree heart block
Only some of the atrial impulses are conducted via the AV node. In Wenckebach (Mobitz type I) heart block, there is progressive widening of the PR interval, culminating in non-conduction through the AV node. The cycle then continues (Fig. 27.15). Mobitz type II heart block is intermittent failure of AV conduction (Fig. 27.16). This is the more serious of the two because the block is below the AV node in the His bundle which may lead to third degree block. The block occurs in the AV node and hence escape rhythms are more stable in Wenckebach block.

Third degree or complete heart block
This is complete dissociation between atria and ventricular contraction (Fig. 27.17). The ventricular rate assumes a slow 'escape' rhythm with a rate between 30–50 b.p.m.. All negatively chronotropic drugs should be stopped. If the patient is symptomatic, atropine can be tried. If this fails, a temporary pacing wire needs to be inserted. Isoprenaline infusion is no longer used routinely. If the patient remains stable or the rhythm problem

Fig. 27.14 Electrocardiogram of first degree heart block.

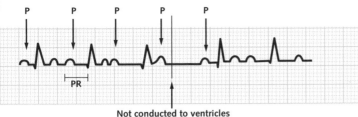

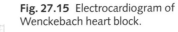

Fig. 27.15 Electrocardiogram of Wenckebach heart block.

does not resolve as they commonly do post MI, then a permanent pacemaker can be fitted as a semi–elective procedure.

In complete heart block, work out the atrial rate and the ventricular rate separately by marking them on a piece of paper. They should both be regular but at different rates

Anti-arrhythmic drugs

Traditionally, anti-arrhythmics are classified according to their effects on the action potential (Vaughan Williams classification; Fig. 27.18). However, this is now of less clinical relevance than a classification based on the site of action in the heart – supraventricular, ventricular, and both. Examples of anti-arrhythmic drugs are given below.

Supraventricular arrhythmias
Adenosine
Adenosine is used for terminating paroxysmal supraventricular tachycardia (SVT). It is a purine nucleoside which causes transient AV block. The half-life is 8–10 seconds but is longer if the patient is taking dipyridamole. It can cause flushing,chest pain and bronchospasm.

Verapamil
Verapamil is an alternative to adenosine and should not be used for wide complex tachycardias unless a supraventricular origin has been established beyond doubt. It should not be used with β-blockers.

Supraventricular and ventricular arrhythmias
Amiodarone
Amiodarone is effective in both types of arrhythmias with little deleterious effect on haemodynamics. This means it is widely used on coronary care units in acute settings (e.g. post MI). In chronic dysrhythmias, its main indication is in prevention of life threatening VF/VT. In this, it is less effective than an implanted defibrillator. Otherwise, it should only be used when other drugs are ineffective or contraindicated, and usually under hospital supervision. It can be used orally or intravenously for rapid effect. The half-life is several weeks. It may therefore take some weeks to achieve steady-state plasma concentration.

It is an iodine containing compound and side effects include hypo- and hyperthyroidism and liver dysfunction. TFTs and liver function tests (LFTs) should therefore be checked at baseline and every 6 months. It may cause pulmonary fibrosis, corneal microdeposits (which are reversible on stopping treatment), and photosensitivity.

β-Blockers
β-Blockers act mainly by attenuating the effects of the sympathetic nervous system on automaticity and conductivity within the heart. Sotalol is a beta blocker which also has class III actions. It is used widely to control paroxysmal AF (PAF).

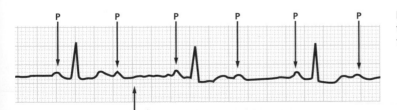

Fig. 27.16 Electrocardiogram of Mobitz type II heart block showing two p waves for each QRS complex (i.e. 2:1 block).

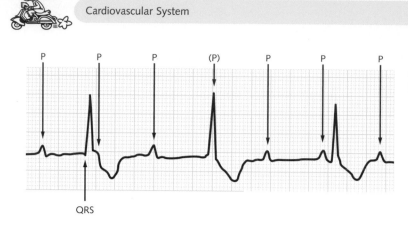

Fig. 27.17 Electrocardiogram of complete heart block. No relationship between atria (P) and venricles (QRS).

Flecainide

Flecainide is used acutely to cardiovert patients in new AF, if there is no structural heart disease or heart failure, with good success rates. It is excellent for the control of PAF. In a trial in which it was successfully used to suppress premature ventricular contractions post MI, it was associated with increased mortality compared to placebo—demonstrating the maxim 'treat the patient not the result'.

Procainamide

Procainamide is used for ventricular arrhythmias and paroxysmal atrial fibrillation. It can cause a syndrome resembling systemic lupus erythematosus with prolonged use.

Ventricular arrhythmias
Bretylium

Bretylium was only used as an anti-arrhythmic drug in resuscitation in unresponsive VT or VF. It can cause severe hypotension, nausea, and vomiting.

Lidocaine (Lignocaine)

Lidocaine was used commonly for VT after an MI but it can only be given intravenously. It can be used in patients with haemodynamically stable VT to attempt to cardiovert to sinus rhythm. In most situations, amiodarone is now preferred. The dose should be decreased with cardiac or liver failure to avoid convulsions, depression of the central nervous system, or depression of the cardiovascular system.

Heart failure

Heart failure occurs when the heart is unable to maintain sufficient cardiac output to meet the demands placed on it by the body. The problem is usually one of failure of myocardium, although excess pre- and after-load plus rhythm disturbances and increased demand beyond that of a normal heart's capacity are possible. The incidence rises with age and almost 1 million adults in the UK have heart failure. It is classified by its severity (Fig. 27.19).

The Vaughan Williams classification of antiarrhythmic drugs	
Class	Features
Ia,b,c	Membrane sodium channel blockers (e.g. quinidine, lidocaine and flecainide, respectively)
II	β-blockers
III	Amiodarone, bretylium, sotalol
IV	Calcium channel blockers (excluding dihydropyridines, e.g. nifedipine)

Fig. 27.18 The Vaughan Williams classification of anti-arrhythmic drugs.

The New York Heart Association classification of heart failure	
Class	Features
I	No limitation of physical activity
II	Slight limitation of physical activity, breathless climbing 2 flights of stairs
III	Marked limitation of physical activity, breathless walking 100m on flat
IV	Inability to carry out any physical activity without discomfort

Fig. 27.19 The New York Heart Association classification of heart failure.

The mortality in severe heart failure is approximately 40% at 1 year. Therapy of systolic heart failure has changed markedly in the last 10 years and prognosis is improving (Fig. 27.20).

Causes of heart failure
High output failure
A normal heart is unable to maintain an increased cardiac output in the face of grossly elevated requirements. It is then unable to meet these requirements. Conditions causing this include:

- Thyrotoxicosis.
- Anaemia.
- AV shunts.
- Beri beri.
- Fever.
- Paget's disease.
- Pregnancy.

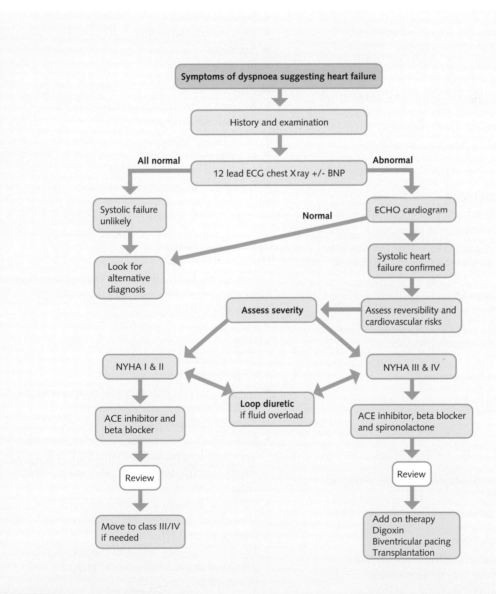

Fig. 27.20 Algorithm for the investigation and management of systolic heart failure. (NYHA, New York Heart Association; BNP, B-type natriuretic peptide; ACE, angiotensin-converting enzyme; ECG, electrocardiogram.)

Such conditions may also cause a previously silent cardiac problem to manifest itself.

Cardiogenic heart failure

Cardiogenic heart failure is due to an abnormality of the heart and can be unmasked when a heart with reduced reserve is unable to cope with the often seemingly minor stresses placed on it. These may manifest at rest or more usually on exertion. Causes include the following:

- Ischaemic heart disease (65% of new UK cases per year).
- Hypertension.
- Valvular heart disease.
- Infectious: viruses, Chagas disease.
- Toxins: alcohol, chemotherapy.
- Nutritional deficiency: beri beri.
- Post partum
- Tachycardia induced: atrial fibrillation, atrial flutter.
- Genetic: hypertrophic obstructive cardiomyopathy, Duchenne muscular dystrophy.

Clinical features

Left heart failure

In systolic heart failure, the inadequate cardiac output leads to elevated left atrial pressures and these combine to give the majority of clinical findings.

Symptoms include:
- Exertional dyspnoea (most common).
- Orthopnoea.
- Paroxysmal nocturnal dyspnoea.
- Fatigue.
- Wheeze ('cardiac asthma').
- Cough.
- Haemoptysis (rare).

Signs include:
- Tachypnoea.
- Tachycardia.
- Pulsus alternans (alternating large and small volume pulse).
- Peripheral cyanosis and low pulse volume.
- Cardiomegaly.
- Third heart sound ('S3 gallop').
- Functional mitral regurgitation secondary to dilatation of the mitral valve annulus.
- Basal crepitations indicating pulmonary oedema.
- Pleural effusions.

Right heart failure

This may occur secondary to chronic lung disease, multiple pulmonary emboli, primary pulmonary hypertension, right heart valve disease, left-to-right shunts, or isolated right ventricular cardiomyopathy. It is commonly associated with LVF, in which case the term congestive cardiac failure (CCF) is used. Elevated right atrial pressures lead to peripheral fluid retention.

Symptoms include:
- Fatigue.
- Nausea.
- Wasting.
- Swollen ankles.
- Abdominal discomfort.
- Anorexia.
- Breathlessness.

The signs include:
- A raised jugulovenous pressure (JVP).
- Smooth hepatomegaly.
- Liver tenderness.
- Pitting oedema.
- Ascites.
- Functional tricuspid regurgitation.
- Tachycardia.
- Right ventricular third heart sound.

Investigations

The cause for the heart failure must always be sought because heart failure itself is an inadequate diagnosis. After the history and examination, investigations include the following:

- FBC: anaemia.
- U&Es: renal dysfunction or electrolyte abnormalities .
- LFTs: liver congestion.
- Cardiac enzymes/troponin: if acute onset, to exclude acute coronary syndromes.
- Thyroid function tests.
- ECG: IHD, arrhythmias, and left ventricular hypertrophy. Finding a normal ECG has a very strong negative predictive value against heart failure.
- CXR: cardiomegaly, alveolar oedema, 'bat's wings shadowing', prominent upper lobe vessels, Kerley B lines, pleural effusions.
- Echocardiography: remains the gold standard investigation and can assess ventricular and valvular function.

Other investigations to consider are:
- Exercise testing: functional severity and prognosis.

- Cardiac catheterisation: assess and treat ischaemic/valve lesions or rarely biopsy myocardium with cardiomyopathy.
- Nuclear techniques: ejection fraction, cardiac function and reversible ischaemia.
- Brain (B-type) natriuretic peptide: this a marker of ventricular dysfunction and may help in the assessment of suspected cardiac failure. A low plasma level makes the diagnosis of heart failure unlikely. In the future it may help to reduce need for echocardiography.

Management

The management of heart failure has two parts:

- Management of chronic cardiac failure is a rapidly growing area as the population ages and management of acute coronary syndromes improves. The drug treatments have evolved rapidly with a large evidence base and improved prognosis for patients.
- Management of acute heart failure is a common scenario for all doctors in general medicine.

When investigating suspected endocarditis, the more sets of blood cultures prior to antibiotics the better the chance of detecting an organism

Chronic cardiac failure

General

The cause of the heart failure should be sought and treated appropriately (e.g. valve lesions). Exacerbating factors such as anaemia and hypertension should be treated. Check the patient's drugs because some may cause fluid retention (e.g. NSAIDs). Patients should be advised to maintain an optimal weight, avoid excessive salt intake and alcohol consumption and stop smoking. Standard cardiac risks should be treated and most patients should be taking antiplatelet drugs and statins.

Drug treatment

These are divided into drugs which improve symptoms of heart failure, namely diuretics and digoxin and those which are improving prognosis namely ACE inhibitors, certain β-blockers and spironolactone. They reduce the risk of MI and increase survival. Treatment is best planned as a stepped care plan in outpatients when stable.

Angiotensin-converting enzyme inhibitors

The renin–angiotensin–aldosterone system is activated in heart failure. ACE inhibitors reduce angiotensin mediated vasoconstriction, reducing afterload, and decrease aldosterone-mediated salt and water retention. This improves the function of the damaged heart. Many studies have been performed using various ACE inhibitors in settings from post acute myocardial infarction to cardiomyopathy in outpatients. Their effects are class effects, and they have revolutionised systolic heart failure treatment by reducing symptoms, hospitalisations and mortality. They should therefore be started early in any patient with heart failure (Fig. 27.21).

Side effects include first dose hypotension, hyperkalaemia and worsening renal function especially in people with bilateral renal artery stenosis. As such, they should be commenced at a low dose and increased gradually with regular electrolyte monitoring. Commonly used examples include ramipril, captopril, perindopril and lisinopril.

β-Blockers

For many years, it was assumed that these were contraindicated in heart failure because the sympathetic nervous system was compensating for the failing heart and that blocking this was deleterious. This remains true in the acute setting where the negatively inotropic and chronotropic effects of β-blockade can be harmful. However, it is thought that high circulating levels of catecholamines

---

Recommendations for inpatient initiation of ACE inhibitors

- Frusemide 80 mg o.d. or more
- Hypovolaemia (check for diarrhoea and vomiting)
- Hyponatraemia (plasma sodium <130 mmol/L)
- Systolic blood pressure <90 mmHg
- Unstable heart failure
- Renal impairment: plasma creatinine >150 mmol/L
- High-dose vasodilator therapy
- Age 70 years or more

Fig. 27.21 Recommendations for inpatient initiation of angiotensin-converting enzyme (ACE) inhibitors. ACE inhibitors are contraindicated in people with known or suspected bilateral renal artery stenosis, in aortic stenosis, or outflow tract obstruction, pregnancy, and porphyria. Common side effects include a dry cough, hypotension, dizziness, and headache.

cause progressive myocardial damage. Indeed, the level appears to correlate with prognosis.

Three β-blockers have shown improved function and survival for patients with moderate to severe heart failure. They are carvedilol, bisoprolol and metoprolol. They can be considered to interfere with the renin–angiotensin–aldosterone axis from the opposite end to ACE inhibitors and spironolactone. These should only be commenced in stable patients by experienced clinicians. The progress should be carefully monitored and the dose increased slowly.

Spironolactone

Spironolactone is an aldosterone antagonist which was more commonly used in ascites as a diuretic. Aldosterone may act directly as a deleterious growth factor on myocytes in addition to its salt and water retaining effects. In a study using low (non-diuretic) doses, it improved morbidity and mortality. Side effects include hyperkalaemia and, because it is usually given with ACE inhibitors, electrolytes need monitoring.

Angiotensin II receptor blockers

Similar to ACE inhibitors, these interfere with the renin–angiotensin–aldosterone system. They are newer and their exact place in therapy is uncertain. The likelihood is that they will have similar effects but the data is awaited. They are usually used in patients who cannot tolerate an ACE inhibitor (e.g. for cough). They may have a role in addition to ACE inhibitors as these do not completely suppress angiotensin II production.

Loop diuretics

Loop diuretics, commonly frusemide and bumetanide, are very effective at reducing symptoms in patients with heart failure both in acute and chronic care. They help manage the fluid balance of patients. Side effects include hypovolaemia and renal impairment if diuresis is excessive, electrolyte disturbance and rarely ototoxicity. Renal function should be monitored regularly. They have not demonstrated improvement in survival in any trial.

Thiazide diuretics

These are rarely used alone in cardiac failure. Metolazone is reserved for severe symptomatic heart failure because, when coupled with a loop diuretic, it can produce very profound diuresis.

Digoxin

As well as its effectiveness in rate control of patients with atrial fibrillation, digoxin is a mild positive inotrope due to its effect in increasing intracellular

calcium. As such, it may have benefits in cardiac failure even in patients with sinus rhythm. It does not improve survival but may reduce symptoms and hospital admissions. Concerns about side effects include rhythm disturbances, nausea and visual disturbances. Therapeutic drug monitoring allows effective dosing to minimise complications. Digoxin should only be added to patients in sinus rhythm with heart failure not responding to accepted best practice. It remains more commonly used in the USA than in the UK.

Hydralazine and nitrates

These are powerful vasodilating drugs which can improve the symptoms of heart failure and may improve prognosis. Their only use currently is in patients who are unable to take ACE inhibiting drugs. They may be more effective in black patients than standard therapy.

Intravenous therapy

In chronic heart failure in the UK, there is little role for intravenous therapy with positive inotropic drugs other than as a bridge to transplantation in end-stage disease. Inotropes used include milrinone, a phosphodiesterase inhibitor, and the β-agonist dobutamine.

Levosimendan, a novel calcium-sensitising drug, produces inotropic benefit which appears to persist for several months; its role in chronic cardiac failure is not known.

Warfarin

Patients with severe heart failure and cardiomyopathy are at risk of thrombus formation and systemic embolisation and, accordingly, warfarin should be considered in patients with poor systolic function regardless of atrial fibrillation.

Non drug therapy

Cardiac rehabilitation

Graded exercise programs and patient education encourage activity and independence, although their long-term effect is unknown.

Transplantation

People who undergo transplantation have very good prognoses with a 1-year survival of more than 80%. The main problem is the extreme shortage of donor organs, coupled with comorbidities.

Biventricular pacemakers

The lack of donor organs has led to much research about improving end-stage cardiac function. It was noted that patients with intraventricular conduction delay (as shown by a widened QRS complex) have poorly coordinated ventricular contraction which further reduces ejection fraction. Resynchronising this using a standard right atrial and right ventricular pacemaker plus a left ventricular pacing wire via the coronary sinus improves cardiac output in some patients. If coupled with first degree heart block, the effect can be further improved. The long-term benefit is uncertain.

Arrhythmias

Patients with cardiomyopathy often have abnormal conduction systems and are at an increased risk of dysrhythmias, in particular ventricular fibrillation and tachycardia. One therapy is long-term amiodarone although its effectiveness is doubted. If the risk is significant, then an implantable defibrillator is the preferred option.

The artificial heart

Despite press reports, the widespread clinical use of a mechanical heart or ventricular assist device that is anything more than a short-term support to patients awaiting transplant is still some way distant.

Acute heart failure

This is an emergency characterised by acute breathlessness, orthopnoea, wheezing, anxiety, and sweating. There may be pink frothy sputum and ischaemic chest pain, as well as signs of pulmonary oedema. The first aim is to relieve symptoms and stabilise the patient, the second is to support other organs with adequate perfusion and the third is to find and treat the cause. If severe, the management should begin before investigations are performed:
- Sit the patient upright.
- Give high-concentration oxygen unless there is coexisting chronic hypercapnia due to long-standing respiratory failure.
- Respiratory support with continuous positive airway pressure to improve oxygenation or non-invasive ventilatory support can be used effectively. If failing, involve an anaesthetist early.

Traditional therapy involves:
- Diamorphine (2.5–5 mg i.v.) slowly with an antiemetic to reduce anxiety and reduce venous capacitance to reduce preload.
- Diuresis with frusemide (40–80 mg i.v if renal function normal). Frusemide may work initially by vasodilatation.
- Give intravenous venodilators (e.g. glyceryl trinitrate) if systolic blood pressure is greater than 100 mmHg. This will reduce preload.

Many cardiologists feel that, in acute cardiogenic shock, where the patient is not overloaded with fluid but where it is merely wrongly distributed due to the failing haemodynamics of the heart, first-line therapy should be with a nitrate, sublingual if needed and that frusemide is of secondary importance.

Treat other conditions that may compromise cardiac function:
- Fast atrial fibrillation: digoxin, orally or intravenously. Other arrhythmias should be treated appropriately. DC cardioversion may be needed.

Further management if the above is inadequate needs to be in a critical care unit (CCU/HDU/ICU).
- Intravenous inotropic agents may be of value if there is hypotension. If pulmonary congestion is dominant, dobutamine is preferred at 5 µg/kg/min, increasing gradually to 20 µg/kg/min if needed. Remember dobutamine has vasodilating properties and so may not have the effect on blood pressure that is expected. It can be combined with low doses of noradrenaline.
- If the pulmonary oedema is not improving, then acute haemofiltration can remove fluid rapidly and prevent intubation.
- Intra-aortic balloon counterpulsation in primary cardiac failure may be available to support the heart whilst therapy is planned.

Hypertension

The prevalence of hypertension differs depending on blood pressure cut-off points, age, sex, and race. It increases with age, and is more common in men and Afro-Caribbeans. Approximately 20% of the UK adult population have blood pressures above 160/95 mmHg. The risk of morbidity and mortality rises continuously with increasing blood pressure, and marginal risk is greater at higher blood pressures. Similarly, the lower the blood pressure achieved with treatment, the lower the risk of complications of hypertension. However, the benefit of lowering diastolic blood pressure to below 90 mmHg is minimal in uncomplicated hypertension in young or middle-aged patients.

Definitions of hypertension differ but whatever the blood pressure thresholds used, the mean of several blood pressure measurements should be taken over time, as an isolated reading predicts cardiovascular risk very poorly. Blood pressure should be taken sitting or lying after 2–3 minutes rest. The air bladder within the cuff should cover at least 80% of the arm circumference, otherwise, in obese patients, artificially high readings are observed. The dial or mercury column should fall slowly, and be read to the nearest 2 mmHg. The diastolic pressure is recorded at the disappearance of sounds (i.e. Korotkoff phase V).

Essential hypertension

In over 90% of people, the diagnosis of hypertension is idiopathic ('essential') (i.e. no cause can be found).

Aetiology

Genetic influences on blood pressure regulation have been suggested by family studies. Factors implicated include defects in the renin–angiotensin–aldosterone axis, problems with sodium handling and increased sympathetic nervous system activation. A number of environmental factors are also associated with the development of hypertension. These include obesity, alcohol, dietary sodium intake, dietary potassium, and smoking.

Vegetarians have less hypertension than meat eaters, although it is difficult to know whether the blood pressure differences are due to diet *per se* or other causes. It is not clear whether psychological factors play a significant part in long-term blood pressure regulation, although there is no doubt that emotional factors can induce pronounced but transient variations in blood pressure.

Obesity

There is a continuous linear relationship between excess body fat and blood pressure levels. Obstructive sleep apnoea is more common although not unique to overweight individuals and appears to be an independent risk factor for hypertension and cardiovascular disease.

Alcohol

Increasing alcohol consumption is related to higher blood pressure levels, and the effects are additive to those of obesity.

Dietary sodium intake

Salt intake has a small effect on population blood pressure levels. Salt restriction may reduce systolic blood pressure by 3–5 mmHg in hypertensives and is most clear-cut in older subjects and those with more severe hypertension.

Dietary potassium

Dietary sodium and potassium intake are generally inversely related. Dietary potassium may have a blood pressure lowering effect.

Smoking

This leads to an acute elevation in blood pressure, which subsides within 15 minutes of finishing a cigarette. Regular smokers can have slightly lower blood pressures than non-smokers, although the small potential benefit is greatly outweighed by the increased cardiovascular and respiratory risks.

Secondary hypertension

A definite underlying cause for hypertension is more common in younger people, and should be looked for specifically in those aged under 35 years:

- Renal disease: chronic glomerulonephritis, chronic pyelonephritis, renal artery stenosis and polycystic kidney disease. Although it only accounts for 1% of all hypertension, the diagnosis of renal artery stenosis is important as it is the commonest curable cause.
- Endocrine disease: Cushing's and Conn's syndromes, phaeochromocytoma, and acromegaly.
- Pregnancy-induced hypertension and pre-eclampsia: associated with oedema and proteinuria.
- Coarctation of the aorta.
- Drugs: oestrogen-containing oral contraceptive pill, NSAIDs, steroids, sympathomimetics in cold cures, carbenoxolone, and liquorice.

History

Patients with hypertension are usually asymptomatic. The history should concentrate on environmental predisposing factors, associated cardiovascular risk factors, and the symptoms of underlying secondary causes. For example, patients with phaeochromocytoma may have symptoms of panic, headache, sweating, nausea, tremor, and pallor. Accelerated hypertension may lead to symptoms secondary to heart failure, renal failure, headaches, nausea and vomiting, visual impairment, or fits.

Examination

The clinical approach to the patient with hypertension is summarised in Fig. 27.22 and Chapter 15. Apart from the blood pressure itself, the examination should focus on complications of hypertension or underlying secondary causes. The patient should be examined for left ventricular

Clinical evaluation of the patient with hypertension	
Causes of hypertension	Drugs causing hypertension? Paroxysmal features? (phaeochromocytoma) Present, past or family history of renal disease? General appearance? (Cushing's syndrome) Radiofemoral delay? (coarctation) Kidney(s) palpable? (polycystic, hydronephrosis, neoplasm) Abdominal or loin bruit? (renal artery stenosis)
Contributory factors	Overweight? Alcohol intake?
Complications	Cerebrovascular disease Left ventricular hypertrophy or cardiac failure Ischaemic heart disease Fundal haemorrhages and exudates (accelerated phase)
Contraindications to drugs	Gout, diabetes (thiazides) Asthma, heart failure, heart block (β-blockers) Heart failure, heart block (verapamil)
Cardiovascular risk	Assessment of other cardiovascular risk factors

Fig. 27.22 Clinical evaluation of the patient with hypertension. Look for the 'five Cs'.

hypertrophy (displaced apex beat), coarctation of the aorta (difference in blood pressure in the arms, weak femoral pulses, radiofemoral delay), renal bruits for possible underlying renal artery stenosis, and palpable kidneys, e.g. in polycystic kidney disease. There may be retinopathy, classified by the Keith–Wagener changes (Fig. 27.23).

Investigation policy

The minimum tests include urinalysis and serum biochemistry for evidence of renal disease, and ECG for evidence of left ventricular hypertrophy or ischaemia.

Consideration should also be given to the following:
- Chest radiograph: cardiac size and signs of heart failure.
- Fasting lipids and glucose: cardiovascular risk.
- Echocardiography: left ventricular hypertrophy and left ventricular function.
- Fundoscopy: indicates end-organ damage.

Further investigations are warranted in young patients where a secondary cause is more likely, in patients with rapidly rising blood pressure or severe hypertension, in patients with hypertension resistant to treatment, and in patients with deranged U&Es. These investigations include urinary catecholamines for phaeochromocytoma and renal tract ultrasound for structural abnormalities; if renovascular disease is suspected, then contrast or magnetic resonance renal arteriography is indicated.

Further investigations depend on clinical suspicion (e.g. aortography for coarctation of the aorta).

Management of hypertension

For secondary hypertension, treatment of the underlying condition may be indicated (e.g. treatment of an underlying endocrine condition or surgical correction of aortic coarctation). In renovascular hypertension, drug treatment may effectively control blood pressure. It is therefore reasonable to consider angioplasty or surgery only for young patients who are more likely to have fibromuscular hyperplasia compared to atherosclerosis, patients with severe hypertension, or patients whose blood pressure is difficult to control medically. Surgery may also be indicated where progressive renal failure in a hypertensive patient is

The Keith–Wagener classification of retinopathy	
Grade	Features
I	Arterial narrowing and increased tortuosity
II	Arteriovenous nipping
III	Haemorrhages and soft exudates
IV	Grades I–III and papilloedema

Fig. 27.23 The Keith–Wagener classification of retinopathy.

due either to bilateral renal artery stenosis or stenosis of an artery to a single kidney.

An algorithm of the decision making process in patients with hypertension is given in Fig. 27.25. The presence of other risks is crucial to proper therapy. The aim is to reduce blood pressure to below 140/90 mmHg. A target of 130/85 mmHg is indicated in very high-risk groups, such as diabetics and patients with nephropathy.

In hypertension, as in many chronic disorders, drugs are best added 'stepwise' until control has been achieved. An attempt can then be made to 'step down' treatment under supervision. Monotherapy controls blood pressure in only 30–50% of patients, and most patients therefore need two or more drugs. In uncomplicated mild hypertension, drugs may be substituted rather than added.

As a rule, it is the response to therapy rather than the class of drugs used which is the most important factor. For uncomplicated hypertension, combining thiazide diuretics with β-blockers is recommended first choice. In specific situations, other choices are best (e.g. ACE inhibitors in diabetes, proteinuria or heart failure).

It has been suggested that hypertension can be divided into two groups; the first is renin-dependent hypertension most common in young white patients. This responds well to ACE inhibitors (A) and β-blockers (B). The second group is low-renin hypertension that is poorly responsive to A and B. Response is better to calcium antagonists (C) or diuretics (D). This has led to the 'AB/CD rule'. This says that combining either A or B with one of either C or D is more likely to be effective and that AC and D should be the first line for resistant disease.

Drug treatment
Thiazide diuretics
Thiazides lower blood pressure mainly by lowering body sodium stores. Initially, blood pressure falls because of a decrease in blood volume, venous return, and cardiac output. Gradually, the cardiac output returns to normal but the hypotensive effect remains because the peripheral resistance decreases. Side effects include impaired glucose tolerance and gout. Low doses (bendrofluazide 2.5 mg) cause little biochemical disturbance without loss of the antihypertensive effect. Higher doses are usually never needed, nor are potassium supplements. Thiazides are better tolerated in women than men, and are more effective in the elderly.

Potassium-sparing diuretics
Potassium-sparing diuretics may be used for the prophylaxis or treatment of diuretic-induced hypokalaemia.

β-Blockers
β-Blockers initially produce a fall in blood pressure by decreasing cardiac output. With continued treatment, the cardiac output returns to normal but the blood pressure remains low because the peripheral resistance is 'reset' at a lower level and renin levels are reduced.

Side effects include negative inotropism, provocation of asthma, and heart block. Less serious side effects include cold hands and fatigue. β-blockers are more effective in young patients and less effective in black patients due to excess renin in the former group.

Calcium channel blockers
Calcium antagonists are a heterogeneous group and work in different ways on both the heart and peripheral vasculature. The dihydropyridines (e.g. nifedipine) are good vasodilating drugs which may cause a reflex tachycardia. Diltiazem also has negatively inotropic and chronotropic effects. They are relatively contraindicated in heart failure. They are effective as monotherapy in 50% of patients and amlodipine (which has demonstrated its safety in heart failure) has become the most common antihypertensive worldwide. Side effects include flushing, headache, oedema, and constipation. The oedema does not respond to diuretics.

Verapamil should not be used with a β-blocker.

Angiotensin-converting enzyme inhibitors
ACE inhibitors act by inhibiting the renin–angiotensin–aldosterone axis with an increase in vasodilating bradykinin. They are more effective in patients with higher renin levels and so are best in young white patients versus black patients. The indications for ACE inhibitors grow yearly as new patient groups to benefit emerge. They are highly effective in heart failure, proteinuric nephropathy and diabetes. As such, they are now often started as monotherapy and are very potent combined with a diuretic or calcium channel blocker.

Side effects include a dry cough, secondary to bradykinin, hyperkalaemia and usually transient, worsening in creatinine (or GFR) as intraglomerular pressure falls. Acute renal failure is uncommon without another pathology (e.g. bilateral renal artery stenosis, sepsis or hypovolaemia). Monitoring of electrolytes is essential as the dose is titrated.

Angiotensin II receptor blockers

These are relatively new drugs (e.g. losartan and irbesartan). They block the renin–angiotensin system producing effects similar to ACE inhibitors. They are probably effective in conditions in which ACE inhibitors have shown benefit although they are usually reserved for people in whom chronic cough limits therapy with ACE inhibitors because they do not affect bradykinin production.

Minoxidil

Minoxidil is a potent vasodilator and decreases peripheral resistance. It may cause a reflex tachycardia, which can be prevented by combination with a β-blocker. It may also cause fluid retention, which responds to a diuretic, and hirsutism. This is its other therapeutic use for men.

α-Blockers

α-Blockers reduce both arteriolar and venous resistance, and maintain a high cardiac output. First dose hypotension can be problematic.

Methyldopa

Methyldopa stimulates α_2-receptors in the medulla and reduces sympathetic outflow. In 20% of patients, it causes a positive Coombs' test and, rarely, haemolytic anaemia. Drug-induced hepatitis with fever may also occur.

Accelerated hypertension

Malignant hypertension or very severe hypertension (diastolic blood pressure over 140 mmHg) requires urgent treatment in hospital. Treatment is normally given orally with β-blockers or calcium antagonists to reduce diastolic blood pressure to 100–110 mmHg within the first 24 hours. Over the next few days, further antihypertensives should be given to lower blood pressure further.

Very rapid falls in blood pressure should be avoided because the reduction in cerebral perfusion may lead to cerebral infarction, blindness, worsening renal function, and myocardial ischaemia. Parenteral antihypertensive drugs such as nitroprusside, GTN or labetalol are rarely required. Sublingual nifedipine is best avoided due to its unpredictable response.

Hypertension in pregnancy

Good blood pressure control in pregnancy is important – oral methyldopa is safe. β-Blockers are effective and safe in the third trimester but may cause intrauterine growth retardation when used earlier in pregnancy. Hydralazine may also be used. Its side effects include drug induced lupus.

Age and hypertension

Factors relating to hypertension associated with advancing age are summarised in Fig. 27.24.

Follow up

Adherence to treatment is an important issue in a chronic, asymptomatic condition such as hypertension where treatment is aimed at reduction of later complications. 25–50% of patients default or discontinue treatment, so an effective recall system is needed. When the blood pressure is satisfactorily controlled, it should be checked once every 3 months. More frequent checks are needed during dose titration if the control is borderline, if compliance is a problem, or if the treatment regimen is complex. On routine visits, the blood pressure and weight should be measured, and the patient should be asked about side effects. The urine should be checked for protein and glucose yearly.

Apart from this, routine re-examination or investigation is unnecessary, and should only be performed if there is a special indication (e.g. variable or borderline blood pressure control, or at the onset of new symptoms).

Prognosis

Patients with untreated malignant hypertension have a 90% mortality in 1 year, and treatment is therefore life saving. The risk of hypertension in other cases depends on the level of blood pressure, the presence of complications (e.g. cardiac or renal

---

Age and hypertension—factors associated with advancing age

- Greater likelihood of hypertension (>50%)
- Greater damage when hypertensive
- Diastolic threshold for treatment 90 mmHg
- As much or more benefit from treatment
- No increase in treatment side effects
- Elderly should be offered treatment unless suffering other life-shortening illness
- Erect pressures should be measured

Fig. 27.24 Age and hypertension-factors associated with advancing age.

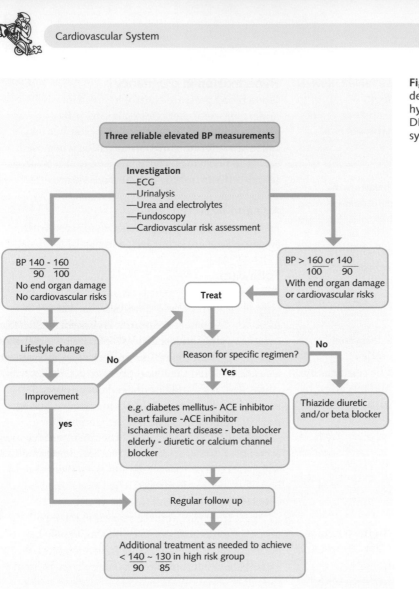

Fig. 27.25 Algorithm for making decisions in systolic and diastolic hypertension. (BP, blood pressure; DBP, diastolic blood pressure; SBP, systolic blood pressure.)

failure), and the presence of other cardiovascular risk factors (e.g. male sex, smoking, diabetes, and older age). Those at highest risk gain most benefit from treatment.

Valvular heart disease

Mitral stenosis

The cause of mitral stenosis is usually rheumatic fever, although only approximately half of all patients give a positive history. It is four times more common than mitral regurgitation in rheumatic fever, and is commoner in women than men.

Progressive stenosis of the mitral valve, via thickening of the cusps and fusion of the commissures, results in a pressure gradient between the left atrium and the left ventricle. As the stenosis worsens, ventricular filling becomes impaired, and

this is compounded by fibrosis of the subvalvar apparatus leading to left atrial dilatation and hypertrophy, atrial fibrillation and thrombus formation. Pulmonary congestion ensues as left atrial pressure rises, and an increase in pulmonary artery pressure may lead to right heart failure.

Management

Maintenance of sinus rhythm confers haemodynamic benefit as ventricular filling is improved. Cardioversion should be considered if atrial fibrillation is present and the chamber dimensions are favourable. Anticoagulation is indicated in patients with atrial fibrillation although some would anticoagulate all patients with mitral stenosis. The risk of emboli is greater with a large left atrium or left atrial appendage.

It may be necessary to add in other rate-controlling drugs such as β-blockers or verapamil.

If symptoms persist, the patient should be considered for mitral valve replacement or valvotomy. If the valve is not calcified and the leaflets are pliable, balloon valvuloplasty may be attempted.

All patients should receive antibiotic prophylaxis before dental and surgical procedures to avoid subacute bacterial endocarditis.

Remember SODOFF for acute heart failure:
- Sit the patient up.
- Oxygen.
- Diamorphine.
- OFFload.

Mitral regurgitation

The incidence of mitral regurgitation is equal in men and women. It is usually secondary to rheumatic fever, floppy prolapsing mitral valve leaflets, papillary muscle dysfunction, rupture after an inferior MI, cardiomyopathy, or secondary to ventricular dilatation or dysfunction. Less common causes include congenital malformations, which may be associated with an ostium primum atrial septal defect, infective endocarditis, rupture of the chordae tendineae, cardiomyopathy, rheumatoid arthritis, or left atrial tumour interfering with mitral valve closure.

The circulatory changes depend on the speed of onset and severity of mitral regurgitation. Acute regurgitation may lead to acute pulmonary oedema whereas chronic regurgitation allows for compensatory left ventricular and atrial dilatation.

Management

Diuretics are used for pulmonary congestion, and vasodilators are helpful in acute regurgitation. Digoxin and anticoagulants are given to patients in atrial fibrillation. Antibiotic prophylaxis is needed prior to dental and surgical procedures.

Mitral valve replacement is indicated if symptoms are severe and uncontrolled by medical treatment, or if pulmonary hypertension develops. Good results are achieved if left ventricular function is preserved, and early referral may allow repair of the valve rather than replacement.

Mitral valve prolapse

This is due to prolapse of the mitral valve leaflets into the left atrium during ventricular systole. Prolapse is common in floppy valves and myocardial disease, and should be distinguished from benign mitral prolapse syndrome. It may affect up to 15% of the population and is three times commoner in women.

Clinical signs and symptoms

It is often asymptomatic and found incidentally. An apical midsystolic click is heard, associated with a late systolic murmur if the valve is regurgitant. It may be associated with palpitations and atypical chest pains, although the latter is more common in people aware of their condition. Systemic emboli and syncope are rare.

Investigations

The ECG may show inferolateral ST/T segment changes. Arrhythmias may be confirmed by Holter monitoring and the commonest rhythm disturbance is ventricular extrasystoles. Echocardiography is diagnostic.

Management

Patients should receive endocarditis prophylaxis. Treatment is only indicated for complications (e.g. anti-arrhythmic drugs for significant rhythm disturbances, or anticoagulants for emboli).

Aortic stenosis

The commonest cause of aortic stenosis is a calcified bicuspid valve, and this is more common in men. In younger patients, the cause may be congenital or due to rheumatic fever but, in older patients, it may be due to senile degenerative calcification, which is commoner in women. Aortic stenosis tends to progress gradually causing obstruction to the left ventricular outflow with resultant hypertrophy. Ventricular dilatation and heart failure are late complications. Conduction defects may result from calcification extending into the ventricular system.

Management

Valve replacement is indicated for severe stenosis because of the risk of sudden death, or for symptomatic aortic stenosis. It should be done whilst left ventricular function is preserved. The management of asymptomatic moderate stenosis is uncertain (i.e. surgery versus medical therapy). Drugs do not alter the progression of the disease though diuretics and digoxin can be given for heart failure. Many cardiovascular drugs are contraindicated in aortic stenosis; these are predominantly vasodilating medications. The decrease in systemic vascular resistance increases the gradient across the valve, increasing the work the ventricle has to perform.

Aortic regurgitation

The more common causes include cusp malformation (e.g. bicuspid valve) and cusp erosion (e.g. infective endocarditis).

Other causes include:
- Cusp distortion (e.g. senile calcification and rheumatic fever).
- Loss of support (e.g. VSD).
- Aortic wall disease due to inflammation (e.g. syphilis).
- Ankylosing spondylitis.
- Reiter's syndrome.
- Psoriatic arthropathy.
- Aortic wall disease due to dilatation (e.g. hypertension with or without dissection).

Management

Valve replacement is indicated for symptomatic patients. In the meantime, diuretics and digoxin may be given to control symptoms of heart failure. The prognosis is good while ventricular function is good but death usually occurs within 2–3 years after the onset of ventricular failure.

Tricuspid regurgitation

This may be functional secondary to right heart failure, commonly as a result of pulmonary hypertension. It may also be rheumatic in association with mitral valve disease, or due to endocarditis in intravenous drug addicts.

Management

Treat any underlying cause, then treat the consequences of right heart failure with diuretics etc. Valve replacement is an option but is often high risk if pulmonary hypertension is present.

Miscellaneous cardiovascular conditions

Cardiomyopathy

Cardiomyopathy is a disorder of heart muscle. It is classified into three types as hypertrophic, dilated, and restrictive. Fig. 27.26 gives examples of aetiology.

Hypertrophic cardiomyopathy

Hypertrophic cardiomyopathy (HCM) follows an autosomal dominant inheritance although half of all cases occur sporadically. There is asymmetrical left ventricular hypertrophy usually of the intraventricular septum, which leads to symptoms of dyspnoea, angina, palpitations, and syncope. On examination, there is a jerky pulse, the apex beat has a double impulse, there may be third and fourth heart sounds, and there is a late systolic murmur best heard at the left sternal edge when upright or performing a Valsalva manoeuvre. There may also be associated mitral regurgitation.

Fig. 27.26 Causes of cardiomyopathy.

Causes of cardiomyopathy	
Cause	**Examples**
Toxic	Alcohol, cyclophosphamide, corticosteroids, lithium, phenothiazines
Metabolic	Thiamine deficiency, pellagra, obesity, porphyria, uraemia
Endocrine	Thyrotoxicosis, acromegaly, myxoedema, Cushing's disease, diabetes mellitus
Collagen diseases	Systemic lupus erythematosus, polyarteritis nodosum
Infiltrative	Amyloidosis, haemochromatosis, neoplastic, sarcoidosis, mucopolysaccharidosis, Whipple's disease
Infective	Viral, rickettsial, mycobacterial
Genetic	Hypertrophic cardiomyopathy, muscular dystrophies
Fibroplastic	Endomyocardial fibrosis, Loeffler's endomyocardial disease, carcinoid
Miscellaneous	Ischaemic heart disease, postpartum

HCM may be complicated by atrial fibrillation, systemic emboli, heart failure, and sudden death, the risk of which is probably increased by strenuous exercise.

Investigation

Electrocardiography shows left ventricular hypertrophy, and sometimes atrial fibrillation and left bundle branch block. The classic echocardiography finding is asymmetrical septal hypertrophy and systolic anterior movement of the mitral valve. 24-hour ECG monitoring may identify silent arrhythmias which are often transient e.g. paroxysmal AF or VT. Cardiac catheterisation shows a small left ventricular cavity with obliteration in systole. There is a systolic outflow tract gradient within the ventricle.

Management

β-blockers help with symptoms and are useful for angina or dysrhythmias. Some treat dysrhythmias prophylactically with amiodarone; implantable defibrillators may be indicated. The patient should be anticoagulated if there is atrial fibrillation. If medical treatment is ineffective, the patient should be considered for dual chamber pacemaker, septal mymectomy, myotomy or cardiac transplantation. Screening of first degree relatives maybe indicated as HCM is a risk for sudden death in young people.

Dilated cardiomyopathy

The ventricles are dilated and contract poorly. Clinically, there are usually signs and symptoms of right and left heart failure, cardiomegaly, and atrial fibrillation with emboli. More dangerous arrhythmias and conduction defects occur.

There are a number of possible heterogeneous causes, which include alcohol, infiltrative disorders, collagen diseases, infective, toxic, metabolic, postpartum and genetic conditions. However ischaemic heart disease remains the leading UK cause. Echocardiography shows a globally hypokinetic and dilated heart. Coronary arteriography is usually normal.

Management

Underlying conditions are treated as appropriate. Heart failure should be treated as for ischaemic cardiomyopathy with diuretics, ACE inhibitors, etc. Anticoagulants and maintenance of sinus rhythm to reduce the risk of emboli are standard. The prognosis is variable. Patients should be considered for cardiac transplantation.

Restrictive cardiomyopathy

This is due to endomyocardial stiffening and includes fibroplastic and infiltrative conditions as shown in Fig. 27.26. The commonest cause in the UK is amyloidosis. It results in impaired diastolic function. The ECG may show small voltage complexes. The differential diagnosis includes constrictive pericarditis. Myocardial biopsy may be indicated. Treatment is that of the cause. There are few effective treatments for symptoms.

Pericarditis and pericardial effusion

Pericarditis is inflammation of the pericardium. Symptoms include a sharp retrosternal pain relieved by sitting forward. It may radiate to the left arm, or inferiorly. It is worse on lying down, with inspiration and coughing. There may be a 'scratchy' friction rub on examination. Pericardial effusion may be present.

The causes of pericarditis are given in Fig. 27.27.

Investigations

In addition to ECG and CXR (below), the following investigations should be considered:
- Blood and sputum culture for bacteria.
- Viral titres and viral culture from throat swabs and stools.
- Autoantibodies if there is evidence of connective tissue disease.
- TFTs.

Electrocardiography

This shows concave (saddle shaped) upwards ST segment elevation; often with PR segment depression. Inverted T waves may also occur.

Causes of pericarditis

- Idiopathic
- Infections—viral (e.g. coxsackie virus B), bacterial (e.g. *Mycobacterium*), parasitic
- Neoplastic (e.g. breast, lung, lymphoma)
- Connective tissue disease (e.g. SLE, RA)
- Uraemia
- Myocardial infarction
- Dressler's syndrome following myocardial infarction or cardiac surgery
- Radiotherapy
- Trauma
- Hypothyroidism

Fig. 27.27 Causes of pericarditis. (RA, rheumatoid arthritis; SLE, systemic lupus erythematosus.)

Chest X-ray

This is usually normal. If there is an associated pericardial effusion, the heart appears large and globular.

Management

The underlying cause is treated. NSAIDs relieve pain.

Clinical features of an associated pericardial effusion include signs of left and right heart failure. Pericardial tamponade means that the intrapericardial pressure increases, with reduced right heart filling and hypotension from reduced cardiac output. Clinically, there is hypotension, Kussmaul's sign (the JVP increases on inspiration), and muffled heart sounds (Beck's triad) plus pulsus paradoxus and tachycardia. The ECG may show low amplitude QRS complexes with electrical alternans. Echocardiography is diagnostic. Management is by pericardiocentesis.

Constrictive pericarditis

This is usually idiopathic or secondary to tuberculosis, although it may follow any cause of pericarditis. The heart is encased within a non-expansile pericardium. Clinically the signs are of right heart failure with ascites, hepatomegaly, and a raised JVP. There may be pulsus paradoxus, hypotension, and auscultation reveals a pericardial 'knock' due to an abrupt end to ventricular filling. The CXR may show pericardial calcification. Management is by pericardiectomy if constriction is severe.

Infective endocarditis

Infective endocarditis is an illness caused by microbial infection of the cardiac valves or endocardium. The annual incidence in the UK is approximately 7 in 10 000. It follows invasion of the bloodstream by micro-organisms from the mouth, gastrointestinal and genitourinary tracts, respiratory tract, or the skin. Platelets adhere to endothelial breaks and form 'vegetations', which are then colonised by circulating bacteria. Common sites of infection are bicuspid aortic valves and mitral valves with prolapse and regurgitation.

Prosthetic valve endocarditis is becoming increasingly important and may occur early postoperatively or late; 50% of patients have no previously known valve disease. In this group, endocarditis tends to follow a more acute course.

Streptococcus viridans is the commonest pathogen; others include *Streptococcus faecalis*, *Staphylococcus aureus*, and *Staphylococcus epidermidis*, especially in drug addicts.

Clinical features

The diagnosis should be suspected in a patient with fever and changing heart murmurs. The clinical features are:

- Infection: malaise and lassitude, sweats, myalgia, arthralgia, weight loss, finger clubbing, anaemia, and splenomegaly. Fever is often low grade.
- Heart disease: listen for murmurs. In tricuspid endocarditis the patient may be murmur free. The patient may present with embolic pneumonia, pleurisy or haemoptysis, or later with a raised venous pressure, jaundice and a pulsatile liver.
- Embolism: this is the most common cause of death in endocarditis. Most emboli are sterile but large fungal mycelia may embolise.
- Immunological phenomena: examples include vasculitic skin lesions, splinter haemorrhages, Roth spots in the retina, and Osler's nodes. They are classic signs of infective endocarditis but are often absent in cases detected relatively early.
- Urine: this is normal in uncomplicated endocarditis. There may be mild proteinuria resulting from fever, or haematuria as a result of embolism with infarction.

Investigations

Numerous sets of blood cultures from different sites at different times are the essential investigation. A positive culture confirms the diagnosis. Other investigations are only supportive.

Inflammatory markers

The erythrocyte sedimentation rate, CRP and white cell count are usually raised. There is a normochromic normocytic anaemia.

Chest X-ray

A CXR with right-sided endocarditis may show multiple shadows due to an embolic pneumonia with infarction.

Electrocardiography

The ECG may show changes of MI due to coronary embolism, or conduction defect due to the development of an aortic root abscess.

Echocardiography

Echocardiography may show vegetations or paravalvular abscess formation. A negative transthoracic echo does not exclude the diagnosis of endocarditis; transoesophageal echocardiography is preferred.

Management

Treatment should be started after blood has been taken for culture, but before obtaining confirmation of a positive culture, because valve destruction can occur rapidly and vegetations may grow and embolise.

Prophylaxis

Prophylactic antibiotics should be given before dental, genitourinary and gastrointestinal procedures for patients with heart valve lesions, septal defects, patent ductus, or prosthetic valves. For the exact regime, a local microbiologist should be consulted.

Treatment

Patients with endocarditis require a prolonged course of intravenous antibiotics. The exact regime depends on the positive cultures plus local resistance patterns. Benzylpenicillin and gentamicin plus flucloxacillin if *Staphylococcus aureus* is suspected is good empirical therapy. If the likelihood of penicillin resistance is high, vancomycin should be given.

Surgery

This is needed for haemodynamic complications with acute severe valvular regurgitation, for valve obstruction by vegetations, for intractable heart failure, cardiac abscess formation, and for resistant infections.

Culture-negative endocarditis

Possible causes of culture-negative endocarditis are given in Fig. 27.28. The addition of broad spectrum antifungal therapy is indicated if continuing sepsis is likely.

Acute rheumatic fever

Acute rheumatic fever is a multisystem immune disease following a group A, β-haemolytic,

---

Possible causes of endocarditis in the event of negative culture

- *Coxiella burnetii* (Q fever)
- Fungi, e.g. aspergillus, histoplasma
- Partially treated bacterial endocarditis
- Systemic lupus erythematosus
- Atrial myxoma
- Non-bacterial endocarditis associated with carcinoma

Fig. 27.28 Possible causes of endocarditis in the event of negative culture.

---

streptococcal infection. Antibodies generated against the bacteria also bind to and damage valvular tissue. The multisystem involvement reflects the vasculitic nature of the underlying disease. It is rare in the developed world due to use of antibiotics for pharyngeal infection. It usually affects children aged 5–15 years but no age or race is immune. Risk factors include crowding and low socio-economic status.

The diagnosis of acute rheumatic fever is based on clinical findings organised by the Jones criteria. The presence of two major or one major and two minor criteria indicates a high probability of rheumatic fever (Fig. 27.29). Evidence of a preceding streptococcal infection greatly strengthens the diagnosis of rheumatic fever.

Major Jones' criteria for rheumatic fever
Carditis (40–50%)

There may be myocarditis (tachypnoea, dyspnoea, pulmonary oedema), endocarditis (listen regularly for transient murmurs—the mitral valve is most commonly affected), or pericarditis (friction rub, effusion). It is more evident in children and may be asymptomatic or result in death in the acute stage, and it can lead to heart failure and chronic valvular heart disease (the classic exam cause of mitral stenosis).

Arthritis (80%)

This is the most common major criterion and usually presents as migratory joint pain affecting larger joints. The onset is sudden with signs of inflammation and

---

Revised Jones' criteria for guidance in the diagnosis of rheumatic fever	
Major criteria	Polyarthritis Carditis Chorea Erythema marginatum Subcutaneous nodules
Minor criteria	Fever Arthralgia Previous rheumatic fever or rheumatic heart disease Raised acute phase reactants (ESR, CRP, WCC) Prolonged PR interval in ECG

Fig. 27.29 Revised Jones' criteria for guidance in the diagnosis of rheumatic fever. For a diagnosis of rheumatic fever, there must also be supporting evidence of preceding streptococcal infection (i.e. increased antistreptolysin O or other streptococcal antibodies, positive throat culture for group A *Streptococcus*, or recent scarlet fever). (CRP, C reactive protein; ESR, erythrocyte sedimentation rate; WCC, white cell count.)

limitation of movement. It responds well to anti-inflammatory drugs and rarely leaves any residual deformity. Symptoms last for 3–6 weeks.

Sydenham's chorea (10%)
Movements are choreoathetoid and involuntary, involving mainly the face and limbs and may be unilateral. It is associated with emotional lability. There can be a latent period of 2–6 months. Symptoms last for approximately 6 months. It is commoner in girls. There may be no other signs of rheumatic fever.

Erythema marginatum (5%)
This is a painless rash appearing as large, pink macules that spread quickly to give a serpiginous edge with a fading centre.

Subcutaneous nodules (rare)
These are round, firm, and painless, ranging from 0.5–2 cm. They are mobile and occur mainly over bony prominences.

Diagnosis of streptococcal infection
Evidence of recent streptococcal infection should be sought and is indicated by either a positive throat swab, increased anti-streptolysin O or anti-DNAse B titres or recent scarlet fever.

Management
This is bed rest for 2 weeks. Painful joints immobilised. Anti-inflammatory drugs relieve the pain and swelling of joints and possibly the later development of valvular heart disease. Treatment is usually for 12 weeks, or longer for severe carditis.

Aspirin or a short course of corticosteroids in severe carditis are the drugs of choice. They reduce the arthritis though effectiveness in changing overall disease progression is lacking. Diazepam is given to control choreiform movements. Intramuscular penicillin G is given in the acute stages, and is followed by continued penicillin for 5 years to prevent recurrence in those patients with carditis.

Prognosis
The initial mortality rate is low at 1%. The long term risk is of structural valve disease, both stenosis and regurgitation. The mitral and pulmonary valves are the most and least affected respectively. Standard prophylaxis and management of valve disease applies.

Atrial myxoma
These are rare, benign, primary tumours usually in the left atrium, which are twice as common in women as men. They present with vague symptoms (e.g. fever, weight loss, general malaise, atrial fibrillation, left atrial obstruction, or systemic emboli). Auscultation may reveal a diastolic 'tumour plop'. The erythrocyte sedimentation rate is characteristically raised. They are diagnosed by echocardiography and treatment is by surgical excision.

Congenital heart disease
Ventricular septal defect
VSD is the most common congenital heart lesion, accounting for approximately one-third of all malformations. Blood moves from the high pressure left ventricle to the right ventricle. If the defect is large, pulmonary flow increases leading to obliterative pulmonary vascular changes and an increase in pulmonary vascular resistance. The pulmonary arterial pressure may then equal the systemic pressure, reducing or reversing the shunt, and central cyanosis may develop (Eisenmenger's syndrome).

Clinical features
A small defect (maladie de Roger) may cause no symptoms but there is a loud pansystolic murmur at the left sternal edge; it may close spontaneously. Larger VSDs produce dyspnoea and fatigue, and the pulse volume may be decreased. The apex beat is prominent due to left ventricular hypertrophy, and there may be a left parasternal heave if there is right ventricular hypertrophy (RVH) with pulmonary hypertension. There is a thrill at the left sternal edge, as well as a pansystolic murmur in the same place. A mitral diastolic flow murmur implies a large shunt.

Investigation
ECG can show no changes in small VSDs and features of right and left ventricular hypertrophy. Chest X-ray may be normal if the defect is small. Prominent pulmonary arteries are present in pulmonary hypertension. There may be left atrial and ventricular enlargement. Echocardiography is diagnostic if the defect can be imaged. Doppler studies identify abnormal flow across the septum. Cardiac catheterisation will show a step-up in oxygen saturation at the right ventricular level due to shunting of oxygenated blood from the left ventricle to the right ventricle. Left ventricular angiography produces opacification of the right ventricle through the defect.

Management
Antibiotic prophylaxis should be advised to prevent endocarditis. Moderate and large defects should be

closed surgically to prevent pulmonary hypertension and Eisenmenger's syndrome.

Atrial septal defect

Atrial septal defect (ASD) accounts for 10% of congenital heart defects, and is more common in women than men. There are two types: ostium secundum (the more common type) and ostium primum. The communication between the atria allows for left-to-right atrial shunting. Atrial arryhthmias are common. In ostium primum defects, there may be involvement of the mitral and tricuspid valves producing regurgitation.

Clinical features

Most patients are asymptomatic; a few have dyspnoea and weakness. The patient may have palpitations secondary to atrial arrhythmias, and right heart failure may develop later in life. Auscultation reveals wide, fixed splitting of the second heart sound. The increased right heart output gives rise to a pulmonary systolic flow murmur. There may be a tricuspid diastolic flow murmur with large defects. There may be a left parasternal heave of RVH.

Investigations

On ECG, there may be evidence of atrial arrhythmias (e.g. atrial fibrillation). In ostium secundum defects, there is right bundle branch block (RBBB), right axis deviation and RVH. In ostium primum defects, there is RBBB, left axis deviation, and RVH. Chest radiography shows prominent pulmonary arteries and the lung fields are plethoric. The right atrium and ventricles are enlarged. Echocardiography reveals dilatation of the right-sided cardiac chambers. Doppler studies allow visualisation of the left-to-right shunt across the atrial septum. Cardiac catheterisation demonstrates a step-up in oxygen saturation at the right atrial level due to shunting of oxygenated blood from the left atrium to the right atrium. The catheter can be directed across the defect into the left atrium.

Management

The defect should be closed surgically if the pulmonary/systemic flow ratio is greater than 2:1.

Patent ductus arteriosus

Patent ductus arteriosus (PDA) accounts for approximately 10% of congenital heart defects and is more common in women. The ductus arteriosus connects the pulmonary artery to the descending aorta but it should close off at birth. Because the aortic pressure is higher than the pulmonary artery pressure throughout the cardiac cycle, the PDA produces continuous shunting from the aorta to the pulmonary artery, leading to increased pulmonary venous return to the left heart and an increased left ventricular volume load.

Clinical features

There are usually no symptoms. Large defects lead to left ventricular failure with dyspnoea. The pulse is collapsing. There may be left ventricular hypertrophy. There is a continuous 'machinery' murmur with systolic accentuation loudest in the first or second left intercostal space.

Investigations

Electrocardiography shows features of left atrial and left ventricular hypertrophy and on chest X-ray the aorta and pulmonary arteries are prominent. The lung fields are plethoric. At echocardiography, there is dilatation of the left-sided cardiac chambers and doppler studies identify the abnormal flow across the ductus. Cardiac catheterisation demonstrates a step-up in oxygen saturation at pulmonary artery level. The catheter can sometimes be passed across the ductus into the descending aorta.

Management

Indomethacin given within the first few days of birth may stimulate duct closure by inhibiting prostaglandin synthesis. If this fails, the duct can be ligated surgically or with an umbrella occlusion device. Antibiotic prophylaxis is advised.

Coarctation of the aorta

This accounts for 5–7% of congenital heart defects. It is twice as common in men, and is associated with Turner's syndrome, Marfan's syndrome and berry aneurysms. There is a narrowing of the aorta at or just distal to the ductus arteriosus; the vast majority are distal to the origin of the left subclavian artery. The condition is a cause of secondary hypertension. It encourages the formation of a collateral arterial circulation involving the intercostal arteries. In 30% of patients, there is an associated bicuspid aortic valve.

Clinical features

In adults, the condition is often asymptomatic until long standing hypertension becomes apparent. When present, symptoms include headache, left ventricular failure, stroke, and endocarditis. On examination, the femoral pulses are weak or absent, and there is radiofemoral delay. The upper limbs may be hypertensive or have unequal blood pressure, and the lower limbs have a low pressure. There may be features of LVH. There is a mid- or late systolic murmur over the upper praecordium or back due to turbulent flow through the coarctation. Collateral murmurs may be heard over the scapulae and there may be an aortic systolic murmur of an associated bicuspid valve.

Investigation

There may be LVH on ECG, and chest radiography shows tortuous and dilated collaterals that may erode the undersurface of the ribs to produce 'rib notching'. There maybe a double aortic knuckle due to stenosis and poststenotic dilatation. Cardiomegaly may indicate left ventricular enlargement. Aortography confirms the diagnosis.

Management

Antibiotic prophylaxis should be advised. Treatment is by surgical resection. Angioplasty is an alternative.

Fallot's tetralogy

This represents 6–10% of cases of congenital heart disease. The four features comprising the tetrad are as follows:
- VSD.
- Right ventricular outflow obstruction (pulmonary stenosis-infundibular or valvar).
- The aorta is positioned over the ventricular septum ('over-riding aorta').
- RVH.

Because there is right ventricular outflow obstruction, the shunt through the VSD is from right to left. This results in central cyanosis.

Clinical features

Children may present with deep cyanosis and syncope. Squatting helps to decrease the right-to-left shunt by increasing systemic resistance. Signs include cyanosis and finger clubbing. There is a parasternal heave and systolic murmur in the pulmonary area (second left intercostal space), P_2 is soft or absent, and there may be growth retardation.

Investigation

ECG features include right atrial and ventricular hypertrophy. The heart is boot shaped ('coeur en sabot') and the pulmonary artery is small with oligaemic lung fields. Echocardiography can be diagnostic but it may be necessary to proceed to cardiac catheterisation studies to confirm the diagnosis.

Management

This is by total surgical correction. There are palliative procedures for the very young as holding measures (e.g. the Blalock shunt), which is anastamosis of a subclavian artery to a pulmonary artery to increase pulmonary blood flow.

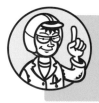 The two most likely murmurs in examinations will be aortic stenosis and mitral regurgitation

- List the most important risk factors for ischaemic heart disease.
- How is the management of ST elevation MI different to non ST elevation MI?
- What drugs are of use for a patient with stable angina in an outpatient clinic?
- What are the ECG characteristics of atrial fibrillation and how do you treat it?
- How has the drug treatment of heart failure changed in the last ten years?
- Which drugs improve survival in systolic heart failure?
- How do you combine drugs to treat hypertension?
- Which class of drug would be best for diabetic patients with hypertension and proteinuria?
- Is valve replacement indicated for all patients with aortic stenosis?
- What is the significance of the onset of left ventricular failure for a patient with aortic regurgitation?
- 'Splinter haemorrhages' indicate what? Do you think a urine dipstick test is indicated?

Further reading

Al-Obaidi, Siva and Noble 2004 *Crash course in Cardiology*, 2nd edn. Mosby

The American College of Cardiology publishes guidelines and reviews on all aspects of cardiology. They are available on its website *www.acc.org*

The British Hypertension Society publishes the UK guidelines on the management of hypertension in the UK. They are available on its website *www.bhsoc.org*

Brown M J, Cruickshank J K, Dominiczak A F et al 2003 Better blood pressure control: how to combine drugs. *Journal of Human Hypertension* **17**: 81–86

Hampton J R 2003 *The ECG made easy* 6th edition Churchill Livingstone

Jessup M and Brozena S 2003 Medical progress: Heart failure. *N Engl J Med* **348**: 2007–2018

Swanton R H 2003 *Cardiology – Pocket Consultant* Blackwell Scientific

Randomised trial of intravenous streptokinase, oral aspirin, both or neither among 17,187 cases of suspected acute myocardial infarction: ISIS-2. *Lancet* 1988; **2**: 349–360

Randomised trial of cholesterol lowering in 4444 patients with coronary heart disease: the Scandinavian Simvastatin Survival Study (4S). *Lancet* 1994; **344**: 1383–1389

Ross R 1999 Atherosclerosis – An Inflammatory Disease. *N Engl J Med* **340**: 115–123

Wang K, Asinger R W, Marriott H J 2003 ST segment elevation in conditions other than acute myocardial infarction. *N Engl J Med* **349**: 2128–2135

Zimetbaum P and Josephson M E 1998 Evaluation of patients with palpitations. *N Engl J Med* **338**: 1369–1373

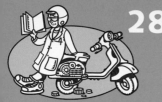

28. Respiratory Disease

Asthma

Introduction

Asthma is a disease of the airways characterised by an increased responsiveness of the tracheobronchial tree to many different stimuli, resulting in variable airflow limitation. It manifests as paroxysms of shortness of breath, cough, chest tightness and wheeze. These symptoms may resolve spontaneously or be relieved by treatment.

Asthma is episodic with acute exacerbations interspersed by symptom-free periods. Typically, most attacks are short (minutes to hours) and, clinically, the patient appears to recover completely after an attack.

In more severe asthma, patients can experience some degree of airway obstruction daily with accompanying symptoms.

Incidence

Asthma is common and occurs in approximately 5% of the population in most Western countries. This figure appears to be increasing for reasons that remain uncertain. Bronchial asthma occurs at all ages but peaks in childhood and is more common in boys. However, in adult asthma, the sex ratio is approximately equal by the age of 30 years. In the UK, 1000–2000 people die from acute asthma attacks every year.

Aetiology

It is helpful to classify asthma by the main factors associated with acute episodes (i.e. into allergic asthma and intrinsic asthma).

Allergic asthma is often associated with a personal or family history of allergy such as hay fever, urticaria, and eczema. There may also be increased levels of immunoglobulin (Ig) E in the serum, and a positive response to provocation tests (e.g. methacholine challenge).

Intrinsic (or idiosyncratic) asthma is a term used to define those patients presenting with no personal or family history of allergy, with negative skin tests, and with normal serum levels of IgE. Many develop typical symptoms following an upper respiratory infection, which, after several days, leads to paroxysms of wheezing and shortness of breath that can last for months.

In general, asthma that occurs in childhood, or early adult life, tends to have a strong allergic component, whereas asthma that develops late tends to be non-allergic.

Despite this, many patients do not fit into either category but fall into a group with a mixture of allergic and non-allergic features.

Pathophysiology

Many theories have been proposed to explain the increased airway reactivity of asthma but the basic mechanism remains unknown.

The relationship between atopy and environment in the airway inflammation of asthma is uncertain. Many theories and mediators are proposed as the mechanisms for asthma. The role of IgE, various cytokines and chemokines, mast cells and histamine, eosinophils and leukotrienes, cell adhesion molecules and activated T lymphocytes—in particular the balance between Th1 and Th2 cells—provides much academic debate.

It has provided potential new therapeutic targets as monoclonal antibodies against IgE and soluble interleukin-4 receptor have been studied in patients.

The clinical features of asthma probably derive from chronic airway inflammation causing denuded airway epithelium, inflammatory cell infiltrate, mast cell activation plus smooth muscle and mucus gland hypertrophy. Acute events produce an intense immediate inflammatory reaction involving bronchoconstriction, vascular congestion, and oedema formation—the pathological hallmarks of asthma.

A number of factors interact with normal airway responsiveness and provoke acute episodes including:

- Allergens (e.g. house dust mites and animal dander).
- Drugs (e.g. β-blockers and non-steroidal anti-inflammatory drugs). The concerns over cardioselective β_1-blockers are probably overestimated.
- The environment (e.g. climatic conditions and air pollution).

- Occupations (e.g. exposure to industrial chemicals, drugs, metals, dusts).
- Infections (e.g. viral and bacterial).
- Exercise.
- Emotion.
- Cigarette smoke.

Clinical features of asthma

The classic symptoms of asthma consist of shortness of breath, chest tightness, cough, and wheezing. In its most typical form, asthma is an episodic disease, and the symptoms coexist.

At the onset of an attack, patients experience a sense of constriction in the chest, often with a non-productive cough. Breathing becomes audibly harsh, speech is difficult, wheezing in both phases of respiration becomes prominent, expiration becomes prolonged as airflow is reduced, and patients frequently have both tachypnoea and tachycardia. If the attack is severe or prolonged, there may be a loss of breath sounds, and the wheeze becomes either very high-pitched or inaudible as airflow is severely compromised. Accessory muscles of respiration are used and pulsus paradoxus can develop.

Less typically, a patient with asthma may present with intermittent episodes of non-productive cough or shortness of breath on exertion. These patients often have a normal physical examination but may wheeze after repeated forced exhalations or may show evidence of airways obstruction with spirometry. Occasionally, a provocation test may be required to make the diagnosis of airway hyper-responsiveness.

Confirming the diagnosis of asthma

Diagnosing asthma is usually not difficult, especially if the patient is seen during an acute attack. In addition, a history of episodic symptoms and a history of eczema, hay fever, or urticaria is valuable. Nocturnal symptoms (e.g. awakening short of breath, coughing or wheezing) are very common features.

Investigations

When well these can be absolutely normal. The diagnosis of asthma is established by demonstrating reversible airways obstruction. Reversibility is traditionally defined as a 15% or greater increase in the forced expiratory volume in 1 second (FEV1) following administration of a β_2-agonist or a greater than 20% diurnal variation on more than 3 days in a week for 2 weeks in a peak expiratory flow rate diary. Peak flow diary may be combined with a two week trial of oral prednisolone. Once the diagnosis is

confirmed, peak expiratory flow rates (PEFR) at home, or the FEV1 in the clinic, can be used to monitor the course of the illness and the effectiveness of therapy. Sputum and blood eosinophilia and measurement of serum IgE levels may be helpful but are not specific for asthma. Similarly, a chest X-ray (CXR) showing hyperinflation is not diagnostic of asthma.

 Causes of a 'coin' lesion on chest X-ray include malignancy, hamartoma, abscess, carcinoid, granuloma, foreign body or a mass outside the thorax

Differential diagnosis

In a small minority of patients the diagnosis can cause some difficulty and differential diagnoses should be considered:

- Upper airway obstruction: tumour or laryngeal oedema.
- Endobronchial disease (e.g. foreign body aspiration, neoplasm, bronchial stenosis).
- Left ventricular failure.
- Carcinoid tumours.
- Recurrent pulmonary emboli.
- Chronic obstructive pulmonary disease (COPD).
- Eosinophilic pneumonias.
- Systemic vasculitis with pulmonary involvement.

Management of asthma

Chronic asthma requires long term management. Ideally, the model of care that characterises all chronic diseases should be applied (i.e. patient education and empowerment, pharmacological therapy and liaison between different professional groups in hospital and the community).

The therapeutic targets of medications used for asthma include:

- Drugs that inhibit smooth muscle contraction (e.g. β_2-agonists, anticholinergics and methylxanthines such as theophylline).
- Drugs that prevent or reverse airway inflammation (e.g. corticosteroids and mast cell stabilising agents).
- Drugs that modify the action of leukotrienes (e.g. leukotriene antagonists or 5-lipoxygenase inhibitors).

In clinical practice, the two most common settings in which patients require treatment are emergency treatment of acute severe asthma and chronic therapy.

Chronic therapy

This is aimed at achieving a stable, asymptomatic state with the best pulmonary function possible and recognising and treating exacerbations appropriately whilst limiting quality of life as little as possible. The first step is to educate patients to function as partners in their management. The severity of the illness needs to be assessed and monitored with objective measures of lung function (PEFR diaries). Asthma triggers should be avoided or controlled, and plans should be made for both chronic management and treatment of exacerbations. Regular follow-up care is mandatory. This should involve doctors, both in hospital and general practitioners, asthma specialist nurses, pharmacists and physiotherapists.

Drug therapy should be kept as simple as possible. Many patients find the division of drugs into 'preventers' and 'relievers' useful to understand their disease and its treatment.

There is consensus worldwide that the stepwise management of asthma is effective. In the UK guidelines are produced by the British Thoracic Society (Fig. 28.1). Treatment is stepped up when symptoms (e.g. nocturnal wakening, exercise induced asthma, morning dips) are not controlled. Short acting β_2-agonists are the first step and then long acting β_2-agonists, inhaled steroid, anticholinergics, oral steroids, leukotriene modifiers and theophyllines added in varying combinations. When control is obtained, the treatment should be reduced to the lowest feasible level.

The PEFR should be monitored and treatment adjusted accordingly, particularly when corroborated by the patient's symptoms.

Emergency treatment

Emergency treatment of acute asthma is one of the most common emergencies seen in medical practice and its life-threatening nature can be underestimated by the less experienced. Senior help should be involved earlier rather than later.

Features indicating severe airway obstruction include the inability to speak in sentences, tachypnoea, tachycardia, much reduced PEFR, poor oxygen saturations, the use of accessory muscles, and marked hyperinflation of the thorax with absent breath sounds, cyanosis, absence of wheeze and a tiring patient. Failure of these signs to remit promptly after aggressive therapy requires objective monitoring of the patient using measurements of arterial blood gases (ABGs) and the PEFR or FEV1.

A checklist for the assessment and treatment of these patients is shown in Fig. 28.2.

Stepped-care plan for the management of chronic asthma	
Step	Measures
1 Mild intermittent asthma	Inhaled short acting β_2 agonist as required.
2 Regular preventer therapy	Start inhaled steroid regularly.
3 Add-on therapy	Add long acting β_2 agonist regularly. Increase dose of regular inhaled steroid. Add third medication, theophylline or leukotriene modifying drugs.
4 Persistent poor control	Trial of high dose of regular inhaled steroid. Addition of medications not used in step 3 and consider oral β_2 agonist.
5 Oral steroid	Add lowest dose of oral steroid to achieve control of symptoms. Continue maximum dose inhaled steroid. Must be under care of a respiratory physician.

Fig. 28.1 Stepped-care plan for the management of chronic asthma (after British Thoracic Society). Treatment is started at the step most appropriate to initial severity, and a 'rescue' course of prednisolone can be given at any time and with any step to cover an exacerbation. Move up the ladder if relief bronchodilators are needed frequently or night-time symptoms occur. Check compliance and inhaler technique, and consider the use of spacer devices.

Generally, there is a direct correlation between the severity of the obstruction with which the patient presents and the time it takes to resolve it. If the patient is drowsy, not tachypnoeic, making little respiratory effort with a silent chest (no wheeze) and a normal pCO_2, they are NOT improving and, in fact, respiratory arrest may be imminent and intubation and intensive care are required.

Chronic obstructive pulmonary disease

COPD is a term used to cover several distinct entities including both chronic bronchitis and emphysema. It is defined by airflow limitation with a reduced FEV1 less than 80% predicted, together with a FEV1 to forced vital capacity (FVC) ratio of less than 70% and limited reversibility. It can be difficult to differentiate from chronic adult onset asthma. It will provide a significant proportion of the junior doctors' on call workload and 10–15% of general medical 'take' admissions.

Definitions
Chronic bronchitis
Chronic bronchitis is a condition associated with excessive mucus production sufficient to cause cough with sputum for at least 3 months of the year for more than two consecutive years, in the absence of another condition known to cause sputum production.

Emphysema
Emphysema is defined as the permanent, abnormal distension of the air spaces distal to the terminal bronchiole with destruction of alveolar septa. It is ultimately a histological diagnosis.

Pathophysiology
The hallmark of chronic bronchitis is hypertrophy of the mucus-producing glands found in the submucosa of large cartilaginous airways. In lungs studied at post-mortem, there is goblet cell hyperplasia, mucosal and submucosal inflammatory cells, oedema, peribronchial fibrosis, intraluminal mucus plugs, and increased smooth muscle in small airways.

Inflammation in chronic bronchitis occurs at the alveolar epithelium and differs from the predominantly eosinophilic inflammation of asthma by the predominance of T-lymphocytes and neutrophils.

Emphysema is classified according to the pattern of involvement of the gas-exchanging units (acini) of the lung distal to the terminal bronchiole. With centriacinar emphysema, the distension and destruction is mainly limited to the respiratory bronchioles with relatively less change peripherally in the acinus; these are the changes found in smokers. They are more prominent in the upper lobes. Panacinar emphysema involves both the central and peripheral portions of the acinus; these changes are those seen in α_1-antitrypsin deficiency and occur more commonly in the lower lobes.

When emphysema is severe, with large emphysematous 'bullous' air spaces, it may be difficult to distinguish between the two types because, most often, they coexist in the same lung.

The chronic airflow limitation which is the hallmark of COPD is a consequence of small airways disease. The airways collapse in expiration due to the loss of elastic recoil and radial traction to balance the positive transmural pressure. This limits airflow and results in the air trapping and hyperinflation seen on CXR and lung function tests.

Aetiology of chronic bronchitis and emphysema
Cigarette smoking
Cigarette smoking is the most commonly identified factor associated with both chronic bronchitis during life and extent of emphysema at post-mortem. Prolonged cigarette smoking impairs ciliary movement, inhibits function of alveolar macrophages, and leads to hypertrophy and hyperplasia of mucus-secreting glands. It is probable that smoke also inhibits antiproteases and causes polymorphonuclear leukocytes to release elastase.

α_1-Antitrypsin deficiency
Patients homozygous for a deficiency of the protease inhibitor α_1-antitrypsin have a greatly increased incidence of emphysema. The gene is on chromosome 14 and the defect is in release from the liver where it is synthesised. Patients with the ZZ genotype having blood levels of 10% of those of normal subjects. They are also at risk of chronic liver disease.

The importance of heterozygosity for this condition in patients, both smokers and non-smokers, is yet to be fully established. Nevertheless, it would seem prudent to advise against smoking.

Air pollution
Air pollution with particulate matter is associated with exacerbations of chronic bronchitis, and the incidence and mortality rates for chronic bronchitis

Assessment and treatment of acute severe asthma	
Tasks to consider	Comment
Assessment	Clinical features indicating severe attack: • Inability to speak sentences in one breath. • Respiratory rate > 25 min⁻¹. • Heart rate > 110 min⁻¹. • Peak flow rate < 50% best or predicted. Features indicating life threatening attack: • Peak flow rate < 33% best or predicted. • Oxygen saturation < 92%. • pO_2 < 8 kPa. • pCO_2 normal or high. • Cyanosis. • Poor respiratory effort and silent chest. • Confusion, coma or exhaustion. • Pulsus paradoxus.
Immediate treatment	High concentration oxygen. Saturations > 92%. Frequent nebulised salbutamol. (2.5–5 mg) with ipratropium bromide (0.5 mg qds) if severe attack. Use oxygen driven nebulisers if possible. Systemic corticosteroids. (Hydrocortisone 200 mg i.v. or prednisolone 40 mg orally). Magnesium sulphate intravenously as a bronchodilator (1.2–2g i.v. over 20 mins). Intravenous bronchodilators (aminophylline or salbutamol).
Criteria for hospital admission	Any life threatening attack All severe attacks which do not respond to initial treatment. If peak flow > 75% best one hour after treatment consider discharge from A & E. Consider short stay observation wards for other patients.
Referral to intensive care	Persisting or worsening hypoxia. Worsening peak flow despite treatment. Exhaustion, poor respiratory effort. Hypercapnia or acidosis on ABG. Coma or respiratory arrest.
Further investigations	CXR (not routine): • if severe or life threatening attack. • if other pathology is considered. FBC, U&Es, ECG (older patients).
Duration of hospital stay	Until symptoms and lung function stable. Peak flow > 75% best or predicted. Peak flow diurnal variation < 25%. No nocturnal symptoms.
Drugs on discharge	Oral steroids for 1–3 weeks. Inhaled steroid therapy. Inhaled short acting β2 agonist. Other medications as per stepwise plan.
Treatment changes on discharge	On inhaled medications (no nebulisers) for 24–48 hours prior to discharge. Inhaler technique reviewed. Appropriate life style advice given. Clinic follow up arranged. Patient action plan to promote self management. Drug level monitoring if needed.

Fig. 28.2 Checklist for the emergency assessment and treatment of asthma. (ABG, arterial blood gases; CXR, chest X-ray; ECG, electrocardiogram; FBC, full blood count; pCO_2, partial pressure of carbon dioxide; pO_2, partial pressure of oxygen; U&Es, urea and electrolytes.)

and emphysema are probably higher in heavily industrialised urban areas.

Occupation

Occupations exposing workers to inorganic or organic dusts, or to noxious gases, result in a higher prevalence of chronic bronchitis among employees.

Acute respiratory infections

These have been hypothesised as a factor associated with both the aetiology and progression of COPD.

199

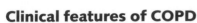

Clinical features of COPD

The clinical presentation of COPD varies in severity from mild airflow limitation without disability to patients with severe disability and chronic respiratory failure. In clinical practice, it is usual to encounter patients with significant COPD. Though most patients will have features of both chronic bronchitis and emphysema, it is traditional to categorise patients as having predominant features of one or other. The usefulness of such classification is limited in clinical practice.

Management of COPD

The management of patients with COPD is based on knowledge of the degree of obstruction, the extent of disability, and any reversibility of the patient's illness.

The extent of the airways obstruction and the potential to reverse this is key as there is a chance that treatment may be effective in improving the overall disability.

Emphysema, however, is an irreversible process and so the prevention of its progression and the avoidance of acute infections are the main approach to management.

Investigations

History, physical examination, and chest radiography should be supplemented by tests of lung function performed during a chronic stable period. Spirometry is essential for diagnosis. In severe disease spirometry, lung volumes, transfer factor and ABGs should be measured. Reversibility should be assessed by spirometry after the administration of bronchodilators.

Long term treatment of COPD

Treatment strategies for COPD are varied and a multidisciplinary approach to the patient is often required. A treatment plan should consider:
- Stopping cigarette smoking.
- Education of the patient about their disease.
- Optimising reversible airflow limitation.
- Treatment of acute exacerbations.
- Treatment of cor pulmonale, if appropriate.
- Home oxygen therapy, when indicated. Domiciliary non-invasive ventilation (NIV) if indicated.
- Nutritional and psychological support.
- Pulmonary rehabilitation.

Smoking cessation

This remains the most important intervention by the health care team to modify the natural course of the disease. It should be reinforced repeatedly. Help from smoking cessation specialists and pharmacological assistance with nicotine replacement or bupropion may improve effectiveness.

Bronchodilators

These are important in symptom relief from COPD, although there is little evidence that they provide long-term survival or lung function benefit. They are commonly given to most patients regardless of objective reversible airflow obstruction. They reduce dynamic hyperinflation and dyspnoea. Patients may still find them useful for symptom relief and often become psychologically attached to them. They include:
- Short acting β-agonists (e.g. salbutamol and terbutaline).

Fig. 28.3 Clinical features to help differentiate COPD and asthma.

Clinical features to help differentiate COPD and asthma		
Features	**COPD**	**Asthma**
Smoker or ex-smoker	Nearly all	Possibly
Chronic productive cough	Common	Uncommon
Symptoms at age < 35	Rare	Often
Dyspnoea	Persistent and progressive	Variable
Nocturnal waking with cough or breathlessness	Uncommon	Common
Significant diurnal or day to day variability of symptoms	Uncommon	Common

- Long acting β-agonists (e.g. salmeterol and formoterol).
- Anticholinergics [e.g. ipratropium and tiotropium (a long-acting once daily drug)].
- Theophyllines.

Corticosteroids

Inhaled corticosteroids in patients whose FEVI is < 50% predicted may reduce airway inflammation, symptoms and reduce exacerbations. They do not alter FEV1 and decline in lung function. Fluticasone and budesonide are examples. Combined use with a long acting β-agonist may be preferred.

Oral steroids are used in exacerbations of COPD and some patients take them long term; this should be discouraged.

Pulmonary rehabilitation

This improves symptoms, exacerbations and can increase exercise ability.

Domicillary oxygen therapy

Many patients have oxygen at home and derive symptomatic relief from it. Long term (>15 hours per day) oxygen use is to be recommended in certain COPD patients as it has a survival benefit. They include:
- Stable non smokers with pO_2 <7.3 kPa and FEV1 <1.5 l.
- Stable non smokers with pO_2 between 7.3 and 8.0 kPa and pulmonary hypertension.

Both groups need repeat blood gases to check that the pCO_2 is stable with oxygen supplementation.

Surgery

Some patients may be suitable for bullectomy or lung volume reduction surgery to improve symptoms. In end-stage disease, lung transplantation is a rare option for some patients.

Other therapies

There is little evidence to suggest that prophylactic antibiotics, either systemic or nebulised alter disease progression or prevent exacerbations. Vaccination against influenza and pneumococcal pneumonia should be offered in patients with COPD. Regular assessment of nutritional and psychological status is recommended.

Acute exacerbation of COPD

This is common and is often ascribed to either a bacterial or viral aetiology though frequently no cause is found. Treatments include nebulised β-agonists, anticholinergics, systemic steroids, controlled oxygen to maintain saturations >90%, chest physiotherapy and theophylline if appropriate. Endotracheal intubation is indicated for severe respiratory failure if a reversible pathology is thought present.

NIV has recently been shown to be extremely effective in certain patients with acute type 2 respiratory failure such as COPD with a benefit over intubation. This may be as a consequence of avoiding the side effects of mechanical ventilation rather than NIV *per se*.

Acute exacerbation of COPD may require admission to hospital. Some less severe patients are managed at home by an intensive community team. This reduces admission rates and the burden on the secondary care provider whilst promoting independence and self-reliance for the patient.

Prognosis

This remains poor, with considerable symptomatic discomfort as the disease process and lung dysfunction become more severe. Only smoking cessation and long term oxygen therapy can be recommended as improving survival at present. Other treatments are aimed at symptom relief only.

Tuberculosis

Tuberculosis (TB) is a chronic granulomatous disease caused by a cell-mediated immune response to bacteria belonging to the *Mycobacterium tuberculosis* complex. The disease usually affects the lungs, although in up to a third of cases other organs are involved. If properly treated, TB caused by drug-susceptible strains is curable in virtually all cases. Transmission usually takes place through the airborne spread of droplets produced by patients with infectious pulmonary TB.

The pathogenic species belonging to the *M. tuberculosis* complex, the most frequent and important agent of human disease is *M. tuberculosis* itself. Closely related organisms that can also infect humans include *Mycobacterium bovis* (the bovine tubercle bacillus, once an important cause of TB transmitted by unpasteurised milk).

Notification of TB in UK, from PHLS	
Year	Notification
1920	73332
1930	67401
1940	46572
1950	49358
1960	23605
1970	11901
1980	9142
1990	5204
1995	5606
2000	6572
2002	6891

Fig. 28.4 Number of notifications for tuberculosis in the UK, from Public Health Laboratory Services.

Mycobacterium tuberculosis is a rod-shaped, non-spore-forming, aerobic bacterium measuring 0.5-3 μm. Though strictly Gram-positive, it may not stain readily and is often neutral on the Gram stain. However, once stained, the bacilli cannot be decolourised by acid alcohol, a characteristic justifying their classification as acid alcohol-fast bacilli (AAFB).

In most developed countries the incidence of TB fell until the 1980s. Since then, it has settled and is now increasing in the UK (Fig. 28.4). It is due to an increase in susceptible groups. These include the elderly, immigrants, people from ethnic minorities, alcoholics, the homeless and immunocompromised groups (both iatrogenic and pathologic; HIV is the most important group of the latter).

Clinical manifestations of tuberculosis

TB is usually classified as pulmonary or extrapulmonary. Before human immunodeficiency virus (HIV) infection, 80% of all cases of TB were limited to the lungs, but now two-thirds of HIV-infected patients with TB may have both pulmonary and extrapulmonary disease, or even extrapulmonary disease on its own.

Pulmonary tuberculosis

Pulmonary TB can be classified as primary or post primary (secondary).

Primary pulmonary tuberculosis

Primary pulmonary TB results from an initial infection with tubercle bacilli. It is commonly asymptomatic. Where TB has a high prevalence, primary disease is often seen in children and is localised to the middle and lower lung zones. The lesion is usually peripheral and associated with hilar or paratracheal lymph node enlargement. In most cases, immunity develops, the lesion heals spontaneously and may later be seen as a small calcified nodule (Ghon focus).

Patients with impaired immunity who develop primary pulmonary TB may progress rapidly to clinical illness. This may result from spread of infection by:

- Pleural effusion: which may lead to tuberculous empyema.
- Necrosis and acute cavitation of the primary lesion: known as progressive primary TB.
- Bloodstream dissemination: resulting in granulomatous lesions in various organs, or even miliary TB with tuberculous meningitis.

Post primary pulmonary tuberculosis

Post primary disease is sometimes termed adult, reactivation, or secondary TB. It results from reactivation of latent infection due to any form of debility or immunocompromise and is usually localised to the apical and posterior segments of the upper lobes. The extent of lung changes can vary from small infiltrates to extensive cavitation. Widespread involvement of the lung with coalescing lesions produces tuberculous pneumonia.

The pathogenicity of TB varies, with a third of untreated patients dying from severe pulmonary TB within weeks or months, while the rest undergo spontaneous remission or proceed along a chronic course often involving lung fibrosis.

Symptoms and signs

Symptoms and signs of early pulmonary TB are often non-specific and include fever, night sweats, weight loss, anorexia, and lethargy. Most patients eventually develop cough with purulent sputum and this may be associated with haemoptysis. Pleuritic chest pain can develop in patients with subpleural lesions or from muscle strain due to persistent coughing. Clinical examination can be of limited use in pulmonary TB but the following features can be present:

- Crepitations: involved areas during inspiration.
- Wheeze: partial bronchial obstruction.

- Classical amphoric breath sounds: areas with large cavities.

Extrapulmonary tuberculosis

This most commonly involves lymph nodes, the pleura, genitourinary tract, bones and joints, meninges and peritoneum.

Diagnostic tests for tuberculosis

The key to the diagnosis of TB is a high index of suspicion especially in at risk groups. It should form part of the differential diagnosis in patients with febrile illnesses, cervical lymphadenopathy, or patients with focal infiltrates on CXR.

The CXR may show the typical picture of upper lobe infiltrates, with or without cavitation. The diagnosis is commonly based on the finding of AAFB by microscopy of a diagnostic specimen such as sputum or tissue (e.g. lymph node biopsy). Laboratory identification depends on either auramine staining and fluorescence microscopy or the more traditional light microscopy of specimens using the Ziehl–Nielsen stain.

Patients with suspected pulmonary TB normally require three sputum specimens for AAFB smear and mycobacterial culture and sensitivity. Specimens are inoculated on to Lowenstein–Jensen medium. Most species of mycobacteria, including *M. tuberculosis*, are slow-growing so that 4–8 weeks may be required before growth is detected and antibiotic sensitivity can be assessed. Newer molecular biological techniques can confirm *M. tuberculosis* more quickly and give drug sensitivities.

Other diagnostic tests for pulmonary TB include:
- Induced sputum by ultrasonic nebulisation of hypertonic saline for patients unable to produce a sputum specimen spontaneously.
- Fibre-optic bronchoscopy with bronchial lavage or transbronchial biopsy (especially with miliary TB).

When extrapulmonary TB is suspected, specimens of involved sites may include:
- Cerebrospinal fluid: tuberculous meningitis.
- Pleural fluid and biopsy samples: pleural disease.
- Bone marrow and liver biopsy culture: good diagnostic yield in disseminated (miliary) TB.
- Early morning urine: renal TB.

In all cases specimens are sent for AAFB microscopy, stain and culture.

Positive tuberculin testing indicates exposure to mycobacteria or vaccination and not active disease per se and is best used in contact tracing and public health screening. The Mantoux and Heaf tests are the two most common methods. They involve intradermal injection of purified protein derivative (PPD) and then observation of the response.

False negatives are possible in active TB especially in miliary TB or if immunosuppressed e.g. HIV (a defect in cell mediated immunity).

Treatment

Uncomplicated TB is treated in the initial phase using at least three drugs for 2 months (rifampicin, isoniazid and pyrazinamide) then a continuation phase using two drugs (rifampicin and isoniazid) for another four months. If drug resistant TB is suspected, ethambutol should be included until sensitivities are known. Treatment of extrapulmonary and drug resistant TB requires specialist involvement. Pyridoxine is usually started to minimise the neurological side effects of isoniazid.

Second-line drugs available for infections caused by resistant organisms, or when first-line drugs cause unacceptable side-effects, include cycloserine, newer macrolides (e.g. clarithromycin), and quinolones (e.g. ciprofloxacin and ofloxacin).

TB is 'notifiable'; you should contact the appropriate public health authorities for contact tracing.

If adherence to treatment is a possible issue, then directly observed therapy in which medications are taken three times per week under supervision should be employed.

Not all patients with TB need to be isolated. All patients with suspected drug resistant TB should be isolated. Most hospitals would also isolate patients with TB positive sputum until 2 weeks of effective treatment has been given. Care should be taken to ensure TB patients do not come into contact with immunocompromised patients.

Monitoring treatment

Isoniazid, rifampicin, and pyrazinamide are associated with liver toxicity, and therefore hepatic function should be checked before treatment with these drugs. Renal function should also be checked before treatment with antituberculous drugs and appropriate dosage adjustments made. Visual acuity should be tested before ethambutol is used because it can cause loss of visual acuity and visual field defects. All TB should be treated by a specialist, usually a respiratory physician.

Control of tuberculosis

By far the best way to prevent TB is the rapid diagnosis of infectious cases with appropriate treatment until cure. Additional strategies include Bacillus Calmette–Guérin (BCG) vaccination and preventive chemotherapy.

Vaccination

BCG was derived from an attenuated strain of *M. bovis* and was first administered to humans in 1921. Many BCG vaccines are now available worldwide, and all are derived from the original strain, but the vaccines vary in efficacy. The vaccine is safe and rarely causes serious complications. It should not be given to HIV positive patients.

BCG vaccination induces PPD reactivity, but the magnitude of PPD skin test reactions after vaccination does not predict the degree of protection afforded. Currently, vaccination is recommended only for PPD-negative infants and children who are at a high risk of intimate and prolonged exposure to patients with TB and who cannot take prophylactic isoniazid. In the UK, BCG is offered to PPD-negative children at the age of 12 years.

Preventive chemotherapy

A major component of TB control involves contact tracing, skin testing, and the administration of isoniazid to contacts at high risk of active disease.

Treatment of lung cancer is different for small cell versus non-small cell cancers

Lung cancer

Lung cancer is the most common malignant disease in first world countries. In the UK, 40 000 new cases are diagnosed every year. More people die from lung cancer than colon, breast and prostate cancer combined. The term 'lung cancer' is usually reserved for primary tumours arising from the respiratory epithelium (bronchi, bronchioles, and alveoli) rather than metastases from distant malignancies. Four major cell types make up 90% of all primary lung neoplasms:

- Squamous cell carcinoma. (35–45%). From the large airways, it grows slowly and spreads late.
- Adenocarcinoma (including bronchioloalveolar cell carcinoma) (20–30%). Peripheral and more common in non-smokers.
- Large cell (anaplastic) carcinoma. (5–10%). Heterogeneous group of undifferentiated tumours.
- Small cell (oat cell) carcinoma. (15–20%). From central airways, it grows rapidly and spreads early.

The first three are commonly grouped together as 'non-small cell lung cancer' as they share common prognoses and treatment strategies.

The remainder includes undifferentiated carcinomas, carcinoids, and rarer tumour types (e.g. mesothelioma arising from the pleura following asbestos exposure). All cell types have different natural histories and responses to therapy, and therefore making a correct histological diagnosis is the mandatory first step to correct assessment and treatment.

Aetiology

The vast majority of lung cancers (non adenocarcinoma) in the UK (approximately 95%) are attributable to cigarette smoking. Cigarette smoke contains numerous well documented carcinogens. There is a clear link to both the quantity smoked and the duration over which it is smoked. The more somebody smokes and the longer the time they smoke it for, the more likely they are to develop lung cancer (Fig. 28.5). The converse is that if smokers stop smoking the risk of cancer steadily declines over time.

The role of passive smoking in cancer risk for non smokers is currently much debated and will remain so. Current wisdom is that there is a small but important increase in the risk of lung cancer if exposed to passive cigarette smoking.

Other risks are much less common and include radon exposure in certain parts of the country (e.g. Cornwall), asbestos exposure and fibrotic lung disease.

Similar to other carcinomas, it is thought that lung cancer is not caused by a single insult but follows the pattern of cellular dysplasia progressing to carcinoma and spread as the burden of genetic damage accumulates and key oncogenes are mutated. This, together with the poor outcome, has led to interest in screening and earlier diagnosis.

Clinical findings in lung cancer

Although 5–15% of patients are detected while asymptomatic, usually on a routine chest radiograph,

Fig. 28.5 The risk of death from lung cancer related to number of cigarettes smoked.

The risk of death from lung cancer related to number of cigarettes smoked		
Pattern of smoking	Death per 100 000 people	Relative risk
Never smoked	14	1
Ex smoker	58	4
Current smoker 1–14 cigarettes day^{-1} 15–24 cigarettes day^{-1} More than 25 cigarettes day^{-1}	105 208 355	7.5 15 25

the vast majority of patients present with signs or symptoms.

Systemic
Anorexia, cachexia and weight loss are common. The patient may have digital clubbing and tar staining of the fingers.

Endobronchial growth of the primary tumour
This may result in cough, haemoptysis, wheeze and stridor, dyspnoea, and post obstructive pneumonitis (fever and productive cough).

Peripheral tumour growth
This could cause pain (pleural or chest wall involvement), cough, dyspnoea, and symptoms of lung abscess due to tumour cavitation.

Regional spread of tumour in the chest
Regional spread of tumour in the chest (by contiguous growth or metastasis to regional lymph nodes). This may lead to tracheal obstruction, oesophageal compression with dysphagia, recurrent laryngeal nerve paralysis with hoarseness, phrenic nerve paralysis with elevation of the hemidiaphragm and dyspnoea, and sympathetic nerve paralysis with Horner's syndrome (ptosis, miosis, enophthalmos, and ipsilateral facial loss of sweating).

Pancoast's tumour growing in the apex of the lung extends locally with involvement of the eighth cervical and first and second thoracic nerves of the brachial plexus. There is shoulder pain which characteristically radiates in the ulnar distribution of the arm, often with destruction of the first and second ribs seen on CXR.

Other problems of regional spread include superior vena cava syndrome from vascular obstruction, pericardial and cardiac extension with resultant effusion or tamponade, lymphatic obstruction with resultant pleural effusion, and lymphangitic spread through the lungs with hypoxaemia and dyspnoea.

Transbronchial spread
Transbronchial spread (especially bronchioloalveolar carcinoma) produces growth along multiple alveolar surfaces with resultant impairment of oxygen transfer, dyspnoea, hypoxia, and the production of copious sputum.

Paraneoplastic syndromes
These syndromes describe symptoms and signs resulting from extrapulmonary organ dysfunction unrelated to space-occupying metastases. They occur in 15–20% of lung cancer patients and are commonly due to tumour secretory products. Important paraneoplastic syndromes associated with lung cancer are listed in Fig. 28.6. Occasionally, resection of the primary tumour may result in resolution of the syndrome.

Investigations
All patients with suspected lung cancer should have a full blood count, liver function tests, and measurement of electrolytes, calcium, and creatinine, in addition to a CXR. However, the diagnosis of lung cancer depends on a histological diagnosis either from cytology or tissue.

Techniques for obtaining a tissue diagnosis are varied and include:
- Fibre-optic bronchoscopy: endobronchial disease.
- Percutaneous needle aspiration: peripheral lesions.
- Mediastinoscopy.
- Lymph node biopsy.
- Biopsy of other metastatic site (e.g. the skin).
- Open lung biopsy via thoracotomy: when simpler investigations are negative.

Important paraneoplastic syndromes associated with lung cancer		
Organ/system	**Syndrome**	**Lung cancer histology**
Endocrine and metabolic	Cushing's	Small cell
	SIADH	Small cell
	Hypercalcaemia	Squamous cell
	Gynaecomastia	Large cell
Connective tissue and bone	Clubbing and HPOA	Squamous cell, adenocarcinoma, and large cell
Neuromuscular	Peripheral neuropathy	Small cell
	Subacute cerebellar degeneration	Small cell
	Eaton–Lambert (myasthenia)	Small cell
	Dermatomyositis	All
Haematology	Anaemia	All
	DIC	All
	Eosinophilia	All
	Thrombocytosis	All
Cardiovascular	Thrombophlebitis	Adenocarcinoma
	Marantic (non-infective) endocarditis	Adenocarcinoma

Fig. 28.6 Important paraneoplastic syndromes associated with lung cancer. (SIADH, syndrome of inappropriate antidiuretic hormone secretion; HPOA, hypertrophic pulmonary osteoarthropathy; DIC, disseminated intravascular coagulation.)

The diagnostic yield of cytological examination of different samples is shown in Fig. 28.7.

Imaging for lung cancer

The CXR is abnormal in most patients (sometimes in retrospect!). Common findings are hilar masses (squamous and small cell), peripheral masses (adenocarcinoma), atelectasis, infiltrates, cavitation (squamous cell) and pleural effusions. These changes are not specific for lung cancer and comparison between an old and current CXR is very important.

Computed tomography (CT) scanning, magnetic resonance imaging (MRI), and ultrasound examination are additional useful investigations in patients with invasion of the lung parenchyma, pleura, or mediastinal disease.

The diagnostic yield of cytology and pleural biopsy in lung cancer		
Cytology/biopsy	**Diagnostic yield**	**Comments**
Sputum cytology	40–60%	Especially for central tumours
Pleural fluid cytology	40–50%	In patients with malignant pleural effusions
Closed pleural biopsy (Abrams' needle)	50–60%	With malignant effusion
Pleural fluid cytology and closed pleural biopsy combined	75–85%	With malignant effusion

Fig. 28.7 The diagnostic yield of cytology and pleural biopsy in lung cancer.

TNM classification for lung cancer		
T/N/M	Stage	Characteristics
Primary tumour (T)	T1	<3 cm diameter surrounded by lung or pleura
	T2	>3 cm diameter and/or collapse extending to hilum, invading pleura and more than 2 cm beyond the carina
	T3	Any size extending to chest wall but not involving mediastinal structures (e.g. heart and great vessels); tumour within 2 cm of carina
	T4	Any size invading mediastinum; malignant pleural effusion
Lymph nodes (N)	N0	No involvement
	N1	Ipsilateral hilar and peribronchial nodes
	N2	Ipsilateral mediastinal and subcarinal nodes
	N3	Contralateral mediastinal or hilar nodes; or any scalene or supraclavicular nodes
Metastases (M)	M0	None known
	M1	Distant metastases outside thorax

Fig. 28.8 Tumour–node–metastasis classification for lung cancer.

Additional imaging may be required to investigate symptoms or signs that suggest the possibility of distant metastatic spread. These include X-rays of suspected bone metastases (or isotope bone scan), and a CT head scan or MRI of the brain for patients with central nervous system abnormalities or liver and adrenal glands if suspicion of metastases exists.

Extent of disease and tumour–node–metastasis (TNM) staging

Eighty percent of patients have inoperable disease at the time of presentation. Small cell cancer is nearly always disseminated at presentation. Diagnosis of this histological type excludes surgical resection, except in very rare circumstances where there is a single, small, peripheral lesion. In all other cell types, surgery is possible and the extent of disease is recorded by the TNM classification as shown in Fig. 28.8. The staging of disease using the TNM classification also helps to estimate the prognosis with treatment.

Assessment of patient before surgery

The patient's general and respiratory status needs to be assessed before surgery can be offered. Many patients have such marked cardiorespiratory disease that surgery is contraindicated. CT scanning remains the most common method of assessing spread and potential resectability of lung cancer. Positron

electron tomography is better but not universally available. A combination of the two is better still.

Treatment

Major treatment decisions are made on the basis of whether a tumour is classified histologically as a small cell carcinoma or as one of the non-small cell varieties. In general, small cell carcinomas have already spread at the time of presentation so that curative surgery cannot be performed, and they are managed primarily by chemotherapy with or without radiotherapy.

In contrast, non-small cell cancers that are found to be localised at the time of presentation should be considered for curative treatment with either surgery (pneumonectomy or lobectomy) or radiotherapy (Fig. 28.9). Traditionally, in the UK, chemotherapy has had a limited role in non-small cell lung cancer. Practice is changing to be more in line with North America as worthwhile survival benefits become apparent.

If inoperable, palliative care is essential as unpleasant dyspnoea and respiratory distress may develop as the disease progresses.

Prognosis

Five-year survival rates in treated lung cancer patients are given in Fig. 28.10. Perhaps due to the nihilistic view of lung cancer they remain poor in the

Treatment strategies for lung cancer		
Histology	**Extent of disease**	**Treatment modality**
Non-small cell lung cancer	Stage 0–IIIa	Surgery and/or postoperative radiotherapy (e.g. for node involvement)
	Stage IIIb–IV	Palliative radiotherapy for local complications or pain from bony metastases
Small cell lung cancer	Proven single peripheral lesion (rare)	Curative surgery attempted
	Limited stage	Combination chemotherapy and radiotherapy
	Disseminated at presentation (usual)	Combination chemotherapy

Fig. 28.9 Treatment strategies for lung cancer.

UK, where overall 5-year survival is approximately 5%, less than half that in the USA.

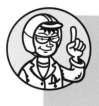

In hospital-acquired pneumonia, the organism and its treatment are often different from that of the community-acquired infection

Pneumonia

Pneumonia is an infection of the pulmonary parenchyma. Various bacterial species, viruses, fungi, and parasites can cause pneumonia. It is not a single disease but a group of specific infections, each with a different epidemiology, pathogenesis, clinical presentation, and clinical course. Identification of the aetiological micro-organism is of primary importance, to enable appropriate antimicrobial therapy. However, because of the serious nature of the infection, antimicrobial therapy generally needs to be started immediately, before laboratory confirmation of the causative agent.

Classification
Community acquired pneumonia
This occurs out of hospital or within 48 hours of admission. Causes include *Streptococcus pneumoniae*

Estimates of 5-year survival of treated patients with lung cancer		
	Stage	**5-year survival**
Non-small cell lung cancer	0 (T1 N0 M0); carcinoma *in situ*	70–80%
	I (T1–2 N0 M0); no nodes or metastases	50%
	II (T1–2 N1 M0); ipsilateral local nodes only	30%
	IIIa (T1–3 N0–2 M0); more than T2 with ipsilateral mediastinal nodes	10–15%
	IIIb (any T, any N, M0); invading vital mediastinal structure, or non-resectable nodes but no extrathoracic spread	<5%
	IV (any T, any N, M1); extrathoracic distant metastases	<2%
Small cell lung cancer	Patients rarely live for 5 years after diagnosis—median survival with combined chemotherapy, e.g. with cisplatin-containing regimens is 40–70 weeks, compared with 6–20 weeks if untreated	

Fig. 28.10 Estimates of 5-year survival of treated patients with lung cancer.

(most common), *Haemophilus*, *Staphylococcus aureus*, and viruses are implicated in approximately 10% of cases. In pre-existing lung disease (e.g. COPD), organisms such as *Pseudomonas* and *Moraxella* are more common.

Atypical pneumonia
Caused by organisms such as *Mycoplasma*, *Legionella* and *Chlamydia*. They can be acquired in the community or in institutions.

Nosocomial pneumonia
New onset pneumonia occurring more than 48 hours after admission to hospital. Can be caused by all of the above agents but Gram-negative organisms such as *Pseudomonas* and *Klebsiella* are much more common.

Aspiration pneumonia
Occurs due to the aspiration of gastrointestinal material due to an inability to protect the airway such as after a stroke or with a decreased conscious level. Anaerobic organisms may be implicated.

Clinical features of pneumonia
Typical
The 'typical' symptoms of pneumonia are sudden onset of fever, tachypnoea, dyspnoea, cough productive of purulent sputum and, in some cases, pleuritic chest pain. Signs of pulmonary consolidation (dullness, increased vocal resonance, bronchial breath sounds, and coarse crepitations) may be found on physical examination and coincide with abnormalities on the CXR.

Atypical
'Atypical' pneumonia traditionally causes a more gradual onset, a dry cough, and extrapulmonary symptoms (headache, muscle aching, fatigue, sore throat, nausea, vomiting, and diarrhoea). Abnormalities on the CXR may be seen despite few signs of pulmonary involvement other than crepitations on physical examination. It is now said that it is the organisms which are 'atypical' and not the symptoms.

Diagnosis of pneumonia
Chest X-ray
A CXR can confirm the presence of the diffuse or lobar pulmonary infiltrates and assess the extent of infection. Air bronchograms may be seen within the areas of consolidation. Other features which may be present include pleural effusions, pulmonary cavitation, or hilar lymphadenopathy. Cavitation

suggests the following infective causes for the pneumonia – oral anaerobic bacteria, enteric Gram-negative bacilli, *Staphylococcus aureus*, *Pseudomonas*, *Legionella*, TB, and fungi.

It should be noted that a normal CXR does not exclude pneumonia, especially early in the disease or in patients unable to mount an inflammatory response because of immunosuppression.

Sputum microscopy and culture
Sputum microscopy and culture is important in severe bacterial pneumonia. Unfortunately, sputum is frequently contaminated by potentially pathogenic bacteria that colonise the upper respiratory tract without causing disease. Contamination reduces the diagnostic specificity of lower respiratory tract specimens and clinical judgement is required when interpreting the results.

Other tests
Full blood count may show a neutrophilia. Urea may be elevated. Eryrthrocyte sedimentation rate (ESR) and C-reactive protein (CRP) may be raised and the CRP can monitor the response to therapy. Blood cultures should be taken prior to antibiotic therapy.

Oxygen saturations and arterial blood gases may show hypoxia with or without ventilatory failure.

Serology for atypical organisms should be taken if clinical suspicion is present and then repeated in 10–14 days.

Pleural effusion, if present and thought to be parapneumonic, should be aspirated to assess for infection or empyema and drained if needed.

The urine can be tested for *Streptococcal* and *Legionella* urinary antigen. These can remain positive even after antibiotics have been commenced.

Fibre-optic bronchoscopy
Fibre-optic bronchoscopy is rarely performed for pneumonia but has become the standard invasive procedure used to obtain lower respiratory tract secretions from seriously ill or immunocompromised patients. Samples are collected with a protected double-sheathed brush, by bronchoalveolar lavage or by transbronchial biopsy at the site of the pulmonary consolidation.

Severity
- Respiratory rate >30 per minute.
- Diastolic blood pressure <60 mmHg.
- Confusion/drowsy.

- White cell count <4 or $>20 \times 10^9$/L.
- Urea >7 mmol/L.
- pO_2 <8 kPa on air.

If present, the above features indicate a worse prognosis and you should consider more intensive monitoring (e.g. in a high dependency unit).

Treatment of pneumonia

This is in two parts. First, general supportive care, namely oxygen, nebulisers, physiotherapy, hydration and respiratory support if the pneumonia is serious enough. Second, the appropriate antimicrobial treatment of pneumonia is shown in Fig. 28.11. However, check with your local microbiology department for their guidelines as local antibiotic sensitivities vary.

Respiratory failure

Definition

Respiratory failure is defined as a dysfunction of gas exchange resulting in abnormalities of oxygenation or carbon dioxide (CO_2) elimination severe enough to impair or threaten the function of vital organs.

Respiratory failure is said to be present in a patient breathing air at sea level when the pO_2 is less than 8.0 kPa as a result of lung disease. If hypoxia is combined with a normal or low pCO_2 (<6.0 kPa), this is type I respiratory failure, but if hypoxia is combined with a raised pCO_2, type II respiratory failure is present. Measurement of the ABGs is essential to the diagnosis of respiratory failure.

Type I respiratory failure

This is hypoxaemia without CO_2 retention. Physiological causes include:
- A low inspired oxygen concentration ((FiO_2) e.g. at high altitude).
- Mismatch of alveolar ventilation (V) to alveolar perfusion (Q).
- Right-to-left shunting of blood bypassing alveoli.

In medical practice, the common causes of type I respiratory failure include:
- Pneumonia.
- Asthma.
- COPD (predominantly emphysema—'pink puffers').
- Pulmonary thromboembolism.
- Acute respiratory distress syndrome.
- Pulmonary oedema.
- Pulmonary fibrosis.

Treatment of type I respiratory failure

The main therapeutic objective in acute hypoxaemic respiratory failure is to ensure oxygen delivery to vital organs. Severe hypoxia is life threatening and oxygen therapy is indicated to maintain saturations of $>90\%$ (>8 kPa). The patient may be cyanosed, confused and delirious.

Drug choice for pneumonia. (This will vary between countries and hospitals)	
Community acquired pneumonia	
Uncomplicated	Broad spectrum penicillin eg. amoxicillin. Macrolide eg. clarithromycin if penicillin allergic or if atypical organism suspected. Flucloxacillin if S. aureus suspected.
Severe	Third generation cephalosporin, eg. cefuroxime or Coamoxiclav i.v. and macrolide for atypical organisms. Flucloxacillin if S. aureus suspected
Atypical pneumonia	Erythromycin or other macrolide. Tetracycline for chlamydia or mycoplasma. Give for 10–14 days.
Hospital acquired pneumonia	Broad spectrum cephalosporin or coamoxiclav plus increased Gram-negative cover eg. aminoglycoside, ciprofloxacin. Vancomycin or teicoplanin if MRSA pneumonia.
Aspiration pneumonia	Cover for anaerobic organisms. Cephalosporin plus metronidazole. Coamoxiclav often sufficient.

Fig. 28.11 Drug choice for pneumonia. This is intended as a guide only.

Whilst high concentrations of inspired oxygen (FiO_2 >50%) are safe in patients with type I respiratory failure, as there is no risk of CO_2 retention, pulmonary oxygen toxicity is a risk if the FiO_2 concentration remains over 60% for more than 48 hours continuously.

Continuous positive airway pressure (CPAP) via a face mask can improve oxygenation and allow intubation to be avoided.

Other therapeutic objectives include:
- Specific therapy of the underlying cause (e.g. antimicrobial therapy for pneumonia, bronchodilators and steroids for asthma, or chest drain insertion for pneumothorax).
- General supportive care: endotracheal intubation if needed, adequate hydration, nutrition, and electrolyte balance.

Type II respiratory failure

In a healthy subject a rise in arterial pCO_2 causes an increase in ventilation by central stimulation of the respiratory centres in the medulla resulting in an increase in breathing to lower the pCO_2. In type II respiratory failure, this mechanism fails and signals that, apart from lung disease, there is also effective alveolar hypoventilation from one of several causes.

Clinical features of type II respiratory failure include central cyanosis (indicating hypoxaemia) but CO_2 retention can only be assessed accurately by the measurement of ABGs. However, there are some clinical signs suggestive of CO_2 retention and these include:
- Tachycardia with bounding pulse.
- A flapping tremor of the outstretched hands.
- Clouding of consciousness.
- Papilloedema (rare).

These are unreliable signs because they can occur from other causes and their absence does not exclude significant CO_2 retention.

Type II respiratory failure is classified as:
- Reduced central drive (e.g. sedation and brainstem disorders).
- Neuromuscular disease (e.g. spinal cord lesions, poliomyelitis, myasthenia gravis and diaphragmatic palsy).
- Thoracic wall abnormalities (e.g. kyphoscoliosis).
- Intrinsic lung disease (e.g. asthma, COPD, pneumonia and lung fibrosis).

Treatment of type II respiratory failure

As in type I failure, the main therapeutic objective is to ensure adequate oxygen delivery to vital organs by administering oxygen therapy. However, in the most common clinical setting (an acute exacerbation of COPD), patients may have chronic CO_2 retention. They are dependent on hypoxia for ventilatory drive, so that with oxygen therapy there is a real risk of inducing hypoventilation, worsening the respiratory dysfunction, and promoting respiratory acidosis. Oxygen therapy must be carefully controlled to ensure that sufficient oxygen is supplied, usually 24% via a 'Venturi' mask, to prevent death from hypoxaemia (remember that saturations of 90% are adequate) but without worsening the respiratory acidosis. This needs repeated monitoring of ABGs.

Other therapeutic objectives include:
- Specific therapy of the underlying cause (e.g. antimicrobial and bronchodilator therapy for an infective exacerbation of COPD).
- General supportive care is as for type I failure.

In certain circumstances, NIV via a face or nasal mask can augment minute ventilation enabling control of CO_2, allowing the underlying disease to be treated and endotracheal intubation and its consequences to be avoided. However, NIV is not a substitute for formal mechanical ventilation if it is needed but cannot be provided. Chemical stimulants to breathing such as doxapram are rarely used now.

Prognosis in acute respiratory failure

The course of the disease and its prognosis depend to a great extent on the underlying pathology. In patients with COPD who do not require mechanical ventilation, the immediate prognosis is good. Patients developing acute respiratory distress syndrome associated with septicaemia have a very poor prognosis with mortality rates of approximately 90%. In general, patients requiring ventilation for respiratory failure have survival rates of approximately 60% to weaning off the ventilator, 40% to discharge from hospital, and approximately 30% 1-year survival.

Pneumothorax

A pneumothorax is the presence of air in the pleural space (i.e. between the lung and chest wall). It has UK hospital admission rates of six in 100 000 and 17 in 100 000 for women and men respectively. Risk factors for pneumothorax include smoking, height, male sex, increasing age and underlying lung disease. The following distinctions are made between the different types of pneumothorax:
- Spontaneous pneumothorax: occurs without trauma to the thorax.

- Primary spontaneous pneumothorax: occurs in the absence of lung disease.
- Secondary spontaneous pneumothorax: occurs in the presence of pre-existing lung disease.
- Traumatic pneumothorax: penetrating or non-penetrating chest injuries.
- Tension pneumothorax: the pressure in the pleural space is positive throughout the respiratory cycle.

Primary spontaneous pneumothorax is usually due to the rupture of an apical pleural bleb that lies within or immediately under the visceral pleura. Approximately 25% of patients with an initial primary spontaneous pneumothorax will have a recurrence.

Clinical features
The patient may be in extremis if a large tension pneumothorax is present or it may be seen on routine chest radiography in a patient with mild chest pain. Clinical features of pneumothorax include:
- Chest pain on the affected side.
- Shortness of breath.
- Tachycardia.
- Decreased expansion, vocal fremitus, hyperresonance and diminished breath sounds may be detected if the pneumothorax is large.

A CXR will confirm the diagnosis by demonstrating a line of visceral pleura with absent lung markings beyond the line. The diagnosis may prove more difficult in secondary pneumothorax, especially if emphysematous bullae are present. In this case lateral X-rays or CT may be indicated. The most recent UK guidelines classify pnemothoraces as large or small, based on the presence of a visible rim of air <2 cm or >2 cm between the lung and chest wall on plain CXR.

Treatment
The treatment for primary spontaneous pneumothorax is aspiration. If the lung does not expand with aspiration, or if the patient has a recurrent pneumothorax, chest drain insertion with underwater seal drainage is indicated. Pleurodesis or surgery by thoracoscopy or thoracotomy plus pleural abrasion is almost 100% successful in preventing further recurrences. Treatment algorithms are shown in Figs 28.13 and 28.14.

Pulmonary embolism
Pulmonary embolism (PE) is a common, potentially fatal and frequently missed cause of death. It results from thrombus formation in the venous circulation which embolises to the lungs, obstructing a major pulmonary artery, causing hypoxia and circulatory collapse.

Risk factors include immobility, including 'economy class syndrome' with air travel, surgery, malignancy, obesity, pregnancy, the contraceptive pill and one of the increasingly described thrombophilic conditions (e.g. Factor V Leiden or the prothrombin 20210A gene mutation).

Clinical features
Dyspnoea is the most frequent symptom and tachypnoea is the most frequent sign in PE. Dyspnoea, syncope, hypotension, or cyanosis indicate a massive PE, while pleuritic pain, cough, or haemoptysis often suggest a small embolism located near the pleura. On examination, young or previously healthy individuals may simply appear anxious but otherwise seem well, even with a large PE.

Investigations
First perform an assessment of the clinical risk of PE e.g. the Well's criteria. Investigations supporting the diagnosis of PE include:
- D-dimer. Remember that its main value is as a negative result to exclude thromboemboli.
- Electrocardiogram: commonly abnormal but no common abnormality. Tachycardia is found most but the S1 Q3 T3 pattern is 'textbook'.
- ABGs: hypoxaemia.
- CXR: usually normal but may show atelectasis or a small wedge shadow.

If these investigations are negative but the clinical suspicion remains high, a search for corroborative evidence of thromboembolism is instigated by looking for the presence of deep vein thrombosis with compression ultrasound or venography.

V/Q scanning looking for the classical mismatch defect is the traditional method of investigating a potential PE. Pulmonary angiography is performed to make a definitive diagnosis in certain circumstances (e.g. pregnancy or acutely ill patients who may require embolectomy). Spiral CT pulmonary angiography is an increasingly common way of diagnosing PE, especially those in the more proximal pulmonary arteries and those with pre-existing lung disease in whom a definitive diagnosis with a V/Q scan may be difficult.

Echocardiography may show evidence of acute right ventricular dysfunction especially in large haemodynamically significant PEs in which thrombolysis is considered.

Common occupational lung diseases		
Disease	**Aetiology**	**Lung injury**
Chronic fibrotic lung disease	Coal workers' pneumoconiosis Silicosis asbestosis	Diffuse nodular infiltrates on CXR
Hypersensitivity pneumonitis	Mouldy hay (farmer's lung) Avian proteins (bird fancier's lung)	Restrictive pulmonary dysfunction
Obstructive airways disorders	Grain dust Wood dust Tobacco Pollen Synthetic dyes Formaldehyde	Occupational asthma
Toxic lung injury	Irritant gases	Pulmonary oedema Bronchiolitis obliterans
Lung cancer	Asbestos	Mesothelioma
	Arsenic	All lung cancer types
	Chromium	All lung cancer types
	Hydrocarbons	All lung cancer types
Pleural diseases	Asbestos	May cause benign effusions and plaques
	Talc	May cause benign effusions and plaques

Fig. 28.12 Common occupational lung diseases.

Treatment

The majority of patients are treated with low molecular weight heparin or intravenous heparin followed by oral warfarin for a period of 6 months; PE is a recurrent disease with an annual relapse rate of approximately 7%. When treatment is continued for only 6 weeks, the relapse rate is twice as high as with 6 months. Monitoring of maintenance warfarin treatment is performed 4-8 weekly in clinical practice, aiming to keep the international normalised ratio in the therapeutic range 2.0–3.0.

Patients who have recurrent or a strong family history of thromboembolic events should be screened for the recognised hypercoagulable states mentioned above. They are also likely to need lifelong anticoagulation and should be considered for a venacaval filter if warfarin fails to prevent further emboli.

Large acute PEs with severe hypoxia and circulatory failure may require inotropic support and thrombolysis. The same contraindications apply as for acute myocardial infarction.

Beware! Patients with type II respiratory failure can stop breathing if given high-dose oxygen

Miscellaneous respiratory conditions

Cystic fibrosis

Cystic fibrosis (CF) is an autosomal recessive disorder that presents as a multisystem disease, and occurs in 1 in 2500 live births in Caucasians and one in 25 is a carrier. Signs and symptoms typically occur in childhood but up to 5% of patients are diagnosed as adults. Improvements in therapy now mean that approximately a third of patients reach adulthood and nearly 10% live beyond 30 years old. The cystic fibrosis transmembrane conductance regulator protein is on chromosome 7; it regulates chloride and water movement across cell membranes.

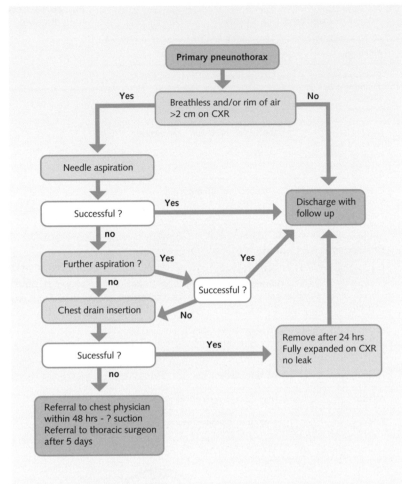

Fig. 28.13 Algorithm for treatment of primary pneumothorax, after British Thoracic Society. (CXR, chest radiograph.)

Whilst there are more than 500 known mutations the Δ508 mutation accounts for over 70% of cases.

CF is characterised by chronic airway infection that ultimately leads to bronchiectasis, exocrine pancreatic insufficiency, intestinal dysfunction, abnormal sweat gland function, and urogenital dysfunction.

Diagnosis

The diagnosis of CF rests on a combination of clinical criteria and analyses of sweat chloride values. Typically in adults a chloride concentration of over 70 mmol/L discriminates between CF patients and patients with other lung diseases.

Treatment

This is best carried out in a specialised centre. The treatment strategies for CF are to promote clearance of secretions and reverse bronchoconstriction (physiotherapy, mucolytics and bronchodilators), control infection in the lung (antibiotics, including prophylactic nebulised ones), vaccination against influenza and pneumococcus, provide adequate nutrition (pancreatic enzyme and fat-soluble vitamin supplements), and prevent intestinal obstruction.

As irreversible complications arise, heart–lung transplantation may be an option for some. Gene therapy remains elusive and far from clinical use.

Allergic bronchopulmonary aspergillosis

Allergic bronchopulmonary aspergillosis (ABPA) occurs in patients with asthma who develop bronchospasm, peripheral blood eosinophilia, aspergillus precipitins and raised IgE levels with pulmonary infiltrates. It can lead on to bronchiectasis. Treatment for exacerbations is with corticosteroids. The cause is the fungus aspergillus fumigatus.

Aspergillus fumigatus can also cause invasive aspergillosis in immunosuppressed patients e.g. neutropenia post chemotherapy or HIV. Treatment is with amphotericin, itraconazole or voriconazole.

In the immunocompetent, pre-existing lung cavities can be colonised to form aspergillomas. Surgical resection remains the most effective treatment.

Aspergillus clavatus causes a type of extrinsic allergic alveolitis. ABPA may resemble hypersensitivity pneumonitis and presents with systemic symptoms and recurrent pulmonary infiltrates, but with eosinophilia. It is the association with asthma and the typical peripheral eosinophilia that distinguishes it from hypersensitivity pneumonitis (or extrinsic allergic alveolitis).

ABPA is the most common example of the allergic bronchopulmonary mycoses and is sometimes confused with hypersensitivity pneumonitis because of the presence of precipitating antibodies to aspergillus fumigatus. However, ABPA is an obstructive rather than a restrictive lung disease, and is associated with allergic (atopic) asthma. The bronchiectasis associated with ABPA is thought to result from a deposition of immune complexes in proximal airways. Adequate treatment usually requires the long-term use of systemic glucocorticoids.

Bronchiectasis

Bronchiectasis is an abnormal and permanent dilatation of the bronchioles. It can be focal, involving airways supplying a limited region of the lung, or diffuse, involving airways in a more widespread distribution. Whatever the distribution, the diagnosis is suggested by the clinical consequences of chronic or recurrent infection in the dilated airways and the associated copious purulent sputum that forms within these airways.

Aetiology

Previously bronchiectasis was often a complication of childhood measles or pertussis but this is now rare as a result of effective immunisation.

It is more common in those with impaired immune systems and mucociliary clearance (e.g. Kartagener's syndrome). Adenovirus and influenza are the main viral causes and infections

with necrotising organisms (e.g. TB or anaerobes) remain important. As other causes decline, cystic fibrosis is increasingly prevalent. Localised bronchial obstruction can lead on to bronchiectasis.

Clinical features

Patients typically present with persistent or recurrent cough and purulent sputum production. Haemoptysis occurs in more than half of cases and can cause massive bleeding. Physical examination of the chest overlying an affected area may reveal any combination of coarse crepitations and wheeze, which reflect the damaged airways containing significant secretions. As with other chronic intrathoracic infections, clubbing may be present.

Patients with severe disease and chronic hypoxaemia may develop cor pulmonale and right ventricular failure. Amyloidosis can result from chronic infection and inflammation, but it is now seldom seen.

Investigation

Chest radiography may show 'tramline shadows' of bronchial wall thickening. High resolution CT has replaced bronchography in diagnosis. Lung function and reversibility should be done by spirometry and sputum culture should guide antibiotic therapy.

Treatment

Treatment strategies are similar to those described for the respiratory complications of CF. Surgery is occasionally effective for localised bronchiectasis. Appropriate treatment should be started when a treatable cause is found (e.g. antituberculous drugs for TB or steroids for ABPA).

Interstitial lung diseases

Fibrotic lung disease is a heterogeneous group of disorders that have been variously classified. Some of the terms used are idiopathic pulmonary fibrosis, cryptogenic fibrosing alveolitis, interstitial pneumonitis and diffuse parenchymal lung disease. They share the fact that damage is as a result of an inflammatory insult to the lung that then leads to cellular proliferation and scarring with chronic loss of lung function.

Aetiology

A way to begin to think about this group of patients is to separate them into those with and without a cause.

215

Known cause

- Environmental agents: asbestosis, silicosis, pneumoconiosis.
- Drugs: sulphasalazine, gold, amiodarone, methotrexate, oxygen, nitrofurantoin.
- Systemic disease: connective tissue disorders (systemic lupus erythematosus, rheumatoid arthritis, systemic sclerosis), neoplasia, vasculitides (Wegener's granulomatosis, Churg-Strauss, microscopic polyangiitis), sarcoidosis, inflammatory bowel disease.

Unknown cause

- Cryptogenic fibrosing alveolitis. (now accurately called usual interstitial pneumonia)
- Cryptogenic organising pneumonia.

Clinical features

Most present with non-productive cough, progressive dyspnoea, fatigue, weight loss and occasionally haemoptysis. The chest radiograph may show reticular nodular shadowing and loss of lung volume. Careful questioning of occupational and environmental risks, travel, medications, past illness, smoking and family history is important to find a cause. Examination may show cyanosis, finger clubbing and bilateral fine end inspiratory crackles. As the disease progresses cor pulmonale may be discernable.

Investigation

These should include full blood count, ESR, urea and electrolytes, calcium, liver function tests, serum ACE and autoantibodies to look for a cause. If any are abnormal they should be followed up.

High resolution CT (HRCT) provides diagnostic and prognostic information. Other tests include pulmonary function tests (usually restrictive pattern) especially transfer factor, DTPA scanning, bronchoalveolar lavage or lung biopsy. Lung biopsy is now considered essential to differentiate between the various subtypes of interstitial pneumonia. Only usual interstitial pneumonia (UIP) can be accurately diagnosed from HRCT.

Treatment

If a disorder is found then the underlying cause must be addressed. If 'honeycomb' changes are seen on the HRCT then fibrosis is permanent. If 'ground glass' changes are seen then high-dose immunosuppression with steroids and cyclophosphamide may be indicated to attempt to prevent irreversible fibrosis. Treatment

of complications is as they develop and when end-stage referral for transplantation may be indicated.

Occupational lung disease

Many acute and chronic lung diseases are directly related to occupational exposure to inorganic and organic dusts. A number of different clinical syndromes may result and these are shown in Fig. 28.12. They are important as they are largely preventable due to increased awareness and improved work-place conditions. Patients with asbestosis, silicosis, pneumoconiosis and mesothelioma may be entitled to compensation.

Many drugs interact with warfarin to enhance or diminish its effect. Ask the patient to report any changes in treatment

Pulmonary embolism is life-threatening and common. If in doubt heparinise and investigate fully

Sleep apnoea

Sleep apnoeas are defined as an intermittent cessation of respiratory airflow during sleep, lasting at least 10 seconds.

Sleep apnoea syndrome

This refers to the coexistence of sleep disordered breathing and excessive daytime sleepiness. The symptoms include snoring, poor concentration, unrefreshing restless sleep, daytime somnolence, morning headaches and nocturia. Risk factors are increasing age, male gender, obesity, sedative drugs and alcohol.

Classification

Sleep apnoeas are classified into three types:

- Central sleep apnoea, where the neural drive to all the respiratory muscles is transiently abolished.

- Obstructive sleep apnoea, in which airflow ceases despite continuing respiratory drive because of occlusion of the oropharyngeal airway.
- Mixed apnoeas, which consist of a central apnoea followed by an obstructive component.

Treatment

Treatment of mild obstructive sleep apnoea is by modest weight reduction, avoidance of alcohol, improvement of nasal patency, intra oral mandibular advancement devices and avoidance of sleeping in the supine posture. Moderate-to-severe cases are treated by nasal continuous positive airways pressure during sleep and rarely with uvulopalatopharyngoplasty.

The top five causes of iatrogenic pneumothoraces are transthoracic needle aspiration, subclavian central line insertion, thoracocentesis, pleural biopsy and mechanical ventilation

If asthma control is poor, do not forget to assess inhaler technique

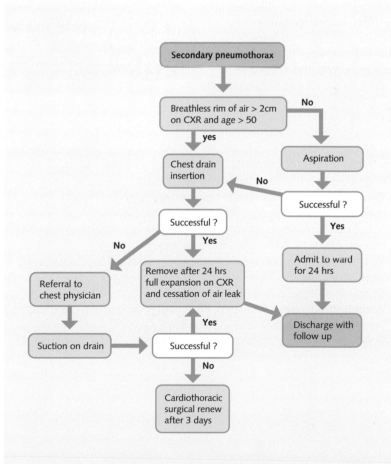

Fig. 28.14 Algorithm for treatment of secondary pneumothorax, after British Thoracic Society. (CXR, chest radiograph.)

Acute respiratory distress syndrome

ARDS represents severe respiratory failure due to a marked lung inflammatory response and capillary leak from a variety of stimuli of which sepsis is the most common cause. Others include trauma, shock, burns, pancreatitis, disseminated intravascular coagulation, cardiac bypass, emboli, near drowning and oxygen toxicity. The hypoxia results from non-cardiogenic pulmonary oedema (i.e. not left ventricular failure, the left atrial pressure is not raised).

It is defined by four criteria:
- Recognised precipitating cause.
- New bilateral infiltrates on chest radiography.
- No evidence of heart failure. Pulmonary artery occlusion pressure <18 mmHg.
- pO_2: FiO_2 ratio <26.6 kPa (i.e. severe hypoxia).

Treatment

This involves treatment of the underlying cause and supportive care, usually mechanically ventilated in an intensive care unit. Recent advances include 'protective' ventilation to minimise tidal volumes and airway pressures; this often means accepting hypercapnia. Positive end expiratory pressure improves oxygenation and allows the FiO_2 to be lowered. Fluid balance is controlled to try and limit the raised extravascular lung water. Other strategies include prone positioning, high frequency oscillatory ventilation and inhaled nitric oxide. The use of long duration methylprednisolone in ARDS which is unresolving after 7 days in the absence of infection has gained widespread acceptance.

Prognosis

This remains poor. It depends on the nature of the precipitating event and the degree to which organ failure develops. Mortality is approximately 40% and, if accompanied by sepsis, it can reach 90%. Most survivors have residual impairment of lung function, both mechanical and diffusing capacity.

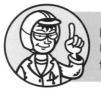

Rifampicin turns urine red. Useful to assess compliance to treatment

Patients with fibrosing alveolitis often appear in examinations as they have good physical signs

- What is meant by 'step wise' treatment of asthma?
- How does bronchitis differ from emphysema?
- Who benefits from long term oxygen therapy?
- How would you investigate suspected tuberculosis?
- What are the four main types of primary lung cancer, how are they more broadly divided and why is this important for treatment?
- What is the difference between community and hospital acquired pneumonia?
- How do you assess the severity of pneumonia?
- Explain how type 1 and type 2 respiratory failures differ?
- When should a pneumothorax be aspirated and when is a chest drain indicated?
- Who are at risk of pulmonary emboli?
- Does asbestosis result in obstructive or restrictive spirometry?

Further reading

Barnes P J 2000 Medical progress: chronic obstructive pulmonary disease. *N Engl J Med* **343**: 269–280

The British Thoracic Society publishes guidelines and reviews on all aspects of respiratory medicine. They are available on its website *www.brit-thoracic.org.uk*

Busse W W and Lemanske R F 2001 Advances in immunology: asthma. *N Engl J Med* **344**: 350–362

Calverley P, Pauwels R, Vestbo J et al for the TRISTAN study group 2003 Combined salmeterol and fluticasone in the treatment of chronic obstructive pulmonary disease: a randomised controlled trial. *Lancet* **361**: 449–455

Corne J, Carroll M and Delany D 2002 *The chest X-ray made easy.* Churchill Livingstone

Fedullo P F and Tapson V F 2003 Clinical practice. The evaluation of a suspected pulmonary embolism. *N Eng J Med* **349**: 1247–1256

Gross T J and Hunninghake G W 2001 Medical progress: idiopathic pulmonary fibrosis. *N Engl J Med* **345**: 517–525

McGowan, Jeffries and Turley 2004 *Crash Course in Respiratory System,* 2nd edn. Mosby

Lung cancer. Thorax ten part review series starting November 2002.

Polkey M I, Green M, Moxham J 1995 Measurement of respiratory muscle strength. *Thorax* **50**: 1131–1135

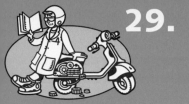

Oesophageal disorders

Hiatus hernia
This is the herniation of part of the stomach into the chest cavity. Hiatus herniae are generally asymptomatic but may be associated with acid reflux causing dyspeptic symptoms (see below and Chapter 7). They rarely require treatment other than symptomatic management for acid reflux. There are two types:

Sliding hiatus hernia
Very common (30% of over-50s). Gastro-oesophageal junction 'slides' through oesophageal hiatus.

Rolling (or para-oesophageal) hiatus hernia
The lower oesophageal sphincter (LOS) remains below the diaphragm, but part of the stomach rolls up into the chest next to the oesophagus. Occasionally, this results in gastric volvulus resulting in severe pain and requiring surgery.

Gastro-oesophageal reflux disease (GORD)
The LOS normally prevents significant acid reflux into the oesophagus. Other anti-reflux mechanisms include the intra-abdominal section of the oesophagus, the diaphragmatic crura and the folds of gastric mucosa. These mechanisms fail in GORD. The factors predisposing to reflux have been outlined in Chapter 7.

Clinical features
These have been described in Chapter 7. It is important to note particularly how the presentation may be difficult to distinguish from that of angina (including non-specific electrocardiogram (ECG) changes), and how atypical symptoms such as nocturnal asthma or laryngeal discomfort may occur. Severe oesophagitis may be associated with micro- and/or macroscopic gastrointestinal bleeding and iron deficiency anaemia.

Investigations
These are outlined in Chapter 7. Endoscopy is useful for demonstrating oesophagitis, peptic strictures and Barrett's oesophagus (see below) and allows biopsies to be taken. 24-hour intra-luminal pH monitoring is the definitive test to confirm the diagnosis, but is not often required, as explained in Chapter 7.

In adhering to the guidelines summarised in Fig. 7.3, a number of patients with GORD (without a firm diagnosis) will receive *Helicobacter pylori* eradication. However, *H. pylori* infection is just as common in the normal population and probably has no specific role in this condition.

Management
Patients should avoid tight clothes, stop smoking, avoid aggravating foods and drinks, and lose weight if overweight. Patients should be advised to prop themselves up in bed with pillows and put a block under the end of the bed to avoid slipping down.

A number of drugs can be used: antacids (including alginate preparations that form a 'foam raft'), H_2 receptor antagonists, proton pump inhibitors, and pro-kinetics such as metoclopramide. Therapy aims to provide symptom relief. Four weeks is a reasonable starting course and then therapy should be titrated to an agent that controls the symptoms at the lowest cost.

Very occasionally, surgical therapy is considered.

Complications
Peptic stricture
Usually occurs in patients aged over 60 years. It causes intermittent dysphagia. The stricture is usually dilated endoscopically but rarely surgery is required. Acid secretion is controlled pharmacologically.

Barrett's oesophagus
This is intestinal metaplasia following longstanding acid reflux and, although visible macroscopically, is confirmed histologically following biopsy. It is particularly significant as it is pre-malignant for oesophageal adenocarcinoma (see below). Whether regular endoscopic screening for cancer in patients with Barrett's oesophagus improves outcome is not clear.

221

Oesophageal motility disorders

These can give rise to dyspepsia (see Chapter 7), pain, dysphagia and odynophagia, and regurgitation. Causes include old age, diabetes mellitus, neurological disorders affecting the brain stem, systemic sclerosis, achalasia and diffuse oesophageal spasm. The diagnosis can be suggested by chest X-ray or barium swallow appearances, but oesophageal manometry is the definitive investigation. Treatment options include balloon dilation, surgery, botulinum toxin injection, and anti-spasmodic drugs.

Oesophageal cancer

Squamous carcinomas occur in the mid-oesophagus. The incidence in the UK is 5–10 in 100 000 but is higher in China and parts of Africa. It is commoner in men, heavy drinkers, and smokers. Predisposing factors include Plummer–Vinson syndrome, achalasia, coeliac disease, and tylosis (hyperkeratosis of the palms and soles).

Adenocarcinoma arises in columnar epithelium of the lower oesophagus. Barrett's oesophagus increases the risk of adenocarcinoma by 40-fold.

Clinical features

The incidence peaks in the seventh decade. General features of malignancy include weight loss, anorexia and lassitude. Local features include retrosternal pain, aspiration pneumonia and dysphagia, progressing from difficulty in swallowing solids to difficulty with liquids. Odynophagia (pain on swallowing) may ensue. Direct invasion of surrounding structures and regional lymph node involvement are common. Metastases to other organs and lymph nodes may occur.

Investigations

Endoscopy with biopsy, and barium swallow are the main diagnostic investigations. Computed tomography (CT) scanning helps with staging.

Management

Surgery is considered depending on the tumour stage/grade and the fitness of the patient but it carries a high morbidity and mortality. Radiotherapy and chemotherapy may play a role. Often palliation is the only option, and this may include endoscopic dilation, stent placement, laser photocoagulation and/or radiotherapy with the aim of maintaining patency of the oesophageal lumen. Overall survival is poor at around 5% at 5 years.

Gastroduodenal disorders

Gastro-duodenitis and peptic ulcer disease (PUD)

Acute gastritis and ulceration can result from non-steroidal anti-inflammatory drug (NSAID) use, steroids, alcohol, or severe stress or burns (Curling ulcer). Chronic gastritis complicates *H. pylori* infection, autoimmune gastritis (e.g. pernicious anaemia) and chronic NSAID use. Most chronic gastritis is asymptomatic, but may be a risk factor for malignant change. Erosive duodenitis is part of the spectrum of duodenal ulcer (DU) disease.

Peptic ulcer disease most commonly occurs in the duodenum, followed by the stomach, oesophagus, and jejunum in Zollinger–Ellison syndrome or after a gastroenterostomy. It may occur in a Meckel's diverticulum with ectopic gastric mucosa. Its prevalence is 15–20% and it is commoner in men. The incidence increases with age.

Duodenal ulceration is associated with *H. pylori* infection in 95% of cases and NSAIDs are implicated in most others. 70% of gastric ulcers are *H. pylori* associated and the remainder are usually due to NSAIDs. It is important to remember that gastric ulceration is a mode of presentation of gastric cancer.

Clinical features

Dyspepsia is the commonest mode of presentation and the symptoms are described in Chapter 7. They are unreliable for separating DU from gastric ulcer (GU). Anorexia, vomiting, and weight loss should lead to the suspicion of gastric carcinoma. If there is persistent and severe pain, complications such as perforation or penetration into other organs should be considered.

Examination reveals epigastric tenderness. A mass suggests carcinoma, and a succussion splash suggests pyloric obstruction.

Investigation

This is described in Chapter 7. Gastroscopy (or barium meal) are the investigations of choice. All GU should be biopsied to exclude malignancy but DUs are nearly always benign; biopsies should be taken for *H. pylori* at endoscopy.

Most gastric carcinomas are on the greater curve and in the antrum. They may have a rolled edge and a translucent halo around them.

Acid secretion status may be assessed if Zollinger–Ellison syndrome is suspected, before and after stimulation with pentagastrin (see p 227).

Management

The patient should be advised to modify exacerbating factors such as smoking, diet, and alcohol. NSAIDs should be stopped if not absolutely necessary and the use of cyclo-oxygenase 2 (COX-2) antagonists may be considered in accordance with national guidelines (see further reading). Antacids, H_2 antagonists and proton pump inhibitors (PPIs) all help with symptomatic relief. Note that anti-secretory therapy can mask diagnoses at endoscopy and should therefore be withheld if endoscopy is planned. More specific therapies aimed at cure are described below:

Duodenal ulcer

Helicobacter pylori eradication should be undertaken using a locally approved regime. If the patient is rendered asymptomatic, no further follow up is required. If symptoms recur the breath test should be repeated; if positive, re-eradication is attempted; treatment failure may indicate poor compliance or antibiotic resistance; if negative, clinical re-evaluation and investigation is required. In the minority of patients who are *H. pylori* negative, culprit drugs such as NSAIDs should be stopped where possible and anti-secretory therapy titrated to symptoms. Low-dose PPI maintenance should only be used in patients who are persistently *H. pylori* positive or who are at risk of NSAID complications where the NSAID cannot be stopped.

Gastric ulcer

If *H. pylori* positive, eradication should be undertaken followed by anti-secretory therapy for 2 months. If *H. pylori* negative, 2 months of anti-secretory therapy should be given. In all cases, NSAID use should be discontinued. If this is not possible, consideration should be given to the use of maintenance therapy with misoprostol (prostaglandin analogue) or PPI, and the use of COX-2 inhibitors (see further reading).

All gastric ulcers should be followed up with endoscopy/biopsy until completely healed due to the risk of an underlying malignancy. If present for longer than 6 months, surgery should be considered.

Surgery

Surgery is usually considered when medical treatment has failed, or for complications that include persistent haemorrhage, perforation, or pyloric stenosis. Operations include partial gastrectomy or now, more commonly, highly selective vagotomy and pyloroplasty. Haemorrhage may be controlled endoscopically by injection with adrenaline or diathermy, laser photocoagulation, or heat probe. Perforations are usually oversewn with an omental plug.

Complications of surgery include:
- Recurrent ulceration.
- Abdominal fullness.
- Bilious vomiting.
- Diarrhoea.
- Dumping syndrome. This is fainting and sweating after eating, possibly due to food of high osmotic potential being dumped into the jejunum and causing hypovolaemia because of rapid fluid shifts. 'Late dumping' is due to hypoglycaemia and occurs 1–3 hours after taking food.

Metabolic complications include:
- Weight loss.
- Malabsorption.
- Bacterial overgrowth (blind loop syndrome).
- Anaemia, usually due to iron deficiency following hypochlorhydria and stomach resection.

Complications

The three main complications secondary to peptic ulceration are bleeding, perforation, and pyloric stenosis. Perforation is commoner in DUs than GUs. Pyloric stenosis may also be prepyloric or in the duodenum. It occurs because of oedema surrounding the ulcer or from scar formation on healing. The patient often has projectile vomiting with food ingested up to 24 hours previously. There may be visible peristalsis and a succussion splash. Vomiting may lead to dehydration and a metabolic alkalosis.

Fluid and electrolyte replacement is needed, as is gastric aspiration with a nasogastric tube. Surgery is indicated if the patient does not settle with conservative management.

Upper gastrointestinal haemorrhage

The haemoglobin concentration will remain normal for several hours after a significant haemorrhage

The differential diagnosis, history, and examination of patients with gastrointestinal (GI) bleeding is given in Chapter 8. Emergency resuscitative

223

measures may be needed before a full assessment is made. All patients with a significant bleed should be admitted to hospital. The vast majority will stop bleeding spontaneously within 48 hours.

Management

It is essential to establish early whether or not the patient is haemodynamically shocked. In the shocked patient fluid resuscitation to correct haemodynamic instability is a priority:

- Ensure the airway is protected and administer high-flow oxygen. Two large bore cannulae should be inserted into large veins (e.g. antecubital fossa) and this enables blood samples to be taken as advised in Chapter 8.
- Intravenous crystalloid or colloid should be given while awaiting cross matched blood. If bleeding is profuse O-negative blood may be used.
- Clotting should be corrected with platelets, vitamin K or fresh frozen plasma as required.
- Insert a urinary catheter to monitor urine output. Consider central venous pressure (CVP) monitoring if the patient is unstable—but be aware of the risks of this procedure if clotting is deranged.
- Fluid resuscitation should be titrated to the pulse rate, blood pressure, urine output, CVP (5–10 cmH$_2$O) and clinical assessment of fluid status.

If there are no signs of shock, and the patient is not anaemic, they may be managed 'conservatively' (i.e. bed rest, nil by mouth, and close monitoring of the pulse, blood pressure, and fluid balance). Blood should be grouped and saved, and normal saline should be given intravenously.

Once the patient is stable, endoscopy should be carried out within 4 hours if variceal bleeding is suspected or within 12–24 hours if the patient was shocked on admission or has significant co-morbidity. Other patients can wait longer. The cause for the bleed will be apparent in over 80% of cases.

If there is active bleeding, adrenaline can be injected, or bleeding vessels coagulated with a heat probe or with laser therapy. Proton pump inhibitors are given to patients with bleeding ulcers and then they are managed as described above.

Surgery is indicated if it is not possible to control the bleeding with medical management, especially for persistent or recurrent bleeding, although this is now becoming less common. It is more often carried out in the elderly and for those with GUs compared to DUs.

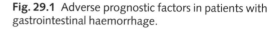

Adverse prognostic factors in patients with gastrointestinal haemorrhage
• Age over 60 years • Recurrent haemorrhage • Initial presentation with shock • More than 6 units of blood needed • An active bleeding vessel seen on endoscopy • Bleeding from oesophageal varices, which can lead to liver failure and hepatic coma

Fig. 29.1 Adverse prognostic factors in patients with gastrointestinal haemorrhage.

Bleeds from GUs carry twice the mortality of bleeds from DUs. Adverse prognostic factors are shown in Fig. 29.1. Patients must be monitored very closely for re-bleeding as this has a mortality of 40% and is often an indication for surgery.

Management of bleeding oesophageal varices

Resuscitative procedures, correction of coagulation and endoscopy should be carried out as above.

- Fluid resuscitation should aim to maintain a systolic blood pressure of 80–90 mmHg (and urine output greater than 30 mL/h). Over-aggressive fluid replacement may increase the chance of a re-bleed.
- Prophylactic antibiotics should be commenced and continued for 1 week.
- Vasoconstrictor therapy is used to reduce splanchnic blood flow and therefore portal pressure. Terlipressin (vasopressin analogue), or octreotide (somatostatin analogue) may be used.
- Urgent endoscopy allows acute variceal sclerotherapy or banding and these are the treatments of choice. This arrests bleeding in 80% of cases and reduces early re-bleeding.
- Measures to prevent hepatic encephalopathy should be started, which include emptying the bowel with enemas or lactulose, and giving neomycin 1 g 6-hourly to reduce the number of bowel organisms.
- If the bleeding continues, a Sengstaken–Blakemore tube can be passed through the oesophagus, with balloons to compress the varices at the oesophago-gastric junction. The patient ought to be intubated and sedated for this, to minimise risks, and its use should be restricted to those in whom massive bleeding is not controlled by initial therapy who are awaiting definitive treatment.
- Options in patients who continue to bleed include transjugular intrahepatic portosystemic shunt,

which is performed by interventional radiologists to lower portal pressure by creating a shunt to the systemic circulation, or surgery. Surgical procedures include oesophageal transection with anastamosis, transthoracic transoesophageal ligation of varices, and gastric transection with reanastamosis.

- To prevent recurrent variceal bleeding, measures include long-term injection sclerotherapy (which may be combined with banding) leading to obliteration of the varices by fibrous tissues. This reduces re-bleeding and mortality. Complications include oesophageal ulceration, mediastinitis, and strictures. Non-selective β-blockers (e.g. propanolol) decrease portal pressures and significantly reduce primary and secondary bleeding and mortality from large varices.

Approximately half of those bleeding from varices for the first time will die. The risk of recurrence is approximately 80% in the next 2 years. Adverse prognostic factors are jaundice, ascites, hypoalbuminaemia, and encephalopathy.

Gastric carcinoma

The incidence of gastric carcinoma is 15 in 100 000, and it is commoner in men and the elderly. There is a link between gastric cancer and *H. pylori*, which may explain the higher prevalence in lower socio-economic groups. Suggested dietary links include alcohol, spicy foods, and nitrates, which are converted to nitrosamines by bacteria. It occurs more often in Japan due to the higher fish intake resulting in a high level of nitrosamines. It is commoner in smokers, in patients with achlorhydria, and in patients with blood group A.

Other predisposing conditions include pernicious anaemia, chronic gastritis with atrophy, areas of intestinal metaplasia, and partial gastrectomy.

Most cancers are adenocarcinomas and affect mainly the pylorus and antrum. They are polypoid or ulcerating lesions with rolled edges. Less common are leather-bottle type adenocarcinomas (linitis plastica).

Clinical features

General features of malignancy may be present (weight loss, anorexia etc.). Local features may include dyspeptic symptoms (see Chapter 7), nausea and vomiting, gastro-intestinal bleeding or iron deficiency anaemia, and a palpable epigastric mass or tenderness. Metastatic features include Virchow's node in the left supraclavicular fossa and metastases to liver, bones, brain and lung. Trans-coelomic spread may occur (e.g. to ovaries, Krukenberg's tumour). Paraneoplastic features include dermatomyositis and acanthosis nigricans.

Investigation

Blood tests include a full blood count (FBC) to look for signs of chronic blood loss, and liver function tests (LFTs) for possible metastases. Diagnosis is made on gastroscopy with multiple biopsies. Computed tomography may help with staging.

Treatment

The 5-year survival is approximately 10% but the 5-year survival with gastrectomy (if found early) is up to 50%. Metastases contraindicate curative surgery in up to 60% of cases and palliation may involve the use of drugs, surgery and radiotherapy.

Small bowel disorders

Malabsorption

Causes of malabsorption are given in Fig. 29.2.

The clinical features of malabsorption have been outlined in Chapter 9 and include anorexia, weight loss and lethargy, abdominal distension and borborygmi, steatorrhoea, wasting, clubbing, petechiae (vitamin K), anaemia (iron, vitamin B_{12}, folate), paraesthesia, bone pain and tetany (hypocalcaemia), oedema, leuconychia and ascites (hypoproteinaemia), and peripheral neuropathy (vitamin B deficiency). There may also be signs of the underlying disease (e.g. jaundice or lymphadenopathy with lymphomas).

The range of investigations to be considered has been dealt with in Chapter 9.

Specific diseases
Chronic pancreatitis

This is a common cause of malabsorption (see 'Diseases of the Pancreas' below).

Coeliac disease

Coeliac disease is a gluten-sensitive enteropathy. In this disease, there is an abnormal jejunal mucosa leading to malabsorption. The condition improves with a gluten-free diet but relapses when gluten is reintroduced.

Gluten is present in wheat, barley, rye, and oats.

225

Fig. 29.2 Causes of malabsorption.

Causes of malabsorption	
Cause	Examples
Biliary insufficiency	Primary biliary cirrhosis, biliary obstruction, cholestyramine, ileal resection (impaired enterohepatic circulation)
Pancreatic insufficiency	Chronic pancreatitis, pancreatic carcinoma, cystic fibrosis, Zollinger–Ellison syndrome (pancreatic enzymes inactive at low pH due to gastric acid hypersecretion)
Small bowel mucosa	Coeliac disease, Whipple's disease, tropical sprue, radiation enteritis, small bowel resection, brush border enzyme deficiency (e.g. lactase deficiency), drugs (e.g. metformin), amyloid, hypogammaglobulinaemia (also predisposes to infection), intestinal lymphangiectasia, lymphoma, abetalipoproteinaemia, ischaemia
Bacterial overgrowth	Especially in diverticula and post-operative blind loops. Also in dilated areas of small bowel in systemic sclerosis
Infection	Giardiasis, diphyllobothriasis, strongyloidiasis, tuberculosis
Intestinal hurry	Post-gastrectomy dumping, post-vagotomy, gastrojejunostomy, short bowel syndrome (multiple resections e.g. Crohn's disease)

Coeliac disease is commoner in Europeans, with an incidence of approximately 1 in 2000 in the UK. It is commoner in females and can occur at any age, but has two peaks in incidence (0–5 years and 50–60 years). There is an increased incidence within families, and it is associated with HLA-B8 and DR3. It is also associated with a blistering subepidermal eruption of the skin (dermatitis herpetiformis). The aetiology is thought to be due to α-gliadin, a peptide present in gluten, which is injurious to the small bowel mucosa. Immunogenic mechanisms and possibly environmental factors (e.g. viral infections) may also play a role.

Clinical features

Symptoms may be non-specific (e.g. lethargy and malaise). There is usually a history of diarrhoea or steatorrhoea, with abdominal discomfort, and there may be weight loss. Other features include mouth ulcers, anaemia, and less commonly tetany, osteomalacia, neuropathies, myopathies and hyposplenism.

There is an increased incidence of autoimmune disease (e.g. thyroid disease and insulin-dependent diabetes). Coeliac disease may be complicated by GI lymphoma and gastric or oesophageal carcinoma.

Investigations

The following investigations are important in the patient with coeliac disease:

- Jejunal biopsy: villous atrophy with chronic inflammatory cells in the lamina propria.
- FBC: may show anaemia (folate or iron deficiency—vitamin B_{12} deficiency is rare as the stomach and terminal ileum are not involved).
- Antireticulin antibodies and anti-endomysial antibodies: usually present.
- Serum albumin: hypoalbuminaemia.
- Prothrombin time: may be prolonged due to vitamin K deficiency.

Management

The condition improves on a gluten-free diet. Deficient vitamins are replaced. If symptoms persist, it may be that the patient is not complying with the diet. A high index of suspicion for the complications mentioned above should be maintained.

Bacterial overgrowth

Although bacterial overgrowth may occur spontaneously, especially in the elderly, it is normally associated with a structural abnormality of the small intestine (e.g. in diverticula or post-operative blind loops). Aspiration of jejunal contents reveals *Escherichia coli* or *Bacteroides* in concentrations greater than 10^6 per mL as part of a mixed flora. The bacteria can deconjugate bile salts, which can be detected in aspirates; this deficiency of conjugated bile salts leads to steatorrhoea. The bacteria also metabolise vitamin B_{12} leading to its deficiency.

Management

Underlying small bowel lesions should be corrected if possible. The condition may respond to intermittent courses of metronidazole 400 mg 8-hourly or oxytetracycline 250 mg 6-hourly.

Tropical sprue

In this condition, there is severe malabsorption usually accompanied by diarrhoea and malnutrition. It occurs in most of Asia and the Caribbean. The aetiology is unknown but it is thought to be infective. Jejunal histology shows partial villous atrophy.

Management

Severe cases may need intravenous fluids and electrolytes, and replacement of nutritional and vitamin deficiencies. Patients often improve when they leave an endemic area. Patients may be helped with tetracycline 250 mg 6-hourly and folic acid.

Whipple's disease

This is a rare cause of malabsorption, usually affecting men over 50 years old. As well as steatorrhoea, there is fever, weight loss, arthralgia, lymphadenopathy, and sometimes involvement of the heart, lung, and brain. Histologically, cells of the lamina propria are replaced by macrophages which contain periodic acid–Schiff positive glycoprotein granules. The organism responsible is *Tropheryma whippelii*. Treatment is with antibiotics (e.g. tetracycline or chloramphenicol).

Endocrine tumours of the gut

Although these are all very rare they are sometimes discussed in examinations. Carcinoid tumours often occur in the small bowel, and the other tumours discussed below arise in the pancreas. They are discussed in this section for convenience, and because they often affect the small bowel.

They arise from APUD (amine precursor: uptake and decarboxylation) cells, which secrete a number of hormones, e.g. gastrin, glucagon, and vasoactive intestinal peptide (VIP). Pancreatic endocrine tumours may occur with other endocrine tumours as part of MEN syndromes (see Chapter 32).

Zollinger–Ellison syndrome

This is usually due to a gastrin-secreting pancreatic adenoma, which stimulates excessive acid production leading to multiple recurrent ulcers in the stomach and duodenum. Approximately half are malignant and 10% are multiple.

Patients commonly get diarrhoea due to the low pH in the upper intestine, and steatorrhoea due to the inactivation of lipase by the low pH. The diagnosis is made by a raised fasting serum gastrin level; the gastric acid output is also raised. Treatment is by removal of the primary tumour (provided there is no evidence of metastases) and omeprazole or octreotide.

Insulinomas

These are tumours of the pancreatic islet β-cells; 5% are malignant and 5% are multiple. The patient presents with recurrent or fasting hypoglycaemia, which may manifest in bizarre behaviour, epilepsy, dementia, or confusion. The diagnosis is confirmed by the demonstration of hypoglycaemia in association with inappropriate and excessive insulin secretion. Treatment is by surgical excision of the tumour. If surgery is not feasible, diazoxide or octreotide are useful. Fasting hypoglycaemia is discussed in Chapter 32.

Vipomas

These tumours release VIP, which produces intestinal secretions leading to watery diarrhoea, hypokalaemia, and sometimes achlorhydria. Diagnosis is by high serum levels of VIP. The tumour should be resected if possible. Octreotide is useful for controlling symptoms.

Glucagonomas

These are tumours of the α-cells of the pancreas, which release glucagon. Symptoms include diabetes, diarrhoea, a necrolytic migratory erythematous rash, weight loss, anaemia, and glossitis.

Carcinoid tumours

These tumours originate from the argentaffin cells of the intestine. They may appear in the appendix, terminal ileum, rectum, or other site in the GI tract. They have malignant potential; 80% of large tumours produce metastases. Presentations include appendicitis (10% of tumours arise in the appendix), GI obstruction and, in 5% of cases, the carcinoid syndrome.

Carcinoid syndrome

This only occurs when liver metastases are present as the level of the metabolites is otherwise controlled by first pass metabolism in the liver. Clinical features include flushing (which may be prolonged and lead to telangiectases), abdominal pain, diarrhoea, bronchospasm, and oedema associated with pulmonary stenosis or tricuspid regurgitation.

Symptoms are due to the release of pharmacologically active mediators [e.g. 5-hydroxytryptamine (5-HT), prostaglandins, and kinins].

Diagnosis is by measurement of 5-hydroxyindoleacetic acid (5-HIAA) in 24-hour urine collection. Abdominal CT scan or laparotomy may be needed to localise the tumour.

Treatment: Food and drink which precipitate flushing should be avoided (e.g. alcohol, coffee). Surgery is best for localised tumours and may be curative. Octreotide alleviates flushing and diarrhoea. Other useful drugs include cyproheptadine (an antihistamine with 5-HT and calcium channel blocking properties), and methysergide (which also blocks 5-HT). Other procedures include enucleation of liver metastases, hepatic artery ligation, embolisation, and 5-fluorouracil injection.

Prognosis: the median survival is 5–10 years after diagnosis.

Inflammatory bowel disease

Extraintestinal manifestations of IBD are A PIE SAC: aphthous ulcers, pyoderma gangrenosum, iritis, erythema nodosum, sclerosing cholangitis, arthritis, and clubbing.

Ulcerative colitis (UC) and Crohn's disease are collectively termed inflammatory bowel disease (IBD). It is likely that these conditions represent a spectrum of disease resulting from a combination of genetic and environmental factors, although they typically differ in their natural history and response to treatment (Fig. 29.3).

Aetiology

The primary cause of ulcerative colitis is unknown, although 10–15% of patients have a first-degree relative with UC or Crohn's disease. It may result from a genetically determined, inappropriately severe, and/or prolonged inflammatory response to a dietary or microbial product. Abnormalities of colonic epithelial cell metabolism have also been reported in ulcerative colitis, and there are associations with certain drugs such as NSAIDs and antibiotics, and with stress, although the significance is uncertain.

There may be a history of atopy, autoimmune disease (e.g. chronic active hepatitis and systemic lupus erythematosus), and the presence of circulating immune complexes and antibodies to colonocytes and neutrophils (pANCA) in ulcerative colitis.

Ulcerative colitis occurs almost exclusively among non-smokers whereas approximately two-thirds of patients who have Crohn's disease smoke cigarettes.

Ulcerative colitis

This is an idiopathic chronic relapsing inflammatory disease which always involves the rectum and extends proximally in continuity to affect a variable length of colon. Although the small bowel is spared there may be some 'backwash ileitis'. It is commoner in the Western world with a prevalence of approximately 150 in 100 000, and an incidence of about 10 in 100 000 annually, and is maximal at 15–40 years of age. There is no major sex difference.

Clinical features

The disease may present with a single mild episode followed by remission for a prolonged period, or progressive symptoms over months with general ill health and chronic diarrhoea, or as an acute severe episode. In general, the severity of diarrhoea and systemic upset depends on the extent of the disease and depth of mucosal ulceration.

Active subtotal or total ulcerative colitis causes frequent bloody diarrhoea, often with fever, malaise, anorexia, weight loss, abdominal pain, anaemia, and tachycardia. With proctitis, characteristic symptoms are rectal bleeding and mucous discharge, but the stool is well formed and general health is maintained. The patient may present with a complication. Between relapses, the patient is usually symptomless.

Complications
Local
Toxic megacolon, perforation, or rarely massive haemorrhage can occur. There is an increased risk of colonic carcinoma in patients with subtotal or total ulcerative colitis. The cumulative incidence is 10–15% at 20 years.

Extraintestinal
Extraintestinal complications of inflammatory bowel disease include the following:
• Skin: erythema nodosum, pyoderma gangrenosum, vasculitis.
• Eyes: uveitis, episcleritis, conjunctivitis.

Features of Crohn's disease and ulcerative colitis		
Feature	**Crohn's disease**	**Ulcerative colitis**
Pathology	Transmural inflammation	Only mucosa and submucosa inflamed
	Fissuring ulcers—cobblestone mucosa	Mucosal ulcers—pseudopolyps
	Non-caseating granulomata	Crypt abscesses
	Can involve whole GI tract. Skip lesions	Continuous involvement proximally from rectum to affect variable length of colon
Clinical	Diarrhoea ± rectal bleeding	Diarrhoea—often with blood and mucus
	Abdominal pain and fever prominent	Abdominal pain less prominent. Fever may be present
	Anal/perianal and oral lesions	
	Stricturing causing obstructive symptoms	
Associations	Increased incidence in smokers	Decreased incidence in smokers
	Cholelithiasis	Increased primary biliary cirrhosis, sclerosing cholangitis, chronic active hepatitis
	Extra-intestinal manifestations of IBD (see below)	Other extra-intestinal manifestations of IBD are less common than in Crohn's
Complications	Fistulae (entero-enteral, -vaginal, -vesical, perianal)	No fistulae
	Strictures causing bowel obstruction	Toxic megacolon (in acute colitis)
	Carcinoma (related to colitis)	Carcinoma
	IDA	
	Abscess formation	
	B_{12} deficiency (terminal ileum commonly involved)	IDA

Fig. 29.3 Features of Crohn's disease and ulcerative colitis (IBD, inflammatory bowel disease; IDA, iron deficiency anaemia.)

- Joints: large joint arthropathy, sacroiliitis, ankylosing spondylitis.
- Liver: pericholangitis, sclerosing cholangitis, cirrhosis, chronic active hepatitis, cholangiocarcinoma.
- Vasculature: arterial and venous thrombosis.
- Renal stones and gallbladder stones: in Crohn's disease.

Investigations

Sigmoidoscopy and rectal biopsy show inflamed mucosa. If the disease is active there may be pus and blood, visible ulceration, and contact bleeding. Other types of colitis should be excluded, and stool microscopy and culture is needed to exclude infection.

Histology shows inflammatory cells infiltrating the lamina propria with crypt abscesses. There is little involvement of the muscularis mucosa, and there is a reduction of goblet cells.

Barium enema shows loss of the normal haustral pattern and the bowel looks like a smooth tube ('leadpipe colon'). Ulcers and pseudopolyps may be seen, oedema of the colonic wall produces widening

229

of the presacral space, and there may be narrowed areas secondary to carcinoma. In the patient with acute colitis a plain abdominal X-ray should be performed to look for colonic dilation and evidence of mucosal oedema.

Management
General measures
A multidisciplinary approach is preferred with gastroenterologists, nursing staff, counsellors, and stoma therapists, in collaboration with primary health-care teams. Support groups are available. Some patients may improve with avoidance of cow's milk, and some with proctitis benefit from fibre supplements. Specific nutritional, haematinic, and electrolyte deficiencies may require correction. NSAIDs and antibiotics should be avoided.

The acute relapse
The mortality of patients with acute colitis climbs sharply if they perforate. Therefore, management is directed at stratifying them in terms of severity (and therefore risk of perforation), treating them accordingly to induce remission, and carefully selecting those patients requiring emergency colectomy, hopefully before they perforate.

The mainstay of therapy in the acute phase is steroids (intravenous, oral, topical as suppository, liquid, foam or enema).

In mild UC (less than five motions/day, systemically well), oral prednisolone 20mg o.d. and daily steroid enemas are given for 4 weeks. In those passing more than eight motions/day, but who remain systemically well, steroid enemas are given and oral prednisolone should be started at 40 mg o.d. and reduced by 10 mg weekly until at 20 mg which is maintained for 4 weeks. If patients are systemically unwell (tachycardia, hypotension, fever, dehydration, tender colon) and passing more than eight motions/day, they should be admitted to hospital:

- Nil by mouth, intravenous fluids, close monitoring of observations, stool chart.
- Daily blood tests and regular plain abdominal X-ray to monitor progress.
- 400 mg intravenous hydrocortisone per day in divided doses with steroid enemas. Prophylactic subcutaneous heparin is given.
- Antibiotics for any accompanying septicaemia (usually Gram-negative).
- If improved at 5 days, commence oral therapy.
- If failing to respond some advocate the careful use of cyclosporin to induce remission.

- Indications for emergency colectomy: continuing deterioration despite medical therapy; toxic dilation of the colon; perforation.

5-aminosalicylic acid (5-ASA) compounds (see below) are also given during the acute phase although their main role is in the prevention of relapse.

Maintaining remission
The aminosalicylates help maintain remission, reducing annual relapse rates from 70% to 30%. They are also available as enemas and suppositories. There are different preparations with different methods of releasing the active component (5-ASA) in the colon. Sulphasalazine is an example. This consists of 5-ASA, linked by an azo bond to sulphapyridine. The 5-ASA is released in the colon by bacterial action. Approximately 20% of patients cannot tolerate sulphasalazine because of adverse effects, mostly related to the sulphapyridine. These include headache and fever, blood dyscrasias, bone marrow suppression, rashes, and oligospermia, making newer compounds preferable in young men.

Mesalazine contains 5-ASA alone and may have fewer side effects. It is a delayed release preparation. Balsalazide is a pro-drug with a diazo bond.

Azathioprine may be used in patients who relapse repeatedly on steroid withdrawal after an acute episode, or in whom aminosalicylates are ineffective for maintaining remission; it may take up to 4 months to effect a noticeable clinical benefit. Serious adverse effects include bone marrow suppression and cholestatic jaundice, necessitating blood checks fortnightly for the first 3 months. Long-term safety data are still awaited.

Surgery
Surgery is curative for colonic disease though not for extraintestinal complications. Options include panproctocolectomy with ileoanal pouch, permanent ileostomy, or rarely subtotal colectomy with ileorectal anastamosis. It may be considered electively for chronic intractable ulcerative colitis, colonic carcinoma, persistent mucosal dysplasia, or growth retardation in children. The emergency indications are summarised above.

Prognosis
Approximately 70% of untreated patients relapse annually, and up to 30% eventually require surgery, although the overall mortality is close to that of the general population. The main risks to life are severe attacks of ulcerative colitis and colonic cancer.

Patients with extensive ulcerative colitis of 10 years' duration or more are offered colonoscopy every 1–2 years to prevent colonic cancer by taking multiple biopsies to look for mucosal dysplasia (i.e. detection of cancer at a curable stage), and by offering elective colectomy if appropriate.

Crohn's disease

Crohn's disease can affect any part of the GI tract from the mouth to the anus. The involvement is not confluent ('skip lesions') (Fig. 29.3). It most frequently presents with ileocaecal disease followed by colonic, ileal alone, diffuse small intestinal, gastric, and oesophageal involvement. The overall prevalence in the Western world is approximately 1 in 1000 and is more common in Caucasians than Afro-Caribbeans.

Clinical presentation

The patient has diarrhoea and abdominal pain. There may be a fever, anaemia, and weight loss. The patient may be clubbed and there may be associated complications (e.g. joint, skin, or eye complications, as with ulcerative colitis).

The presentation depends on the site of disease, and on the tendency to perforate or fistulate rather than to fibrose and stricture, which is probably determined by genetic factors. Terminal ileal disease presents with right iliac fossa pain, often with an associated mass. This may present acutely, mimicking appendicitis, or chronically, mimicking irritable bowel syndrome.

Colonic Crohn's disease is distinguishable from ulcerative colitis by the presence of skip lesions (multiple lesions with normal bowel in between), rectal sparing, perianal skin tags, or fistulae with or without granulomata on biopsy, although the distinction is unclear in up to a third of patients.

Complications
Local
Strictures cause partial or complete gastrointestinal obstruction. Entero-enteric, -vesical, -vaginal and perianal fistulae may develop. Prolonged disease increases the risk of small and large bowel cancer. Abscesses may form. Iron, folate and vitamin B_{12} deficiency can all occur.

Extraintestinal
As for UC above. Fig. 29.3 summarises the few differences between UC and Crohn's in terms of their extraintestinal manifestations.

Investigations
Diagnosis is made by endoscopy and biopsy of lesions. Histology demonstrates transmural inflammation with an inflammatory cell infiltrate and non-caseating granulomata (in 30%). Barium imaging of the small and large bowel is performed. This shows skip lesions, a coarse cobblestone appearance of the mucosa and, later, fibrosis producing narrowing of the intestine ('string sign') with proximal dilatation.

Serum C-reactive protein is raised in approximaterly 95% of cases with active disease.

Magnetic resonance imaging (MRI) is useful for evaluation of fistulas and abscesses.

Management
In most cases of active Crohn's disease, there are three therapeutic alternatives: drugs, diet and surgery. These options should be discussed with the patient.

Medical management
Some patients manage on symptomatic therapy alone (e.g. loperamide or codeine phosphate) provided there is no evidence of obstruction. Cholestyramine (ion exchange resin) is useful for diarrhoea due to terminal ileal disease or resection as it prevents conjugated bile acids from entering the colon. However, it should not be given at the same time as other medications as it impairs their absorption. Haematinics may require replacement although anaemia often improves as disease activity falls.

Acute attacks are often treated with corticosteroids (e.g. prednisolone 30–60 mg o.d.), but these have no effect on reducing the rate of relapse. Their inappropriate use must be avoided due to their side effect profile. Budesonide is a corticosteroid analogue with rapid hepatic conversion and therefore reduced systemic side effects that is useful in mild attacks. Azathioprine (or its active metabolite 6-mercaptopurine) is often started during the acute attack. It is helpful in maintaining the steroid induced remission but takes several weeks to be effective.

Patients with colonic involvement may benefit from a 5-ASA compound (see above). Antibiotics also have a role. Metronidazole is effective in colonic and perianal disease and in prevention of recurrence following bowel resection. If used for longer than 3 months, there is a risk of peripheral neuropathy. Other antibiotics are also used.

Elemental diets are useful for inducing remission in small bowel disease but are expensive and unpalatable, therefore compliance is often poor.

Some patients can be maintained in remission without drug therapy—the importance of stopping smoking to Crohn's disease patients must be emphasised. However, some patients require immunosuppressive therapy—azathioprine and other agents are used. The National Institute of Clinical Excellence (NICE) supports the expert use of infliximab (monoclonal antibody against tumour necrosis factor alpha) in severe cases without fistula formation resistant to other drugs.

Surgery
80% of patients will require an operation at some stage but surgery should be avoided if possible. It is indicated for:
- Failure of medical therapy with acute or chronic illness causing ill-health.
- Complications—abscess, obstruction, perforation, toxic dilation, fistulae not responding to conservative treatment with antibiotics.
- Failure to grow (children).

Small bowel strictures can be widened (stricturoplasty) whereas those elsewhere need resection. Post-operative fistulas used to be a common complication but are now rare, partly due to perioperative antibiotics, particularly metronidazole. After surgical resection, approximately half the patients remain symptom free for 5 years and half require further surgery within 10 years.

Prognosis
A minority of patients have extensive disease or frequent recurrences, and account for most of the 10% who ultimately die of the disease. Around 10–20% of patients remain asymptomatic for 20 years after the first or second episode of symptomatic disease. Most patients need surgery within the first few years and further resections at intervals of 10–15 years but have a good quality of life for most of this time.

Colorectal disease

Colorectal neoplasia
Colonic polyps are common and often found incidentally during investigation of coincidental GI symptoms such as pain, altered bowel habit, or bleeding haemorrhoids. They may be non-neoplastic or neoplastic (commoner) and may be sessile or pedunculated, vary from a few millimetres to up to 10 cm in diameter, and they may be solitary or multiple.

Peutz–Jeghers' syndrome consists of mucocutaneous pigmentation and hamartomatous polyps (non-neoplastic) anywhere along the GI tract, most commonly in the small bowel. It has a Mendelian dominant inheritance.

Adenomatous polyps (neoplastic) are usually asymptomatic. They may bleed and lead to iron-deficiency anaemia. Sessile villous adenomas of the rectum may present with profuse diarrhoea and hypokalaemia. Most colonic carcinomas originate from adenomas. Once a polyp is found, it is therefore removed endoscopically, and as further polyps may develop a programme of continuous colonoscopic surveillance every 3–5 years is recommended.

Familial adenomatous polyposis (FAP) is Mendelian dominant. Patients have multiple polyps throughout the GI tract. In high-risk patients, colectomy with ileorectal anastamosis may be performed, with continued surveillance of the rectal stump.

Colonic adenocarcinoma is the second commonest tumour in the UK with a lifetime incidence of approximately 1 in 27. It is commoner in the elderly and less common in Africa and Asia. It may be related to low fibre and high animal fat diets. Predisposing conditions include colitis in inflammatory bowel disease and FAP. Genetic factors also play a role, with a two- to three-fold increased risk of developing colon cancer with one first-degree affected family member. At the upper end of this risk spectrum is hereditary non-polyposis colon cancer. This is a dominantly inherited mutation of a DNA mismatch repair gene. Affected family members develop right sided cancers at an early age and therefore colonoscopic surveillance is commenced from 25–35 years.

90% of colon cancer occurs in patients without a strong family history. Over half of these tumours occur in the recto-sigmoid area. Two-thirds of tumours occur with ulceration, and spread by direct infiltration, invading the lymph nodes and blood vessels, leading to metastases.

Clinical features
General features of malignancy include weight loss, anorexia and lethargy. Local features depend on the location of the tumour. Left-sided tumours present with altered bowel habit and abdominal pain.

Rectosigmoid tumours commonly bleed. Right-sided carcinomas can become large and remain asymptomatic (as the stool has a liquid consistency here). They may present with iron deficiency anaemia alone. The elderly often present with bowel obstruction. Any change in bowel habit or rectal bleeding must be investigated—especially in the elderly.

Examination should always include a digital rectal examination and sigmoidoscopy. A mass may be detected and with liver metastases hepatomegaly is felt.

Investigation

FBC for anaemia, and urea and electrolytes (U&Es) for electrolyte abnormalities with diarrhoea. Colonoscopy and barium enema will identify most tumours. Ultrasound and computed tomography is useful for staging—modified Duke's classification (Fig. 29.4). Biopsy is essential for tissue diagnosis and tumour grading.

Treatment

Over 90% of primary tumours can be resected surgically. Adjuvant radiotherapy and chemotherapy may be used for more advanced disease. The prognosis is summarised in Fig. 29.4.

Diverticular disease

A diverticulum is an outpouching of the wall of the gut. Diverticula can occur anywhere in the gut but are most common in the colon, especially the sigmoid colon. Diverticulosis implies the presence of diverticula, and diverticulitis implies that there is inflammation within a diverticulum. They are due to high intracolonic pressure with weakness of the colonic wall. The mucosa therefore herniates through the muscle layers of the gut. The incidence increases with age and affects up to a third of the population although most people are asymptomatic. It is more common in women then men.

Clinical features

There may be colicky left-sided abdominal pain and tenderness, nausea, and flatulence. The pain may be relieved with defecation and there may be a change in bowel habit with constipation or diarrhoea. With diverticulitis, pain is more severe, and the patient is pyrexial. Diverticula may perforate and lead to localised or generalised peritonitis or fistula formation. Fistulae may communicate between the colon and bladder (vesicocolic fistula) leading to pneumaturia and recurrent urinary tract infection. They may also form between the colon and vagina or small bowel. Rectal bleeding may occur and is usually sudden and painless. Subacute obstruction may occur due to stricture formation.

Management

In acute diverticulitis, treatment is with bed rest, analgesia, and antibiotics. The patient may have to be kept nil by mouth and given intravenous fluids. Abscesses may need to be drained, and peritonitis following perforation or obstruction may necessitate resection and colostomy. Patients with profuse rectal bleeding may require transfusion and colonic resection. Treatment of fistulae is surgical.

For diverticulosis, a high-fibre diet is recommended, and bran supplements and bulk-forming agents can be prescribed. Antispasmodics may provide symptomatic relief when colic is a problem. Drugs which slow intestinal motility (e.g. codeine and loperamide, could exacerbate symptoms and are contraindicated).

Modified Duke's classification of colorectal carcinoma			
Tumour stage	Definition	Percentage of cases	Five-year cancer-related survival (%)
A	Confined to bowel wall	10	90–100
B	Beyond bowel wall/no metastases	35	65–75
C	Involves lymph nodes	30	30–40
D	Distant metastases/residual disease after surgery	25	<5

Fig. 29.4 Modified Duke's classification of colorectal carcinoma.

Pseudomembranous colitis

Pseudomembranous colitis is caused by colonisation of the colon with *Clostridium difficile*, which produces toxins. It usually follows antibiotic therapy and should be suspected in patients in hospital who develop diarrhoea after a period of antibiotics. It is usually of acute onset but may run a chronic course. The most frequently implicated antibiotic is clindamycin but few antibiotics are free of this side effect. Clinical features include diarrhoea, fever and abdominal cramps. As with all causes of colitis, if severe, toxic dilation of the colon can occur.

Diagnosis

Diagnosis is by identification of the toxin in stool specimens. Sigmoidoscopy reveals an erythematous, ulcerated mucosa, which is covered by a membrane. However, the appearances are not essential for the diagnosis.

Management

Suspected antibiotics should be stopped and patients should be isolated for infection control. Oral vancomycin or metronidazole are used as specific treatments. Careful attention should be paid to fluid and electrolyte management.

Lower gastrointestinal bleeding

The differential diagnosis of lower GI bleeding is shown in Fig. 29.5.

Resuscitation should be carried out as for upper GI bleeds, and further investigations are carried out when the patient is stable. Examination should include a rectal examination to exclude carcinoma, sigmoidoscopy, and colonoscopy. Barium enema may add to information,

---

Differential diagnosis of lower gastrointestinal bleeding

- Anal fissure
- Haemorrhoids
- Inflammatory bowel disease
- Infective colitis
- Gastrointestinal carcinoma: sigmoid, caecum, rectum
- Ischaemic colitis
- Diverticulitis
- Intestinal polyps
- Vascular abnormalities: angiodysplasia, arteriovenous malformations
- Meckel's diverticulum
- Peutz–Jeghers' syndrome
- Osler–Weber–Rendu syndrome
- Endometriosis

Fig. 29.5 Differential diagnosis of lower gastrointestinal bleeding

---

and angiography can be carried out if vascular abnormalities are suspected. Stool samples must also be sent to microbiology to exclude an infectious cause.

Lower GI bleeding may be occult and chronic, presenting with iron-deficiency anaemia, and general lethargy and fatigue. If the history does not suggest a particular site in the GI tract responsible for the blood loss, a sensible working plan is upper GI endoscopy followed by colonoscopy or barium enema. If no diagnosis is apparent, a small bowel follow-through (or enteroscopy) is next performed, followed by angiography if needed. Isotope-labelled red blood cells may localise the site of bleeding. Note that both angiography and isotope labelled red blood cell studies require active bleeding in order to provide useful information (see Chapter 8).

Ischaemic colitis

Acute ischaemia of the bowel may occur and is often embolic (e.g. due to atrial fibrillation). This is a surgical emergency. It is suggested by severe abdominal pain, haemodynamic shock, and a relative absence of clinical signs with a metabolic acidosis.

Chronic intestinal ischaemia usually relates to low flow in the inferior mesenteric artery and therefore affects the descending colon. Severe post-prandial pain occurs ('gut claudication') with rectal bleeding and diarrhoea. There is often a pyrexia, tachycardia and leucocytosis. It usually settles with conservative management. Diagnosis is difficult but revascularisation may be attempted following angiography. Occasionally gangrene of the affected gut segment occurs—surgical resection is necessary and mortality is high.

Irritable bowel syndrome and non-ulcer dyspepsia

Irritable bowel syndrome

Irritable bowel syndrome is the commonest diagnosis made in GI clinics, although there is no accepted definition. It occurs mainly in young women. There is intermittent colicky abdominal pain which is relieved by bowel action, diarrhoea or frequent passage of small amounts of stool, and bloating. The diarrhoea may alternate with periods of constipation. Some people have a sense of incomplete evacuation or 'rectal dissatisfaction'. Symptoms may be precipitated by certain foods, drugs (e.g. antibiotics) or stress. Note that rectal bleeding is not a feature and that prominent nocturnal symptoms point away from the diagnosis.

Investigation

The diagnosis is one of exclusion. It is important not to miss more serious disease, e.g. inflammatory bowel disease or malignancy. It is prudent to check the FBC and erythrocyte sedimentation rate, faecal occult blood, and perform a sigmoidoscopy. Older patients, or patients in whom colonic carcinoma is suspected, warrant a barium enema.

Treatment

Symptoms may improve with a high-fibre diet, with bran or with other agents which increase stool bulk. Specific aggravating foods should be avoided. In some patients there may be important psychological aggravating factors which respond to reassurance. Antimotility drugs such as loperamide may relieve diarrhoea, and antispasmodic drugs (e.g. mebeverine 135 mg t.d.s.) may relieve pain. Opioids with a central action such as codeine are best avoided because of the risk of dependence. Some patients derive benefit from low doses of tricyclic antidepressant drugs.

Non-ulcer dyspepsia

This term encompasses a heterogeneous group of patients with dyspeptic symptoms (see Chapter 7) and no macroscopic mucosal abnormality. Only a minority of them actually undergo endoscopy (see Fig. 7.3).

The cause of their symptoms is unclear but is likely to be multi-factorial and include acid, dysmotility, *Helicobacter pylori* infection and depression. Management is often unsatisfactory. Lifestyle advice is given regarding smoking, alcohol, obesity, etc. Culprit drugs such as NSAIDs should be withdrawn if possible. Anti-secretory therapy is used and is titrated to the lowest cost preparation that achieves symptom control. Those who are *H. pylori* positive should receive eradication and patient reassurance is an important part of their management.

Diseases of the gallbladder

Gallstones

Courvoisier's law: 'if the gallbladder is palpable in painless jaundice, the cause will not be gallstones' (because gallstones cause fibrosis and shrinkage of the gallbladder)

Gallstones are most common in people with the 'six Fs':
- Fair.
- Fat.
- Fertile.
- Female.
- Forty.
- (Low) fibre diet.

The incidence of gallstones rises with age, and is greater in women on the oral contraceptive pill.

Bile contains cholesterol, bile pigments, and phospholipids, and it is the relative concentrations of these that determines the kind of stone that is formed. Pigment stones are small and radiolucent, and they are occasionally associated with haemolytic anaemia due to increased formation of bile pigment from haemoglobin.

Cholesterol stones are large, often solitary, and are radiolucent. Mixed stones contain calcium salts, pigment, and cholesterol; 10% are radio-opaque. (Compare with renal stones, of which approximately 90% are radio-opaque.)

Gallstones are often asymptomatic but may cause acute or chronic cholecystitis (see below), biliary colic (stone impacted in neck of gallbladder or cystic duct), or obstructive jaundice. Other presentations include cholangitis (infection of the bile ducts causing right upper quadrant pain, jaundice, and fever with rigors), pancreatitis, empyema, and gallstone ileus where the gallstone perforates the gallbladder, ulcerates into the duodenum, and passes on to obstruct the terminal ileum. The long-term presence of gallstones may be associated with gallbladder carcinoma.

Investigations
- Liver function tests may show a cholestatic picture (see Chapter 11).
- Prothrombin time prolongation may occur over a longer period due to vitamin K (fat soluble) malabsorption.
- Ultrasound examination may demonstrate stones in the gallbladder or bile ducts.
- In the presence of duct dilation or stones, endoscopic retrograde cholangiopancreatography (ERCP) is usually performed. This can be both diagnostic and therapeutic, allowing sphincterotomy and the removal of stones.

- Magnetic resonance cholangiopancreatography (MRCP) and endoscopic ultrasound (EUS) help to image the biliary tree but have no therapeutic use. Hepatic iminodiacetic acid scintigraphy can demonstrate a blocked cystic duct.
- Haemolysis screen: if pigment stones are suspected or found operatively.

Management

Stones in the gallbladder itself can cause various syndromes (see above). If the patient is symptomatic of gallstones (and this is not always easy to ascertain—see 'chronic cholecystitis' below) treatment is by cholecystectomy which may be performed acutely or after a delay (see 'acute cholecystitis' below). Gallstones may be treated conservatively by medical dissolution (with ursodeoxycholic acid given for up to 2 years) or shockwave lithotripsy -these methods are of limited efficacy.

Stones in the biliary tree can cause obstructive jaundice, cholangitis and pancreatitis. These patients require resuscitation and intravenous antibiotics for infection – notably in cholangitis. Sphincterotomy via ERCP may release stones in the common bile duct pre-operatively if these are present. Other options include exploration of the ducts at open operation or laparoscopic exploration in the case of laparoscopic cholecystectomy if there is a reason to suspect stones in the duct.

Acute cholecystitis

This disease is most common in overweight, middle-aged women, but may occur at any age. It usually follows the impaction of a stone in the cystic duct which causes right upper quadrant or epigastric pain. It is distinguishable from biliary colic by the presence of inflammation leading to fever, rigors, vomiting, local peritonism, or a gallbladder mass. If the stone moves to the common bile duct, jaundice may occur. Murphy's sign may be positive; this is pain on inspiration when two fingers are placed over the right upper quadrant, due to an inflamed gallbladder impinging on the examiner's fingers.

Differential diagnosis

The differential diagnosis of acute cholecystitis includes the following:
- Appendicitis in a highly-situated appendix.
- Right basal pneumonia.
- Perforated peptic ulcer.
- Pancreatitis.
- Myocardial infarction.

Investigations

The white cell count is elevated and inflammatory markers raised (unlike in biliary colic). A chest X-ray (CXR), ECG, serum amylase and cardiac enzymes should be taken to help exclude differential diagnoses. Ultrasound will show a thickened gallbladder wall and stones.

Management

Management is usually initially conservative, unless complications ensue (e.g. perforation of the gallbladder). The patient should be on bed rest, nil by mouth with intravenous fluids, and analgesia and antibiotics (e.g. cefuroxime or cefotaxime) should be given. Cholecystectomy is either performed after 48 hours, or the inflammation is allowed to settle and the gallbladder is removed after 2–3 months.

Chronic cholecystitis

Recurrent episodes of cholecystitis are usually associated with gallstones, leading to intermittent colic and chronic inflammation. There is abdominal discomfort, bloating, nausea, flatulence, and intolerance of fats.

The differential diagnosis includes myocardial ischaemia, hiatus hernia and oesophagitis, peptic ulcer disease, irritable bowel syndrome, chronic relapsing pancreatitis, and tumours of the GI tract. It can be very difficult to be sure that the symptoms relate to the gallbladder and stones and therefore the decision to perform a cholecystectomy should be made cautiously.

Diseases of the pancreas

Carcinoma of the pancreas

The incidence of pancreatic carcinoma is increasing. Risk factors include smoking and possibly diabetes. Approximately three-quarters of tumours occur in the head, the rest occurring in the body or tail. Secondary diabetes is uncommon. Pancreatitis may occur due to obstruction of the pancreatic duct.

Clinical features

General features of malignancy include anorexia, weight loss and lethargy. Local features are dyspepsia or epigastric pain radiating to the back and obstructive jaundice with an enlarged gallbladder. There may be hepatomegaly from biliary obstruction or metastases. Thrombophlebitis migrans is a paraneoplastic feature in 10% of patients. Fever may occur.

Investigations

Ultrasound and CT scan may show the tumour and help to stage it. ERCP may confirm the diagnosis, and needle biopsy can be performed under CT control. MRCP and EUS can provide valuable information.

Management

A minority of patients may be suitable for operative treatment although survival is not usually greater than 1 year, even after surgery. Patients with ampullary carcinoma often present early with jaundice, and surgical removal may therefore be more successful.

Without treatment, survival is usually only a few weeks after diagnosis. Palliative procedures may include bypass surgery for obstructions (e.g. gastrojejunostomy to bypass duodenal obstruction) or stent insertion to relieve obstructive jaundice (either percutaneously or by ERCP).

Acute pancreatitis

The causes of pancreatitis can be recalled from the mnemonic GET SMASHED: **g**allstones, **e**thanol, **t**rauma, **s**teroids, **m**umps, **a**utoimmune diseases, **s**corpion stings, **h**ypertriglyceridaemia, **E**RCP and **d**rugs, e.g. azathioprine or diuretics

Aetiology

Most cases are secondary to gallstones or alcohol. It may be also be idiopathic.

Clinical features

There may be a history of cholecystitis or other complications of gallstones. Alcohol intake should be ascertained. The patient complains of severe abdominal pain radiating to the back or shoulder, which may be relieved by sitting forward. There may be associated vomiting.

On examination, there is abdominal tenderness with guarding and rebound tenderness. There may be a tachycardia, fever, jaundice, hypotension, and sweating. There may be bruising around the umbilicus (Cullen's sign) or in the flanks (Grey–Turner's sign).

Differential diagnosis

This includes any cause of an acute abdomen (e.g. cholecystitis, mesenteric ischaemia, and intestinal perforation). Myocardial infarction and dissecting aortic aneurysm should also be excluded.

Investigations

The following investigations are important in the patient with acute pancreatitis:

- Serum amylase: markedly raised (over 1000 IU/mL). Amylase is also raised with cholecystitis and perforated peptic ulcer, but usually to a lesser extent.
- Abdominal X-ray: gallstones, pancreatic calcification indicating previous inflammation, an absent psoas shadow due to retroperitoneal fluid, and a distended loop of jejunum ('sentinel loop').
- Serum calcium: may be low.
- White cell count: usually raised.
- Serum glucose: raised in pancreatitis.
- ECG: to exclude myocardial infarction.
- Arterial blood gases: metabolic acidosis.
- CXR: widened mediastinum in aortic dissection; gas under the diaphragm in perforated peptic ulcer.

Management

Management is usually conservative. Intravenous fluids should be given to maintain the circulating volume, and a central venous catheter may be helpful for assessing the volume of fluid required. If the patient is shocked, plasma expanders will be required.

Pain relief is with intravenous or intramuscular opiates (e.g. pethidine 50–150 mg 4-hourly or pentazocine 30–60 mg 4-hourly, with an antiemetic such as prochlorperazine 12.5 mg 8-hourly). A nasogastric tube should be inserted. Blood tests, especially U&Es, glucose, and calcium should be monitored.

Surgery should be considered for suspected haemorrhagic necrosis of the pancreas. Some give H_2-receptor antagonists, prophylactic antibiotics, or peritoneal lavage, although these measures are of unproven value.

Prognosis

Mortality is 5–10% but recurrence is uncommon in patients who recover. Death may be from shock, renal failure, sepsis, or respiratory failure. Other complications include hypocalcaemia due to the formation of calcium soaps, transient hyperglycaemia, pancreatic abscess requiring drainage, and pseudocyst (i.e. fluid in the lesser sac presenting as a palpable mass), persistently raised serum amylase or liver function tests, and fever. Patients should be investigated to exclude gallstones, and alcohol should be avoided.

Chronic pancreatitis

The main cause of chronic pancreatitis is chronic excessive alcohol intake. Other causes include gallstones, cystic fibrosis, and haemochromatosis. The patient is generally ill with weight loss and has recurrent abdominal pain radiating to the back. Steatorrhoea is secondary to malabsorption from pancreatic insufficiency. Diabetes may occur due to involvement of pancreatic islet β-cells, and there may be intermittent or persistent obstructive jaundice.

Investigations

These are similar to those for acute pancreatitis although serum amylase is not helpful in the diagnosis as it is usually only slightly raised. In addition the following investigations should be performed:

- Plasma glucose: raised in diabetes.
- CT scan: may show dilated ducts.
- ERCP: outlines the anatomy of the ducts and shows calculi.

Investigations of consequences or complications of pancreatitis should also be carried out (e.g. tests of malabsorption, jaundice, and pancreatic exocrine function).

Management

Alcohol should be avoided, and the patient should be advised to follow a low-fat diet because of malabsorption. Fat-soluble vitamins, calcium, and pancreatic enzymes are given. Insulin is required if the patient develops diabetes, and gallstones should be removed.

For recurrent attacks causing unremitting pain, pancreatectomy should be considered. Patients often have chronic persistent pain and can become addicted to opiates.

Acute viral hepatitis

Hepatitis A
Epidemiology

Hepatitis A virus (HAV) is a member of the picornavirus family. The incubation period varies from 3–6 weeks. Transmission is by the faecal–oral route. Clinical disease with jaundice is uncommon in infants and young children, and the infection may go unnoticed. It may be acquired by eating partially cooked shellfish from estuaries contaminated by sewage.

Spread amongst drug smugglers by faecal contamination of condom-borne drugs has also been reported.

Serology

At the onset of symptoms, immunoglobulin (Ig)M anti-HAV antibody is present in serum. High titres persist for 3–12 months, so a positive test in a patient with acute hepatitis indicates recent acute infection. Previous infection, and therefore immunity, can be diagnosed by the presence of IgG anti-HAV without IgM anti-HAV.

Outcome

Relapses and cholestatic jaundice may occur but hepatitis A does not progress to chronic hepatitis.

Prevention and control

Prophylaxis can be obtained by immune serum immunoglobulin or active immunization. The latter induces higher levels of anti-HAV.

Hepatitis B
Epidemiology

The complete infectious virion (Dane particle) consists of the following:

- Hepatitis B surface antigen (HBsAg): the outer lipoprotein 'surface' envelope.
- Hepatitis B core antigen (HBcAg): the internal core, which surrounds the viral genome of DNA.
- Hepatitis B e antigen (HBeAg): a subunit of HBcAg; it can be detected in serum and is a useful marker of circulating virions and infectivity.

Transmission is parenteral through cutaneous and mucosal routes, across breaks in the skin or mucous membranes, and the mean incubation period is 75 days. In developed countries hepatitis B occurs sporadically.

Risk factors are male homosexuality, low socio-economic status, intravenous drug abuse, ethnic group, sexual promiscuity, residence in institutions, mental handicap, and employment in health professions. In endemic areas such as China and southern Africa, the disease is often acquired in childhood, and can occur by inoculation of infectious blood during the birth process. Infection is characteristically anicteric, asymptomatic, and chronic.

Serology

Following exposure to hepatitis B virus (HBV), HBsAg can be detected throughout the prodromal phase and is not usually cleared from the serum until convalescence. Other early markers include anti-HBc and HBeAg. A positive IgM anti-HBc test typically distinguishes acute from chronic hepatitis B. The presence of HBeAg implies high infectivity but it is often no longer detectable by the time the patient consults the physician.

The loss of HBeAg is a good prognostic sign, indicating that the patient will clear HBsAg and will not develop chronic infection. The disappearance of HBeAg is usually followed by the appearance of serum anti-HBe. Anti-HBs is the last marker to appear in serum.

Outcome

Acute infection rarely leads to fulminant hepatic failure. The disease may progress to chronic hepatitis, particularly in males and older people. Progression to chronic hepatitis occurs in less than 5–10% of people with clinically apparent hepatitis B. Cirrhosis and hepatocellular carcinoma are complications of chronic hepatitis.

Prevention and control

Infection can be prevented by active immunization.

Hepatitis C
Epidemiology

Hepatitis C (HCV) is an RNA virus, and can be divided into many major types and subtypes. Transmission is most common after transfusion of whole blood products, and the mean incubation period is 9 weeks. There is a high prevalence in haemophiliacs, thalassaemics, haemodialysed patients, transplant recipients, and intravenous drug abusers.

Serology

Anti-HCV develops 1–3 months after the onset of clinical illness and, in some patients, will not be detected for up to 1 year afterwards. Identification of the viral RNA in serum is possible using the polymerase chain reaction. HCV antigens cannot be detected in serum.

Outcome

The acute disease is often asymptomatic and leads to chronic infection in over 50% of patients. In about 20% of patients, cirrhosis may develop insidiously within 10 years, and patients may develop a clinical picture resembling autoimmune hepatitis. Systemic manifestations include cryoglobulinaemia, porphyria cutanea tarda, and membranous glomerulonephritis. Hepatocellular carcinoma is recognised with chronic infection.

Prevention and control

Blood bank screening for anti-HCV, and genetically engineered factor VIII preparations for haemophiliacs limit the occurrence of hepatitis C.

Hepatitis D
Epidemiology

Hepatitis D (delta) virus (HDV) is an RNA virus. The virion particle is encapsulated by the coat protein of HBV (i.e. HbsAg). Thus infection by HDV only occurs in patients affected by hepatitis B. Transmission is similar to HBV and the incubation period is 35 days. In developed countries, infection occurs mainly in drug addicts, haemophiliacs, and institutionalised persons.

Serology

IgM anti-HD, IgG anti-HD, and HDAg can be detected.

Outcome

The disease is not usually progressive but outbreaks of fulminant hepatitis caused by HBV plus HDV are described. Chronic infection can occur.

Prevention and control

The prevention of HBV infection will also prevent HDV infection as HDV cannot replicate in the absence of HBsAg.

Hepatitis E
Epidemiology

This RNA virus is transmitted via the faecal-oral route with a peak of epidemic infection 6–7 weeks after primary exposure and low secondary attack rate.

Serology

Serological tests are still in development.

Outcome

This is usually self-limiting and progression to chronic hepatitis does not occur. There is a high mortality (20%).

Prevention and control

This is dependent on high standards of public sanitation and sewage elimination.

Clinical features

The clinical features of the various forms of acute viral hepatitis are similar. In the pre-icteric phase, the main symptoms include malaise, fatigue, listlessness, and lack of energy. Anorexia, nausea, and vomiting occur, which may be induced by fatty food. There is often a distaste for cigarettes. There may be right upper quadrant pain, change in bowel habit, myalgia, fever, and headaches.

In 10% of patients, acute hepatitis B may be accompanied by a serum sickness-like syndrome, which is characterised by low-grade fever, urticarial rash, and arthralgia.

The prodromal symptoms become less severe as jaundice appears. The urine darkens and the stools are pale. During the first week, the jaundice may deepen, and anorexia and fatigue may worsen in this period. There may be accompanying weight loss.

During recovery, symptoms gradually resolve although malaise and fatigue may persist and mild relapses can occur in 1–5% of patients. Exercise tolerance is generally depressed for some weeks; depression may be a prominent symptom.

Physical signs are usually minimal. Common findings are jaundice, hepatic tenderness, hepatomegaly, splenomegaly, and occasionally lymphadenopathy. Skin rashes may be noted.

Fulminant hepatitis leads to hepatic encephalopathy with severe jaundice, ascites, and oedema, and is usually accompanied by haemorrhage caused by coagulopathies. The disturbance of consciousness reflects a combination of hepatic coma, hypoglycaemia, and cerebral oedema.

Investigations

The following investigations are important in the patient with acute viral hepatitis:

- Liver enzymes, alanine aminotransferase (ALT), and aspartate aminotransferase: these are markedly elevated. Bilirubin concentration is also increased. During recovery, liver enzymes return to normal. A persistently raised ALT 6 months after the acute onset of hepatitis usually indicates progression of the disease.
- Prothrombin time: may be prolonged if fulminant hepatic failure occurs.
- Serum albumin concentrations: may fall slightly during the course of hepatitis, and serum globulin may rise.

- Hypoglycaemia: may occur with fulminant hepatic failure.
- Serum α-fetoprotein values: increased transiently in patients with acute viral hepatitis.

Management

Most patients can be cared for at home although hospital admissions may be required for diagnosis, social reasons, or if complications occur. Patients should be barrier nursed in hospital. All unnecessary drugs should be stopped. Paracetamol is the preferred analgesic, and is not hepatotoxic in low doses. Cholestyramine may alleviate itching.

For uncomplicated acute viral hepatitis, no specific treatment is required. Rest is recommended and alcohol should be avoided.

Chronic liver disease

Chronic hepatitis

Clinically, chronic hepatitis is defined as any hepatitis lasting 6 months.

Chronic hepatitis may follow viral hepatitis, or develop with alcohol or drug use (e.g. isoniazid and methyldopa). Clinical features may include general malaise and lethargy, anorexia, hepatosplenomegaly, and signs of chronic liver disease. There may be remissions and exacerbations, and either complete recovery or progression to cirrhosis.

Management of chronic liver disease

The principal problems in severe chronic liver disease are the degree of hepatocellular failure and the complications of portal hypertension. Hepatocellular dysfunction causes hypoglycaemia (failure of synthesis of clotting factors) and hypoalbuminaemia. It may also cause hepatic encephalopathy. Portal hypertension may be complicated by ascites, splenomegaly and varices.

Management of variceal bleeds

This is described on p. 224.

Ascites

Ascites is the presence of free fluid within the peritoneal cavity. Factors leading to the formation of ascites include salt and water retention as a result of cirrhosis, hypoalbuminaemia resulting in decreased plasma colloid pressure, portal hypertension, and increased hepatic lymph production.

Clinically, there may be abdominal distension, shifting dullness, and a fluid thrill, if the ascites is tense. Associated features include hernias, divarifaction of the recti, abdominal wall venous distension, ankle oedema, and distension of the neck veins.

Investigations include diagnostic paracentesis. The ascites is clear and yellow unless it is infected, when it appears turbid. If the tap is non-traumatic, blood signifies intra-abdominal malignancy. The protein content is usually less than 15 g/L. Higher values indicate infection, hepatic venous obstruction, or malignancy. Fluid should be sent for cytology to look for malignant cells and for culture.

The patient should be on bed rest with restricted salt and fluids. The first choice of diuretic is spironolactone 100–200 mg per day. This can cause painful gynaecomastia in men, and amiloride can be substituted. If there is a poor response to spironolactone, frusemide is added. Fluid balance, weight, and U&Es should be monitored daily. Ascites can also be treated with therapeutic paracentesis and albumin infusion.

Overdiuresis may result in dehydration, uraemia, and hyponatraemia, and may precipitate hepatic encephalopathy, oliguria, and hepatorenal syndrome.

Hepatic encephalopathy

Encephalopathy can either be reversible and episodic, or lead to coma and death (Fig. 29.6). Liver failure results in diminished hepatic metabolism of substances derived from the gut, which can cause neurotoxicity. Clinical features include impaired conscious level, personality disturbances, inversion of the normal sleep pattern, slurred speech, constructional apraxia, flapping tremor (asterixis), hepatic fetor, brisk tendon reflexes, increased muscle tone and rigidity, and hyperventilation in deep coma.

Management

Initial treatment aims to correct or remove the precipitating cause. These may include electrolyte abnormalities, sepsis, hypovolaemia, hypoxia, bleeding, and constipation. Diuretics, sedatives, and opiates should be stopped, and intracranial pathology should be excluded, especially in alcoholic patients. CT scanning of the brain is useful to exclude subdural haematomas.

Measures should then be instituted to remove nitrogenous material, and bacteria from the bowel. Oral laxatives and neomycin are used. The patient is put on a low-protein, high-calorie diet. In alcoholics, intravenous thiamine is given to treat possible Wernicke's encephalopathy.

Once over the acute phase, routine measures include lactulose to ensure two soft bowel motions per day. Protein intake is restricted, and the patient is educated to avoid precipitating causes, including alcohol. In difficult cases of chronic encephalopathy, a trial of bromocriptine is required. Recurrent acute-on-chronic encephalopathy is an indication for liver transplantation.

Haemochromatosis

Haemochromatosis is due to excess iron in the tissues. The presence of skin discolouration and diabetes mellitus have led to it being called 'Bronze Diabetes' in the past.

Classification

Haemochromatosis may be classified as hereditary ('primary') or secondary.

Hereditary haemochromatosis is autosomal recessive. Secondary haemochromatosis may result from excessive iron administration (e.g. blood transfusion or iron tablets).

Clinical features

Affected organs are the liver, endocrine system, heart, and joints. Most patients are asymptomatic or have non-specific symptoms such as arthralgia and lethargy, until the effect of iron overload becomes apparent in the fifth or sixth decade. Joints are involved by chondrocalcinosis.

In the early stages, pain and swelling of the second and third metacarpophalangeal joints is

Grading of conscious level in hepatic encephalopathy	
Grade	Features
1	Confusion, altered behaviour, psychometric abnormalities
2	Drowsy, altered behaviour
3	Stupor, obeys single commands, very confused
4	Coma responding to painful stimuli
5	Coma unresponsive to painful stimuli

Fig. 29.6 Grading of conscious level in hepatic encephalopathy.

characteristic. There is slate-grey skin, due to melanin, and iron deposition. Symptoms include asthenia, abdominal pain, impotence, arthralgia, and amenorrhoea. Signs include hepatomegaly, splenomegaly, jaundice, and gynaecomastia. The disease may lead on to cirrhosis.

The prevalence varies from 1 in 200 to 1 in 2000, and men are five to 10 times more likely to be affected than women, indicating that environmental and genetic factors modify disease expression. Women are usually affected at a later age partly due to loss of iron during pregnancy or menstruation. Alcohol may exacerbate the problem by influencing iron metabolism and absorption.

Pathology
Total body iron is increased in haemochromatosis from 4 g up to as much as 60 g. There is cellular damage and fibrosis, leading to a rusty colour of the liver, pancreas, spleen, and abdominal lymph nodes. The liver is usually enlarged and may be cirrhotic. Iron is found in all liver cell types and in cardiac myocytes, the adrenals, pituitary, pancreas, and testes. Chondrocalcinosis in the joints is associated with synovial haemosiderin and loss of intra-articular space.

Investigations
- Serum iron is elevated and saturation of plasma transferrin is high. Serum iron is reduced in inflammatory conditions and is subject to diurnal variation.
- Serum ferritin is usually high.
- Definitive diagnosis of haemochromatosis depends on histology of liver biopsies.
- CT scanning and MRI can be used to detect increased tissue iron but are not routine.
- Genetic testing can be performed to look for the most common mutations (C282Y and H63D).

Course and prognosis
Complications include diabetes mellitus, cirrhosis, heart disease with arryhthmias, and liver cancer.

Life expectancy and hepatic and cardiac function in primary haemochromatosis are improved by iron depletion. The 5-year survival rate increases from 18% to 66%. Removal of iron does not prevent the development of cancer in patients with established cirrhosis.

Venesection does not improve endocrine failure or joint disease.

Treatment
Patients should be venesected regularly (e.g. 500 mL weekly), until they develop a mild microcytic anaemia. Care is needed in patients with severe hepatic disease because vigorous bleeding may be complicated by hypoproteinaemia. Folate supplementation may be needed to optimise erythropoiesis. Seriously ill patients with overt cardiac haemochromatosis may require high-dose parenteral chelation therapy with desferrioxamine to reverse life-threatening disease.

Patients with established haemochromatosis should be investigated for cardiac involvement and pituitary as well as target organ endocrine failure, and replacement therapy should be instituted when necessary. Patients should be reviewed to monitor diabetic control, to care for joint disease, and to search for the development of complications (e.g. hepatocellular carcinoma).

Physical examination and screening tests to search for disordered iron metabolism should be carried out in family members to identify presymptomatic individuals so that iron can be removed before cirrhosis and other complications occur. Genetic studies may be of help.

Primary biliary cirrhosis
Primary biliary cirrhosis (PBC) is a disease of unknown aetiology primarily affecting the middle-sized intrahepatic bile ducts as a non-suppurative, destructive cholangitis leading to bile duct damage, cholestasis, fibrosis, cirrhosis, and death from liver failure. It is more common in Europe than Africa and Asia with a prevalence of 3–35 per 100 000 and an incidence of 6-15 million per year.

Clinical features
The disease is nine times more common in women. It usually presents in middle age with lethargy and pruritus. Pigmentation and xanthomata may be present, jaundice may develop, and portal hypertension may lead to ascites or oesophageal varices. There may be stigmata of chronic liver disease. Approximately 80% have hepatomegaly at presentation, and 50% have splenomegaly. The patient may be asymptomatic at presentation, or present with liver failure.

The average life expectancy is 10 years from diagnosis. If the serum bilirubin is greater than 180 µmol/L, the life expectancy is 18 months.

PBC is associated with autoimmune conditions (e.g. Sjögren's syndrome, thyroid disease, Addison's disease, Raynaud's syndrome, systemic sclerosis, and coeliac disease). It is also associated with malabsorption, extrahepatic malignancies, particularly of the breast, and hepatocellular carcinoma.

Investigations

LFTs show an obstructive pattern with elevated serum alkaline phosphatase and gamma-glutamyl transpeptidase (GGT). As the disease progresses, serum bilirubin rises.

With regard to immunology, HLA-B8 and C4B2 are associated with a threefold increase in the risk of PBC. Serum immunoglobulins are raised, especially immunoglobulin M. Antimitochondrial antibody is positive in approximately 90%.

Ultrasound of the liver is important to exclude obstruction. It can also show evidence of portal hypertension and splenomegaly.

Histology of the liver will confirm the diagnosis. Initially, there is asymmetrical destruction of middle-sized bile ducts and surrounding lymphocytic infiltrate. Granulomas may be present. Increasing fibrosis, and eventually cirrhosis, develops.

Differential diagnosis

This includes autoimmune hepatitis, sarcoidosis, and drug reactions (e.g. phenothiazines).

Treatment

Immunosuppressive agents may have a small effect. Bile salts (e.g. ursodeoxycholic acid) may help with cholestasis. Antifibrotic agents (e.g. colchicine) may be of help. Liver transplantation is indicated for intractable symptoms or end-stage disease.

Itching can be treated with cholestyramine. Alternatives include enzyme inducers, e.g. phenobarbitone, and opiate antagonists (e.g. naloxone or propofol). Patients with jaundice should receive supplementation with fat-soluble vitamins A, D, and K. Diarrhoea is treated with a low-fat diet and pancreatic supplements.

Hepatolenticular degeneration (Wilson's disease)

This is an autosomal recessive disorder of copper metabolism leading to deposition of copper in the following:

- Liver: cirrhosis with its ensuing complications.
- Basal ganglia: tremor and choreoathetosis.
- Cerebrum: dementia and fits.
- Eyes: Kayser–Fleischer rings (a brown pigmentation of the periphery of the iris best seen with a slit lamp).

- Renal tubules: renal tubular acidosis.
- Bones: osteoporosis and osteoarthritis.
- Red blood cells: haemolytic anaemia.

Clinical features are usually due to hepatic or central nervous system involvement.

Investigations

There is a high concentration of copper in the blood, and low caeruloplasmin, the copper binding protein.

Management

The dietary intake of copper should be reduced, and penicillamine is given to aid the elimination of copper ions. Regular blood counts are mandatory due to potential agranulocytosis and thrombocytopenia with treatment. Other side effects include oedema, proteinuria, haematuria, rashes, loss of taste, and muscle weakness. Relatives should be screened. The prognosis is generally good.

Alcoholic liver disease

Men who drink over 80 g of alcohol per day, or women who drink over 40 g per day have a significant risk of developing cirrhosis. However, cirrhosis is not inevitable. Only 10–20% of chronic alcoholics develop cirrhosis even though they drink the same amount of alcohol over the same period as other alcoholics. Risk factors for developing cirrhosis include genetics, gender (women develop alcoholic hepatitis and cirrhosis younger, and after less intake, than men), nutrition (alcohol is better tolerated under optimal dietary conditions), and a synergistic effect with hepatotropic viruses.

Pathology

Initially there are fatty changes within the liver. With alcoholic hepatitis, there is liver cell necrosis and an inflammatory reaction. Cells contain alcoholic hyaline or Mallory's bodies. Later there is deposition of collagen around the central veins, which may spread to the portal tracts.

Cirrhosis may result, which is initially micronodular. Extensive fibrosis contributes to the development of portal hypertension. With continued cell necrosis and regeneration, the cirrhosis may progress to a macronodular pattern.

Clinical features

The patient may initially be asymptomatic. With alcoholic hepatitis, there may be fatigue, anorexia, nausea, and weight loss. There may be signs of chronic liver disease (see Chapter 11). Ascites may develop, and complicating hypoglycaemia can precipitate coma.

Hepatic decompensation leads to encephalopathy and liver failure, and can be precipitated by the factors listed in Fig. 29.7.

With advanced cirrhosis, there may be signs of malnutrition, ascites, encephalopathy, and a tendency to bleed. Signs include bilateral parotid enlargement, palmar erythema, Dupuytren's contractures, and multiple spider naevi. Men develop gynaecomastia and testicular atrophy. Portal hypertension develops, leading to splenomegaly and distended abdominal wall veins.

Factors that can precipitate hepatic decompensation
• Constipation
• Vomiting and diarrhoea
• GI bleeding
• Intercurrent infection
• Alcohol
• Morphine
• Surgery
• Electrolyte imbalance

Fig. 29.7 Factors that can precipitate hepatic decompensation.

There may be signs of alcohol damage in other organs (e.g. peripheral neuropathy, cardiomyopathy, proximal myopathy, or pancreatitis).

Investigations

The mean corpuscular volume (MCV) and GGT are sensitive indices of alcohol ingestion. Important variables for predicting outcome include the prothrombin time, serum albumin, serum bilirubin, and haemoglobin.

Ultrasound will demonstrate fatty liver, and histology of liver biopsy will show the pathological changes discussed above.

Management

Patients should abstain from alcohol. General measures for the management of chronic liver disease should be instigated. Patients may need nutritional support including vitamins B and C.

Prognosis

Fatty liver alone carries a good prognosis if the patient abstains from alcohol. If the patient is encephalopathic and malnourished, the mortality is up to 50%. Ascites, peripheral oedema, persistent jaundice, uraemia, and the presence of collateral circulation are unfavourable prognostic signs.

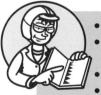

- What are the complications of gastro-oesophageal reflux disease?
- What are the differences in the management of gastric and duodenal ulcers, and why?
- Describe the emergency management of a patient with a large haematemesis.
- What are the complications of coeliac disease?
- What are the differences between Crohn's disease and ulcerative colitis?
- Do genetic factors have a role to play in the development of colorectal cancer?
- What clinical syndromes may result from the presence of gallstones?
- What are the causes of acute pancreatitis?
- How would you manage a patient with hepatic encephalopathy?

Further reading

www.bsg.org.uk/clinical_prac/guidelines/dyspepsia.htm

Rhodes J M and Tsai H H, 1995 *Clinical Problems In Gastroenterology* Mosby-Wolfe

www.nice.org.uk—guidelines on the use of COX-2 inhibitors

www.nice.org.uk—guidelines on the use of infliximab for Crohn's disease

Crash Course in Gastroenterology Mosby

30. Genitourinary Disease

Renal disease is traditionally confusing for the student. Here, glomerular disorders are discussed first as they apply to both acute and chronic renal failure, which then follow on.

Glomerular disease

Glomerular disease is seemingly complicated because there are no simple relationships between the clinical findings and the histology. Glomerular disease can be both primary and secondary i.e. systemic disorders that can involve the glomerulus: they are listed in Fig. 30.1.

Clinical features

Presenting clinical features of glomerular disease include the following:

- Proteinuria (see also Chapter 14): up to 150 mg of proteinuria daily is normal. Diabetic microalbuminuria is a level less than this but indicates damage to the glomerulus that may progress if not treated.
- Haematuria: isolated microscopic haematuria or more usually with proteinuria. Frank haematuria is rare.
- Raised blood urea and/or creatinine.
- Hypertension.
- Nephritic syndrome: this is a combination of proteinuria, haematuria and impaired renal

function, often in association with oliguria and hypertension. It best describes acute renal impairment from a yet to be clarified glomerular disease. Systemic features may be present.
- Nephrotic syndrome: this is a combination of proteinuria >3 g per day, hypoalbuminaemia <20 g/L and peripheral oedema.

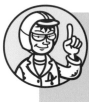

The causes of secondary nephrotic syndrome (i.e. not of direct renal origin) are DAVID: **d**iabetes mellitus, **a**myloidosis, **v**asculitis, **i**nfections, and **d**rugs

History

The history should include asking about haematuria and proteinuria (e.g. is there frothy urine? See Chapter 14). There may also be a history of previous nephritis. Ask about associated systemic diseases (e.g. arthritis, diabetes, hypertension or evidence of malignancy). A full drug history should be taken including exposure to toxins.

Hearing impairment is present in Alport's syndrome, and there may be a family history of renal disease. Ask about recent upper respiratory tract infections (post streptococcal glomerulonephritis) and valvular heart disease.

Investigations

The following investigations are important in the patient with glomerular disease:

- Urine dipstick: to detect proteinuria and haematuria.
- Urine microscopy for red blood cell casts and dysmorphic red cells indicating glomerular disease.
- 24-hour urinary protein excretion and creatinine clearance (inaccurate if renal function is changing rapidly) serve as a baseline, and can be used to monitor response to treatment.
- Urine for Bence-Jones protein.
- Full blood count, urea and electrolytes, liver function tests and bone profile.

Systemic disorders that can involve the glomerulus

- Diabetes
- Amyloidosis
- Systemic lupus erythematosus
- Rheumatoid arthritis
- Ankylosing spondylitis
- Neoplasia
- Myeloma
- Vasculitic syndromes
- Liver disease
- Sarcoidosis
- Partial lipodystrophy

Fig. 30.1 Systemic disorders that can involve the glomerulus.

- Fasting blood glucose: to exclude diabetes mellitus (DM).
- Erythrocyte sedimentation rate (ESR) and C-reactive protein (CRP).
- Antineutrophil cytoplasmic antibodies (ANCA) are present in microscopic polyangiitis and Wegener's granulomatosis.
- Anti-dsDNA and antinuclear antibodies in systemic lupus erythematosus (SLE).
- Antiglomerular basement membrane (anti-GBM) antibodies for the diagnosis of anti-GBM 'Goodpasture's' disease.
- Hepatitis B and C serology.
- Antistreptolysin O titre and anti-DNase: recent streptococcal infection.
- Serum immunoelectrophoresis to exclude myeloma.
- Tests for rheumatoid arthritis (e.g. Rose–Waaler and Latex tests).
- Cryoglobulins.
- Blood cultures.
- Serum complement levels: C3 and C4 are classically reduced in active SLE.
- Chest X-ray (CXR): this may show pulmonary oedema, malignancy, pulmonary haemorrhage or cavitation in Wegener's granulomatosis or anti GBM disease.
- Renal ultrasound scan: exclude structural lesion and assess renal size.
- Renal biopsy: the ultimate investigation clarifies the lesion and guides treatment.

Histological classification

As there is a wide spectrum of pathologies, biopsy is indicated for most people with acute nephritis. The interpretation is highly specialist and not expected of the student; however, certain principles apply. The terms 'focal' and 'diffuse' refer to the kidney as a whole, i.e. some or all of the glomeruli are involved respectively. 'Segmental' and 'global' refer to individual glomeruli, i.e. part or all of each glomerulus is involved respectively.

General principles of management

When a specific cause has been found, the appropriate treatment should be initiated. All patients should be referred to a nephrologist. In most patients, immunosuppression is needed to halt the nephritic process, for example a combination of high dose corticosteroids and cyclophosphamide. Whilst the response to treatment is assessed, hypertension, renal failure and fluid balance should be managed with careful supportive care and dialysis if needed.

Important primary and secondary glomerular diseases
ANCA positive vasculitis

This is typically either Wegener's granulomatosis (cANCA against proteinase-3) or microscopic polyangiitis (pANCA against myeloperoxidase). They are both small-vessel vasculitides causing pulmonary and renal disease though other sites can be affected. Wegener's causes granulomatous lesions and commonly has upper airway involvement. Both can cause a rapidly progressing glomerulonephritis (RPGN) and acute renal failure.

Symptoms include malaise, fever, haemoptysis, sinusitis and epistaxis. CXR may show transient shadowing due to pulmonary haemorrhage and resolution. They are considered together as treatment is the same, namely aggressive immunosuppression. Most enter complete remission with treatment; if the response is incomplete long term renal support may be needed.

Antiglomerular basement membrane disease

There is the even and linear deposition of immunoglobulin (Ig)G along the glomerular basement membrane, with a variable inflammatory response. At its most destructive, this produces a neutrophilic cell infiltrate, heavy fibrin deposition, and extensive crescent formation.

Goodpasture's syndrome is anti-GBM disease associated with pulmonary haemorrhage. Other 'pulmonary-renal syndromes' include SLE, Henoch-Schönlein purpura, Wegener's granulomatosis, and microscopic polyangiitis. Goodpasture's syndrome is six times more common in men than women.

Treatments with plasma exchange and immunosuppressive drugs remove and suppress the antibody, together with the reversal of its renal and pulmonary effects.

IgA Nephropathy

IgA nephropathy (Berger's disease) is the most common acute glomerulonephritis worldwide. The classic presentation is of a young man with macroscopic haematuria 1–2 days after an upper respiratory tract infection. Other presentations include microscopic haematuria, proteinuria and renal impairment. Biopsy shows mesangial proliferation and IgA deposition in the mesangium on immunofluorescent staining.

The cause is unknown. Proteinuria >1 g/day and hypertension are poor prognostic signs. Steroids and immunosuppression are not very effective. Angiotensin-converting enzyme (ACE) inhibitors are the mainstay of treatment though recent studies have shown the possible benefit of omega-3 fish oils. Approximately 25% of patients will go on to require dialysis. Henoch-Schönlein purpura has much in common with IgA nephropathy and can be thought of as its systemic cousin.

Lupus nephritis

SLE is a multisystem disease and the kidneys are commonly affected. The changes are classified by the World Health Organisation from I to V based on histology. The different types lead to presentations varying from nephritis to nephrotic syndrome. Typically, the anti-double-stranded DNA titres and ESR are raised with a normal CRP and C3 and C4 levels are low in active lupus. If treatment is indicated, steroids and cyclophosphamide are the mainstay.

Minimal change nephropathy

This accounts for 80% of children and 20% of adults in the UK who present with nephrotic syndrome. Renal biopsy is therefore not always indicated in children. Light microscopy is normal but electron microscopy reveals retraction and fusion of the epithelial foot processes at the glomerular basement membrane. There are no deposits of immunoglobulin or complement on immunofluorescence. There is usually severe and selective proteinuria, which remits with corticosteroid therapy. In patients with frequently relapsing disease, a course of cyclophosphamide can be considered.

Focal segmental glomerulosclerosis (FSGS)

Histology shows a proliferation of sclerotic lesions but electron microscopy and immunofluorescence findings are variable. Nephrotic syndrome is the usual presentation with features of nephritis. It can be idiopathic but is associated with a wide range of systemic diseases. HIV associated nephropathy is increasingly common and causes a characteristic 'collapsing' FSGS.

Treatment with high-dose steroids can induce remission but progression to end-stage renal failure is likely.

Rapidly progressive glomerulonephritis

RPGN or crescentic GN is usually an aggressive process, and presents with renal failure, haematuria, oliguria, and hypertension. The biopsy shows severe acute inflammation in the glomerulus with necrotising 'crescent' formation. It may occur in SLE, anti-GBM disease, and vasculitides, but often occurs in the absence of underlying disease. It is a medical emergency. Treatment is with immunosuppression. The prognosis is usually poor unless treatment is instituted sufficiently early.

Nephrotic syndrome

This is the combination of heavy proteinuria, hypoalbuminaemia and oedema due to damage to the integrity of the GBM. A minority of patients have a causative systemic disease (e.g. diabetes, amyloid, HIV and SLE). The majority have primary nephrotic syndrome. Other clinical features include hyperlipidaemia due to increased hepatic synthesis, a prothrombotic tendency due to urinary loss of antithrombin III, protein C and protein S, and increased risk of infection due to urinary loss of immunoglobulins. Renal biopsy is indicated in most adults.

Treatment of the cause is then required. Supportive therapy includes salt and fluid restriction plus diuretics if not intravascularly deplete to produce a gradual negative fluid balance plus an adequate oral protein intake. The hyperlipidaemia should respond to treatment of the cause; if not, statins are the drug of choice. Anticoagulation should be started with heparin and continued long term if required. As for all proteinuria ACE inhibitors are beneficial unless contraindicated. Prognosis depends on cause and response to treatment.

Acute renal failure

Acute renal failure (ARF) is a rapid decline in glomerular filtration rate (GFR). Deranged urea and creatinine levels and/or oliguria (below 500 mL per day) are the usual presenting features. Non-oliguric renal failure can occur, particularly in patients with nephrotoxic damage or patients with oliguric renal failure that has been converted to non-oliguric renal failure by aggressive management with fluids, diuretics, and other agents.

Aetiology

It is conventional to classify ARF into prerenal, renal, and postrenal causes (Fig. 30.2). The single most common cause for the house officer will be prerenal hypovolaemia. This may progress to acute tubular

247

Causes of acute renal failure	
Prerenal failure (ischaemic)	Extracellular volume loss: gastrointestinal loss (e.g. severe diarrhoea or vomiting), urinary loss (polyuria with salt-losing kidneys), burns Intravascular volume loss or redistribution: sepsis, haemorrhage (e.g. postpartum or at operation), hypoalbuminaemia Decreased cardiac output: heart failure (e.g. postmyocardial infarction), cardiac tamponade, cardiac surgery Miscellaneous: hepatorenal syndrome
Renal failure	Postischaemic acute tubular necrosis: shock, trauma, sepsis, hypoxia Nephrotoxic acute tubular necrosis: antibiotics, analgesics, contrast media, heavy metals, solvents, proteins Glomerulonephritis Acute pyelonephritis Acute interstitial nephritis: antibiotics, analgesics, leptospirosis, *Legionella*, viral infections Vasculitis Intratubular obstruction: myeloma (Bence–Jones protein), urate, rhabdomyolysis Coagulopathies: acute cortical necrosis, haemolytic uraemic syndrome, thrombotic thrombocytopoenic purpura, postpartum renal failure Miscellaneous: malignant hypertension, hypercalcaemia
Postrenal failure	Renal tract obstruction: stones, tumour (prostatic or pelvic), prostatic hypertrophy, surgical mishap (e.g. accidental ligation of ureters), periureteric fibrosis, bladder dysfunction Major vessel occlusion: renal artery thrombosis, renal vein thrombosis

Fig. 30.2 Causes of acute renal failure.

necrosis (ATN) if the renal perfusion remains poor. However, the aetiology is often multifactorial. For example, in postsurgical ARF, fluid depletion, systemic infection, and nephrotoxic drugs may all play a role. ARF may also complicate chronic renal failure (CRF).

Clinical features

The clinical features depend on whether there is pre-existing chronic renal impairment, and whether the cause is pre-, intrinsic-, or post-renal failure. A full history should be taken focusing on previous renal disease, a history of diabetes, hypertension, analgesic and ACE inhibitor use, symptoms of prostatism, recent diarrhoea, vomiting or blood loss and recent operations. The symptoms of acute renal failure are often non specific and it is detected with routine urea and electrolytes. If a new presentation of chronic renal failure, then the symptoms of CRF may be present.

The examination should focus on the cause and consequences of the renal failure. The most important initial assessment is to gauge the patient's volume status. Skin turgor, JVP, postural blood pressure, heart rate and the presence of peripheral or pulmonary oedema should be noted. If in hospital, the patient's fluid balance chart may be available. There may be palpable kidneys with polycystic kidney disease or hydronephrosis. There will be a palpable bladder with outflow obstruction. If present, a rectal exam for prostatic disease and vaginal exam for masses is indicated. Vasculitic changes can be seen in the skin.

Complications of ARF should be elicited as they may indicate the need for dialysis. Uraemia manifests as pericarditis, twitching, hiccoughs, and uraemic frost. Kussmaul's deep sighing respiration may indicate acidosis. Respiratory exam may show pulmonary oedema.

Investigations

Urine should be dipstick tested and then sent for microscopy, culture, and sensitivity. Casts may be normal or indicate glomerulonephritis, interstitial disease or ATN.

In prerenal failure the kidney avidly retains salt and water, hence urinary sodium is below 20 mmol/L; the urine is concentrated (osmolality over 500 mmol/L) with a urine/plasma osmolality ratio over 1.5 : 1.

Patients with established acute tubular necrosis cannot concentrate the urine or conserve sodium. Consequently, urinary sodium is over 40 mmol/L; the urine is dilute (osmolality below 350 mmol/L) with a urine/plasma osmolality ratio below 1.1 : 1.

Urea, creatinine, and electrolytes should be assessed. This will confirm renal impairment and serve as a useful baseline for monitoring the patient's progress. If the patient is acidotic, serum bicarbonate will be low. It is crucial to check the potassium as hyperkalaemia can be life threatening, and immediate measures to lower the potassium need to be taken.

Electrocardiogram (ECG) can show the precipitating cause (e.g. myocardial infarction), or complications such as pericarditis or hyperkalaemia.

Other tests to consider, depending on the circumstances, include:
- Arterial blood gases.
- Full blood count, liver and bone profiles, creatine kinase, ESR and CRP.
- Blood cultures.
- Serum autoantibodies, complement, antistreptolysin O titres and immunoglobulin levels.
- Urine for Bence–Jones protein or myoglobin levels.
- Chest radiograph if fluid overload suspected.

If the patient is truly anuric, especially if signs of sepsis are present or if volume depletion is not likely, then an urgent ultrasound scan of the renal tract is indicated. It will show urinary tract obstruction and kidney size and structure.

Management

Immediate thoughts should be to treat life-threatening complications, correct hypovolaemia and hypotension, exclude obstruction, and assess the presence of previous intrinsic renal disease. Fluids should be replaced and electrolytes should be corrected quickly. A urinary catheter is mandatory to monitor output and may be therapeutic in bladder outflow tract obstruction. A central venous pressure line is useful for proper assessment of fluid balance; it is not required in the fluid resuscitation of the patient. Appropriate antibiotics should be given for septicaemia or other infections. Bilateral nephrostomy tubes will relieve obstruction. Ureteric stents can then be placed later.

Inotropes and vasopressors (e.g. dobutamine and noradrenaline) may be necessary to achieve a renal perfusion pressure which is appropriate for the patient's age and history. Low-dose dopamine is still widely used though there is little evidence it alters outcome even if it produces increased urine output. Correction of hypoxia and acidosis may also improve cardiac and renal function.

If oliguria persists after an adequate circulation is achieved, or if the patient has established renal failure and is volume overloaded, intravenous frusemide should be given, either as slow boluses or as an intravenous infusion. Similar to low-dose dopamine, there is little evidence for this, although it may make fluid balance easier and indicate those with less severe impairment. Strict fluid balance should be kept with daily weights and regular assessment of fluid, electrolyte, and nutritional requirements. In general, patients should be given 500–1000 mL of fluid per 24 hours plus the volume of urine output from the previous 24 hours. In patients with fluid retention, a weight loss of 1 kg per day should be aimed for.

Note, however, that fluid overload may occur in patients without any change in weight, as negative nutritional balance may cause a loss of 1–2 kg per day. Careful examination is necessary to detect fluid accumulation, which should be counteracted by further sodium and water restriction.

Treatment of hyperkalaemia

This may be life threatening and so the reduction of potassium should be the first priority if it is over 7 mmol/L, particularly if ECG changes are present. These ECG changes can be reversed temporarily by boluses of calcium chloride. The patient should also be on a cardiac monitor.

Potassium can be temporarily redistributed into cells using an infusion of 50% dextrose and insulin. This can be repeated if needed. If acidotic the use of bicarbonate can help this. These treatments allow control of serum potassium whilst total body potassium is reduced (e.g. by restoration of urine flow). Calcium resonium resin orally or rectally will help excrete potassium over a period of days.

Indications for renal replacement therapy in acute renal failure

Indications for dialysis or haemofiltration in acute renal failure are as follows:
- Persistent hyperkalaemia (e.g. serum potassium above 6.5 mmol/L).
- Severe acidosis (e.g. bicarbonate below 15 mmol/L).
- Symptomatic uraemia (e.g. pericarditis, confusion and hiccoughs).
- Pulmonary oedema or progressive fluid retention not responding to medical therapy.

It should be noted that the level of creatinine is not an indication for emergency dialysis.

Prognosis

The prognosis of patients with ARF depends on the cause, other organ failure and pre morbid state. Prerenal and postrenal aetiologies usually respond well to prompt treatment and appropriate support and regain independent renal function. Intrinsic renal disease is less predictable. Patients with non-oliguric ARF have a lower mortality.

Do not give calcium chloride i.v. through the same cannula as sodium bicarbonate—it forms chalk!

Chronic renal failure

CRF is an irreversible reduction in glomerular filtration rate (GFR); it can be classified as follows:
- Mild: GFR 30–50 mL/min.
- Moderate: GFR 10–30 mL/min.
- Severe: GFR less than 10 mL/min.
- End stage: renal replacement therapy is needed

It can be difficult to differentiate between a new presentation of severe chronic renal failure and acute renal failure. Much of the initial assessment is common to both. Features that suggest chronic rather than acute renal failure include a long history of urinary symptoms and chronic ill health, anaemia, osteodystrophy, and small kidneys on imaging.

Aetiology

Finding the cause of CRF is important because in some treatment can delay or prevent progression to end-stage renal failure (ESRF). In addition, the prognosis can be better determined, risks of recurrence with renal transplantation can be assessed, and diagnosis of familial disease may benefit other family members. Common causes include the following:
- Diabetes mellitus: both insulin-dependent and non-insulin-dependent diabetes can lead to ESRF.
- Hypertension: the incidence of ESRF seems to be decreasing due to better identification and treatment of hypertension. It is more common in the black population.

These two are responsible for more than half of all patients entering dialysis programs; others include:

- Glomerular disease: both primary and secondary.
- Chronic or recurrent infection: mainly due to obstruction or vesicoureteric reflux.
- Obstruction: most cases are due to prostatic hypertrophy and stones.
- Renovascular causes: renovascular atheroma and consequent ischaemia is becoming increasingly recognised, reflecting the ageing population. Risk factors are the same as for all vascular disease. Consider if there is a marked decline in GFR with ACE inhibitors.
- Drugs: analgesic nephropathy; HIV associated nephropathy is increasingly common.
- Interstitial nephritis: this may be idiopathic but also secondary to non-steroidal anti-inflammatory drugs (NSAIDs) and chronic frusemide use.
- Inherited disease: the two most common conditions are polycystic kidney disease and Alport's disease.
- Less common causes are amyloidosis, myeloma, SLE, gout, hypercalcaemia, and retroperitoneal fibrosis.

Clinical features

The symptoms of CRF can be very nebulous. They include fatigue, malaise, thirst, anorexia, nausea, itching, confusion and poor urine output. It is often found on routine blood tests performed to investigate non-specific illness.

Specific questions in the history are the same as when investigating ARF or haematuria and proteinuria.

There may be signs of anaemia from CRF. Uraemic skin is classically 'lemon yellow' and there may be bruising due to platelet dysfunction. A pericardial rub, peripheral oedema, neuropathy, and hyperventilation secondary to acidosis may be present. Hypertension is common as both a cause and consequence of CRF. Examine for signs of obstruction (e.g. a palpable bladder) and perform a rectal examination for prostatic hypertrophy or pelvic masses. The kidneys are large in polycystic disease.

Investigations

The following are important in the patient with chronic renal failure:
- Urine: microscopy for casts and culture to exclude infection. A 24-hour urinary protein and creatinine clearance should be measured.
- Urea and electrolytes will help determine the degree of renal dysfunction and acidosis.

Remember that the relationship between GFR and creatinine is not a linear one and that GFR can fall by approximately 50% before the serum creatinine rises outside the normal range. GFR can be estimated from the creatinine value via the Cockcroft–Gault equation. Serum calcium may be low secondary to hyperphosphataemia or acquired vitamin D resistance. The acidosis protects the patient from tetany by increasing the ionised portion of the reduced calcium. Serum phosphate is high and plasma uric acid is often raised although clinical gout is uncommon.

- A cause should be sought and the tests are common to acute renal failure.
- Once chronic renal failure is established the following are needed to check for complications and progress. These include regular blood pressure checks, urinary protein estimation, and control of diabetes plus haemoglobin, calcium, phosphate, parathyroid hormone (PTH) levels, haematinics and lipid profile.
- X-rays of the chest and hands may show evidence of secondary hyperparathyroidism.
- Renal biopsy should be considered once prerenal and postrenal disease have been excluded, especially if renal size and structure is normal on ultrasound scan suggesting more acute disease.

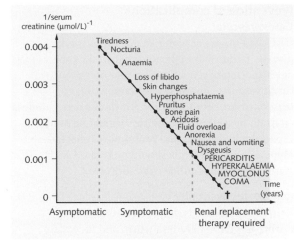

Fig. 30.3 Inverse creatinine plot with typical progressive onset of the non-specific symptoms and signs of chronic renal failure.

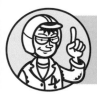

More than 50% of glomeruli may be lost before the U&Es become abnormal

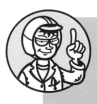

In severe CRF, creatinine clearance overestimates GFR as the tubular secretion of creatinine is a larger percentage of that excreted

Management

The aims of treatment are to minimise further deterioration in renal function, and to prevent or treat the complications of renal failure. Renal function can be monitored with reciprocal plots of serum creatinine (Fig. 30.3), calculated or measured GFR. Whenever an abrupt decline in the slope is noted, its cause must be determined and rectified.

Possible causes include uncontrolled hypertension, infection, systemic illness, hypovolaemia or fluid overload, urinary tract obstruction and drugs. Always question whether the drugs that the patient is on are necessary, in particular NSAIDs, and ACE inhibitors in patients with renovascular disease. Other drugs to avoid include tetracycline, nitrofurantoin, aminoglycosides, and potassium-sparing diuretics.

Prevention of decline in renal function

Hypertension should be tightly controlled (130/85 mmHg) with ACE inhibitors or angiotensin II receptor blockers (ARB) unless contraindicated. Cholesterol should be aggressively reduced.

The diet of patients with renal failure can be severely restricted. The total fluid intake may be restricted if urine output is low. Restriction of dietary phosphate intake may delay the decline in renal function, although it is difficult to achieve as it is often accompanied by a concomitant decrease in calcium intake, which can accelerate the development of renal osteodystrophy. Low protein diets have been advocated to slow loss in renal function. It is not clear how effective this is and which patients benefit most. Potassium restriction may be necessary to prevent hyperkalaemia, and sodium restriction to prevent fluid retention.

In diabetic nephropathy tight control of glycaemia plus ACE inhibitors or ARBs (even if normotensive) slow down the decline in renal function.

Prevention of complications

Cardiovascular

CRF patients are at high risk of cardiovascular disease. Control of hypertension can slow the deterioration of renal function and prevent cardiovascular complications. High doses of frusemide are often required for fluid balance; unless contraindicated ACE inhibitors should be used, especially in diabetes and proteinuric renal failure. Hypercholesterolaemia should be treated with statins and other cardiac risks addressed.

Renal osteodystrophy

Renal bone disease is due to a combination of disturbed vitamin D metabolism and secondary hyperparathyroidism. Serum alkaline phosphatase is raised. Management is by the normalisation of serum phosphate by diet and oral phosphate-binding agents such as calcium carbonate. Serum calcium should be maintained in the normal range and PTH levels controlled with synthetic vitamin D analogues. Frequent monitoring of serum calcium is required for the early detection of hypercalcaemia, which will further decrease renal function. Parathyroidectomy may be required.

Systemic acidosis

Systemic acidosis accompanies declining renal function. It increases myocardial excitability, encourages renal bone disease and may contribute to increased potassium levels. Sodium bicarbonate supplements will help to maintain serum bicarbonate levels within the normal range.

Anaemia

In renal failure there is a normochromic normocytic anaemia. Evidence of blood loss should be sought if there is an inappropriately low haemoglobin. Ferritin, vitamin B_{12} and folate deficiency should be corrected with diet and supplements if needed. Recombinant human erythropoietin has improved the management of anaemia and will increase the haemoglobin and improve symptoms attributable to anaemia, but it can cause hypertension.

Nausea and vomiting

This often responds to protein restriction or antiemetics. Dialysis should be considered if these measures are unsuccessful.

Pruritus

This can lead to excoriation of the skin, bleeding and secondary infection. The correction of serum calcium and phosphate may help, and antipruritic agents such as chlorpheniramine may also be of value.

Peripheral neuropathy

Dialysis should produce an improvement.

Hyperuricaemia

Treatment with allopurinol may be required.

End-stage renal failure

End-stage renal failure is identified on biochemical and clinical grounds as that point when, despite conservative measures, the patient will die without the institution of renal replacement therapy. Specific indications for dialysis in ESRF include symptomatic uraemia, hyperkalaemia, metabolic acidosis, peripheral neuropathy, pericarditis, central nervous system disorders, and poor control of ESRF by conservative treatment. The need for dialysis should be predictable, allowing for the creation of vascular access and education of the patient well before it is required. Renal replacement can be done through continuous ambulatory peritoneal dialysis (CAPD) using a catheter placed into the abdomen to allow fluid in and out and the dialysis membrane is the peritoneum. The most common method is thrice weekly haemodialysis via an arteriovenous fistula or indwelling dual lumen central venous catheter. Problems with dialysis include loss of vascular access, infection, hypotension, and the maintenance of fluid and electrolyte balance.

Renal transplantation is increasingly common and successful. Patients are on immunosuppressive drugs (e.g. cyclosporin, prednisolone, and mycophenolate mofetil or azathioprine), which have their own problems such as susceptibility to opportunistic infections, skin malignancies, and cyclosporin-induced nephrotoxicity.

Other complications of transplantation include acute rejection, obstruction of the ureteric anastamosis, and gradual loss of function with time (chronic allograft nephropathy).

Urinary tract infection

Urinary tract infections (UTIs) are one of the most common infections encountered in medical practice. Women are more prone to UTIs than men, except during the first few months of life, and in old age. Approximately 25–35% of all women describe symptoms of a UTI at some stage in their lives.

UTI is a general term referring to the presence of micro-organisms in the urine. Significant bacteriuria is defined as urine that yields a pure growth of more than 100 000 organisms per mL on culture. Predisposing factors for UTI are given in Fig. 30.4.

Lower urinary tract infections

Lower UTIs may take the following forms:
- Cystitis: a symptomatic infection of the bladder with significant bacteriuria.
- Asymptomatic bacteriuria: the patient has no symptoms, but urine culture yields a growth of over 100 000 per mL.
- Acute urethral syndromes: symptomatically similar to cystitis but the urine culture may be sterile.

Upper urinary tract infections

Upper UTIs may take the following forms:
- Acute pyelonephritis: an inflammatory process within the renal parenchyma, most commonly caused by bacterial infection.
- Chronic pyelonephritis: this is usually the result of long-standing or recurrent bacterial infection with eventual parenchymal scarring characteristic of chronic pyelonephritic kidneys. Vesicoureteric reflux and obstruction also contribute. Hypertension and chronic renal failure may ensue. It is more common in children.

Infection usually occurs by ascent of the invading organism from the urethra into the bladder. Colonisation of the ureters may occur, and from there to the kidneys. The haematogenous route of infection is less common but may occur secondarily to bacteraemia, septicaemia, or endocarditis.

The commonest pathogen is *Escherichia coli*. Other organisms include *Proteus*, *Klebsiella*,

coagulase negative staphylococci, and enterococci. Pseudomonas may be present after catheterisation. In patients with long-term catheters, mixed infections can be a significant problem.

Clinical features

Symptoms of lower UTI are suprapubic pain, frequency, nocturia, dysuria (classically 'burning'), and strangury. Upper UTIs such as acute pyelonephritis or renal abscesses present with fever, rigors, loin pain, vomiting, and weight loss. Macroscopic haematuria can occur in one-third of severe cases. In the elderly, the presentation may be very non specific with mild cognitive, behavioural and mobility changes.

Investigations

A clean urine sample should be obtained and a dipstick test done for blood, protein, leucocytes and nitrites; subsequently it should be sent for microscopy and culture. White cell count and CRP will be raised in infection. Urea and electrolytes may demonstrate poor renal function. Obvious predisposing factors such as pregnancy, diabetes or indwelling catheter should be considered. Indications for further investigations include recurrent infections, childhood onset, male sex, urological symptoms, persistent haematuria especially if aged over 40 years, unusual organisms (such as pseudomonas), and recurrence of infections.

Initial investigations should involve an ultrasound scan, which will determine renal size, cysts, obstruction, and residual urine; abdominal X-rays involving the kidneys, ureters, and bladder will detect radio-opaque stones.

An intravenous urogram (IVU) often complements the above investigations, and gives a better demonstration of parenchymal scars and calyceal clubbing. A micturating cystogram is used to detect vesicoureteric reflux, and bladder and urethral abnormalities, especially in children. Scarring may also be demonstrated on isotope and computed tomography (CT) scanning.

Management

Treatment is usually started after urine has been sent for culture and antibiotic sensitivities, but before results are available. Antibiotics may then be changed if necessary according to the results. High fluid intake should be encouraged. More than 80% of lower UTIs respond to a short course of an antibiotic such as trimethoprim or amoxicillin. If the urinary

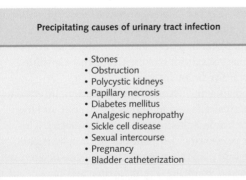

Precipitating causes of urinary tract infection

- Stones
- Obstruction
- Polycystic kidneys
- Papillary necrosis
- Diabetes mellitus
- Analgesic nephropathy
- Sickle cell disease
- Sexual intercourse
- Pregnancy
- Bladder catheterization

Fig. 30.4 Precipitating causes of urinary tract infection.

tract is structurally abnormal, a 5–10 day course of therapy is indicated. Follow-up microscopy and culture should be carried out to ensure eradication of organisms and pyuria.

Patients with acute pyelonephritis usually require admission to hospital for intravenous fluids and antibiotics. Paracetamol will reduce the temperature but stronger analgesia may be required. Antibiotic resistance is increasing in UTIs, so be guided by local policies. Other antibiotics include cephalosporins, co-amoxiclav and quinolones.

Patients with recurrent infections require a high fluid intake; frequent and complete voiding should be encouraged. Long-term, low-dose prophylaxis using antibiotics such as trimethoprim may be of benefit, but the need for continued treatment should be reassessed after 6 months.

If infection is related to sexual intercourse, the patient should void after intercourse and may benefit from a single dose of an antibiotic.

Miscellaneous genitourinary conditions

Adult polycystic kidney disease

This is an autosomal dominantly inherited disease, the genes lying on chromosomes 4 and 16 (PKD2 and PKD1). Patients are usually between the ages of 30 and 50 years. Cysts develop in the kidney and lead to progressive renal failure. Approximately 40% of patients also have cysts in the liver. Haematuria, infection, stones or abdominal pain are common presenting features. If due to a new mutation, established renal failure may be the first sign. There is an association with subarachnoid haemorrhage due to intracranial aneurysms. Examination reveals large irregular palpable kidneys, and the patient is often hypertensive. Mitral valve prolapse, diverticular disease and herniae are also increased in frequency. Ultrasound shows multiple cysts. CT provides greater detail. Blood pressure should be controlled and infections treated. Renal failure is progressive and may necessitate dialysis or renal transplantation. Screening of first degree relatives and genetic counselling is recommended.

Hepatorenal syndrome

Hepatorenal syndrome (HRS) is defined as renal failure in patients with severe liver disease for which no other cause can be found. Hence the exclusion of sepsis, hypovolaemia, nephrotoxic drugs and

nephritis is paramount, not least because they may be easily remediable. It is divided into

- HRS 1: rapidly progressive renal failure often in acute liver failure, alcoholic hepatitis or decompensation of chronic disease.
- HRS 2: more slowly progressive renal failure, often over months.

The aetiology is unknown. It is characterised by renal vasoconstriction and decreased perfusion pressures and peripheral and splanchnic vasodilatation. If the kidney is biopsied it is structurally normal. This is emphasised in treatment as it is mainly supportive and renal function recovers if the liver recovers, including after liver transplantation. Combinations of octreotide, vasopressin analogues, midodrine and dopamine have all been tried to improve renal haemodynamics but no treatment is especially advantageous. Prognosis is usually poor.

Haemolytic uraemic syndrome

Haemolytic uraemic syndrome is a disorder characterised by microangiopathic haemolytic anaemia, renal failure, thrombocytopenia, normal coagulation and no neurological changes. These separate it from disseminated intravascular coagulopathy and thrombotic thrombocytopenic purpura (with which it shares many features, see Chapter 34). It may follow diarrhoea in children (especially from *Escherichia coli* 0157:H7) though this is less common in adults. In adults the prognosis is worse. Treatment includes plasma exchange, steroids and renal support. A large proportion of patients will need long term dialysis even with treatment.

Renal stones

Renal stones are common. Men are more likely to be affected than women, with the initial presentation usually in the third and fourth decades of life. Most are composed of calcium and most are radio-opaque (80%). They include calcium oxalate, calcium oxalate/phosphate, calcium phosphate and triple phosphate staghorn stones. Urate and xanthine stones are radiolucent.

Predisposing factors are dehydration, infection, hypercalcaemia and hypercalciuria, gout and high oxalate intake (chocolate, tea and spinach). The classic presenting complaint of renal colic is pain; severe loin pain radiating to the groin associated with nausea and vomiting. Frank haematuria may occur. Diagnosis rests on history, the presence of blood on urinary dipstick and possible visualisation on an abdominal X-ray. Computerised tomography is more sensitive. Urgent intravenous urography if present leads to rapid diagnosis. Acute treatment is analgesia with NSAIDs, fluids and antibiotics if indicated. Urinary tract obstruction needs urological intervention especially if infection is a possibility. Most stones pass spontaneously; if they do not then they can be crushed endoscopically or fragmented with lithotripsy. To avoid future stones, the patient should avoid dehydration and excess dietary calcium oxalate or phosphate.

Urinary tract malignancies
Renal cell carcinoma

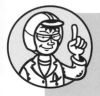

Tumours presenting with polycythaemia include renal cell carcinoma, hepatoma and cerebellar haemangioblastoma

The causes of sterile pyuria (a common exam question) include:
- Tuberculosis of the urinary tract.
- Analgesic nephropathy.
- Partially treated UTI.
- Neoplasia.
- Intra-abdominal inflammation.

Renal cell carcinoma (hypernephroma) is the commonest renal tumour in adults and is twice as common in men. The peak age of onset is between 50 and 60 years of age. It may be solitary, multiple, or occasionally bilateral. The classic triad of haematuria, loin pain and a palpable mass is found in only 10% of patients. Other features may include cough, pyrexia, polycythaemia, anaemia, bone pain with hypercalcaemia, and left-sided varicocele associated with left renal vein obstruction. A tendency to grow into the inferior vena cava (IVC) is a typical characteristic. About a quarter of patients present with metastases.

Investigations include urinalysis for red cells, ultrasound then CT scan of the kidneys, CXR (cannon ball metastases), bone scan for metastases

and magnetic resonance imaging of the abdomen to assess IVC spread.

Treatment is by nephrectomy if possible. Metastases may regress after the primary tumour is removed. This can be enhanced with interferon alpha and interleukin-2 administration. No chemotherapy or radiotherapy is very effective. The overall 5-year survival is approximately 40% but is better if the tumour is confined to the renal parenchyma and worse if there are metastases or lymph node involvement.

Transitional cell carcinoma
This occurs mainly in those aged over 40 years and most commonly affects the bladder, though the ureter and renal pelvis are other sites. It is three times more common in men than women. Predisposing factors include cigarette smoking, exposure to industrial carcinogens, exposure to drugs (e.g. cyclophosphamide), and chronic inflammation (e.g. schistosomiasis).

Patients usually present with painless haematuria although pain may occur. There may be symptoms similar to UTI. Investigations include urine cytology, IVU, cystourethroscopy, abdominal CT scanning.

Treatment options include local resection with follow-up cystoscopy, cystectomy, radiotherapy and local or systemic chemotherapy.

Prostatic carcinoma
Prostatic carcinoma is the second most common malignancy in men. The incidence increases with age and may be very indolent. Patients are often asymptomatic, but may present with symptoms of 'prostatism' (e.g. hesitancy, frequency, nocturia and postmicturition dribbling), or with symptoms arising from metastatic spread, especially to bone. There is a hard irregular prostate on rectal examination.

Investigation includes prostate-specific antigen (PSA), transrectal ultrasound, and prostatic biopsy, which shows an adenocarcinoma. Evidence of metastases should also be sought.

Treatment for local disease may be observation alone, transurethral resection of the prostate, radical prostatectomy, or radiotherapy. Testosterone is a growth factor for prostate cancer and therefore it responds well to antagonising its effect. This can be achieved with orchidectomy, luteinising hormone-releasing hormone analogues (e.g. goserelin) and antiandrogens (e.g. cyproterone acetate).

Prognosis even with metastases may be excellent if the tumour responds to hormonal treatment.

The PSA is very useful as a tumour marker to allow the response to therapy to be assessed when prostate disease is present. However, how to screen for prostate cancer and how to follow up abnormal PSA tests is a cause of much debate for urologists and public health authorities.

Fluid and electrolyte balance

In a 70 kg man, the total fluid volume is 42 L (i.e. 60% of the body weight). The intracellular fluid volume is 28 L or two-thirds of the total body fluid, and the extracellular fluid volume is 14 L or a third of the total body fluid. The intravascular component is 3 L (plasma contributing to 5 L of blood).

The average total fluid intake in 24 hours is 2500 mL (1500 mL drunk, 800 mL in food, and 200 mL via the metabolism of food). The output matches this via urine, insensible loss, and stool.

Sodium ingestion is approximately 80 mmol in 24 hours and potassium is also 80 mmol in 24 hours.

Salt and water balance
Disorders of sodium homeostasis are common.

Hyponatraemia
New onset hyponatraemia is frequent in hospital practice. It is rarely due to the legion of potential causes especially the syndrome of inappropriate antidiuretic hormone production (SIADH). It is usually the result of neurohumoral changes in acute illness and the type, volume and route of fluid administered. To evaluate chronic hyponatraemia three questions should be answered:

- Is the patient hypo or euvolaemic?
- What is the plasma osmolality? (normal 285–295 mOsm/kg) True water excess decreases the osmolality. Pseudohyponatraemia can result from hyperproteinaemia or hyperlipidaemia; with this the osmolality remains normal. Hyperglycaemia causes a shift of water to the extracellular space resulting in hyponatraemia but the osmolality is raised.
- What is the urinary sodium value? For example, in hypovolaemia secondary to dehydration or diarrhoea, the kidneys retain salt and water resulting in low (<20 mmol/L) urinary sodium. Diuretics or mineralocorticoid deficiency will

cause hypovolaemia with a high urinary sodium (>20 mmol/L).

With this information the diagnostic algorithm shown in Fig 30.5 can be followed.

Treatment depends on the cause. If dehydrated then volume replacement with normal saline is required. Fluid restriction for SIADH is correct. Beware of diagnosing it in hospital patients admitted for other reasons because fluid-restricting a dehydrated patient is a well recognised cause of acute renal failure. The sodium level should not rise at more than 1 mmol/L per hour as central pontine myelinolysis can ensue. This is osmotically induced demyelination. Severe hyponatraemia (<115 mmol/L) can cause confusion and seizures. It is an emergency and treatment with 0.9% or 1.8% saline to raise the levels to >120 mmol/L is indicated.

SIADH is characterised by hyponatraemia, low plasma osmolality, inappropriately increased urine osmolality (>500 mOsm/kg, urinary sodium >20 mmol/L without hypovolaemia, cardiac, renal, adrenal and hepatic disease. Causes are shown in Fig. 30.6.

Hypernatraemia
Hypernatraemia usually results from reduced intake or increased loss of water. Causes include dehydration and diabetes insipidus (Fig. 30.7). Excess saline replacement can be the cause in hospital.

Treatment is again that of the cause and appropriate fluid replacement. The sodium level should be reduced at 1 mmol/L per hour to avoid rapid fluid shifts and cerebral oedema. Normal saline can be used as it may have a lower osmolality than the blood and will not abruptly lower the sodium level.

Hypokalaemia
The causes of hypokalaemia are given in Fig. 30.8. The clinical features of hypokalaemia are muscle weakness, confusion, ileus, increased cardiac excitability, augmented digoxin toxicity, thirst, polyuria, renal lesions (e.g. Fanconi's syndrome), interstitial inflammation, and fibrosis in severe prolonged depletion. The ECG changes are described in Chapter 40.

Management
The underlying cause should be identified and treated. If hypokalaemia is mild, oral potassium

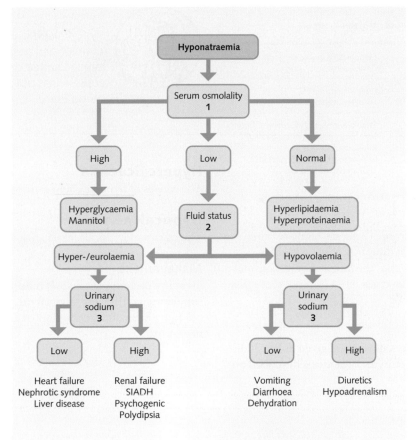

Fig. 30.5 Algorithm for investigation of hyponatraemia. (SIADH, syndrome of inappropriate antidiuretic hormone secretion.)

Fig. 30.6 Causes of the syndrome of inappropriate antidiuretic hormone release.

Causes of syndrome of inappropriate antidiuretic hormone (SIADH) secretion	
Groups	**Examples**
Central nervous system	Stroke Subarachnoid haemorrhage Head trauma Brain tumour
Pulmonary	Neoplasms Tuberculosis Pneumonia
Malignancies	Small cell lung cancer Pancreas Lymphoma
Drugs	Antidepressants Neuroleptics Chlorpropamide Carbamazepine

Causes of hypernatraemia	
Low total body sodium	Extrarenal, e.g. sweating, diarrhoea renal—osmotic diuresis
Normal total body sodium	High temperatures Diabetes insipidus
High total body sodium	Steroid excess, e.g. Cushing's, Conn's Iatrogenic, e.g. hypertonic sodium Infusions Self-induced, e.g. ingestion of Sodium chloride tablets

Fig. 30.7 Causes of hypernatraemia.

Hyperkalaemia causes large T waves on the ECG, hypokalaemia causes small ones—large pot, lots of tea; small pot, no tea

supplements are given. These are rarely required for patients on thiazide diuretics. If the patient is severely hypokalaemic, the infusion of intravenous potassium should be considered (but not more than 20 mmol per hour).

Hyperkalaemia
The causes of hyperkalaemia are given in Fig. 30.9. The management of hyperkalaemia is described on p. 249.

Hypercalcaemia
The causes of hypercalcaemia are given in Fig. 40.19.

Hypocalcaemia
The causes of hypocalcaemia are given in Fig. 30.10.

Management
Treat the underlying cause. If mild, give oral calcium supplements. If severe, give 10 mL 10% intravenous calcium gluconate over 3 minutes and repeat as necessary.

Fig. 30.8 Causes of hypokalaemia. (ACTH, adrenocorticotrophic hormone; SVT, supraventricular tachycardia.)

Causes of hypokalaemia	
Cause	**Examples**
Losses	Gastrointestinal: chronic laxative abuse, diarrhoea and vomiting, villous papilloma of the colon Renal: diuretics (e.g. thiazides and frusemide), hyperaldosteronism, glucocorticoid excess (including treatment with steroids, and ACTH-secreting tumours), renal tubular acidosis, Bartter's syndrome Inadequate replacement: postoperative, diuretic phase of acute renal failure
Redistribution of potassium	Alkalosis Insulin overdose Familial periodic paralysis
ACTH-secreting tumour	
Secretion of atrial natriuretic peptide	Paroxysmal SVT

Causes of hyperkalaemia	
Cause	Examples
Excessive oral intake	Potassium supplements
Diminished renal excretion	Renal failure Potassium sparing diuretic in combination with renal failure, e.g. amiloride, spironolactone
Redistribution of potassium	Haemolysis, e.g. incompatible blood transfusion, DIC acidosis Tissue necrosis, e.g. burns
Artefact	Delay in separation of plasma or serum, improper storage conditions

Fig. 30.9 Causes of hyperkalaemia. (DIC, disseminated intravascular coagulation.)

Causes of hypocalcaemia	
Cause	Examples
Hypoproteinaemia	Nephrotic syndrome
Renal disease	Chronic renal failure
Inadequate intake of calcium or vitamin D	Malabsorption
Hypoparathyroidism	—
Target organ resistance	Pseudohypoparathyroidism
Neonatal hypocalcaemia	—
Others	Acute pancreatitis, cystinosis, cytotoxic drugs

Fig. 30.10 Causes of hypocalcaemia.

- Give 5 different ways in which renal disease may present?
- Classify acute renal failure?
- What changes are seen on light microscopy of a glomerulus in a patient with minimal change glomerulonephritis?
- What tests are important in acute renal failure?
- What are the long term complications of chronic renal failure?
- What is the most common organism causing urinary tract infections?
- Further investigation is required for which patients with urinary tract infections?
- Renal cell carcinoma presents with what triad?
- How is adult polycystic kidney disease inherited?
- What features are required to diagnose SIADH?
- How would you recognise hyperkalaemia on ECG and how is it managed?

Further reading

Andrews P A 2002 Recent developments: renal transplantation. *BMJ* **324**; 530–534

Adrogue H J and Madias N E 2000 Hyponatremia. *N Engl J Med* **342**; 1581–1589

Dagher L and Moore K 2001 The hepatorenal syndrome. *Gut* **49**; 729–737

Datta, Mirpuri and Patel 2003 *Crash Course in Renal and Urinary Systems*, 2nd edn. Mosby

Madaio M P and Harrington J T 2001 The diagnosis of glomerular disease. *Arch Intern Med* **161**: 25–34

O'Callaghan C A and Brenner B M 2000 *The Kidney at a Glance*. Blackwell Publishing

Parmar M S 2002 Clinical review. Chronic renal failure. *BMJ* **325**; 85–90

The Renal Association is the professional body of UK Nephrologists. It has published guidelines on renal failure; they can be seen on its website *www.renal.org*.

Short A and Cumming A 1999 Clinical review. Renal support. *BMJ* **319**; 41–44

Williams A J 1998 Assessing and interpreting arterial blood gases and acid-base balance ABC of Oxygen. *BMJ* **317**: 1213–1217

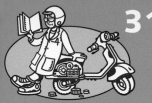

Cerebrovascular disease

Stroke

A stroke is a focal neurological deficit due to a vascular lesion that lasts for more than 24 hours. Approximately 80% are due to infarction secondary to thrombosis or embolism, and 20% are due to intracerebral haemorrhage. The overall incidence is about 150 in 100 000 but rises with age so that the incidence at 75 years is 1000 in 100 000.

Risk factors for stroke are summarised in Fig. 31.1. The main causes of ischaemic strokes are thromboembolism from arteries and emboli from the heart. Uncommon causes of cerebral infarction are vasculitis, arterial dissection, venous sinus thrombosis (which may also cause haemorrhage), polycythaemia , and meningovascular syphilis. Thrombus *in situ* may also occur following hypotension.

Cerebral haemorrhage is usually due to rupture of microaneurysms in perforating arteries or intracerebral vessels (primary intracerebral haemorrhage). Rarely, cerebral haemorrhage is secondary to other pathologies (e.g. arterio-venous malformations, tumour, abscess or blood dyscrasias).

The sudden onset of any symptom usually suggests a vascular aetiology

Clinical features

Signs and symptoms usually appear rapidly whereas a gradual progression over days suggests another pathology (e.g. tumour). The commonest presentation is hemiplegia due to infarction of the internal capsule.

The Bamford classification is now widely used in clinical practice and is also a useful guide to prognosis (Fig 31.2). The diagnosis of stroke is made clinically and the physical findings are interpreted to predict which part of the cerebral circulation has been affected. Motor signs are upper motor neurone. Lacunar strokes result from small areas of infarction affecting the basal ganglia, thalamus and pons.

Investigations

The following investigations should be performed in patients who have suffered a stroke:

- Full blood count (FBC): polycythaemia or thrombocytopenia.
- Electrolytes: dehydration.
- Clotting screen: bleeding disorders.
- Erythrocyte sedimentation rate (ESR): giant cell arteritis.
- Blood glucose: hyper- or hypoglycaemia may lead to impaired consciousness.
- Chest X-ray (CXR): primary tumour; aspiration pneumonia.
- Computed tomography (CT) scan: this will distinguish between haemorrhagic and ischaemic infarction if performed within 2 weeks; also aids diagnosis of other conditions in cases of uncertainty, such as tumour or subdural haematoma; should always be performed in cerebellar stroke as haematoma requires urgent evacuation. It MUST be performed urgently if consciousness is impaired or fluctuating, the patient is anticoagulated or if there has been trauma. In these situations there may be

Risk factors for stroke	
Major risk factors	Hypertension Atrial fibrillation Previous transient ischaemic attacks Diabetes mellitus Ischaemic heart disease Peripheral vascular disease Oral contraceptive pill
Other risk factors	Smoking Obesity Excessive alcohol intake Polycythaemia Arteritis Bleeding disorders Hyperlipidaemia* Low cholesterol†

Fig. 31.1 Risk factors for stroke. *Hyperlipidaemia is associated with cerebral infarction. †Low cholesterol may be associated with cerebral haemorrhage.

The Bamford classification of stroke sub-types				
Stroke sub-type	Clinical features	Risk of recurrence in 1 year	Patients independent after 1 year	Mortality at 1 year
TACI	Homonymous visual field defect, *and*	6%	4%	60%
	Unilateral motor and/or sensory deficit, *and*			
	Higher cerebral dysfunction (e.g. dysphasia, neglect)			
PACI	2 of 3 components of TACI syndrome	17%	55%	16%
LACI	Unilateral pure motor defect	9%	60%	11%
	Unilateral pure sensory defect			
	Unilateral mixed motor/sensory defect			
	Ataxia and hemiparesis			
POCI	Ipsilateral CN palsy with contralateral motor and/or sensory deficit	20%	62%	19%
	Disordered conjugate eye movement			
	Cerebellar dysfunction (without long tract deficit)			
	Isolated homonymous visual field defect			

Fig. 31.2 The Bamford classification of stroke sub-types. (TACI, total anterior circulation infarct; PACI, partial anterior circulation infarct; LACI, lacunar infarct; POCI, posterior circulation infarct; CN, cranial nerve.)

haemorrhage requiring urgent neurosurgical intervention.

- Echocardiogram: especially if suspect a cardiac embolic source (e.g. bilateral infarcts) and the patient is suitable for anti-coagulation.
- Carotid duplex scan: for anterior circulation events where the patient makes a good recovery and is suitable for carotid surgery if a significant stenosis is found (e.g over 70%).
- Thrombophilia screen: for patients <55 years, in the absence of other risk factors, following multiple episodes (see Chapter 34).
- Autoimmune screen: if suspect vasculitis
- Magnetic resonance (MR) angiography: if suspect arterial dissection or venous sinus thrombosis.

Management
Treatment
- Aspirin: evidence of (small) prognostic benefit if given in first 48 hours. Ideally, should be delayed until CT scan excludes haemorrhage but can be given empirically while awaiting scan.

- Swallow assessment: i.v. fluids if necessary. Reduce risk of aspiration pneumonia.
- Stroke unit: management in a specialised unit has been shown to improve outcome.
- Supportive therapy: hydration; monitoring of pressure areas, for infection and complications like hydrocephalus; nutrition; physiotherapy; occupational therapy; speech and language therapy.
- Neurosurgical review for brain haemorrhages, especially posterior fossa.

If the patient is unconscious or severely impaired, a decision on the most appropriate degree of intervention needs to be taken in liaison with relatives, and the patient if possible. Factors to consider include prognosis, quality of life, and the patient's wishes.

Prevention
- Aspirin following ischaemic stroke.
- Warfarin for cardioembolic strokes, those associated with atrial fibrillation, occurring less

than 3 months after myocardial infarction (presumed cardio-embolic) and possibly those occurring despite aspirin. The risks and benefits of anticoagulation need to be considered and discussed with the patient. Anticoagulation is avoided in the 10–14 days following infarction due to the risk of bleeding into friable, infarcted brain.

- Blood pressure fluctuates initially and should not be lowered acutely as cerebral autoregulation of blood flow is impaired and thus cerebral hypoperfusion may result. There is now evidence to support the lowering of blood pressure in all patients with an angiotensin-converting enzyme-inhibitor and thiazide diuretic 2 weeks after stroke, even if normotensive at the time of the stroke (PROGRESS study).
- Lipids: treatment has been controversial in stroke prevention. However, many patients with cerebrovascular disease die of ischaemic heart disease and one should be guided by the patient's overall cardiovascular risk (see Chapter 32). A recent trial in a population at high risk for cardiovascular disease suggests that treatment with a statin can reduce the risk of vascular events, including stroke, even if the absolute cholesterol level is not elevated (Heart Protection Study).
- Carotid endarterectomy: for patients with anterior circulation ischaemic strokes (or TIAs—see below) who make a good recovery and have a stenosis >70% in the culprit artery.
- Advice and help with smoking cessation and other lifestyle measures should be given.

Prognosis

Prognosis is variable and is influenced by stroke subtype (Fig. 31.2). Features associated with a poor prognosis include impaired consciousness, severe hemiplegia, incontinence, a defect in conjugate gaze, and increasing age. Approximately 20–25% of patients with thromboembolic infarction and 75% of patients with intracerebral haemorrhage die at 1 month. Recurrent strokes are common. Approximately a third of survivors make a complete recovery and a third are left with severe disability.

Attempts should be made to assess the prognosis in order to set appropriate rehabilitation goals and to allow appropriate counselling of the patient and family.

Transient ischaemic attacks

These are focal neurological deficits due to vascular events that settle within 24 hours with a complete clinical recovery. They are usually due to emboli from the carotid or vertebrobasilar arteries, but emboli may also arise from the heart or other vessels. The annual incidence is approximately 50 per 100 000.

Other possible causes are arteritis (e.g. giant cell arteritis), polyarteritis nodosa (PAN), systemic lupus erythematosus (SLE), syphilis, arterial trauma, and haematological causes (e.g. polycythaemia rubra vera and sickle cell disease).

Clinical features

There is a sudden focal neurological deficit, which gradually resolves over minutes or hours, leading to complete recovery within 24 hours. The neurological deficit is dependent on the vascular territory affected (Fig. 31.2).

Events occurring in different vascular territories suggest a cardio-embolic source. Recurrent events in the same carotid artery territory may be due to an unstable carotid plaque. Recurrent TIAs in close succession of this nature may be labelled as 'crescendo TIAs'.

Sources of emboli should be sought. Risk factors are the same as for stroke, and should be identified and managed appropriately.

Differential diagnosis

This includes all conditions that may cause transient neurological symptoms. Epilepsy is usually distinguished by features such as jerking, and migraine is usually associated with headache, which is rare in TIAs. Hypoglycaemia, multiple sclerosis (MS) and intracranial lesions should be excluded. Occasionally, phaeochromocytoma or malignant hypertension may mimic TIAs.

Investigations

Investigations are directed at the causes and risk factors for cerebrovascular disease as described above. The diagnosis itself is a clinical one.

CT scanning is not usually performed as haemorrhages causing TIAs are very rare. However, further imaging may be indicated if a space-occupying lesion is suspected or in the case of crescendo TIAs where the patient may be anticoagulated (under specialist supervision).

Treatment

- Aspirin 75–300 mg o.d. The addition of dipyridamole MR may provide an additional benefit.

- Address risk factors and consider the use of warfarin and carotid endarterectomy as described above.

Prognosis

Patients with TIAs in the carotid distribution fare worse than those in the vertebrobasilar territory. The risk of stroke and myocardial infarction are significantly increased (approximately 5% per year each).

Extracerebral haemorrhage

Subarachnoid haemorrhage

Subarachnoid haemorrhage (SAH) is due to bleeding into the subarachnoid space. The annual incidence is 15 in 100 000. Most cases are due to rupture of a congenital berry aneurysm in the circle of Willis and its adjacent branches (Fig. 21.2); 15% are multiple.

Berry aneurysms are associated with coarctation of the aorta, polycystic kidneys, and Ehlers–Danlos syndrome. Approximately 5–10% of SAHs are due to arteriovenous malformations but, in 15% of patients, no cause is found.

Bleeds may occasionally be due to ruptures, mycotic aneurysm from endocarditis, and bleeding diatheses.

Clinical features

The classic history is of a feeling like a sudden blow to the back of the neck. This is usually followed by faintness, nausea, vomiting, and sometimes loss of consciousness.

On examination, there is photophobia and neck stiffness, and a positive Kernig's sign. If bleeding continues, the level of consciousness deteriorates. There may be signs of raised intracranial pressure, or pressure effects on surrounding structures (e.g. cranial nerve palsies). There may be a bruit over the skull due to an arteriovenous malformation.

Investigations

A CT scan shows blood in the subarachnoid space in 95% of cases, and it can also identify arteriovenous malformations. A lumbar puncture shows raised pressure, uniform blood staining in consecutive samples, and xanthochromia (yellow colour) which develops after approximately 12 hours and persists for several days. It is present in all cases. Angiography will show the aneurysm, and is carried out if surgery is considered.

Approximately 5% of subarachnoid haemorrhages are missed by CT scan and therefore an appropriately timed lumbar puncture for xanthochromia is necessary to exclude the diagnosis

Management

Immediate treatment is bed rest, analgesia, and supportive measures. The neurosurgeons should be consulted early. Approximately a third of patients rebleed, most commonly about a fortnight after the initial event. Angiography should therefore be performed before then if the aneurysm is to be clipped. Blood pressure should be monitored and lowered if severely raised.

Nimodipine 60 mg 4-hourly is used to prevent vascular spasm following SAH, and reduces mortality. It is related to nifedipine but the smooth muscle relaxant effect preferentially acts on cerebral arteries. It should be started within 4 days and continued for 21 days.

Prognosis

Nearly half of patients with SAH are dead or moribund before reaching hospital. A further 30% will rebleed in the next few days.

Patients who have severe neurological deficits have a poor prognosis. Of patients who survive 1 year, approximately a third will have made a full recovery.

Subdural haematoma

These are due to bleeding from bridging veins between the cortex and venous sinuses. An initial small haemorrhage gradually enlarges by absorbing fluid osmotically from the cerebrospinal fluid (CSF). It is more common in the elderly, epileptics, and alcoholics. Although it is often secondary to trauma, the initial event may not be recalled.

Symptoms develop insidiously. They include headache, confusion, a fluctuating level of consciousness, and sometimes a personality change. There may be focal neurological signs (which may develop many days after the initial insult), signs of raised intracranial pressure, or secondary epilepsy.

A CT scan should show the haematoma, which may be bilateral. Treatment is by removal of the haematoma, which often leads to a full recovery if performed early.

Haematomas may resolve spontaneously, and in the very elderly they can be monitored with serial CT scans.

Extradural haematoma

This results from tearing of the middle meningeal artery or its branches following head injury. The classic picture is of a sudden brief loss of consciousness followed by a lucid interval. The patient's conscious level then deteriorates and the ipsilateral pupil dilates, followed by bilateral fixed dilated pupils and death. Treatment is by evacuation of the clot through burr holes.

Management of conditions causing headache

The differential diagnosis of headache is given in Chapter 16. Headache is a common symptom, which may either be of trivial significance or the expression of serious disease. The clinical approach to headache depends on a detailed analysis of symptoms and a thorough general and neurological examination.

Acute headache

The differential diagnosis of acute headache and facial pain is summarised in Fig. 16.1. In clinical practice, it is important to maintain a high index of clinical suspicion for SAH and meningitis as these are diagnoses one does not want to miss. CT scanning is usually the first investigation used to exclude a mass lesion, haematoma, or hydrocephalus. Lumbar puncture may be necessary to examine the CSF for SAH and meningitis. Occasionally acute migraine can produce a meningitic picture.

Progressive headache
Brain tumours and other space-occupying lesions

These present with headaches in approximately 50% of patients but are uncommon causes of headache overall. The following symptoms may be present:

- Raised intracranial pressure: headache, vomiting, and papilloedema.
- Generalised or focal epilepsy.
- Progressive focal signs: hemiparesis, hemianopia, and dysphasia.
- Mental changes: depression, apathy, dementia, and hallucinosis.

Headaches often occur in the mornings and are worse with coughing, exertion, or a change in posture. Focal signs are suggestive of tumours. Investigations should include CT scanning to show primary or secondary tumour.

Benign intracranial hypertension

This is also known as pseudotumour cerebri. The aetiology is often unknown but it may be related to steroids in some patients. The condition occurs mainly in overweight young women, and there may be a history of menstrual irregularities or recent pregnancy. Symptoms include headache and vomiting. There is marked papilloedema which, if long standing, can lead to optic atrophy and infarction of the optic nerve causing blindness. Therefore, the condition is not entirely 'benign'.

A CT scan shows no mass lesion, and the ventricles are of normal or small size. Thiazides or frusemide may reduce the intracranial pressure, and repeated lumbar puncture may induce a remission. In resistant cases, or if visual acuity deteriorates, a ventriculoperitoneal CSF shunt may be necessary.

Cranial (giant cell) arteritis

This disease usually occurs in patients aged over 60 years old. The classical features include engorged, reddened, tender, non pulsatile temporal arteries (Fig. 31.3) but this is not invariably present. The headache is severe and often worse at night, and may be accompanied by sweats, fever, malaise, and pain in the jaw during eating ('masseter claudication'). It may be associated with polymyalgia rheumatica. Involvement of the vertebral arteries may lead to TIAs or stroke, and disease of the ophthalmic arteries may lead to retinal ischaemia or infarction, which is irreversible.

Investigation

The ESR is usually raised at around 100 mm per hour, although a normal ESR does not exclude the diagnosis. A biopsy of the temporal artery should be taken within 24 hours of starting steroid therapy. 'Skip lesions' may lead to false negatives, and a long biopsy specimen should be obtained. Inflammatory cells infiltrate the tunica, and the internal elastic lamina is commonly destroyed or disrupted and intraluminal thrombosis may be found.

Treatment

Treatment is with high doses of prednisolone (60 mg daily). This relieves the headache within 24 hours and averts the risk of blindness, which occurs in up to 50% of patients if untreated. The prednisolone is gradually reduced to a maintenance level, and the

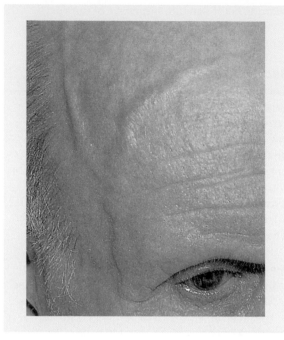

Fig. 31.3 Temporal arteritis with typical thickening of the right temporal artery. This patient presented with temporal pain and sudden visual impairment in the right eye but responded to prompt treatment with systemic steroid. (Courtesy of Dr C.D. Forbes and Dr W.F. Jackson, *Color Atlas and Text of Clinical Medicine*, Mosby, 1993.)

dose is monitored by symptoms and serial ESRs. Treatment may have to be continued for many years, and itself carries a significant morbidity from side effects.

Episodic headache
Migraine
Migraine affects approximately 10% of the population, and is slightly commoner in women than men (ratio of 1.5 : 1). Approximately 75% of people have their first attack before the age of 20 years.

Clinical features
The frequency of headaches varies from one to two each week to a few attacks scattered over a lifetime. The prodrome may consist of yawning, euphoria, or depression, and sometimes a craving for, or a distaste of, food in the 24 hours before the headache.

This is followed by an aura 30–60 minutes before the headache. It is usually visual, consisting of teichopsiae (flashes of light), scotomata, and fortification spectra (zigzag castellations). There may be micropsia and metamorphosia. Circumoral

tingling and paraesthesiae in the hands may also occur. In hemiplegic migraine, a hemiparesis, sometimes with dysphasia, occurs. Other focal neurological phenomena have been described.

The headache is commonly unilateral. It usually starts in the day and is classically throbbing or pulsating. Associated features include nausea and vomiting, diarrhoea, chills, faintness, and fluid retention. There may be photophobia and sonophobia. The headache is usually worse with movement, and lasts for 24–48 hours.

Occasionally, especially in older people, the aura may occur without the headache—'migraine sine cephalgia'. Conversely, the headache may occur without an aura ('common migraine'). Migraine is a risk factor for stroke.

Pathology
The mechanisms of migraine attacks are not well understood but a reduction in cerebral blood flow leads to the aura. This is followed by an increased blood flow associated with vasodilatation leading to headache. The process involves neurohumoral triggers including 5-hydroxytryptamine (5-HT) and noradrenaline.

The cerebral mechanism is responsive to mood, emotions, tiredness, relaxation, hormonal changes, and peripheral stimuli (e.g. bright lights and noise). There is often a seasonal and/or diurnal pattern.

Management
Precipitating factors should be identified and avoided, such as certain foods including cocoa, cheese, citrus fruits, and alcohol. Acute attacks should be treated with simple analgesia (e.g. aspirin, paracetamol, or codeine), combined with an antiemetic (e.g. domperidone or metoclopramide).

Sumatriptan and other 5-HT antagonists are of value for treatment of acute attacks, although experience is still relatively limited. They should not be given to patients with ischaemic heart disease or previous myocardial infarction, coronary vasospasm, or uncontrolled hypertension.

Ergotamine is used occasionally in patients who do not respond to analgesics. It relieves migraine headache by constricting cranial arteries but the aura is not affected and vomiting can be made worse. Common side effects include nausea, vomiting, abdominal pain, and muscular cramps. It should not be used for hemiplegic migraine, in patients with peripheral vascular disease, or in coronary heart disease. The frequency of administration should be limited to no more than twice a month to avoid habituation.

Prophylaxis

Prophylactic drugs are indicated in patients who have two or more attacks each month, and include pizotifen, β-blockers, and tricyclic antidepressants. The need for continuing therapy should be reviewed every 6 months.

β-Blockers, such as propanolol, are effective but their use is limited by contraindications and interaction with ergotamine.

Pizotifen is an antihistamine and serotonin antagonist related to the tricyclic antidepressants. It may cause weight gain and drowsiness, which can be avoided by starting with low doses at night and gradually increasing the dose.

Tricyclic antidepressants, such as amitriptyline, can be effective in low doses, even in patients who are not depressed.

Cyproheptadine can be tried in refractory cases. It is an antihistamine with serotonin antagonist and Ca^{2+}-channel-blocking properties.

Cluster headache

Cluster headaches are 10 times more common in men than women. Attacks usually start in adulthood. Headaches are of agonizing severity around one eye, and often occur at night. Attacks last for 30–120 minutes and usually occur every day for 4 weeks to 3 months. There is then usually a total remission until the next cluster ensues a year or two later.

The pain may radiate to the face, jaw, neck, and shoulder, and the eyes may water and become red. The nostrils may also run or feel blocked. Meiosis occurs in 20% of attacks, and in approximately 5% a permanent partial Horner's syndrome occurs. Attacks can be precipitated by vasodilators, e.g. alcohol, nitrites, and Ca^{2+} channel blockers.

Treatment is with ergotamine given in anticipation of the attacks or with pizotifen or verapamil for the duration of the cluster. Oxygen affords prompt relief in some patients. Sumatriptan will stop attacks in 5–10 minutes in 70% of patients.

Trigeminal neuralgia

This condition of unknown cause is seen most commonly in the elderly and is more common in women. In young patients, MS should be suspected. It is unilateral in 96% of patients, and consists of paroxysms of stabbing pain in the distribution of the trigeminal nerve. The face may screw up with pain, hence the alternative name of *tic douloureux*. If motor or sensory deficits are present consider underlying structural disease (e.g. atrioventricular malformation, cerebellopontine angle tumour, or MS).

The pain may be brought on by touching a specific trigger zone such as the side of the nose, and is thus provoked by factors such as eating, shaving, or talking. If left untreated, the condition usually progresses with shorter periods of remission.

Treatment is with carbamazepine, phenytoin, or occasionally clonazepam or baclofen. Surgical procedures such as sectioning of the sensory root or thermocoagulation of the ganglion are reserved for failure of medical therapy.

Other neuralgias include glossopharyngeal neuralgia and auriculotemporal neuralgia, which are precipitated by swallowing. Postherpetic neuralgia occurs in patients with previous herpes zoster.

Atypical facial pain

This refers to episodes of prolonged facial pain for which no cause can be found. It is commoner in women, and is often bilateral. It is associated with depression and may respond to tricyclic antidepressants.

Chronic headache
Tension headache

Tension headaches are extremely common and classically present as intermittent attacks of diffuse tightness, pressure or heaviness over the vertex, or in the neck or occiput. It may occasionally be unilateral. The headache may be relieved by analgesics but is not accompanied by vomiting or visual disturbance. When the headaches are constant and occur daily, analgesics are ineffective, and excessive medication, when withdrawn, may itself induce headache (analgesic rebound headache). Tension headaches are commonest in middle-aged women.

Enquiries should be made for the common and often concealed fear of a brain tumour or stroke.

Glaucoma

Localized pain in the eye and forehead may be a recurrent source of headache, and glaucoma should be considered in hypermetropic, middle-aged or elderly patients. In acute attacks, there may be vomiting, blurred vision, cloudiness of the cornea, and discoloration of the iris with a dilated pupil and circumorbital injection. Tonometry will confirm the elevated intraocular pressure.

Standard treatments include miotics, acetazolamide, and iridectomy, which should be supervised by an ophthalmologist.

Paget's disease of the skull

This is a common condition presenting with diffuse headaches, somnolence, deafness, and enlargement of the skull. Headaches result from local bony changes with vascular hyperaemia. Hydrocephalus may later be an additional factor of importance.

Parkinsonism

Parkinsonism comprises the syndrome of tremor, rigidity, and bradykinesia; Parkinson's disease is only one type of parkinsonism.

First described by James Parkinson in 1817, it is now known to be due to degeneration in the basal ganglia primarily affecting dopaminergic neurones in the substantia nigra causing a relative deficiency of dopamine. Eosinophilic inclusion bodies (Lewy bodies) are characteristic pathological features. The cause of the degeneration is unknown.

People with Parkinson's disease are less likely to be smokers. The incidence increases with age, and affects 1 in 200 people aged over 70 years old. It affects men and women equally and there does not appear to be a genetic predisposition.

Clinical features

Early on the patient may complain of fatigue, muscular discomfort, or restlessness. Fine movements may be difficult.

Tremor

Initially, this is intermittent and may only appear when the patient is tired. It commonly affects one hand, spreading to the leg on the same side, and later to the other limbs. The frequency of the tremor is 3–6 beats per second and is most marked at rest (whereas a cerebellar tremor is more marked on intention). There is a 'pill rolling' movement of the thumb over the fingers.

Rigidity

There is resistance to passive movement, which may be smooth throughout its range ('lead pipe' rigidity). When combined with tremor, resistance to passive movement is jerky and termed 'cogwheel' rigidity.

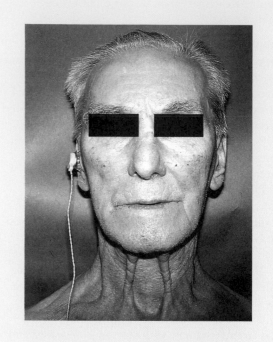

Fig. 31.4 Parkinson's disease is characteristically associated with a mask-like face which is devoid of emotion. The patient often drools and has monotonous speech. (Courtesy of Dr C.D. Forbes and Dr W.F. Jackson, *Color Atlas and Text of Clinical Medicine*, Mosby, 1993.)

Bradykinesia

Bradykinesia means difficulty in initiating movements and varying posture. It may be difficult rising from a chair. Writing becomes small (micrographia), spidery, and cramped. The face is expressionless and mask-like (Fig. 31.4), and the voice is monotonous and unmodulated. There is a shuffling, 'festinant' gait, and the patient stoops (Fig. 31.5). The arms do not swing, and the frequency of spontaneous blinking reduces.

To examine for bradykinesia, ask the patient to unbutton and button his or her shirt

Other features

Due to a disorder of the normal pattern of swallowing, saliva gathers and drips from the half-open mouth. Constipation and urinary difficulties are common. Rigidity may be accompanied by pain in

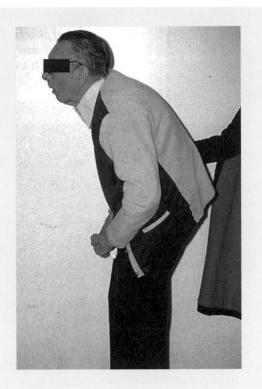

Fig. 31.5 Typical posture in Parkinson's disease. (Courtesy of Dr Kamal, St George's Hospital, Lincoln.)

the muscles. Late on in the disease, dementia may occur. Depression is common.

Other causes of parkinsonism

Other causes of parkinsonism include the following:
- Drugs (e.g. neuroleptics., anti-emetics; domperidone is best because it does not cross the blood–brain barrier)
- Arteriosclerotic pseudoparkinsonism: look for symptoms and signs of atherosclerosis in other regions (e.g. TIAs or intermittent claudication).
- Postencephalitis: following outbreaks of encephalitis lethargica (as in 1917–25).
- 'Parkinsonism plus' syndromes: rare disorders in which there is evidence of parkinsonism and other pathology (e.g. progressive supranuclear palsy—a symptom complex comprising a parkinsonism-like illness, dementia, and a failure of upward gaze; Shy-Drager syndrome—parkinsonism with evidence of autonomic failure).
- Poisoning with heavy metals or carbon monoxide.
- Wilson's disease (hepatolenticular degeneration).
- 'Punch drunk' syndrome: brain damage in boxers.

Management

The disease is treated symptomatically. Physiotherapy can improve the gait and help build confidence. Physical aids such as high chairs and rails may help with daily activities. Patient and carer information, education and support are very important.

Drugs

The aim of drug therapy is to correct the neurohumoral imbalance. This may greatly improve the quality of life but does not prevent progression of the disease. Ten to twenty percent of patients are unresponsive to treatment.

Drugs may cause confusion in the elderly, and it is important to start treatment with low doses, and use small increments.

Levodopa

Levodopa is the amino acid precursor of dopamine, and acts mainly by replenishing depleted striatal dopamine. It helps bradykinesia and rigidity more than tremor. It is generally administered with an extracerebral dopa decarboxylase inhibitor (e.g. benserazide or carbidopa). These prevent the peripheral breakdown of levodopa to dopamine, but unlike levodopa do not cross the blood–brain barrier. Effective brain concentrations of dopamine can thus be achieved with lower doses of levodopa.

The reduced peripheral formation of dopamine decreases peripheral side effects (e.g. nausea, vomiting, and cardiovascular effects). There is less delay in the onset of therapeutic effect and a smoother clinical response. However, there is an increased incidence of abnormal involuntary movements.

Levodopa is the treatment of choice for idiopathic Parkinson's disease. It is less helpful for older patients or those with longstanding disease who may not tolerate the high doses required to overcome their deficit. Side effects of levodopa include nausea and vomiting which may be limited by domperidone. Late side effects include the sudden unpredictable swings of the 'on–off' syndrome', dyskinesia, and 'end-of-dose' deterioration. In the latter example, the duration of benefit after each dose becomes progressively shorter. This may be improved with modified-release preparations.

Dopamine agonists

These act at the endogenous neuroreceptor. They may be used as an adjunctive therapy after motor complications have arisen from the long term use of

L-dopa, but may also be used as monotherapy before starting L-dopa, especially in young patients.

The most common side effect of these agents is nausea due to stimulation of the area postrema in the medulla. This can be alleviated with domperidone. Drugs in this group include bromocriptine, pergolide, ropinirole and apomorphine (which may be given by a continuous subcutaneous infusion).

Monoamine oxidase B (MAO B) inhibitors
Selegiline is the drug of this type in use. It inhibits the breakdown of dopamine. It is used in severe parkinsonism in conjunction with levodopa to reduce end-of-dose deterioration. Early treatment with selegiline may delay the need for levodopa therapy but does not delay disease progression.

Amantadine
Its mechanism of action is unclear. It improves bradykinesia and rigidity more than tremor. It may be helpful in the late stages of disease.

Anticholinergics
Examples include benzhexol and procyclidine. Tremor and rigidity are improved more than akinesia. They are best avoided in the elderly due to their side effects.

Catechol-O-Methyltransferase (COMT) inhibitors
These reduce the peripheral breakdown of L-dopa and thus reduce the fluctuation in plasma levels and prolong the benefit from each dose. Entacapone is an example.

Other therapy
Stereotactic surgery may help with severe tremor. There is ongoing work in the transplantation of dopamine containing cells—either foetal or autologous adrenal medulla.

Multiple sclerosis

MS, also called disseminated sclerosis, is an inflammatory, demyelinating disorder. It is the most common cause of neurological disability in young adults in the UK. The prevalence of MS varies worldwide and is much higher in temperate zones. The overall prevalence in the UK is 100 in 100 000, rising to as high as 300 in 100 000 in the Shetland and Orkney islands.

There is a female preponderance with a male:female ratio of 1 : 1.5. The mean age of onset is 30 years but there is a bimodal distribution with a major peak at 21–25 years and a lesser peak at 41–45 years.

Aetiology
The cause of MS is unknown. Evidence suggests that in a genetically susceptible individual an environmental agent is responsible. The causative agent is likely to be a virus and it is possible that a range of viruses may be involved. First-degree relatives have an increased chance of developing MS.

Pathology
The hallmark of MS is the presence of multiple lesions disseminated in site and time. These are characterised by demyelination with relative preservation of the axons, gliosis, and varying degrees of inflammation. Sites of predilection include the optic nerve, spinal cord, periventricular areas, and the brainstem. Each small lesion is orientated around a venule, which, in the acute stages, shows perivascular cuffing with lymphocytes and plasma cells.

Axonal loss is seen in established lesions and may result in an expansion of the extracellular space. Chronic lesions show marked astrocytic gliosis. There are also a number of immunological abnormalities.

Clinical features
The diagnosis depends on the demonstration of physical signs that can only be explained by lesions in at least two sites in the central nervous system (CNS). There is a wide spectrum of disease activity, and the course of the disease is extremely variable. The onset is monosymptomatic in 85% of patients, while in the remainder there is clear evidence of involvement at a number of sites. Common presentations include optic neuritis, symptoms referable to the brainstem and cerebellum (including diplopia and ataxia), sensory disturbance of the limbs, and leg weakness.

Optic neuritis
The patient develops increasingly blurred vision in one eye, which may progress to complete uniocular blindness during a period of a few hours or 2–3 days. Central vision is usually more severely affected. The affected eye may be painful, and colour vision is almost always affected. The optic nerve head appears normal unless the plaque is very anterior, when the disc may be swollen. Vision usually improves after 3–4 weeks and often returns to normal within

2 months. Transient blurring of vision lasting minutes, associated with exercise or raised body temperature (Uthoff's phenomenon), may occur. Following an episode of optic neuritis optic atrophy may ensue with pallor of the disc on fundoscopic examination.

Diplopia

This is a common symptom caused by a brainstem plaque involving fibres of the third, fourth, or sixth cranial nerves, or by a lesion in the medial longitudinal bundle causing an internuclear ophthalmoplegia.

Motor weakness

Motor weakness is more common in the arms than in the legs, reflecting involvement of the thoracic spinal cord.

Sensory symptoms

These include paraesthesia and dysaesthesia, proprioceptive disorders resulting in sensory ataxia and incoordination, and diminished vibration sense. Flexion of the neck may lead to an electric shock sensation in the back and limbs (Lhermitte's sign), and is associated with a lesion in the cervical cord.

Cerebellar signs

Cerebellar signs include nystagmus, dyssynergia (fragmentation of voluntary movements resulting in intention tremor), dysdiadochokinesia, incoordination of the heel-shin test, titubation (continuous rhythmical tremor of the head and trunk), and dysarthria.

Cerebellar lesions lead to VANISH'D: **v**ertigo, **a**taxia, **n**ystagmus, **i**ntention tremor, **s**lurred speech, **h**ypotonic reflexes, and **d**ysdiadochokinesia

Other manifestations

Other manifestations include the following:
- Cognitive impairment: especially of memory, sustained concentration, and abstract conceptual reasoning.
- Psychiatric abnormalities: most commonly depression; about 10% of patients suffer psychotic symptoms; euphoria may be present in severely disabled patients.
- Pain: this occurs in up to 50% of patients; trigeminal neuralgia is 300 times more common in patients with MS than in the general population.
- Paroxysmal symptoms: these include tonic seizures, and rapid flickering contraction in the facial muscles (myokymia).
- Bladder disturbance: this occurs in 50–75% of patients and is the presenting symptom in 10%; frequency, urgency, and incontinence are the most common symptoms; sexual dysfunction is common.
- Uncommon manifestations: 'useless hand' syndrome (an upper limb ataxia), lower motor neurone signs, swallowing and respiratory problems, and extrapyramidal movement disorders.

Diagnosis and differential diagnosis

The diagnosis of MS is based on clinical findings, and the exclusion of conditions producing a similar clinical picture.

Initially, individual plaques may cause diagnostic difficulty and must be distinguished from compressive, inflammatory, and mass or vascular lesions. Inflammatory conditions include isolated angiitis of the CNS, SLE, primary Sjögren's syndrome, Behçet's disease, and PAN.

The differential diagnosis also includes infectious diseases (e.g. Lyme disease and brucellosis), multiple emboli, and granulomatous disorders (e.g. sarcoidosis and Wegener's granulomatosis).

Investigations

The following investigations are important in the patient with MS:
- Examination of CSF shows a pleocytosis, raised protein, and immunoglobulin (Ig)G. Oligoclonal IgG is seen in 90% of patients with clinically definite MS but is not specific for MS as it is also seen in a wide range of inflammatory and infectious disorders.
- Delay in the visually evoked response follows optic neuropathy, which may be subclinical. It is useful in providing evidence of a second lesion in patients whose neurological deficits are only attributable to a single lesion. Delays may also occur in auditory or somatosensory evoked potentials depending on the site of the lesions.
- MR imaging (MRI) is very useful and can show plaques in the vast majority of patients with clinically definite disease.

Prognosis

The progression of MS is very variable. There are four distinctive clinical presentations:

- Relapsing-remitting MS: intermittent relapses followed by remissions. With each ensuing attack, the remissions are less complete so that, within 10–20 years, the patient is physically disabled.
- Secondary progressive MS: rapid deterioration with numerous relapses and only partial remissions in the first year or two of illness.
- Benign MS: infrequent attacks with long periods of remission.
- Primary progressive MS: continuous deterioration without remission.

Once the particular pattern has been established, the disease tends to develop along its declared path. After 5 years, 70% of patients are still employed. After 20 years, only 35% are employed, and 20% are dead from complications.

Management

No cure for MS has been found. Adrenocorticotrophic hormone or corticosteroids have an established role in acute relapses but do not alter the course of the disease. Intravenous pulses of steroids may be effective in acute disease, but there is no justification for subjecting patients to the hazards of long-term corticosteroid therapy.

Symptomatic treatment is of great importance. Physiotherapy and occupational therapy maintain maximum function. Spasticity may respond to baclofen, dantrolene, or vigabatrin. The intention tremor resulting from the involvement of the cerebellum may respond to isoniazid and pyridoxine, or to β-blockers. Trigeminal neuralgia and paroxysmal symptoms may respond to carbamazepine, and chronic dysaesthetic pain may respond to tricyclic antidepressants.

The management of patients with bladder disturbance has been revolutionised by the introduction of clean intermittent self-catheterisation. Anticholinergic agents, particularly oxybutynin, may alleviate urinary frequency. In men with erectile dysfunction, intracorporeal papaverine may be helpful.

β-Interferon and glatiramer acetate have been shown to reduce the relapse rate in the relapsing-remitting form of the disease (by about 1 relapse per 2.5 years). However, NICE has concluded that it cannot recommend the use of the drugs following a cost–benefit analysis.

Meningitis

Meningitis is inflammation of the membranous coverings of the brain and spinal cord. It may be caused by the following:

- Infection: bacteria, viruses, and fungi.
- Malignant cells.
- Blood following SAH.
- Air, drugs or contrast media during encephalography.

The term 'meningitis' is usually reserved for infection of the meninges by organisms.

Causative organisms

This is likely to vary with the patient's age:

- In neonates: *Escherichia coli* and β-haemolytic streptococci are common.
- In children: *Haemophilus influenzae* and meningococcus predominate.
- Young adults: prone to meningococcus.
- Older adults: prone to pneumococcus (*Streptococcus pneumoniae*).
- Immunocompromised patients and the elderly: prone to pneumococcus, *Listeria*, Gram-negative organisms, and cryptococcus.

Pathophysiology

In acute bacterial meningitis, a dense exudate forms over the base of the brain and extends towards the convexity along the sulci. It may affect emerging cranial nerves giving rise to ocular palsies. Sulcal pockets of the exudate may become encysted or it may occlude the foramina of Magendie and Luschka with consequent hydrocephalus.

In tuberculous meningitis, the meninges over the base of the brain are most severely affected. A tough gelatinous exudate often involves the cranial nerves and the blood vessels. The subsequent arteritis may lead to occlusion of the vessel and infarction of the tissues which it supplies. In the case of miliary dissemination, choroidal tubercles can often be found in the optic fundus.

Viral meningitis consists mainly of a lymphocytic inflammatory reaction in the CSF without the formation of pus or adhesions.

Predisposing factors

Outbreaks of meningitis tend to occur with overcrowding, poverty, and malnutrition. Infection may spread in institutions such as prisons or universities. Secondary meningitis can occur after head injury, sinusitis, mastoiditis, or extension of infection from the ears and nasopharynx. Immunocompromised patients such as those with acquired immunodeficiency syndrome (AIDS), carcinoma, or those on cytotoxic drugs, and following splenectomy are at increased risk. People with congenital meningeal defects or CSF shunts are also prone to infection.

Clinical features
Meningism
The features of meningism are headache, neck stiffness, and Kernig's sign (Fig. 31.6) may be positive (i.e. pain on passively extending the knee with the hips fully flexed).

Sepsis
The patient may describe malaise and arthralgia. Any rash may occur although a petechial rash is strongly suggestive of meningococcal disease. Pyrexia, rigors, tachycardia and hypotension may occur.

Raised intracranial pressure
Headache, vomiting, reduced consciousness, fits may all occur. Later bradycardia and hypertension can occur.

In tuberculous meningitis, symptoms may initially be non-specific with malaise, anorexia, headache, and a variable mild pyrexia. These symptoms may persist for days but gradually an unremitting deterioration occurs. There may be personality changes and intermittent dulling of consciousness before signs of meningism are obvious. The appearance of focal neurological signs suggests a complication (e.g. venous sinus thrombosis, cerebral oedema, or hydrocephalus).

Differential diagnosis
Any cause of headache (Chapter 16) or infection should be considered. Of particular note are severe migraine, acute encephalitis, and SAH.

Investigations
Although it is useful to gather diagnostic and microbiological information this process must not be allowed to delay therapy—particularly if meningococcal meningitis is suspected.

Blood should be taken for FBC, urea and electrolytes (U&Es), glucose , and culture. Cultures should also be taken from the urine and nose.

Lumbar puncture is the key investigation and should be performed as soon as possible. If the patient is profoundly ill, intravenous antibiotics should be given first. A CT scan should be performed first if there is any evidence of raised intracranial pressure: reduced consciousness, fits, focal neurology. Proceed to an LP if the scan is normal.

CSF changes in meningitis are summarised in Fig. 31.7 (see also Ch. 23).

Treatment
High doses of appropriate antibiotics should be given immediately a lumbar puncture is performed, or before it if the patient is very ill.

If outside a hospital, give 1.2 g i.m. of benzylpenicillin. Therapy in hospital is usually empirical initially (consult local policy) [e.g. i.v. ceftriaxone for patients <50 years and i.v. ceftriaxone and ampicillin (to cover *Listeria*) in patients >50 years]. Aciclovir i.v. should also be given if encephalitis is suspected (see below). These treatments may subsequently be modified depending on the results of microbiological analysis.

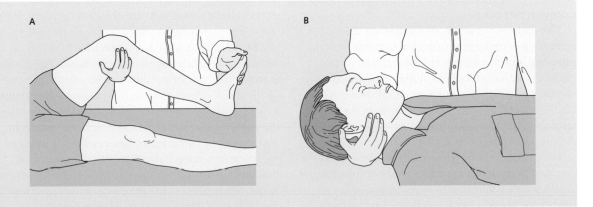

Fig. 31.6 (A) Eliciting Kernig's sign. (B) Testing for neck stiffness.

Changes in the cerebrospinal fluid in meningitis				
	Normal	Viral	Bacterial	Tuberculous
Appearance	Clear	Clear/turbid	Turbid	Turbid/fibrinous
Predominant cell	<5 mononuclear cells/mL	10–100 mononuclear cells/mL	200–3000 polymorphs/mL	10–300 mononuclear cells/mL 0–300 polymorphs/mL
Protein	0.2–0.4 g/L	0.4–0.8 g/L	0.5–5 g/L	0.5–5 g/L
Glucose	>2/3 plasma level	>2/3 plasma level	<2/3 plasma level	<2/3 plasma level

Fig. 31.7 Changes in the cerebrospinal fluid in meningitis.

Analgesia and careful monitoring of the patient's haemodynamic status and urine output are important. In cases of meningococcal disease, treatment in an intensive care unit is most appropriate.

Always remember that meningitis is a notifiable disease and cases must be reported to the Department of Public Health. Close contacts of the index case may require antibiotic therapy.

Encephalitis

This is inflammation of the brain parenchyma. There is usually some inflammation of the meninges in encephalitis and conversely some inflammation of the parenchyma in meningitis.

Encephalitis can be caused by viruses (most commonly herpes simplex—HSV), *Listeria* and toxoplasma if immunocompromised, and by bacteria where there may be associated abscess formation.

The patient may present with headaches, depressed consciousness, meningism, fits, focal neurology, or psychiatric features, and a high index of suspicion is required.

The diagnosis depends on knowledge of local epidemics, unreliable radiological features (such as temporal lobe swelling in HSV encephalitis) and electroencephalogram (EEG) findings (periodic complexes in HSV encephalitis), CSF findings (see Ch. 23), and demonstration of viruses in the CSF by serology or polymerase chain reaction (PCR). Often, the diagnosis is not confirmed.

HSV encephalitis is potentially treatable and therefore if there is any suspicion of encephalitis give i.v. aciclovir (in addition to other empirical treatments for meningoencephalitis) and send the CSF off for HSV PCR.

Epilepsy

Epilepsy refers to a group of conditions in which paroxysms of abnormal electrical activity of cerebral neurones result in seizures. As many as 1 in 20 of the general population have a fit at some time in their lives and, at any one time, around 200 000 people in the UK are taking antiepileptic drugs.

Classification

Seizure disorders can be divided into two main groups: idiopathic generalised epilepsies, and partial epilepsies. There may be a prodrome lasting hours to days before a seizure where there is a change in mood or behaviour. This is not part of the seizure, unlike an aura (see below).

Idiopathic generalised epilepsies

These are mostly genetic in origin and are often associated with a characteristic spike and wave on EEG.

Tonic-clonic (grand mal) fits

Before the fit, the patient may be irritable and experience minor disturbances such as myoclonic jerks. There may be a strange feeling (aura) before the fit, which has a sudden onset. The tonic phase involves powerful muscular contractions. The patient is struck unconscious and falls rigidly to the ground. Teeth are clenched; cyanosis may occur. After about a minute, the clonic phase starts, consisting of violent convulsive movements. There may be tongue biting and urinary or faecal incontinence. Tongue biting is more specific to epilepsy than incontinence. The patient then becomes drowsy or will sleep for several hours. The reflexes are depressed, with a positive Babinski sign. The patient may be confused on waking (post-ictal confusion).

Absence attacks (petit mal)

These start in childhood and are accompanied by a characteristic EEG pattern of three spike-and-wave discharges per second. It is due to a congenital neuronal instability. There are brief interruptions of consciousness, sometimes accompanied by rhythmical blinking of the eyelids. To an observer, the child may appear to be dazed or daydreaming. Recovery is immediate and there are no sequelae.

Myoclonic epilepsy

This is a form of idiopathic epilepsy developing in early childhood. Various types of generalised fits occur including sudden jerking movements of the limbs (myoclonus).

Partial epilepsy

The features of partial seizures can be referred to a single hemisphere and are therefore suggestive of underlying structural problems. They may lead to generalised tonic-clonic seizures. The nature of the attack varies according to the primary site of the lesion. In simple partial seizures, consciousness is preserved (e.g. focal motor or sensory attacks). In complex partial seizures, there is clouding of consciousness—usually temporal lobe epilepsy (see below).

Focal motor attacks

These arise in the precentral motor cortex and consist of clonic movements in localised groups of muscles such as the hand or face. They may continue for hours, in which case it is called epilepsia partialis continuans. The discharge may spread along the precentral gyrus causing a march of clonic movements throughout the body (Jacksonian seizure). After the seizure, there may be a short-lived weakness of the affected parts of the body (Todd's paresis).

Focal sensory attacks

These start in the postcentral sensory cortex, and either localised or spreading paraesthesiae occur.

Temporal lobe epilepsy

This may consist of hallucinations of any of the five senses and of memory. Gustatory and olfactory hallucinations are usually unpleasant. *Jamais vu* is a sudden feeling of unfamiliarity while the patient is in his or her own environment and *déjà vu* is a vivid sense of familiarity with the current situation.

In automatism, the patient remains conscious but 'dreamy' and may continue with normal activities.

The patient cannot remember these events after the attack.

Aetiology

Although most fits are idiopathic, a cause for the seizures and precipitating factors should be looked into. These include the following:

- Metabolic causes: hypoxia, hyper- or hypoglycaemia, hypocalcaemia, uraemia, alcoholism, hypo- and hypernatraemia, liver failure, pyridoxine deficiency.
- Drugs and toxins: alcohol, lead, and drugs (e.g. phenothiazines, monoamine oxidase inhibitors, tricyclic antidepressants, amphetamines, lidocaine, nalidixic acid).
- Trauma and surgery (e.g. perinatal trauma or head injury).
- Space-occupying lesions.
- Cerebral infarction.
- Other organic brain diseases: SLE, PAN, sarcoidosis, vascular malformations.
- Infections: encephalitis, syphilis, and human immunodeficiency virus.
- Degenerative brain disorders: Alzheimer's disease, Creutzfeldt–Jacob disease.

Precipitants of epilepsy

Fits may be precipitated by flashing lights. Other possible precipitants include fever, irregular meals, menstruation, hyperventilation leading to alkalosis, lack of sleep, emotional disturbances, and pregnancy.

Differential diagnosis

Seizures can be difficult to distinguish from other causes of collapse. This is discussed in Chapter 19.

Investigations

After a careful history and examination to consider differential diagnoses, blood tests include FBC, U&Es, serum calcium, liver function tests, and glucose. A CXR and ECG should be performed. The diagnosis is a clinical one and a good witness account of the 'seizures' is vital.

The diagnosis should not be based solely on the EEG because 10–15% of the general population may have an 'abnormal' EEG, and approximately 15% of people with epilepsy never have specific epileptiform discharges.

CT scanning as the sole basis of diagnosis is also unreliable. The frequency of abnormalities found in CT scans in people with epilepsy varies greatly. A CT scan is indicated in a patient with late-onset epilepsy who has focal seizures, because it may detect a tumour. However, a single normal CT scan does not exclude a lesion and other imaging modalities such as MRI and MR angiography may be used.

Treatment

It is important to be as certain as possible of the diagnosis as there are significant lifestyle implications, associated stigma and the need to take potentially toxic drugs for long periods of time. Specialist advice should always be considered prior to labelling a patient epileptic. Many centres reserve therapy until after at least two seizures.

UK advice on epilepsy and driving is as follows.
First/solitary fit:
- 1 year off driving (must be fit-free) with medical review before restarting. If another fit occurs during this time, the patient must wait a year from that fit before review.

Loss of consciousness without known cause:
- As above.

Seizures during sleep:
- After one seizure, regulations as above. If all attacks for at least 3 years have been during sleep, and the patient has never had an attack while awake, driving is allowed.

Withdrawal of antiepileptic medication:
- Advise patient not to drive (but this is not a legal obligation on the patient's part) for 6 months from the time of withdrawal. Clearly, if further seizures occur, the above regulations apply.

The aims of drug treatment are to prevent seizures whilst keeping the patient free of side effects. Antiepileptic drugs should be prescribed singly using the lowest dose to obtain complete seizure control with minimum side effects. A single drug will suffice in approximately 80% of patients, the remainder needing a second drug to achieve acceptable control. Partial epilepsy is more likely to be refractory.

Having chosen a drug the dose is gradually increased until control is achieved, the maximum dose is reached, or toxic effects supervene. In the latter two cases, alternatives need to be considered (see below).

Carbamazepine, phenytoin, and barbiturates all induce hepatic enzymes and therefore speed up the metabolism of oestrogens and progestogens making the oral contraceptive pill unreliable. Sodium valproate does not affect oral contraceptive efficacy.

First-line drugs
Idiopathic generalised epilepsy
Sodium valproate is often recommended as the treatment of choice because carbamazepine is ineffective for the treatment of absence or myoclonic seizures. They are equally as effective for idiopathic generalised tonic-clonic seizures. Common unwanted effects of sodium valproate include weight gain, hair thinning, and tremor. Hepatotoxicity, thrombocytopenia, and pancreatitis may occur. Ethosuximide is a useful alternative in children with absence seizures only.

Partial epilepsies
Carbamazepine is the first-line therapy. Sodium valproate may also be used. Carbamazepine may cause CNS side effects (e.g. dizziness, nausea, headaches, and drowsiness), which may be avoided by slowly increasing the dose. It induces hepatic microsomal enzymes and so increases the metabolism of phenobarbitone, sodium valproate, lamotrigine, corticosteroids, oral contraceptives, theophylline, and warfarin. It also inhibits the metabolism of phenytoin. Idiosyncratic reactions include the Stevens–Johnson syndrome, exfoliative dermatitis, and hepatitis.

Second-line drugs
Phenytoin is useful but often difficult to use because of its unpredictable pharmacokinetics and so the best dose is difficult to determine. Vigabatrin, lamotrigine, and gabapentin are used as add-on therapies for partial or secondarily generalised seizures. Benzodiazepines may also be used as add-on therapy rarely. These agents may be started by specialists as alternative or add-on therapy and they also have important interactions and side-effects.

Changing drugs
This may be performed in cases of treatment failure or due to side effects. The new drug is commenced at

its starting dose and gradually increased. The old drug is withdrawn over 6 weeks.

Withdrawing drugs

Most patients are seizure free within a few years of starting therapy and 60% remain so after drug withdrawal. Therefore drug withdrawal is considered in some patients after a period of therapy if neurological examination is normal, EEG is normal prior to withdrawal and the patient has been seizure free for >2 years. In cases of juvenile myoclonic epilepsy, drugs are not withdrawn.

Epilepsy and pregnancy

There are several important issues to be considered when an epileptic patient wants to become, or becomes, pregnant. It is important to enlist specialist help in this situation.

There are several different concerns to balance: are anti-epileptic drugs necessary, and what are their effects on the fetus? What is the effect of pregnancy on maternal seizures and what risk is there to the fetus from maternal seizures? It is imperative to counsel the patient regarding these issues so that informed choices can be made.

If it is felt that anti-epileptic therapy must continue during pregnancy it is important to try to use a single agent in the lowest possible dose.

Status epilepticus

This is a medical emergency and is defined as seizures lasting >30 minutes or repeated seizures without intervening recovery of consciousness. Both the risk of permanent brain damage and mortality are related to the length of the attack and therefore seizures must be stopped as soon as possible.

- Priority is Basic Life Support and ABC.
- Lay in the recovery position, remove false teeth and insert an oral airway. The patient may require intubation.
- Administer 100% oxygen and suction.
- Gain i.v. access and check FBC, glucose, U&Es, liver function test, calcium, toxicology screen and drug levels if on anticonvulsant.
- Give 50 ml 50% dextrose unless confident that glucose is normal. Note that this can precipitate Wernicke's encephalopathy in alcoholics and therefore also give i.v. thiamine if patient may be alcoholic (or malnourished).
- Give slow i.v. bolus of lorazepam 4 mg.
- If seizures persist commence a phenytoin infusion (with cardiac monitor) or a diazepam infusion.

- If seizures still persist consider paralysis, ventilation and an urgent EEG.

Intracranial tumours

Cerebral tumours represent about 10% of all malignancies. They may be primary or secondary mainly from the bronchus, breasts, kidneys, colon, ovary, prostate, or thyroid. The main sites of origin of brain tumours are shown in Fig. 31.8. Other tumours are rare.

Clinical features

Symptoms arise from the direct effects of the mass on surrounding structures, the effects of raised intracranial pressure, or by provoking seizures. Similar symptoms may be produced by any mass lesion (e.g. haematomas, aneurysms, abscesses, tuberculomas, granulomas, and cysts).

Direct effects depend on the site of the tumour:
- Frontal lobe: personality changes, apathy, and impairment of intellectual function. There may be anosmia, contralateral hemiparesis, or dysphasia (Broca's area).
- Parietal lobe: contralateral homonymous field defects and hemisensory loss. There may be apraxia, spatial disorientation, and dysphasia if the temporoparietal region is affected. Signs include 'parietal drift' or falling of the outstretched contralateral arm, astereognosis (inability to recognize an object placed in the hand), and sensory inattention.
- Temporal lobe: symptoms and signs are those of temporal lobe epilepsy (see p. 275).
- Occipital lobe: contralateral hemianopia.

The origins of brain tumours	
Site	**Example of tumour derived**
Glia	Gliomas (50%), oligodendrogliomas, ependymomas
Meninges	Meningiomas (25%)
Blood vessels	Angiomas, angioblastomas
The Schwann cells of the cranial nerves	Acoustic neuromas
Pituitary gland	Craniopharyngioma

Fig. 31.8 The origins of brain tumours.

- Cerebellopontine angle: there is progressive ipsilateral perceptive deafness, numbness of the ipsilateral side of the face, facial weakness, vertigo, and ipsilateral cerebellar signs.

Raised intracranial pressure

Symptoms include a throbbing headache (which is worse in the morning and with stooping, coughing, and sneezing), nausea and vomiting, and papilloedema. A shift of intracranial contents produces symptoms similar to direct mass effects. There may be impairment of consciousness progressing to coma, respiratory depression, and 'false localising signs' (e.g. a sixth nerve lesion, as it is compressed on the petrous temporal bone).

Investigations

The main investigations are a skull X-ray, EEG, CT brain scan, and MRI. If metastases are suspected, investigations for the primary neoplasm should be carried out. Lumbar puncture is contraindicated because of the risk of herniation of the cerebellar tonsils through the foramen magnum ('coning'). Biopsy should be considered, especially if an abscess is suspected.

Management

This is by surgical excision if possible. Radiotherapy is usually recommended for gliomas and for radiosensitive metastases. Dexamethasone will reduce cerebral oedema. Epilepsy is treated with anticonvulsants.

Prognosis

The overall 1-year survival for patients with primary intracerebral tumours is less than 50%. There may be complete recovery from meningiomas if they are removed completely.

Miscellaneous neurological disorders

Horner's Syndrome

Interruption of the sympathetic nerve supply to the face causes the following: miosis, enophthalmos (sunken eye), partial ptosis and ipsilateral loss of sweating (anhydrosis). The sympathetic nerves may be disrupted anywhere along their course:
- brainstem – demyelination, vascular disease
- cervical cord – syringomyelia
- thoracic outlet – Pancoast's tumour
- carotid artery – aneurysm

Motor neurone disease

This is a disease of unknown cause involving progressive degeneration of the anterior horn cells, lower cranial nuclei (hence the external ocular movements are normal), and neurones of the motor cortex and pyramidal tracts. Both upper and lower motor neurones can be affected but there are no sensory abnormalities.

It is slightly more common in men with a peak incidence between the ages of 50 and 70 years. The prevalence in the UK is about 6 in 100 000. Clinically there are three classical patterns of disease:
- Amyotrophic lateral sclerosis (50%): combined lower motor neurone wasting and upper motor neurone spasticity and hyperreflexia. Weakness starts in the legs and spreads to the arms.
- Progressive muscular atrophy (25%): anterior horn cell involvement leading to lower motor neurone weakness, wasting, and fasciculation of distal muscles, which spreads proximally.
- Progressive bulbar palsy (25%): lower motor neurone weakness and wasting of the tongue and pharynx leading to dysarthria and dysphagia.

Combinations of the above may occur.

Management

Management is symptomatic. The aim is to help the patient with activities of daily living and to reduce symptoms. Opiates should be considered for joint pains and distress. Difficult decisions regarding nasogastric or percutaneous endoscopic gastrostomy feeding and tracheostomy insertion and artificial ventilation may arise. These interventions may prolong life but also the process of dying. Riluzole, an anti-glutamate drug, is licensed in motor neurone disease and offers a small increase in length of life but is expensive. Death usually occurs 2–5 years after diagnosis.

Bulbar and pseudobulbar palsy

These two conditions affect the function of the brainstem motor nuclei therefore causing weakness of the tongue, muscles of chewing/swallowing (and therefore there is an increased risk of aspiration) and facial muscles.

Bulbar palsy is a lower motor neurone problem with a flaccid, fasciculating tongue, normal or absent jaw jerk and quiet nasal speech. It is caused by motor neurone disease, Guillain–Barré syndrome, polio, syringobulbia and brain stem tumours.

Pseudobulbar palsy refers to bilateral upper motor neurone lesions affecting the brainstem motor nuclei. The tongue is spastic, jaw jerk increased, speech is like 'Donald Duck' and there is emotional lability. Pseudobulbar palsy is more common and is usually due to bilateral strokes. Other causes are multiple sclerosis and motor neurone disease.

Peripheral neuropathy

The causes of peripheral neuropathy are summarised in Chapter 23. The four most common causes are DM, malignancy, vitamin B_{12} deficiency, and drugs (notably alcohol). Treatment is aimed at the underlying cause.

Bell's palsy

This is an idiopathic unilateral lower motor neurone palsy of the VII nerve. Other causes must be excluded (see Fig. 38.29).

Rapid onset of facial weakness occurs and may be accompanied by pain below the ear. The characteristic physical signs are described in Chapter 38.

Most patients recover fully in a few weeks. Approximately 15% have axonal degeneration and recovery may only begin after about 3 months and it may be incomplete. Occasionally aberrant reconnections are formed (e.g. eating may stimulate unilateral lacrimation—'crocodile tears').

High-dose prednisolone may reduce damage and speed recovery if given within a few days (ideally <24 hours) of onset. Some studies support the use of aciclovir as some cases of Bell's palsy may be due to herpes viruses. The eye must be protected when closure is incomplete: patches and artificial tears are useful initially and if a longer-term solution is required, lateral tarsorrhaphy is performed (eyelids sutured together at their lateral edge).

Guillain-Barré syndrome

This condition (also called acute postinfective polyneuropathy) affects motor nerves more than sensory nerves, and follows days or weeks after an infectious illness such as *Campylobacter*, cytomegalovirus or Epstein–Barr virus. There is inflammation, oedema, and demyelination of peripheral nerves and roots. Clinically, there is paraesthesia and numbness followed by a flaccid paralysis, which is progressive and ascending, but may come on rapidly and affect all four limbs simultaneously. The trunk, respiratory, and cranial nerves may be affected. Complications include

respiratory failure, pulmonary embolism, cardiac dysrhythmias due to autonomic dysfunction and aspiration due to bulbar palsy.

Investigations

The CSF shows a very high protein concentration (up to 10 g/L) with a normal cell count. The vital capacity should be measured 4–6-hourly to anticipate respiratory depression. In addition, the swallow should be monitored closely as should the postural blood pressure drop (as an indicator of autonomic funtion).

Management
Supportive

Attention should be paid to fluid balance and nutrition, and prevention of pressure sores, deep vein thrombosis, and pneumonia (physiotherapy). Ventilation may be necessary if respiratory failure occurs.

Specific

Steroids are not of benefit. However, intravenous immunoglobulin and plasma exchange have been shown to improve outcome.

Around 90–95% of patients recover within 3–6 months.

Muscle disorders

For more on muscle disorders, see polymyositis on pp. 326.

Myasthenia gravis

This is an autoimmune disease with a reduction in the number of functioning postsynaptic acetylcholine receptors leading to muscle weakness. Approximately 90% of patients have detectable antiacetylcholine receptor antibodies. It is associated with thymic tumours, hyperthyroidism, rheumatoid arthritis, and SLE.

Clinical features

The condition affects young adults and women twice as commonly as men. There is painless muscle weakness, which worsens on repetitive contraction. It is usually most marked in the face and eyes producing ptosis, diplopia, and a 'myasthenic snarl' on smiling. The voice may weaken on continued speaking and dysphagia may occur. Proximal muscles and upper limbs are more often affected than distal muscles and lower limbs. Reflexes tend to be brisk.

Investigations

Edrophonium (Tensilon®) 10 mg is given intravenously (with cardiac monitoring and resuscitation facilities). This improves muscle power for 3–4 minutes. It is an anticholinesterase, which enhances neuromuscular transmission in myasthenia gravis. It prolongs the action of acetylcholine by inhibiting the action of the enzyme acetylcholinesterase. There is raised antiacetylcholine receptor antibody.

Management

Symptomatic control is with a longer-acting anticholinesterase (e.g. pyridostigmine or neostigmine). The dose is slowly titrated against muscle power. Side effects include nausea, vomiting, increased salivation, diarrhoea, and abdominal cramps. In overdosage there may be excessive bronchial secretions and sweating, involuntary defecation and micturition, bradycardia, agitation, and weakness eventually leading to fasciculation and paralysis. Thymectomy increases the percentage of patients in remission.

Immunosuppression with prednisolone on alternate days may achieve remission. If there is no remission and weakness is severe, azathioprine may be helpful. In intractable cases, plasmaphoresis gives approximately 4 weeks of benefit. The condition is usually relapsing or slowly progressive, and respiratory muscle involvement can lead to death. The 5-year survival with a thymoma is approximately 30%.

Myotonic dystrophy (myotonia dystrophica)

This is an autosomal dominant condition characterised by myotonia, i.e. the inability of the muscles to relax normally after contraction. The peak onset is between the ages of 20 and 30 years, and the incidence in the UK is approximately 5 in 100 000. There is muscle wasting and weakness of the facial muscles with frontal balding, ptosis, a wry smile or 'sneer' and a 'hound dog' appearance.

There is also weakness of the shoulder girdle and quadriceps, cataracts, testicular or ovarian atrophy, cardiomyopathy with conduction disturbances, and mental impairment. Reflexes are lost. The myotonia is often revealed by shaking the patient's hand (slow to release grip) or by asking them to repetitively open and close their eyes or fists. It may be elicited by percussing the thenar eminence—the induced depression is slow to fill ('percussion myotonia'). It increases with fatigue, cold, and stress and may improve with procainamide or phenytoin. There may be associated DM.

Muscular dystrophies

These are a group of genetically determined diseases characterised by progressive degeneration and weakness of certain muscle groups.

Duchenne muscular dystrophy (pseudohypertrophic)

This is the commonest type and is sex-linked recessive. The incidence is 25 in 100 000 male births. The condition presents at around 5 years of age with clumsiness in walking and difficulty in climbing stairs. Examination reveals a lordotic posture and 'waddling' gait due to proximal muscle weakness. The calves are hypertrophied. Investigations show a markedly raised creatine kinase concentration. Electromyography and muscle biopsy show characteristic changes. Death usually occurs before the age of 20 years from intercurrent illnesses (e.g. chest infection). There is no specific treatment.

Fascioscapulohumeral dystrophy (Landouzy–Dejerine syndrome)

This is autosomal dominant. The onset is around puberty with wasting and weakness of the upper limb girdle and face. Life expectancy is normal.

Limb girdle dystrophy (Erb's syndrome)

This is autosomal recessive and presents at around 20–40 years. The shoulders and muscles of the pelvic girdles are affected, and the condition is progressive with death in middle age.

Disorders of the spinal cord
Syringomyelia

This is due to a longitudinal cyst in the cervical cord. As it enlarges it may extend into the dorsal horns and white matter. Clinical features are insidious and include the following:

- Weakness and wasting of the small muscles of the hand.
- Dissociated sensory loss in the hand: loss of pain and temperature sensation only. This may involve the trunk and arm.
- Trophic changes (e.g. ulceration and scarring, and swollen fingers due to subcutaneous hypertrophy).
- Loss of tendon reflexes.
- Pain in the arm.
- Spastic paraplegia: upper motor neurone signs.
- Charcot's joints in the upper limbs: destruction of the joints by too great a range of movement when normal sensation is lost.

Treatment is by surgical decompression or aspiration.

Syringobulbia

This is usually due to the extension of the cyst into the midbrain. It may involve the trigeminal nerve root, the motor nuclei of the lower cranial nerves, and the cervical sympathetic tract. Symptoms include the following:

- Facial pain or sensory loss: fifth cranial nerve.
- Vertigo and nystagmus: eighth cranial nerve.
- Facial, palatal, or laryngeal palsy: seventh, ninth, tenth, and eleventh cranial nerves.
- Wasting of the tongue: twelfth cranial nerve.
- Horner's syndrome: sympathetic tract.

Subacute combined degeneration of the cord

This is due to vitamin B_{12} deficiency and refers to demyelination of the posterior and lateral columns. The onset is usually insidious and associated with a sensory peripheral neuropathy. Clinical features include the following:

- Loss of vibration and proprioception senses, and positive rombergism: posterior columns.
- Weakness, hypertonia, and extensor plantars: upper motor neurone.
- Absent knee jerks and reduced touch sensation: peripheral neuropathy.

Treatment is with vitamin B_{12} injections intramuscularly.

Spinal cord compression

Spinal cord compression is a medical emergency. Symptoms include root pain often precipitated by movement or straining, spastic paraparesis with upper motor neurone signs below the level of the lesion, lower motor neurone signs at the level of the lesion, sensory loss with a characteristic 'sensory level', and sphincter disturbances at a later stage. It is important to note that there is a gap between the level of the root lesion and that of the sensory level and spastic paraparesis. This discrepancy arises because the spinal cord is shorter than the spinal column (it ends at the second lumbar vertebra in the adult). For example, the spinal cord segment at the level where the T_{12} nerve root exits through its foramen will be from the lumbosacral region. Compression lower down in the spinal canal of the cauda equina causes root pain and lower motor neurone weakness in the legs with saddle anaesthesia and sphincter disturbances.

Investigation is by X-ray of the spine, and CT or MRI to show the spinal cord. These must be done urgently as early intervention may prevent irreversible paraplegia. Therefore the neurosurgeons must also be informed promptly. Investigations should also include those of the underlying cause.

Treatment is by decompression, which should be performed as soon as possible to prevent irreversible damage. Radiotherapy may be useful in malignant disease. If the patient has a known or suspected malignancy dexamethasone should be given.

Causes of spinal cord compression are summarised in Fig. 31.9.

Causes of spinal cord compression	
Cause	**Example**
Vertebral (extradural)	Collapsed vertebrae, e.g. metastatic cancer (bronchus, breast, thyroid, kidney, prostate), osteoporosis, myeloma Spondylosis with disc prolapse Pott's disease (tuberculosis) Paget's disease Abscess Reticuloses
Intradural, extramedullary	Meningioma Neurofibroma
Intramedullary	Glioma

Fig. 31.9 Causes of spinal cord compression.

- How would you define 'stroke'?
- What are the options to be considered for secondary prevention following a stroke or TIA?
- What are the clinical features of a subdural haemorrhage?
- Describe the clinical features and complications of giant cell arteritis. How would you investigate and treat it?
- What are the causes of parkinsonism? Describe its characteristic clinical features.
- How would you investigate a patient with suspected multiple sclerosis?
- How would you investigate and treat a patient with suspected encephalitis?
- What are the causes of seizures (other than epilepsy)?

Further reading

Iain Wilkinson 1999 *Essential Neurology* Blackwell Publishing

www.dvla.gov.uk/drivers/dmed1.htm—guidance on driving and medical conditions

www.rcplondon.ac.uk/college/ceeu_stroke_home.htm—Royal College of Physicians guidance on stroke

www.nice.org.uk—NICE guidance on multiple sclerosis

PROGRESS Collaborative Group. Randomised trial of a perindopril-based blood-pressure-lowering regimen among 6105 individuals with previous stroke or transient ischaemic attack. *Lancet* 2001; **358**: 1033–1041

Heart Protection Study Collaborative Group. MRC/BHF Heart Protection Study of cholesterol lowering with simvastatin in 20536 high risk individuals: a randomised placebo controlled trial. *Lancet* 2002; **360:** 7–22

Munchau A and Bhatia K P. Pharmacological treatment of Parkinson's Disease. *Postgrad Med J* 2000; **76:** 602–610

Bahra A and Cikurel K 1999 *Crash Course in Neurology*, Mosby

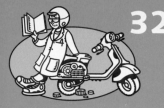

32. Metabolic and Endocrine Disorders

Diabetes mellitus

Diabetes mellitus (DM) is a persisting state of hyperglycaemia due to diminished availability or effectiveness of insulin. It affects approximately 2% of the population but type II diabetes is becoming commoner as levels of obesity rise (see below).

The WHO criteria are used for the diagnosis of DM. A fasting venous plasma glucose ≥7 mmol/L or a random venous plasma glucose >11.1 mmol/L in the presence of symptoms are diagnostic. A fasting level between 6–7 mmol/L implies impaired fasting glycaemia and should be further investigated with an oral glucose tolerance test (OGTT). To perform an OGTT, the fasted patient is given 75 g of glucose in 300 mL of water to drink. The venous plasma glucose is determined at the start and after 2 hours. A 2-hour level >11.1 mmol/L is diagnostic of DM; a fasting level of <7 mmol/L but with a 2-hour level ≥7.8 mmol/L and <11.1 mmol/L is diagnostic of impaired glucose tolerance. Impaired fasting glycaemia and impaired glucose tolerance refer to fasting and post-prandial abnormalities of glucose metabolism respectively; the terms are not interchangeable. In both cases, patients have an elevated risk of progression to frank DM and have increased macrovascular disease (see below).

Classification

Type I DM usually starts in young people who are thin and have an abrupt onset of signs and symptoms associated with low circulating insulin. Type I DM is due to autoantibodies to pancreatic β-cells causing a low concentration of circulating insulin. Therefore, these patients always require insulin replacement therapy and there is an association with other autoimmune diseases.

Patients with type II DM are usually older and overweight, and the onset is more insidious. Type II DM is due to reduced insulin production and reduced sensitivity of peripheral tissues to circulating insulin. Patients may require insulin if hyperglycaemia persists despite maximal doses of oral hypoglycaemic agents and in times of stress such as severe infections or after myocardial infarction. There is almost 100% concordance between identical

twins for non-insulin-dependent diabetes mellitus suggesting that inherited factors have a significant role to play.

Fig. 32.1 demonstrates some of the differences in presentation between type I and type II DM.

Secondary DM may be caused by:
- Drugs (e.g. steroids).
- Gestational DM: patients develop impaired glucose tolerance or frank diabetes during pregnancy.
- Pancreatic disease (e.g. pancreatectomy, carcinoma of the pancreas, pancreatitis, cystic fibrosis, haemochromatosis).
- Endocrine causes: Cushing's syndrome, acromegaly, phaeochromocytoma.

Clinical presentation

Diabetes may be asymptomatic and discovered on routine screening where elevated levels of glucose are found in the blood or urine but approximately half of all diabetics are undiagnosed.

Patients may present with non-specific symptoms such as weight loss and lethargy, and they are more prone to infection (e.g. carbuncles and thrush). Polyuria and polydipsia are characteristic and relate to the osmotic diuresis caused by the filtered glucose load in the nephrons overcoming their ability to reabsorb it.

The patient may present for the first time with a diabetic emergency (i.e. diabetic ketoacidosis, DKA) in the case of type I DM or hyperosmolar non-ketotic coma (HONK) in the case of type II DM.

Some patients, particularly type II diabetics with an insidious onset of disease, may present with chronic complications of their diabetes (see below). Fig. 32.1 summarises the characteristic presenting features in DM.

Complications

The chronic complications of DM are summarised in Fig. 32.2. They can be considered in two broad groups: macro- and micro-vascular. 'Macrovascular' refers to complications related to larger blood vessels (e.g. coronary artery, cerebrovascular and peripheral vascular disease). 'Microvascular' refers to complications related to smaller blood vessels

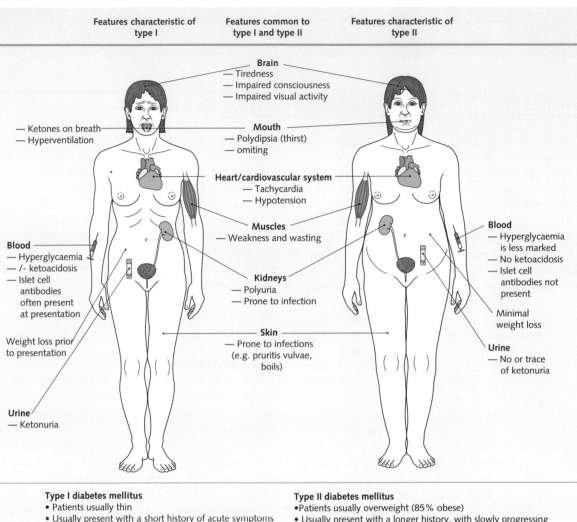

Features characteristic of type I	Features common to type I and type II	Features characteristic of type II

Brain
— Tiredness
— Impaired consciousness
— Impaired visual activity

— Ketones on breath
— Hyperventilation

Mouth
— Polydipsia (thirst)
— omiting

Heart/cardiovascular system
— Tachycardia
— Hypotension

Blood
— Hyperglycaemia
is less marked
— No ketoacidosis
— Islet cell
antibodies not
present

Muscles
— Weakness and wasting

Blood
— Hyperglycaemia
— /- ketoacidosis
— Islet cell
antibodies
often present
at presentation

Minimal
weight loss

Kidneys
— Polyuria
— Prone to infection

Weight loss prior
to presentation

Urine
— No or trace
of ketonuria

Skin
— Prone to infections
(e.g. pruritis vulvae,
boils)

Urine
— Ketonuria

Type I diabetes mellitus
• Patients usually thin
• Usually present with a short history of acute symptoms
• Treat with insulin

Type II diabetes mellitus
• Patients usually overweight (85% obese)
• Usually present with a longer history, with slowly progressing symptoms or with chronic complications
• May be asymptomatic, or have less severe but slowly progressing symptoms similar to type I diabetes, e.g. increasing tiredness.
• Many cases are discovered only by routine testing
• Treat with diet and oral hypoglycaemic agents initially (may need insulin subsequently)

Fig. 32.1 Acute symptoms and signs of diabetes mellitus (types I and II).

(e.g. diabetic retinopathy, nephropathy and neuropathy).

In a patient with gangrene and a palpable dorsalis pedis pulse, think of microvascular disease

Macrovascular disease

This is a cause of significant morbidity and mortality among diabetics. A diabetic's risk of myocardial

infarction is equivalent to that of a patient who has already suffered an infarction. Therefore, it is of paramount importance to assess and address all cardiovascular risk factors when managing diabetic patients (see below).

Eyes

Blindness occurs in up to 20% of patients with type I DM. The stages of diabetic retinopathy are shown in Fig. 38.27. Patients with maculopathy and pre-proliferative changes must be referred to an

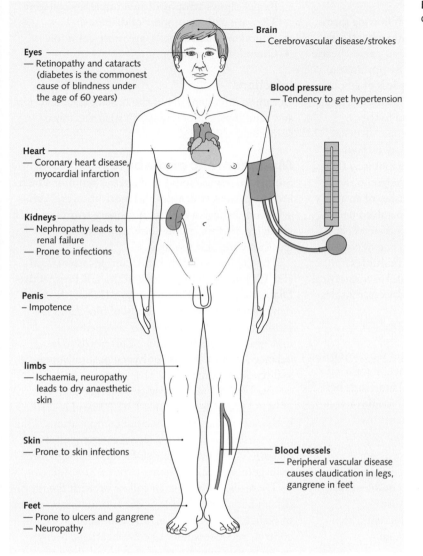

Fig. 32.2 Chronic complications of diabetes mellitus.

Brain
— Cerebrovascular disease/strokes

Eyes
— Retinopathy and cataracts (diabetes is the commonest cause of blindness under the age of 60 years)

Blood pressure
— Tendency to get hypertension

Heart
— Coronary heart disease, myocardial infarction

Kidneys
— Nephropathy leads to renal failure
— Prone to infections

Penis
– Impotence

limbs
— Ischaemia, neuropathy leads to dry anaesthetic skin

Skin
— Prone to skin infections

Blood vessels
— Peripheral vascular disease causes claudication in legs, gangrene in feet

Feet
— Prone to ulcers and gangrene
— Neuropathy

ophthalmologist; those with proliferative retinopathy require urgent referral for laser therapy.

Diabetics are also at elevated risk of early cataract formation. Rubeosis iridis is a late complication related to new vessel formation on the iris and may result in glaucoma.

Kidneys

The first sign of renal involvement is microalbuminuria (30–300 mg albumin per 24 hours). A negative dipstick test does not exclude microalbuminuria and therefore more sensitive tests must be used to screen diabetics for it (e.g. a timed urine collection or estimation of the albumin :

creatinine ratio in an early morning specimen). Microalbuminuria affects 20–40% of diabetics 10–15 years after diagnosis. These patients can progress to frank nephropathy (albumin excretion >300 mg per 24 hours) and the renal function then declines at a rate varying from patient to patient. Diabetic nephropathy is almost always associated with the presence of retinopathy and its absence should prompt a search for an alternative renal diagnosis.

The pathological hallmark of diabetic nephropathy is the Kimmelstiel–Wilson lesion.

Neuropathies

Diabetic neuropathy can take several forms:

Somatic neuropathies

Somatic neuropathies may take the following forms:

- Peripheral neuropathies: this commonly affects the lower limbs, with numbness and paraesthesiae of the feet, spreading up the leg. Symptoms are predominantly sensory with early loss of vibration sense and absent ankle jerks. In advanced cases, the loss of pain sensation may lead to the development of punched-out chronic ulcers at pressure points, in areas of thick callus. Foot pulses may be easily palpable; the foot may then become infected and eventually gangrenous.
- Mononeuritis: this is due to occlusion of an artery supplying the nerve. Commonly involved nerves include the third cranial nerve, ulnar nerve, and lateral popliteal nerve. More than one nerve can be involved, hence mononeuritis multiplex.
- Diabetic amyotrophy: this is painful asymmetrical weakness and wasting of the quadriceps muscles. It may recover.

Autonomic neuropathies

This may lead to symptoms of postural hypotension (i.e. dizziness on standing, impotence, nocturnal diarrhoea, and urinary retention). There may be lack of awareness of symptoms of hypoglycaemia, which is also more frequent in patients on β-blockers.

Diabetic feet

Diabetic foot problems are due to a combination of neuropathy and peripheral vascular disease. Diabetics are also predisposed to infection which may affect the soft tissue and even bone (osteomyelitis) of ulcerated feet.

Sensory neuropathy causes ulcers over pressure points (e.g. metatarsal heads) and can cause joint deformity due to the lack of pain and proprioception (e.g. pes cavus, Charcot joint). Peripheral vascular disease, which may be due to small and/or large vessel occlusion, affects the toes primarily.

Skin

Complications occurring in the skin include the following:

- Lipoatrophy: this is fat necrosis at insulin injection sites. The patient should be advised to vary the injection sites because the absorption of insulin at sites of atrophy is unpredictable. Transfer to human insulin may help.
- Necrobiosis lipoidica diabeticorum: these are yellowish areas on the skin with telangiectasia.

Biopsy shows atrophy of subcutaneous collagen. They are pathognomonic of diabetes.

- Infections, such as boils, are more common.
- Granuloma annulare.

Infections

Common infections are of the urinary tract and skin, and candidiasis. Tuberculosis (TB) is also more common in diabetics.

Management of diabetes

Successful management of diabetics requires a high level of patient education and motivation and this is achieved through a multi-disciplinary team approach involving doctors, nurses, ophthalmologists, dieticians and chiropodists.

The Diabetes Control and Complications Trial (DCCT) in type I diabetics and the UK Prospective Diabetes Study (UKPDS) in type II diabetics have demonstrated that tight control of blood glucose (aiming for an HbA1c of 6.5–7.5%) reduces microvascular complications. This needs to be balanced against the risk of hypoglycaemic episodes and rendering the patient obsessional.

The UKPDS also demonstrated that tight control of blood pressure (aim for <130/70 mmHg) reduces both macro- and micro-vascular complications. This emphasises the need for a global assessment of a diabetic's cardiovascular risk factors and aggressive management of all of them.

There should be regular follow up with the multi-disciplinary team. The aims of continued assessment of diabetics are education, assessment of glycaemic control, and assessment of complications. Many patients now monitor their own blood glucose concentrations using blood glucose strips, preferably with an electronic meter. These records should be examined, together with any hypoglycaemic symptoms, and HbA1c. Visual acuity should be checked, together with an examination of the optic fundi (after dilatation of the pupils with tropicamide) for retinopathy. The feet should be examined for neuropathy, ischaemic changes, and infection. Nephropathy should be looked for by monitoring the urea and electrolytes and by testing for albuminuria.

Diet

Calorie intake should be adjusted to achieve or maintain an ideal body weight. The diet should be low in fat (to help delay the progression of atherosclerosis), low in refined sugars but high in complex carbohydrates like starch, and high in fibre which, among other benefits, helps to lower postprandial hypoglycaemia.

Oral hypoglycaemic agents
These drugs should be used in addition to, not instead of, diet. The two main classes are sulphonylureas and biguanides, although other classes have recently been introduced, with more in development.

Sulphonylureas
These act mainly by augmenting insulin secretion and therefore some residual pancreatic β-cell activity is required. There are several sulphonylureas but all are probably equally effective. Elderly patients are particularly prone to the dangers of hypoglycaemia when long-acting sulphonylureas are used, and so chlorpropamide and glibenclamide should be avoided and replaced by shorter-acting drugs.

The sulphonylureas tend to encourage weight gain and this can be a problem in obese patients whose insulin resistance is worsened as a consequence.

Biguanides
Metformin is the only available biguanide. It exerts its effect mainly by decreasing gluconeogenesis and by increasing peripheral utilisation of glucose. Some residual islet cell function is required. It is usually reserved for people with type II DM who are overweight and in whom diet and sulphonylureas fail to control diabetes adequately, but it may be used as a first-line agent in obese patients. The UKPDS demonstrated a survival benefit in these individuals; hypoglycaemia is not usually a problem. Gastrointestinal (GI) side effects are common and lactic acidosis may also occur, although usually only in patients with renal impairment, in whom it should not be used.

Thiazolidinediones
These agents increase insulin sensitivity. National Institute of Clinical Excellence (NICE) guidelines suggest that they may be used if the combination of metformin and sulphonylurea is not tolerated or fails to adequately control the glucose level.

Acarbose
Acarbose, an inhibitor of intestinal α-glucosidases, delays the digestion of starch and sucrose and hence the increase in blood glucose levels which follow a carbohydrate-containing meal. It may be used as an adjunctive therapy but often causes intolerable flatulence.

Insulin
Approximately 25% of diabetics require treatment with insulin (a polypeptide hormone). It is inactivated by GI enzymes and must therefore be given by injection, usually subcutaneously. Mixtures of available insulin preparations may be required to maintain good control, and these will vary for individual patients. Requirements may be affected by variations in lifestyle, infections, and concomitant drugs.

Patients should aim for blood glucose concentrations between 4–10 mmol/L for most of the time, while accepting that on occasions they will be above or below these values. They should be advised to look for 'peaks' and 'troughs' of blood glucose, and to adjust their insulin dosage only once or twice weekly. The insulin preparations may be short, intermediate, or long-acting. Most patients are best started on insulins of intermediate action twice daily; a short-acting insulin can later be added to cover any hyperglycaemia which may follow breakfast or evening meals (Fig. 32.3).

Diabetes and surgery
Diabetic patients should be first on the operating list, and fasted on the morning of surgery. Oral agents should be stopped 24 hours before surgery, and restarted post-operatively unless the patient is ill or the blood glucose is very high, necessitating a period on insulin.

For patients already on insulin, the usual insulin should be given the night before the operation. An intravenous infusion of 500 mL of 5% glucose with 10 mmol KCl should be started early on the day of the operation and run at a constant rate to the patient's fluid requirements. A 1 unit/mL solution of soluble insulin in 0.9% saline should also be infused intravenously using a syringe pump. The rate varies according to the patient's blood glucose concentration, which should be measured every 2 hours until stable and every 6 hours thereafter.

When the patient starts to eat and drink, he or she may be restarted on the normal insulin regimen.

Diabetic coma
Hypoglycaemia
Symptoms of hypoglycaemia include sweating, hunger, and tremor. Very low glucose concentrations may cause drowsiness, fits, transient neurological symptoms, and loss of consciousness.

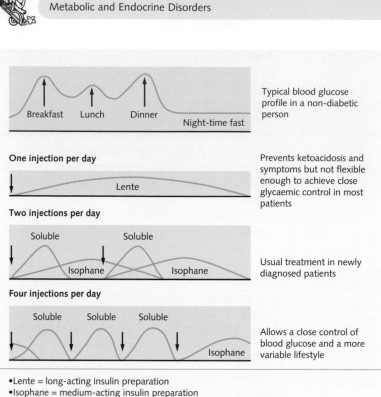

Fig. 32.3 Examples of different insulin regimens.

- Lente = long-acting insulin preparation
- Isophane = medium-acting insulin preparation
- Soluble insulin = short-acting insulin preparation

Aetiology

Hypoglycaemia may occur after a meal or after a fast. The aetiology of fasting hypoglycaemia includes the following:

- Drugs: excessive insulin or sulphonylureas (especially chlorpropamide). Large doses may be taken deliberately, particularly by medical and paramedical staff. Alcohol binges, especially with decreased food intake, may also lead to hypoglycaemia.
- Endocrine causes: pituitary insufficiency, Addison's disease, and insulinomas.
- Post-gastrectomy and functional hypoglycaemia.
- Liver failure.
- Inherited enzyme defects.
- Neoplasms (e.g. retroperitoneal fibrosarcomas).
- Immune hypoglycaemia (e.g. anti-insulin receptor antibodies in Hodgkin's disease).
- Malaria.

Investigations

Blood glucose and simple tests to exclude possible causes (e.g. liver function tests, LFTs). Consider a short Synacthen test for Addison's disease and thick and thin blood films for malaria.

Insulin is secreted as proinsulin from the pancreas and this is broken down to insulin and C-peptide.

Insulinoma can be confirmed by infusing intravenous insulin and measuring C-peptide. Normally insulin suppresses C-peptide but this suppression does not occur in patients with insulinomas.

Management

If the patient is conscious, three or four lumps of sugar should be given with a little water, and this should be repeated as necessary. If unconscious, 50 mL of 50% glucose should be given intravenously. Glucagon intramuscularly can be given as an alternative – this is a polypeptide hormone produced by the α-cells of the pancreatic islets of Langerhans. It increases plasma glucose by mobilising glycogen stored in the liver.

For patients who have taken a long-acting preparation, a continuous intravenous glucose infusion for 24 hours may be required. If an underlying cause is found it should be treated on its own merits.

Diabetic ketoacidosis

Diabetic ketoacidosis occurs in type I diabetics and may the mode of presentation or may be precipitated by an inadequate insulin dose or an intercurrent illness (e.g. infection or myocardial infarction). There is usually a gradual deterioration over hours to days.

The patient may describe polyuria, polydipsia, abdominal pain and vomiting. There may be evidence of the underlying cause. They often hyperventilate to compensate for the metabolic acidosis (Kussmaul respiration) and their breath smells of ketones (like nail varnish remover). There are physical signs of dehydration.

Investigations
- Urea and electroytes, arterial blood gases, full blood count, glucose, blood cultures.
- Urine dipstick and midstream urine. Test urine for ketones.

The diagnosis of DKA requires the demonstration of ketosis and acidosis. It is important to look for and treat the underlying cause.

Management
Correction of dehydration takes precedence. These patients are potassium depleted overall but the serum concentration may be normal or high as the acidosis causes potassium to move out of the intracellular compartment. Therefore the serum potassium concentration can fall precipitously as acidosis is corrected and it must be monitored closely and replaced.

Some 6–9 L of intravenous normal saline may be required and the first 2 L can be given over the first hour. An intravenous infusion of insulin titrated to the blood glucose is commenced. Once the blood glucose drops to around 15 mmol/L, the fluid replacement may be modified to include dextrose until the patient is eating and drinking.

A nasogastric tube should be inserted to reduce the risk of aspiration from the gastric stasis that occurs in this condition. Prophylactic heparin is commenced as there is a significant risk of venous thromboembolism.

Broad spectrum antibiotics are used and attempts made to identify the precipitant. The patient should be observed very closely in a high dependency or intensive care unit.

Hyperglycaemic hyperosmolar non-ketotic coma
The onset of this is gradual over days and it occurs in type II diabetics. The patient is often elderly and may not be a known diabetic. Polyuria leads to dehydration. The blood glucose is very high and plasma osmolality is increased. There is no acidosis or ketonuria because there is no change to ketone metabolism. Patients require small doses of intravenous insulin. Rehydration is usually with normal saline. If the sodium concentration is very high it may be tempting to use hypotonic saline. However, this can cause cerebral oedema by lowering the osmolality too quickly and, because these patients are so volume depleted, their total body stores of sodium are low and require replacement. Central venous pressure monitoring may be required. Patients are at a very high risk of venous thromboembolism and therapeutic dose anticoagulation with heparin is used. The mortality rate is up to 50%.

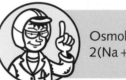

Osmolality can be calculated: $2(Na + K) + glucose + urea$

Obesity

This is defined as a body mass index (BMI) greater than 30. The normal range is 19–25 and it is calculated by dividing the weight in kilograms by the square of the height in metres (kg/m^2).

In 1980, 6% of adult males and 8% of adult females were obese. In 1998, these figures had increased to 17% and 21%, respectively. It is currently estimated that approximately 50% of the adult population is overweight or obese and there is certainly a growing problem amongst children as well. This trend constitutes an enormous Public Health issue with widespread changes in dietary and exercise patterns required.

Although there has been little change in the number of calories consumed since 1980, an increasing proportion of these are now in the form of fat and people are exercising less than before. Obesity is associated with significant mortality and morbidity. It increases the incidence of type II DM, dyslipidaemia and hypertension and therefore cardiovascular disease. It also causes musculoskeletal and psychological problems and there is some evidence to suggest that there may also be an increased incidence of cancer.

Management
Patients should be given lifestyle and dietary advice and support. Those patients with a BMI >28 with

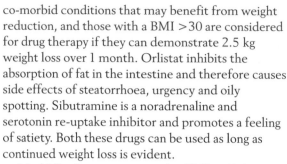

co-morbid conditions that may benefit from weight reduction, and those with a BMI >30 are considered for drug therapy if they can demonstrate 2.5 kg weight loss over 1 month. Orlistat inhibits the absorption of fat in the intestine and therefore causes side effects of steatorrhoea, urgency and oily spotting. Sibutramine is a noradrenaline and serotonin re-uptake inhibitor and promotes a feeling of satiety. Both these drugs can be used as long as continued weight loss is evident.

Morbidly obese patients with a BMI >40 (or >5 with co-morbidity) in whom there has been a failure to lose weight despite all conservative measures at a specialist clinic may be considered for surgery. This takes two forms: malabsorptive surgery where bypass procedures are performed or restrictive surgery where the size of the stomach is reduced.

Lipid disorders

Hypercholesterolaemia is widely prevalent in Western societies, particularly in the UK, where over 50% of the population aged older than 45 years have serum total cholesterol concentrations above 6.5 mmol/L. There is a positive association between serum cholesterol and coronary heart disease, although cholesterol concentration alone is of limited predictive value. Of more importance is the patient's overall coronary risk, of which cholesterol is one risk factor. Hence some patients will have 'normal' cholesterol concentrations but may be at high coronary risk by virtue of additional risk factors such as diabetes or left ventricular hypertrophy. Conversely, some patients, notably young women, will be at low coronary risk even with 'high' cholesterol concentrations.

There is now good evidence that lowering serum cholesterol in high-risk patients leads to a reduction in coronary events, and these people should therefore be targeted for treatment. Drug treatment of people at low risk is undesirable as the adverse effects of treatment may outweigh any potential benefits.

Lipids are insoluble in water, and so cholesterol and triglyceride are transported in the bloodstream bound to proteins as lipoproteins. There are five principal types of protein in the blood, and they can be separated in the laboratory by their density and electrophoretic mobility.

Chylomicrons are very large particles, mainly containing triglyceride. They provide the main mechanism for transporting the digestion products of dietary fat to the liver and peripheral tissues. Very low density lipoproteins are synthesised and secreted by the liver and contain most of the endogenously synthesised triglyceride. As they pass round the circulation, triglyceride is progressively removed by lipoprotein lipase leaving a particle called an intermediate density lipoprotein (IDL).

IDLs can bind to the hepatocyte and be catabolised, or have further triglyceride removed, producing low density lipoprotein (LDL) particles.

LDLs are the main carrier of cholesterol, and deliver it to both the liver and to peripheral cells. The LDL concentration correlates strongly with coronary risk.

High density lipoproteins (HDLs) are produced in both the liver and intestine. They take up cholesterol from cell membranes in peripheral tissues to the liver by 'reverse cholesterol transport'. HDL cholesterol therefore has a cardioprotective effect and concentrations are inversely proportional to coronary risk.

Classification of hyperlipidaemia

The most common form of hyperlipidaemia is polygenic with high serum cholesterol concentrations and normal triglyceride concentrations. Other forms are much less common.

Primary hyperlipidaemia

Familial combined hyperlipidaemia has a prevalence of 1 in 200 and is associated with high cholesterol and triglyceride concentrations.

Familial hypercholesterolaemia has an autosomal dominant inheritance and is due to LDL receptor deficiency resulting in an increase in LDL particles in the circulation. The prevalence is approximately 1 in 500. Homozygotes can have serum cholesterol levels of up to 30 mmol/L or more and may develop coronary artery disease in their teenage years.

Familial hypertriglyceridaemia is also an autosomal condition and can cause pancreatitis. Patients may have eruptive xanthomata. Triglyceride may also be raised in diabetes, alcoholism, and obesity.

Other classes of dyslipidaemia are rare. Cases of primary hyperlipidaemia are generally managed by lipid specialists.

Secondary hyperlipidaemia

Causes include DM, excess alcohol, hypothyroidism, cholestasis, chronic renal impairment, nephrotic syndrome, and synthetic oestrogens.

Management

Causes of secondary hyperlipidaemia should be treated. Where there is no secondary cause, dietary measures should be tried first. However, the average fall in total cholesterol concentration with a general lipid lowering diet is only 2%. Drug treatment is aimed at high-risk patients. For every 1% reduction in total cholesterol concentration (by diet or drug treatment), coronary heart disease risk is reduced by 1–2%.

Drugs

Statins

The statins competitively inhibit HMG-CoA reductase, an enzyme involved in cholesterol synthesis, especially in the liver. They are usually first-line therapy. There is evidence that statins produce important reductions in coronary events in high-risk patients, and their use is outlined below. They should be used with caution in those with a history of liver disease. Side effects include reversible myositis.

Treatment should be stopped if there are symptoms of myopathy and creatinine phosphokinase is markedly elevated. Patients should therefore be advised to report unexplained muscle pain, tenderness, and weakness. Other side effects include headache, altered LFTs and GI effects (e.g. abdominal pain, nausea, and vomiting).

Fibrates

Their main action is to decrease serum triglyceride but they also tend to reduce LDL cholesterol and raise HDL cholesterol. They can all cause a myositis-like syndrome, especially in patients with impaired renal function and those on a statin. They are usually used as second-line therapy or when there is persistent elevation of triglycerides despite a statin.

Anion-exchange resins

These drugs are rarely used. They include cholestyramine and colestipol, and act by binding bile acids, preventing their reabsorption; this promotes hepatic conversion of cholesterol into bile acids. They reduce LDL cholesterol but can aggravate hypertriglyceridaemia. Anion-exchange resins interfere with the absorption of fat-soluble vitamins. Supplements of vitamins A, D, and K, and of folic acid may be required when treatment is prolonged.

Side effects are mainly GI effects, and include change in bowel habit, nausea, vomiting, and abdominal pain. Other drugs should be taken at least 1 hour before, or 4–6 hours after cholestyramine or colestipol to reduce possible interference with absorption.

Nicotinic acid group

The value of nicotinic acid is limited by its side effects, especially vasodilatation. In high doses it lowers both cholesterol and triglyceride concentrations by inhibiting synthesis. It also increases HDL cholesterol. It is rarely used.

Fish oils

These may be useful in hypertriglyceridaemia. However, they can aggravate hypercholesterolaemia.

Ispaghula

Ispaghula husk is a form of soluble fibre and can be used as an adjunct to a lipid-lowering diet in patients with mild hypercholesterolaemia. It probably acts by reducing reabsorption of bile acids. Plasma triglycerides remain unchanged.

The use of statins

Before considering treatment with statins, other methods to reduce the risk of coronary heart disease should be instigated. This includes stopping smoking, dietary advice to control weight and lower lipids, advice on regular physical activity, control of hypertension, and other pharmacological measures, such as aspirin therapy, where appropriate. Although recent trials such as the Heart Protection Study suggest that individuals at risk of cardiovascular disease may benefit from lipid lowering regardless of their baseline lipid profile, current guidelines continue to target those patients at highest risk in whom the potential gains are greatest. There would be enormous cost implications if everybody who may benefit was treated. This is an area of controversy.

Secondary prevention

Patients with coronary artery disease (angina or acute myocardial infarction), peripheral vascular disease, or a history of ischaemic stroke are treated if they have a cholesterol >5 mmol/L or LDL >3 mmol/L. The aim is to achieve a 30% reduction or better these targets (whichever is lower).

Primary prevention

The patient's cardiovascular risk should be estimated using a method such as that in Fig. 32.4 that takes into account multiple risk factors. Statin therapy is targeted at those individuals with a coronary heart disease risk of 30% or greater over 10 years in whom the cholesterol is >5 mmol/L or LDL is >3 mmol/L.

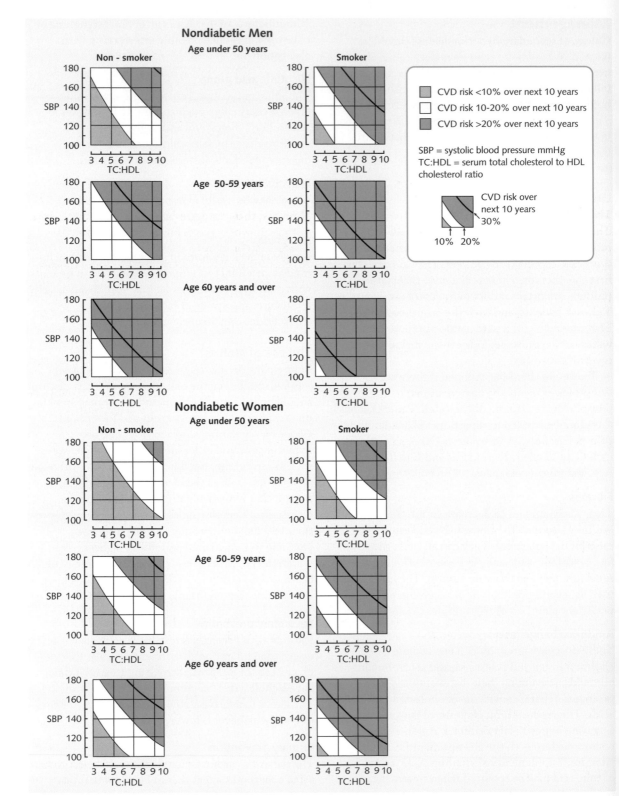

Fig. 32.4 Cardiovascular Disease Risk Prediction Charts for Primary Prevention (see below for an explanation of its use). Reproduced with kind permission from the British Heart Foundation.

Therapy should be adjusted to achieve a cholesterol concentration <5 mmol/L (or a reduction of 20–25% if that is greater), or an LDL concentration <3 mmol/L (or a reduction of 30% if that is greater).

How to use the cardiovascular disease risk prediction charts for primary prevention

These charts are for estimating cardiovascular disease (CVD) risk (non-fatal myocardial infarction [MI] and stroke, coronary and stroke death and new angina pectoris) for individuals who have not already developed coronary heart disease (CHD) or other major atherosclerotic disease. They are an aid to making clinical decisions about how intensively to intervene on lifestyle and whether to use antihypertensive, lipid lowering medication and aspirin.

- The use of these charts is not appropriate for the following patients groups. Those with:
  - CHD or other major atherosclerotic disease
  - Familial hypercholesterolaemia or other inherited dyslipidaemias
  - Chronic renal dysfunction
  - Type 1 and 2 diabetes mellitus
- The charts should not be used to decide whether to introduce antihypertensive medication when blood pressure (BP) is persistently at or above 160/100 or when target organ damage (TOD) due to hypertension is present. In both cases antihypertensive medication is recommended regardless of CVD risk. Similarly the charts should not be used to decide whether to introduce lipid-lowering medication when the ratio of serum total to high density lipoprotein (HDL) cholesterol exceeds 7. Such medication is generally then indicated regardless of estimated CVD risk.
- To estimate an individual's absolute 10 year risk of developing CVD choose the table for his or her gender, smoking status (smoker/non-smoker) and age. Within this square define the level of risk according to the point where the coordinates for systolic blood pressure (SBP) and the ratio of total cholesterol to HDL-cholesterol meet. If no HDL cholesterol result is available, then assume this is 1.00mmol/l and the lipid scale can be used for total serum cholesterol alone.

- Higher risk individuals (red areas) are defined as those whose 10 year CVD risk exceeds 20%, which is approximately equivalent to the CHD risk of >15% over the same period indicated by the previous version of these charts. As a minimum those at highest CVD risk (greater than 30% shown by the line within the red area) should be targeted and treated now. When resources allow, others with a CVD risk of >20% should be progressively targeted.
- The chart also assists in the identification of individuals whose 10 year CVD risk moderately increased in the range 10-20% (orange area) and those in whom risk is lower than 10% over 10 years (green area).
- Smoking status should reflect lifetime exposure to tobacco and not simply tobacco use at the time of assessment. For example, those who have given up smoking within 5 years should be regarded as current smokers for the purposes of the charts.
- The initial BP and the first random (non-fasting) total cholesterol and HDL cholesterol can be used to estimate an individual's risk. However, the decision on using drug therapy should generally be based on repeat risk factor measurements over a period of time.
- Men and women do not reach the level of risk predicted by the charts for the three age bands until they reach the ages 49, 59, and 69 years respectively. Everyone aged 70 years and over should be considered at higher risk. The charts will overestimate current risk most in the under forties. Clinical judgement must be exercised in deciding on treatment in younger patients. However, it should be recognised that BP and cholesterol tend to rise most and HDL cholesterol to decline most in younger people already possessing adverse levels. Thus untreated, their risk at the age 49 years is likely to be higher than the projected risk shown on the age-less-than 50 years chart.
- These charts (and all other currently available methods of CVD risk prediction) are based on groups of people with untreated levels of BP, total cholesterol and HDL cholesterol. In patients already receiving antihypertensive therapy in whom the decision is to be made about whether to introduce lipid-lowering medication or vice versa the charts can act as a guide, but unless recent pre-treatment risk factor values are available it is generally safest to assume that CVD risk is higher than that predicted by current levels of BP or lipids on treatment.

- CVD risk is also higher than indicated in the charts for:-
  - Those with a family history of premature CVD or stroke (male first degree relatives aged <55 years and female first degree relatives aged <65 years) which increases the risk by a factor of approximately 1.5
  - Those with raised triglyceride levels
  - Women with premature menopause
  - Those who are not yet diabetic, but have impaired fasting glucose (6.1-6.9mmol/l)
- In some ethnic minorities the risk charts underestimate CVD risk, because they have not been validated in these populations. For example, in people originating from the Indian subcontinent it is safest to assume that the CVD risk is higher than predicted from the charts (1.5 times).
- The charts may be used to illustrate the direction of impact of risk factor intervention on estimated level of CVD risk. However, such estimates are crude and are not based on randomised trial evidence. Nevertheless, this approach maybe helpful in motivating appropriate intervention. The charts are primarily to assist in directing intervention to those who typically stand to benefit most.

Metabolic bone disease

Vitamin D metabolism is shown in Fig. 32.5.

Osteoporosis

Bone normally consists of 60% mineral and 40% matrix or organic matter. In osteoporosis, there is a loss of bone matrix and reduction in bone mass, although the deposition of calcium salts, or mineralisation, occurs normally. There is therefore a reduction in the amount of bone mineral per unit volume of anatomical bone. The World Health Organisation (WHO) has defined osteoporosis as a bone mineral density (BMD) ≥ 2.5 standard deviations below the mean value for young adults (T score less than -2.5). Osteopenia is defined as a BMD T score between -1.0 and -2.5.

The prevalence of osteoporosis in White women aged 50–59 years is 4% and the prevalence in those aged 80 years or over is 52%. Osteoporosis predisposes patients to hip, vertebral and wrist fractures. These are associated with considerable morbidity and mortality. The cost attributable to these fractures annually in England and Wales is £1.7 billion and this indicates the scale of the problem.

Pathogenesis

Involutional or primary osteoporosis
Involutional bone loss commences at age 35–45 years in both sexes but is accelerated in women following the loss of sex steroids at the menopause. This explains the higher incidence in post-menopausal women. Age related bone loss is increased by smoking, alcohol, inactivity, low body mass index and impaired vitamin D production.

Secondary osteoporosis
Causes include steroid therapy, hypogonadism, alcohol abuse, hyperthyroidism, multiple myeloma and anticonvulsants.

Clinical features
Osteoporosis itself is painless unlike the fractures with which it is associated. The risk of fracture is related to the BMD but also to conditions predisposing to falls (e.g. stroke, parkinsonism, dementia, visual impairment). These must also be assessed.

Investigations
- Blood tests including a bone profile should be normal.
- BMD is estimated by bone densitometry. There is no evidence for population based screening. It is performed if there are risk factors and therapy is being considered (e.g. premature menopause, steroid therapy). It may also be done following a fragility (low trauma) fracture, an X-ray demonstrating osteopenia or for monitoring the effect of therapy.
- Thyroid function, luteinizing hormone (LH), follicle-stimulating hormone (FSH) and testosterone should be measured to exclude secondary causes. 50% of males with hip fractures are hypogonadal.

Prevention and treatment
A holistic approach to the reduction of fracture risk is important. Falls risk should be assessed and interventions implemented, alcohol excess and smoking should be discouraged and a good diet with regular activity encouraged.

Patients with osteopenia are given lifestyle advice and monitored unless they have had a fracture, in which case therapy is instituted. All those with osteoporosis are treated.

Treatment options include bisphosphonates, raloxifene (a selective oestrogen receptor

Fig. 32.5 Metabolism of vitamin D.

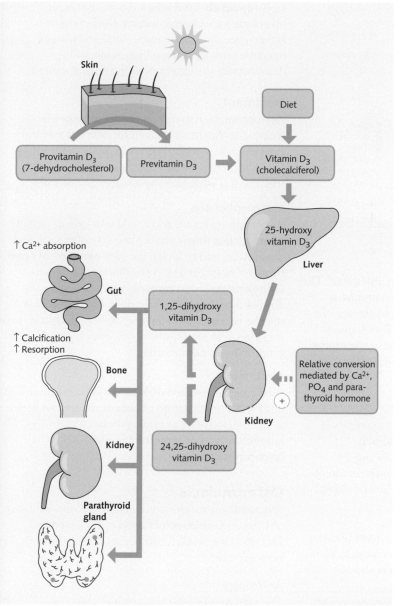

modulator), calcitonin and intermittent parathyroid hormone. Bisphosphonates are the mainstay of therapy in most cases. It was thought that hormone replacement therapy (HRT) should be given around the time of the menopause for at least 8–10 years. However, recent data suggest that this may be associated with a significantly increased risk of breast cancer, venous thromboembolism and cardiovascular disease. Therefore, HRT is no longer recommended as a first-line therapy. The institutionalised elderly, in whom diet and sunlight exposure may be limited,

should receive calcium and vitamin D supplementation.

Patients on long-term steroids are particularly at risk and a low threshold for therapy is needed.

Paget's disease

In Paget's disease, there is uncontrolled bone turnover with local excessive osteoclastic resorption. This is followed by disordered osteoblastic activity, leading to new bone formation, which is structurally abnormal and weak (Fig. 32.6). The aetiology is

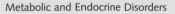

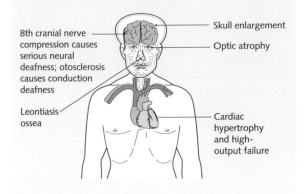

8th cranial nerve compression causes serious neural deafness; otosclerosis causes conduction deafness

Leontiasis ossea

Skull enlargement

Optic atrophy

Cardiac hypertrophy and high-output failure

Fig. 32.6 General features of Paget's disease of the bone.

unknown although viruses have been implicated. The incidence increases with age—it is uncommon in individuals aged under 40 years but, by the age of 90 years, approximately 10% of the population in temperate climates is affected. It is also commoner in Anglo-Saxons and there appears to be a familial incidence.

Clinical features

The axial skeleton and femur are most commonly affected. The condition is most commonly asymptomatic but can cause bone pain and tenderness, and there may be deformities of affected bones, such as an enlarged skull and bowed (sabre) tibia.

Complications include:

- Progressive occlusion of the foramina of the skull (e.g. deafness due to nerve compression, basilar invagination, and cervical cord stenosis with paraparesis).
- Conductive deafness due to involvement of the ossicles.
- Optic atrophy.
- Fractures of long bones.
- Hypercalcaemia: if the patient is immobile.
- High-output cardiac failure from shunting.
- Osteogenic sarcoma.
- Osteoarthritis of related joints.

Investigations

Serum alkaline phosphatase is markedly raised but serum calcium and phosphate are normal; 24-hour urinary hydroxyproline output is raised and reflects the increased bone turnover. There may be mild hypercalcaemia in immobile patients.

X-rays of affected bones show a mosaic of osteolytic and sclerotic lesions, thickening of trabeculae, and thick cortices with an enlarged irregular outline. Isotope bone scans will demonstrate the extent of skeletal involvement.

Treatment

Asymptomatic patients do not require specific treatment. Analgesia is given for pain but specific treatment is given for bone pain, bone deformities, hypercalcaemia, or for complications. Drug treatment is with bisphosphonates or calcitonin.

Bisphosphonates

Bisphosphonates are adsorbed on to hydroxyapatite crystals, thus slowing both their rate of growth and dissolution, and reducing the increased rate of bone turnover associated with the disease. Disodium etidronate is most commonly used. A single daily dose of 5 mg/kg is given for up to 6 months. This may be repeated after an interval of 3 months if there is evidence of reactivation. Side effects include focal osteomalacia and fractures.

Calcitonin

Calcitonin is involved with parathyroid hormone (PTH) in the regulation of bone turnover and hence in the maintenance of calcium balance and homoeostasis. It is less effective than bisphosphonates.

Osteomalacia

Osteomalacia results from inadequate mineralisation of bone and occurs after fusion of the epiphyses. Rickets is the result if this occurs during the period of bone growth.

Aetiology

The aetiology of osteomalacia includes:

- Lack of dietary vitamin D.
- Ineffective conversion of 7-dehydrocholesterol (provitamin D_3) to previtamin D_3 by ultraviolet light in the dermis. This is due to lack of sunlight and, in the UK, is most commonly seen in Asians.
- Intestinal malabsorption (e.g. gluten-sensitive enteropathy and postgastrectomy states).
- Vitamin D resistance: chronic renal disease most commonly due to ineffective conversion of 25-hydroxyvitamin D_3 to 1,25-dihydroxyvitamin D_3, inherited deficiency of renal 1α-hydroxylase, or end-organ receptor abnormality (rare).

- Drug induced: chronic anticonvulsant therapy may induce liver enzymes, leading to the breakdown of 25-hydroxyvitamin D_3.
- Excessive renal phosphate loss due to Fanconi's syndrome or a specific defect in renal phosphate handling.

Clinical features

In patients with osteomalacia, there may be bone pain and tenderness. Fractures may occur, especially of the femoral neck. There is a proximal myopathy resulting in a waddling gait and difficulty in rising from a chair.

In rickets, there are deformities of the legs (bow-legs and knock-knees), the chest (ricketic rosary), and the skull. There may also be features of hypocalcaemia (e.g. tetany).

Investigations

Biochemistry

- Serum calcium and phosphate: tend to be decreased.
- Serum alkaline phosphatase activity: increased.
- Urinary calcium excretion: low.
- Plasma 25-hydroxyvitamin D_3: low except in resistant cases.
- 1,25-dihydroxyvitamin D_3: low in renal failure.
- Parathormone is high because of secondary hyperparathyroidism due to hypocalcaemia.

X-rays

X-rays of bone in rickets show cupped, ragged metaphyseal surfaces. In osteomalacia, there is loss of cortical bone, and pseudofractures (Looser's zones), which are small translucent bands perpendicular to the bone and extending inwards from the cortex. They are best seen on the lateral border of the scapula, the femoral neck, and in the pubic rami.

Bone scan

A bone scan shows a generalised diffuse increase in uptake of isotope.

Treatment

Dietary vitamin D deficiency can be prevented by taking an oral supplement of 10 μg of ergocalciferol daily. Vitamin D deficiency caused by intestinal malabsorption or chronic liver disease usually requires vitamin D in pharmacological doses, such as calciferol tablets up to 1 mg (i.e. 10 000 units) daily.

The newer hydroxylated vitamin D derivatives – alfacalcidol and calcitriol – have a shorter duration of action, and therefore have the advantage that problems associated with hypercalcaemia due to excessive dosage are shorter lived and easier to treat.

In patients with chronic renal impairment, alfacalcidol or calcitriol should be prescribed. All patients receiving pharmacological doses of vitamin D should have their serum levels of calcium checked at intervals, and whenever nausea and vomiting are present.

Breast milk from women taking pharmacological doses of vitamin D may cause hypercalcaemia if given to an infant.

Renal osteodystrophy

The term 'renal osteodystrophy' is used to cover the various forms of bone disease that develop in chronic renal failure. These include:

- Delayed epiphyseal closure in children and young adults.
- Rickets or osteomalacia.
- Osteitis fibrosa cystica (brown tumours) due to secondary or tertiary hyperparathyroidism.
- Generalised or localised osteosclerosis.

The kidney does not excrete phosphate effectively as its function drops. This hyperphosphataemia stimulates PTH secretion. The impaired hydroxylation of 25-hydroxyvitamin D causes osteomalacia and also hypocalcaemia. The hypocalcaemia further stimulates the release of PTH.

Management

Dietary phosphate intake is reduced and oral phosphate binders are used to help control the hyperphosphataemia. Calcium and hydroxylated vitamin D supplements can be given when the phophate levels are controlled (reducing the risk of ectopic calcification) to help normalise the calcium and reduce the level of PTH further. Renal replacement therapy in the form of haemodialysis, peritoneal dialysis or transplantation will help restore calcium and phosphate metabolism in end-stage renal failure.

In cases of tertiary hyperparathyroidism, subtotal parathyroidectomy is required.

Hypercalcaemia

The causes of hypercalcaemia are given in Fig. 40.20. The two commonest pathological causes are primary hyperparathryroidism and malignant disease. However, the commonest cause of borderline hypercalcaemia is probably faulty technique (i.e. excessive venous stasis when collecting blood samples). An abnormally high result should therefore be repeated without a tourniquet (uncuffed sample).

The physiologically relevant measurement is of ionised calcium. This can be determined by correcting serum total calcium levels for serum protein or albumin concentrations. The higher the protein concentration, the more calcium is protein bound, and the lower the proportion of ionised calcium. Add 0.1 mmol/L to calcium concentration for every 4 g/L that albumin is below 40 g/L and perform a similar subtraction for high albumin.

Clinical features

 For the clinical features of hypercalcaemia, remember *bones* (bone pain), *stones* (renal stones), *groans* (peptic ulcer), and *moans* (psychiatric disease)

These include abdominal pain, constipation and vomiting. Polyuria, polydipsia and dehydration are common. Depression and confusion may occur. Renal stone formation and renal failure can occur and, if severe, cardiac arrest. There may also be features of the underlying cause.

Investigations

- Full blood count, electrolytes, calcium profile and PTH, liver and thyroid function tests. PTH should be suppressed unless hyperparathyroidism is the cause.
- Chest X-ray—any evidence of malignancy or sarcoidosis?
- Other investigations will be determined by the differential diagnosis (e.g. isotope bone scan, myeloma screen, etc.).

Management

Severe hypercalcaemia is a medical emergency. In the acute phase, it is essential to rehydrate with normal saline as the renal excretion of calcium is dependent on exchange with sodium ions in the nephron. 4–6 L

may be given over 24 hours. Intravenous bisphosphonate therapy (usually a single dose of pamidronate) is given. Frusemide was previously given after adequate hydration to induce a calciuresis. High-dose prednisolone is effective for hypercalcaemia secondary to myeloma, sarcoidosis, and excess vitamin D but otherwise is of little value. Calcitonin is now rarely used.

After the acute phase, it is important to elucidate the cause of the hypercalcaemia and treat it.

Hyperparathyroidism

Hyperparathyroidism results from excess circulating PTH, which increases serum calcium by increasing calcium absorption from the gut, increasing mobilisation of calcium from bone, and reducing renal calcium clearance.

Primary hyperparathyroidism is usually due to a single benign adenoma but may less commonly be due to multiple adenomas, carcinoma, or hyperplasia. It may be associated with other endocrine abnormalities as part of the multiple endocrine neoplasia (MEN) syndromes. Ectopic PTH production may be produced by carcinoma from the lung and kidney.

Secondary hyperparathyroidism occurs when PTH levels are persistently and appropriately raised to maintain calcium concentrations in the face of a disorder that lowers calcium levels. Causes include chronic renal failure and deficiency of vitamin D (e.g. due to inadequate intake or malabsorption).

Tertiary hyperparathyroidism is the continued secretion of excess PTH after prolonged secondary hyperparathyroidism. The parathyroids act autonomously and cause hypercalcaemia, despite the absence of the original cause of the secondary hyperparathyroidism.

Clinical features

Symptoms may be due to hyperparathyroid bone disease and can result in fractures. In addition the features of hypercalcaemia discussed above may be present.

Investigations

In primary hyperparathyroidism, serum calcium is raised. Fasting blood samples should be taken without venous compression. Serum phosphate is low and alkaline phosphatase is high, reflecting increased bone turnover. There is a mild renal tubular acidosis with a high serum chloride level, and serum PTH is raised. In secondary hyperparathyroidism of renal failure, serum calcium is low or normal and phosphate is normal or high. Both of these metabolic abnormalities stimulate the secretion of PTH.

X-rays show subperiosteal resorption, being most marked in the hands, and evidence of osteitis fibrosa cystica. A chest X-ray (CXR) should be performed to look for a carcinoma producing PTH. A skull X-ray shows a 'pepperpot' appearance.

Treatment

Parathyroidectomy is indicated for persistent hypercalcaemia above 2.8 mmol/L or for symptomatic hypercalcaemia. The parathyroid glands may be localised by computed tomography (CT) scan or isotope scans. All four glands should be biopsied; single adenomas can be removed.

If the glands are hyperplastic, three and a half are removed, leaving the last half *in situ*. Serum calcium and magnesium should be checked frequently post-operatively as removal of the glands may lead to rapid and prolonged hypocalcaemia and hypomagnesaemia as the 'hungry bones' recover the minerals lost during the period of hyperparathyroidism.

Hypoparathyroidism

Hypoparathyroidism is usually secondary to thyroid surgery. Primary (idiopathic) hypoparathyroidism is an autoimmune disorder associated with vitiligo, Addison's disease, pernicious anaemia, and other autoimmune diseases. The DiGeorge syndrome is a familial condition with parathyroid agenesis. It is associated with intellectual impairment, cataracts, and calcified basal ganglia.

Pseudohypoparathyroidism is a syndrome of end-organ resistance to PTH. It is associated with intellectual impairment, short stature, a round face, and short metacarpals and metatarsals.

Pseudopseudohypoparathyroidism describes the appearance present in pseudohypoparathyroidism but without the calcium abnormalities.

Other causes of hypocalcaemia include chronic renal failure and osteomalacia. In acutely ill patients acute pancreatitis and rhabdomyolysis can cause hypocalcaemia.

Clinical features

Circumoral paraesthesiae, cramps, anxiety, and tetany are followed by convulsions, laryngeal stridor, dystonia, and psychosis. Trousseau's sign may be present – carpopedal spasm when the brachial artery is occluded with a blood pressure cuff. Chvostek's sign may also be present – twitching of the facial muscles when the facial nerve is tapped.

Investigations

Serum calcium is low, phosphate is high, and alkaline phosphatase is normal. Additional tests include serum urea and creatinine, serum PTH level, parathyroid antibodies, and vitamin D metabolite levels.

X-rays of the hands show short fourth metacarpals in pseudohypoparathyroidism.

Treatment

Emergency treatment is with 10 mL 10% intravenous calcium gluconate, repeated as necessary. Intravenous magnesium chloride may also be required if there is hypomagnesaemia.

Long-term treatment is with alfacalcidol or calcitriol. Serum calcium should be monitored to prevent hypercalcaemia.

Crystal arthropathy

Gout

Gout is a result of the deposition of sodium urate crystals in joints and soft tissues due to an abnormality of uric acid metabolism. It affects approximately 1 in 500 people in the UK. It is commoner in men, drinkers, and in higher socio-economic classes, and about a third have a positive family history. The underlying biochemical abnormality is an overproduction or underexcretion of uric acid resulting in hyperuricaemia. The main causes are given in Fig. 32.7.

Clinical features
Acute gout

This typically starts in the first metatarsophalangeal joint with an acute onset of a red, hot, swollen, extremely painful big toe (Fig. 32.8). It may be precipitated by alcohol, diet, starvation, diuretics, or after surgery. Other commonly affected joints include the ankle, wrist, knees, and bursae. The patient may have high blood pressure, renal impairment, or peripheral vascular disease. The renal disease may be secondary to uric acid stones.

Causes of gout
• Idiopathic
• Drugs: diuretics, low-dose aspirin
• Chronic renal impairment
• Hypertension
• Primary hyperparathyroidism
• Hypothyroidism
• Alcohol
• Glucose-6-phosphate deficiency
Rapid cell turnover:
• Myeloproliferative disorders, e.g. polycythaemia rubra vera
• Lymphoproliferative disorders, e.g. leukaemia
• Severe psoriasis

Fig. 32.7 Causes of gout.

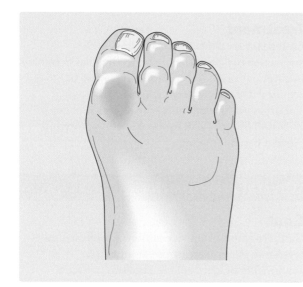

Fig. 32.8 Acute gout of the first metatarsophalangeal joint.

Chronic tophaceous gout

This leads to joint erosion and disruption leading to chronic disability. There are tophi in the ear lobes or around joints (particularly hands and elbows), which are soft tissue deposits of urate.

Investigations

The following investigations are important in patients with gout:

- Joint aspiration is the definitive test and allows exclusion of septic arthritis in the single hot swollen joint. Synovial fluid examined under polarised light microscopy shows needle-shaped, negatively birefringent crystals.

- X-rays may be normal in acute gout but show punched-out erosions and joint disruption in chronic gout.
- Serum uric acid may be high but there are a large number of false positive and false negative results. It is more useful for monitoring treatment.

Management

Acute attacks

These are normally treated with high doses of non-steroidal anti-inflammatory drugs (NSAIDs) such as naproxen 500 mg b.d. or ibuprofen 400 mg t.d.s. They should be used with care in patients with peptic ulcer disease, heart failure, hypertension, and renal impairment.

Colchicine is probably as effective as NSAIDs but excessive doses cause diarrhoea. If colchicine and NSAIDs cannot be tolerated, steroids may be used. Intra-articular injection of steroid into an affected joint often provides symptomatic relief.

Prophylactic treatment

The patient should be advised on weight reduction, reducing alcohol consumption, avoiding precipitating foods such as red meat, and avoiding precipitating drugs if possible.

If the patient suffers recurrent attacks, has tophi or has a documented state of uric acid over-production (e.g. myeloproliferative disease), uric acid-lowering drug therapy is indicated. The initiation of treatment may precipitate an acute attack, therefore colchicine or NSAIDs should be used prophylactically for at least 1 month after the hyperuricaemia has been corrected.

Allopurinol inhibits xanthine oxidase, which catalyses the conversion of hypoxanthine to xanthine, and of xanthine to uric acid. It is especially useful in patients with renal impairment or urate stones where uricosuric agents cannot be used. It is usually given once daily (initially 100 mg after food) and gradually increased to a maintenance dose of about 300 mg daily. Lower doses are given in patients with renal impairment. It may cause skin rashes.

Uricosuric drugs include probenecid and sulphinpyrazone. They may be used instead of allopurinol or with it in cases that are resistant to treatment. Aspirin antagonises the effect of uricosuric drugs. It is important to ensure a good urine output as they may lead to crystallization of urate in the urine.

Pituitary disorders

Hypopituitarism

There are six anterior pituitary hormones—adrenocorticotrophic hormone (ACTH), growth hormone (GH), FSH, LH, thyroid stimulating hormone (TSH) and prolactin (PRL). Hypopituitarism may be associated with loss of all or some of these hormones. The clinical and biochemical presentation will depend on which hormones are deficient and to what extent. The most common cause includes the mass effect of pituitary adenomas (if these are functional there may be features of hypersecretion of a particular hormone—see below), with additional loss of pituitary function after surgery and pituitary irradiation. Other causes include hypothalamic tumours and cysts, peripituitary tumours (e.g. gliomas and meningiomas, craniopharyngiomas), infiltrative diseases (e.g. sarcoidosis), and vascular and metastatic lesions in and around the pituitary fossa.

Clinical features

These can be worked out from knowledge of the effects of the various pituitary hormones:

- GH: fatigue, loss of energy, increased abdominal adiposity, and reduced muscle strength and exercise capacity.
- LH and follicle-stimulating hormone (FSH): in women, there is oligomenorrhoea, infertility, dyspareunia, breast atrophy, loss of pubic and axillary hair, and hot flushes; in men, there is loss of libido, impotence, infertility, flushes, regression of secondary sexual characteristics, soft testicles, and fine wrinkles on the face.
- TSH: fatigue, muscle weakness, sensitivity to cold, constipation, apathy, weight gain, and dry skin.
- ACTH: fatigue, anorexia, weight loss, pallor, weakness, nausea and vomiting, hypoglycaemia, apathy, and loss of pubic and axillary hair.
- Vasopressin (posterior pituitary): polyuria and polydipsia with nocturia.

Investigations

- Basal thyroxine, TSH, LH/FSH, PRL, testosterone and short synachten test.

Previously, a triple stimulation test was performed: thyroid releasing hormone was used to assess the TSH response; gonadotrophin releasing hormone was used to assess the response of LH and FSH; insulin was given to induce hypoglycaemia and the GH and cortisol response to this was assessed (both should increase). However, T4/TSH now reliably diagnoses TSH deficiency; testosterone/LH/FSH in men and LH/FSH/menstrual history are as reliable as a GnRH test; the short synachten test provides enough information about ACTH deficiency.

- A water deprivation test is performed if diabetes insipidus is suspected (see Chapter 13).
- CT/MRI/visual field assessment—see below.

Management

Hormone replacement involves the use of multiple hormones. Hydrocortisone is given for adrenal failure, thyroxine for hypothyroidism and testosterone for men and oestrogen for pre-menopausal females. Some patients are given growth hormone. Careful instruction and patient compliance are mandatory for long-term recovery.

Pituitary tumours

Pituitary tumours may be non-functioning or may secrete hormones. The incidence of pituitary tumours varies from 0.2–3 in 100 000 population, and the prevalence is about 9 in 100 000. PRL- and ACTH-secreting tumours occur most commonly in 25–35-year-olds, GH-secreting tumours in those aged 35–50 years, and non-functioning tumours usually present after the age of 60 years.

Clinical features

The clinical features relate to (i) pressure effects from the tumour mass, (ii) the effects of hypersecretion of any hormone and (iii) the suppression of other pituitary hormones (hypopituitarism).

Pressure effects cause headaches and there may be compression of the optic chiasm causing bitemporal hemianopia. Seizures may occur and other focal cranial nerve signs. Extension into the hypothalamus affects appetite, sleep and temperature regulation.

The effects of functioning tumours depend on the hormone secreted. They may cause acromegaly via GH, amenorrhoea-galactorrhoea syndrome via PRL, or Cushing's disease via ACTH. Secondary thyrotoxicosis is rare. The features of hypopituitarism have been described above.

Investigations

As described above, endocrinological assessment is performed.

CT and MRI scans assess the anatomy of the tumour and visual field assessment is important as many of these tumours have effects on the visual pathways, particularly at the optic chiasm.

Management

Management may be medical, surgical or with radiotherapy. The surgical approach may be trans-sphenoidal or trans-frontal. Drug therapy includes dopamine receptor agonists (e.g. bromocriptine which inhibits PRL release and induces shrinkage of PRL-secreting adenomas). Somatostatin analogues inhibit GH release and induce a lesser degree of tumour shrinkage in most GH-secreting adenomas.

Acromegaly

Acromegaly is an insidious disease resulting from excessive circulating levels of GH in adults. The incidence is approximately 5 per million per year, and the prevalence is 50 per million.

Acromegalic gigantism results from acromegaly in young individuals before epiphyseal fusion, and is very uncommon.

Aetiology

The commonest cause is a benign pituitary tumour secreting GH. Pituitary carcinoma is an uncommon cause. Carcinoid tumours which secrete hypothalamic GH-releasing hormone are another uncommon cause.

Clinical features

The clinical features of acromegaly are summarised in Fig. 32.9.

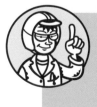

The diagnosis of acromegaly may become more obvious by comparing old photographs of the patient with their present appearance

Cardiovascular problems are often the cause of mortality. Coronary artery disease, hypertension, and diabetes are more common than in the normal population. Cardiomyopathy may occur.

Headaches, visual field defects, and cranial nerve palsies may occur due to the effects of the pituitary tumour. Hyperprolactinaemia (due to compression of the pituitary stalk and therefore loss of tonic inhibitory dopamine from hypothalamus—see below) is common and hypopituitarism can also occur.

Diagnosis

GH levels are elevated although they may rise with stress. Therefore, GH is measured during a glucose tolerance test. In healthy individuals, GH is undetectable during the test. In some centres, insulin-like growth factor-1 levels are used to provide an estimate of growth hormone levels over the previous 24 hours.

Other investigations include the following:
- Assessment of visual fields: bitemporal hemianopia.
- Skull X-ray, and CT or MRI of the brain.
- Hand X-ray: tufting of the terminal phalanges and increased joint spaces due to hypertrophy of the cartilage. The heel pad is usually thickened.
- Glucose tolerance test.
- CXR and electrocardiogram (ECG): left ventricular hypertrophy secondary to hypertension.

Management

The aim of treatment is to relieve symptoms, reverse somatic changes, and reverse metabolic abnormalities. Treatment is by surgery, radiotherapy, or drugs.

Surgery

The trans-sphenoidal route is usually used. Up to 90% of microadenomas are cured. The success rate is lower for larger tumours. Complications include hypopituitarism, meningitis, intra-operative bleeding, and death.

Radiotherapy

This is often used if attempts at surgery do not reduce GH levels sufficiently. Hypopituitarism may occur, and regular tests of pituitary function should be performed.

Medical therapies

The most effective treatment is with octreotide, a somatostatin analogue. Somatostatin inhibits GH secretion. Side effects include colicky abdominal pain and diarrhoea but this usually settles with continued treatment. Gallstones occur in

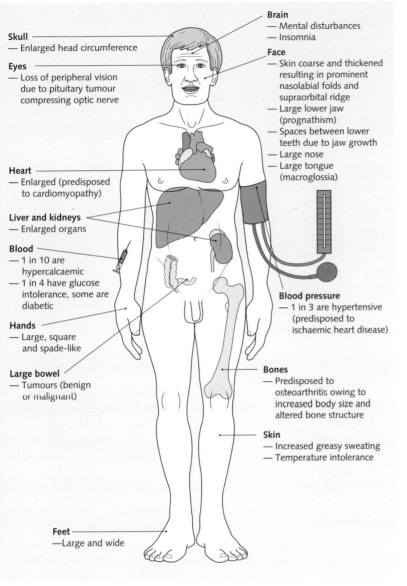

Fig. 32.9 Signs and symptoms of acromegaly (caused by excessive growth hormone secretion in adults).

Skull
— Enlarged head circumference

Eyes
— Loss of peripheral vision due to pituitary tumour compressing optic nerve

Heart
— Enlarged (predisposed to cardiomyopathy)

Liver and kidneys
— Enlarged organs

Blood
— 1 in 10 are hypercalcaemic
— 1 in 4 have glucose intolerance, some are diabetic

Hands
— Large, square and spade-like

Large bowel
— Tumours (benign or malignant)

Feet
— Large and wide

Brain
— Mental disturbances
— Insomnia

Face
— Skin coarse and thickened resulting in prominent nasolabial folds and supraorbital ridge
— Large lower jaw (prognathism)
— Spaces between lower teeth due to jaw growth
— Large nose
— Large tongue (macroglossia)

Blood pressure
— 1 in 3 are hypertensive (predisposed to ischaemic heart disease)

Bones
— Predisposed to osteoarthritis owing to increased body size and altered bone structure

Skin
— Increased greasy sweating
— Temperature intolerance

approximately a third of patients. Bromocriptine also reduces GH and PRL levels.

Prognosis
Untreated, mortality is more than twice that in healthy individuals. Death is secondary to cardiovascular and cerebrovascular disease.

Prolactin disorders
PRL is the hormone most commonly secreted by pituitary tumours. Secretion of PRL is constantly negatively controlled by the action of dopamine produced in the hypothalamus and transported down the pituitary stalk, such that interruption produces

hyperprolactinaemia. The causes of hyperprolactinaemia are summarised in Fig. 32.10. It is commoner in women.

Clinical features
In women, the commonest symptoms are oligomenorrhoea, galactorrhoea, infertility, and occasionally hirsutism. In men, symptoms include reduced libido, impotence, infertility, and galactorrhoea. Symptoms caused by large tumour size are more common in men and include headache, visual field defects, and cranial nerve palsies. Varying degrees of hypopituitarism may be present.

Causes of hyperprolactinaemia	
Cause	**Examples**
Physiological	Pregnancy, lactation, stress
Drugs	Antiemetics, e.g. metoclopramide, prochlorperazine Phenothiazines Tricyclic antidepressants
Primary hypothyroidism	—
Pituitary tumours	Prolactinoma Growth-hormone secreting tumours Non-functioning tumours
Polycystic ovary syndrome	—
Uncommon	Sarcoidosis
Hypothalamic lesions	Langerhans' cell histiocytosis Hypothalamic tumours
Chest wall stimulation	Repeated self-examination of breasts Post herpes zoster
Liver or renal failure	—

Fig. 32.10 Causes of hyperprolactinaemia.

Investigations
Elevated prolactin levels should be confirmed on repeat testing. Other blood tests include thyroid function tests (TFTs) and a pregnancy test in women. A careful drug history should always be taken.

Radiological assessment of the pituitary tumour should be carried out with skull X-rays, and MRI or CT scans of the brain. Full assessment of pituitary function should be undertaken if a macroadenoma is suspected, and visual fields should be assessed.

Management
Microprolactinomas are <10 mm on MRI. Trans-sphenoidal surgery is usually successful but there is a small recurrence rate. The alternative is dopamine agonist drug therapy such as bromocriptine which should be stopped in pregnancy. Prolactin levels are monitored and scans are repeated if there is evidence of tumour growth e.g. headache, visual field defects.

Macroprolactinomas are >10 mm on MRI. They can be treated with drugs but if there are pressure effects, visual symptoms or pregnancy is considered (25% expand in pregnancy), surgery is usually performed.

Diabetes insipidus
This rare disease is due to deficiency of vasopressin – cranial diabetes insipidus. The differential diagnosis includes nephrogenic diabetes insipidus (i.e. a lack of renal response to adequate circulating vasopressin), and primary polydipsia or excessive drinking. Clinically, the patient presents with polyuria, nocturia, and polydipsia. Investigation is outlined in Chapter 13.

Causes of diabetes insipidus
Cranial diabetes insipidus
Familial cranial diabetes insipidus is inherited as autosomal dominant or as part of the DIDMOAD syndrome (diabetes insipidus, diabetes mellitus, optic atrophy, and deafness).

Causes of acquired cranial diabetes insipidus are given in Fig. 32.11.

Causes of acquired cranial diabetes insipidus	
Cause	**Examples**
Trauma	Head injury and neurosurgery
Tumours	Craniopharyngioma or secondary tumours
Granulomas	Tuberculosis, sarcoid, histiocytosis
Infections	Encephalitis or meningitis

Fig. 32.11 Causes of acquired cranial diabetes insipidus.

Causes of acquired nephrogenic diabetes insipidus

- Metabolic: hypokalaemia, hypercalcaemia
- Chronic renal failure
- Lithium toxicity
- Postobstructive uropathy
- Diabetes mellitus

Fig. 32.12 Causes of acquired nephrogenic diabetes insipidus.

Nephrogenic diabetes insipidus
Familial nephrogenic diabetes insipidus is X-linked recessive and autosomal recessive.

Causes of acquired nephrogenic diabetes insipidus are given in Fig. 32.12.

Treatment
For cranial diabetes insipidus, desmopressin is the treatment of choice because it has minimal pressor activity but prolonged antidiuretic potency compared to native vasopressin. It may be administered orally, intranasally, or parenterally.

Metabolic and electrolyte disturbances should be corrected if they are responsible for nephrogenic diabetes insipidus. In familial forms, thiazide diuretics or indomethacin can reduce urine output by up to 50%.

For patients with primary polydipsia, water restriction and treatment of any associated psychiatric disorder is required.

Thyroid disorders

For a diagram of the hypothalamus–pituitary–thyroid axis, refer to Fig. 40.17.

Hypothyroidism
Hypothyroidism results from deficiency of thyroxine (T_4) or tri-iodothyronine (T_3). The prevalence is 15 in 1000 females and 1 in 1000 males.

Aetiology
Primary thyroid failure may take the following forms:
- Idiopathic atrophic hypothyroidism: incidence increases with age and is 10 times commoner in women than men. The aetiology is probably autoimmune.
- Autoimmune (Hashimoto's thyroiditis): this is 15 times commoner in women than men, and tends to affect the middle aged and elderly. Patients may present with a firm, non-tender goitre, hypothyroidism, or both. It is associated with vitiligo, pernicious anaemia, insulin-dependent diabetes mellitus, Addison's disease, and premature ovarian failure.
- Previous treatment for hypothyroidism: operative or radioiodine.
- Congenital hypothyroidism: the prevalence in the UK is 1 in 3500–4000 infants and is diagnosed in the first week of life by routine screening, measuring TSH or T_4. It is usually due to thyroid agenesis or dyshormonogenesis, which are both due to autosomal recessively inherited enzyme defects. The commonest is Pendred's syndrome, characterised by congenital hypothyroidism, goitre, and nerve deafness in homozygotes.
- Iodine-deficient hypothyroidism: this is a major cause of hypothyroidism and goitre worldwide, although most iodine-deficient people are euthyroid even though they have a goitre.
- Iatrogenic hypothyroidism: long-term iodine therapy, for example in expectorants, may result in hypothyroidism. Other drugs include amiodarone and lithium carbonate.

Secondary thyroid failure is caused by diseases of the hypothalamus or pituitary. These are very rare.

Clinical presentation
The onset is insidious and the symptoms often non-specific and vague. Common presenting symptoms include tiredness, lethargy, weight gain, cold intolerance, hoarseness, and dryness of the skin. However, virtually any organ system can be affected (Fig. 32.13).

Investigations
The following investigations are important in patients with hypothyroidism:
- Free or total T_4 are reduced, and serum TSH is high.
- T_4 may be normal with a high serum TSH. This indicates subclinical hypothyroidism.
- If secondary hypothyroidism is suspected, the free and total T_4 are reduced and the TSH is also low. This picture is also obtained in sick people without thyroid disease, and patients on steroids and anticonvulsants.
- Antibodies to thyroglobulin or thyroid peroxidase (microsomal antibodies): typically strongly positive in Hashimoto's thyroiditis.
- Cholesterol: raised.
- FBC: anaemia and raised mean corpuscular volume.
- ECG: sinus bradycardia, low voltage complexes.

Effects of hypothyroidism by body system	
Body system	**Effects**
Cardiovascular	Bradycardia, hyperlipidaemia, angina, heart failure, pericardial and pleural effusions
Neuromuscular	Aches and pains, carpal tunnel syndrome, deafness, cerebellar ataxia, depression and psychoses, delayed relaxation of reflexes
Haematological	Macrocytic anaemia, iron deficiency anaemia (due to menorrhagia)
Dermatological	Dry skin, myxoedema (which is local infiltration of the skin with mucopolysaccharides), erythema ab igne, vitiligo, alopecia
Gastrointestinal	Constipation, ileus, ascites
Reproductive	Infertility, menorrhagia, galactorrhoea
Developmental	Growth retardation, mental retardation, delayed puberty

Fig. 32.13 Effects of hypothyroidism by body system.

Treatment

Thyroxine sodium is the treatment of choice for maintenance therapy. Usual maintenance doses are between 100–200 μg daily. The initial dose is usually 50 μg, increased as necessary over a few weeks, and even lower doses (25 μg) are started in elderly patients or patients with cardiac disease to avoid worsening angina or precipitating a myocardial infarction. Treatment is monitored by serum TSH and serum T_4 and is nearly always lifelong except in cases of subacute or silent thyroiditis.

Myxoedema coma

This is uncommon. It is typically seen in the elderly and precipitated by infection, treatment with sedatives, or inadequate heating in cold weather. Most patients have hypothermia and are hypotensive with heart failure, hyponatraemia, hypoxia, and hypercapnia.

Treatment is with T_3 intravenously because of its rapid action. Intravenous hydrocortisone is also given, particularly if pituitary hypothyroidism is suspected. Supportive measures are also needed including intravenous fluids, antibiotics, ventilation, and slow rewarming. T_4 can be substituted after 2–3 days if there is a clinical improvement.

Thyrotoxicosis

Thyrotoxicosis results from an excess of circulating free T_4 and free T_3. It affects approximately 10 in 1000 women and 1 in 1000 men. Hyperthyroidism indicates thyroid gland overactivity, resulting in thyrotoxicosis.

Aetiology
Primary hyperthyroidism
Graves' disease

This accounts for 70–80% of all cases of hyperthyroidism. It is caused by the production of autoantibodies that stimulate the TSH receptor. There is a painless diffuse goitre in more than 90% of patients. In addition to the general features of thyrotoxicosis, pathognomonic features include ophthalmopathy, pretibial myxoedema, and thyroid acropathy.

The ophthalmopathy includes grittiness and increased tear production, periorbital oedema, conjunctival oedema (chemosis), proptosis, diplopia, impaired visual acuity, and corneal ulceration. It is clinically obvious in 60% of patients with Graves' disease but subclinical ophthalmopathy can be detected in more than 90% by CT scan or MRI, revealing fusiform enlargement of the extraocular muscles caused by lymphocytic infiltration, oedema, and later fibrosis.

Pretibial myxoedema occurs in 1–5% of patients with Graves' disease and comprises of painless thickening of the skin in nodules or plaques, generally over the shin.

Thyroid acropathy occurs in less than 1% of patients and resembles finger clubbing.
Other causes of primary hyperthyroidism

Toxic multinodular goitre and toxic adenoma account for most of the remaining causes. Less common causes include metastatic thyroid cancer, genetic causes such as the McCune–Albright syndrome and TSH receptor mutations, and ectopic thyroid tissue (e.g. struma ovarii).

Secondary hyperthyroidism

This is very uncommon. Causes include pituitary adenoma-secreting TSH, and trophoblastic tumours secreting human chorionic gonadotrophin.

Thyrotoxicosis without hyperthyroidism

This may occur with destructive thyroiditis such as in postpartum thyroiditis, subacute (de Quervain's) thyroiditis, and amiodarone-induced thyroiditis, and with excessive thyroxine administration, or self-administered thyroxine, particularly in doctors and nurses.

Clinical presentation

The symptoms and signs of thyrotoxicosis are shown in Fig. 32.14. General symptoms include:

- Weight loss.
- Increased appetite.
- Heat intolerance and sweating.
- Fatigue and weakness.
- Hyperactivity, irritability.
- Tremor.

Less common symptoms include:
- Depression.
- Oligomenorrhoea.
- Pruritus.
- Diarrhoea and vomiting.
- Polyuria.

Signs include:
- A goitre possibly with a murmur over it.
- Tremor.

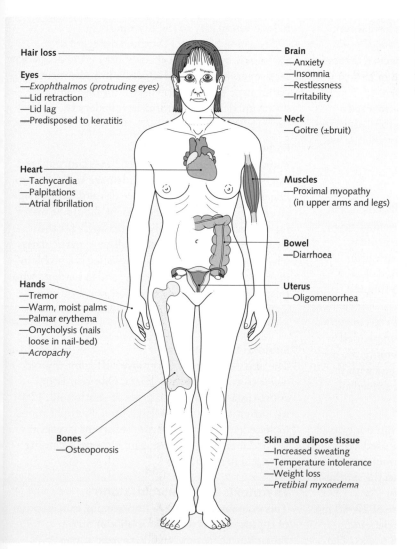

Fig. 32.14 Symptoms and signs of thyrotoxicosis (caused by hyperthyroidism). The features shown in italics are exclusive to thyrotoxicosis caused by Graves' disease.

Hair loss

Eyes
—*Exophthalmos (protruding eyes)*
—Lid retraction
—Lid lag
—Predisposed to keratitis

Heart
—Tachycardia
—Palpitations
—Atrial fibrillation

Hands
—Tremor
—Warm, moist palms
—Palmar erythema
—Onycholysis (nails loose in nail-bed)
—*Acropachy*

Bones
—Osteoporosis

Brain
—Anxiety
—Insomnia
—Restlessness
—Irritability

Neck
—Goitre (±bruit)

Muscles
—Proximal myopathy (in upper arms and legs)

Bowel
—Diarrhoea

Uterus
—Oligomenorrhea

Skin and adipose tissue
—Increased sweating
—Temperature intolerance
—Weight loss
—*Pretibial myxoedema*

- Tachycardia and atrial fibrillation.
- Warm moist skin.
- Lid retraction and lid lag.
- Muscle weakness.
- Proximal myopathy.
- Cardiac failure.

Investigations

In thyrotoxicosis, TSH is suppressed. It can also be suppressed in euthyroid patients with Graves' ophthalmopathy, large goitres, recent treatment for thyrotoxicosis, or severe non-thyroid illness.

T_4 is raised although excess oestrogens, protein-losing states, drugs, and hereditary abnormalities can alter the binding of T_4 to thyroxine-binding globulin, making total T_4 levels inaccurate in these situations. Free T_4 assays are therefore preferable.

If the TSH is suppressed and free T_4 is normal, T_3 should be measured to diagnose T_3 toxicosis.

In Graves' disease, 80% of people have serum autoantibodies against thyroglobulin and thyroid peroxidase/microsomal antigen. However, these also occur in autoimmune thyroiditis, and in 15% of healthy women and 5% of healthy men.

If a toxic nodule or thyroiditis is suspected a radioisotope thyroid scan may be performed. In the case of thyroiditis no uptake is seen by the thyroid; a toxic nodule appears as a 'hot spot'.

Treatment

Treatment options include drugs, radioiodine, and surgery. Most patients under 50 years old receive a course of antithyroid drug as initial treatment. Patients with large goitres usually relapse after antithyroid drugs. Relapse after a period of drug therapy should be treated with ^{131}I or subtotal thyroidectomy; ^{131}I is generally given to older patients in whom recurrent thyrotoxicosis may be dangerous. Subtotal thyroidectomy is often recommended in young patients with large goitres to remove the neck swelling. All options should be discussed with the patient and a joint decision should be arrived at.

Antithyroid drugs

In the UK, carbimazole is the most commonly used drug. Propylthiouracil (PTU) may be used in patients who suffer sensitivity reactions to carbimazole. Both drugs act primarily by interfering with the synthesis of thyroid hormones.

Carbimazole is given in a daily dose of 20–60 mg and maintained at this dose until the patient becomes euthyroid, usually after 4–8 weeks. The dose may then be progressively changed to a maintenance dose of 5–15 mg daily, adjusted according to response. Rashes are common and PTU may then be substituted. Pruritus and rashes can also be treated with antihistamines without discontinuing therapy, although patients should be advised to report any sore throat immediately because of the rare complication of agranulocytosis.

PTU is given in a dose of 300–600 mg daily and maintained at this dose until the patient becomes euthyroid. The dose is then lowered to a maintenance dose of 50–150 mg daily.

A combination of carbimazole 20–60 mg daily with thyroxine 50–150 µg daily may be used in a 'block and replace' regimen. Treatment is usually for 18 months—this regimen is not suitable during pregnancy.

Iodine may be given 10–14 days before surgery in addition to carbimazole to assist control and to reduce vascularity of the thyroid.

Propanolol is useful for the rapid relief of thyrotoxic symptoms because antithyroid drugs may take several weeks to produce an improvement in symptoms. They are also useful for the control of supraventricular arrhythmias secondary to thyrotoxicosis.

Radioiodine

Radioactive sodium iodide ($Na^{131}I$) is concentrated by the thyroid and causes cell damage and cell death. Hypothyroidism may therefore develop at any stage after treatment, and so the patient should be under regular follow up. It is used increasingly for the treatment of thyrotoxicosis at all ages, particularly where medical therapy or compliance is a problem, in patients with cardiac disease, and in patients who relapse after thyroidectomy. Contraindications include pregnancy and breastfeeding. Pregnancy is safe 4 months or more after treatment.

Subtotal thyroidectomy

The aim of surgery is to remove sufficient thyroid tissue to cure hyperthyroidism. One year later, approximately 80% of patients are euthyroid, 15% hypothyroid, and 5% have relapsed. Complications include hypoparathyroidism, recurrent laryngeal nerve damage, and bleeding into the neck causing laryngeal oedema.

Thyrotoxic crisis (thyroid 'storm')

This is an uncommon, life-threatening exacerbation of thyrotoxicosis with a mortality of 50%. Precipitating factors include thyroid surgery, radioiodine, withdrawal of antithyroid drugs, iodinated contrast agents, and acute illnesses (e.g. stroke, infection, trauma, and diabetic ketoacidosis). It requires emergency treatment with oxygen, intravenous fluids due to profuse sweating, propanolol (5 mg i.v.) for control of tachycardia, hydrocortisone (100 mg 6-hourly i.v.), which inhibits T_4 conversion to T_3 in the tissues, as well as oral iodine solution, which may need to be administered by nasogastric tube.

Subacute (de Quervain's) thyroiditis

Various viruses (e.g. enterovirus or coxsackievirus) can cause subacute thyroiditis. Patients present with a small, tender goitre and initially thyrotoxicosis caused by release of stored thyroid hormones. There may be a history of preceding 'influenza-like' illness. Some weeks later, there is a period of hypothyroidism followed by the recovery of normal thyroid function 3–6 months after onset.

The erythrocyte sedimentation rate is raised and there is low radioisotope uptake by the thyroid. Treatment is with NSAIDs for mild symptoms, and with high-dose prednisolone for moderate or severe thyroiditis. The dose is gradually tailed off in subsequent weeks.

Goitre and thyroid cancer

'Goitre' means an enlarged thyroid gland.

Clinical assessment

Most patients are asymptomatic. The history should include the following:

- Duration of goitre: long-standing goitres suggest benign disease.
- Goitrogenic drugs (e.g. lithium).
- Prior exposure to radiation: risk factor for benign and malignant thyroid nodules.
- Age: increased risk of cancer in those aged over 65 years.
- Sex: thyroid cancer is more common in men than women.
- Family history: if positive for goitre, this suggests autoimmune thyroiditis. A positive family history for thyroid cancer suggests familial thyroid cancer or MEN.
- Tenderness: subacute thyroiditis.
- Local symptoms: dysphagia, dyspnoea, and hoarseness; all are uncommon.

Physical examination should look for the following:

- The patient's thyroid status.
- Is the goitre smooth or nodular?
- Are there multiple nodules or a single nodule?

Differential diagnosis

- Smooth toxic goitre—Graves' disease.
- Smooth non-toxic goitre—congenital, physiological, thyroiditis, iodine deficiency.
- Multi-nodular goitre—usually euthyroid although a nodule may become autonomous and cause thyrotoxicosis.
- Single thyroid lump—approximately 10% are malignant. Causes include cyst, adenoma, malignancy, a single palpable nodule within a goitre.

Investigations

The following investigations are important in patients with goitre and thyroid cancer:

- TFTs: hyper- or hypothyroidism.
- Calcitonin secretion: increased in medullary thyroid cancer, and should be measured in patients with a positive family history.
- Thyroid size: assessed using plain X-rays, which may show tracheal deviation, or CT scan.
- Respiratory function tests: upper airways obstruction.
- Radionuclide imaging: can distinguish 'hot nodules' (high uptake of radioisotope) from 'cold nodules' (due to lack of concentration of radioisotope). Unfortunately, there are no specific features that indicate the benign or malignant nature of a thyroid nodule. Malignant nodules are more likely to be cold than hot, although most cold nodules are benign. Even so, the presence of a hot nodule does not exclude malignancy.
- Ultrasound scan: differentiation of solid from cystic lesions of the thyroid; it cannot distinguish benign from malignant nodules, although a solid nodule is more likely to contain malignant cells.
- Fine-needle aspiration cytology: can be performed in outpatients and is well tolerated; cytology is not completely reliable as false positive and false negative results occur.

Thyroid malignancy
Papillary thyroid carcinoma

This accounts for 70–80% of thyroid malignancies and is more common in women; the peak age of onset is 20–30 years. It may be locally invasive or multifocal, treatment is by surgical excision, and the 10-year survival rate is 95%.

The most common thyroid carcinoma is P-apillary (P-opular). It also has P-sammoma bodies on histology. It causes P-alpable lymph nodes (lymphatic spread)

Follicular thyroid carcinoma

This occurs in older people. Distant metastases develop in 20% of patients. Treatment is by thyroidectomy and radioiodine ablation of the thyroid remnant. The 10-year survival rate is 20%.

Anaplastic carcinoma

Anaplastic carcinoma is uncommon. The peak incidence is at 60–70 years. The mean survival is only 6 months from diagnosis.

Medullary thyroid carcinoma

This is rare. It secretes calcitonin and other hormones. It may be associated with phaeochromocytoma. The prognosis is poor. Family members should be screened.

Lymphoma

Lymphoma may be primary or as part of a systemic disease. There is an increased risk in patients with autoimmune thyroiditis. Radiotherapy is the treatment of choice.

Disorders of the adrenal glands

Histologically, the adrenal glands are divided into the medulla, which secretes adrenaline and noradrenaline, and the cortex, which is divided into three zones:

- The inner zone or zona reticularis produces sex hormones.
- The middle zone or zona fasciculata produces cortisol. Production is stimulated by ACTH produced by the pituitary gland. In turn, cortisol influences, by negative feedback, both corticotropin-releasing hormone production in the hypothalamus and pituitary release of ACTH.
- The outer zona glomerulosa produces aldosterone which is regulated through the renin–angiotensin system.

Cushing's syndrome

Cushing's syndrome is the result of chronic exposure to excess glucocorticoid. This is most commonly iatrogenic secondary to glucocorticoid administration given to treat inflammatory diseases. Other causes include the following:

- As a result of ACTH hypersecretion by a pituitary corticotrophic adenoma (60–70%). This is cushing's disease.
- Primary adrenocortical tumours (30%).
- Ectopic ACTH syndrome caused by a variety of ACTH-secreting non-pituitary tumours (5–10%) (e.g. small cell lung carcinoma).

The annual incidence of spontaneous Cushing's syndrome is approximately 1 in 100 000 and is three to five times more common in women than men.

Clinical features

The clinical features of Cushing's syndrome are demonstrated in Fig. 32.15.

Investigations

Investigations for Cushing's syndrome are discussed in Chapter 40. They include 24-hour urinary free cortisol measurement, dexamethasone suppression tests, assessment of corticotrophic function, and imaging techniques. 24-hour urinary free cortisol measurement or an overnight dexamethasone suppression test are the best screening tools, but may give false positives in obesity, depression, alcoholism and if the patient is on a hepatic enzyme-inducing drug (as this increases the metabolism of dexamethasone).

Management
Cushing's disease

Trans-sphenoidal surgery is the first line of treatment and is curative in approximately 80% of patients. Drugs are used if surgery fails. Metyrapone inhibits steroidogenesis and is the drug of choice. Ketoconazole may be used.

Rarely, bilateral adrenalectomy is necessary although this has a risk of leading to Nelson's syndrome resulting in hyperpigmentation from excess β-lipotrophin activity (melanocyte-stimulating hormone and ACTH) which is not suppressed by a high blood cortisol.

Adrenocortical tumours

Surgical removal of an adrenocortical tumour is curative. Bilateral adrenalectomy necessitates replacement therapy with cortisol 20–40 mg daily and fludrocortisone 0.1 mg daily.

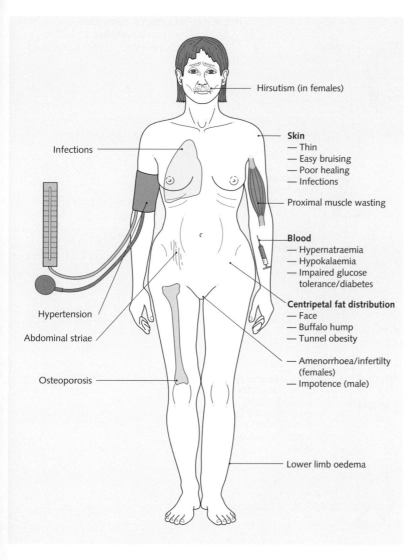

Fig. 32.15 Symptoms and signs of Cushing's syndrome.

Hirsutism (in females)

Infections

Skin
— Thin
— Easy bruising
— Poor healing
— Infections

Proximal muscle wasting

Blood
— Hypernatraemia
— Hypokalaemia
— Impaired glucose tolerance/diabetes

Hypertension

Abdominal striae

Osteoporosis

Centripetal fat distribution
— Face
— Buffalo hump
— Tunnel obesity

— Amenorrhoea/infertilty (females)
— Impotence (male)

Lower limb oedema

Ectopic ACTH syndrome

Surgical resection of the tumour cures the hypercortisolism, although this is often not possible and medical therapy has to be used.

Addison's disease

Addison's disease is primary adrenocortical failure. The prevalence is approximately 100 per million per year, and the incidence is approximately 5 per 1 million per year.

Causes

Causes of Addison's disease include the following:
- Autoimmune adrenal destruction: this accounts for up to 90% of cases. Women are affected 2–3 times more often than men. Patients may have other autoimmune endocrine deficiencies.

- Infections: especially tuberculosis; cytomegalovirus and fungal infections associated with AIDS are now becoming common.
- Adrenal haemorrhage/infarction: this may be associated with sepsis, particularly meningococcal septicaemia – the Waterhouse–Friderichsen syndrome. The presentation is usually acute.
- Metastatic carcinoma: especially from the breast.
- Inherited disorders: there are several familial disorders of adrenal function which are all rare.

Clinical features

Symptoms and signs of Addison's disease are predominantly caused by cortisol deficiency, although deficiencies of aldosterone and adrenal androgen will also be present to varying extents (Fig. 32.16). The main symptoms are insidious and

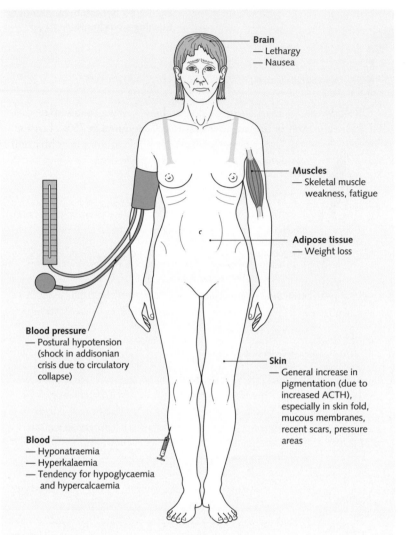

Fig. 32.16 Symptoms and signs of adrenal insufficiency. (ACTH, adrenocorticotrophic hormone.)

non-specific: fatigue, weight loss, orthostatic dizziness, and anorexia. Patients may present with GI symptoms (e.g. abdominal pain, nausea, vomiting, and diarrhoea). Hyperpigmentation of the skin and mucous membranes may occur as a result of high ACTH concentrations.

Investigations

The following are important investigations in patients with Addison's disease:

- Serum cortisol concentration: low.
- Adrenal autoantibodies are detected in approximately 50% of patients.
- Serum ACTH levels: raised in Addison's disease and low in secondary failure.

- Serum electrolytes: usually normal but in an impending crisis there may be hyponatraemia, hyperkalaemia, and raised blood urea.
- Short and long Synacthen tests: described in Chapter 40.
- TFTs: may show low thyroxine and raised TSH.
- Screening for other autoimmune diseases.

Management

In emergencies, intravenous saline and glucose are required. Intravenous hydrocortisone 100 mg 6-hourly is given. Underlying infection must be treated.

Maintenance therapy is with hydrocortisone, usually 20 mg in the mornings and 10 mg in the evenings. The dose of hydrocortisone should be increased during intercurrent illnesses and during surgery. Enzyme inducing drugs (e.g. phenytoin and rifampicin) may also increase patient requirements for hydrocortisone. Fludrocortisone is used to replace aldosterone because aldosterone taken orally undergoes first pass metabolism through the liver. The dose is adjusted to maintain blood pressure and potassium levels. The usual dose is about 0.1 mg daily.

Phaeochromocytoma

This is a rare tumour arising from the chromaffin tissues of the sympathetic nervous system, producing catecholamines. It may be associated with medullary carcinoma of the thyroid, parathyroid adenoma, and neurofibromatosis.

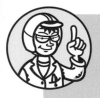

In phaeochromocytoma 90% are benign, 90% are in the adrenal medulla, and 90% of these are unilateral

Clinical features

Symptoms and signs are due to the release of adrenaline and noradrenaline, and include episodic hypertension, cardiomyopathy, weight loss, and hyperglycaemia. During a period of crisis, there may be pallor, palpitations, panic, sweating, nausea, tremor, pain (headache or chest pain), and rarely paroxysmal thyroid swelling. The blood pressure may rise to very high levels and may precipitate a cerebrovascular accident or myocardial infarction.

Investigations

Urine is collected for 24 hours for measurement of adrenaline and noradrenaline, or of their metabolites vanillylmandelic acid or hydroxymethylmandelic acid. An abdominal CT scan may show the tumour.

Treatment

This is by surgical removal of the tumour. The patient must be fully α-blocked with phenoxybenzamine or phentolamine, and β-blocked with propanolol before surgery to prevent the consequences of release of catecholamines during operation. Changes in pulse and blood pressure should be monitored closely.

α-Blockade must be achieved before β-blockade to prevent unopposed α-agonism causing severe hypertension.

Conn's syndrome (primary hyperaldosteronism)

This is a very rare condition, which is due to a unilateral adrenocortical adenoma in 75% of cases. Other causes include adrenal carcinoma or bilateral hyperplasia of the zona glomerulosa.

Clinical features

The clinical features are due to excess production of aldosterone. Hypokalaemia and muscle weakness occur during attacks, and polyuria and polydipsia are secondary to hypokalaemia. The diagnosis should be suspected in a patient with hypertension and hypokalaemia when not on a diuretic. Sodium tends to be mildly raised but there is usually no oedema.

Investigation

Serum potassium is low and should be measured whilst the patient is not on drugs. Urinary potassium is increased for serum blood level. There is usually a metabolic alkalosis. Serum sodium is raised.

Serum renin is low and 24-hour urinary aldosterone and serum aldosterone are raised.

Secondary hyperaldosteronism is a result of high circulating renin. Causes include nephrotic syndrome, heart failure, hepatic failure, and bronchial carcinoma.

Management

Tumours should be resected. Spironolactone is an aldosterone antagonist, which can be given in primary or secondary aldosteronism.

Miscellaneous endocrine conditions

Multiple endocrine neoplasia

There are two main syndromes, both autosomal dominant and both rare. Tumours originate from two or more endocrine glands which produce peptide hormones.

MEN type I refers to benign adenomas of parathyroid, pancreatic islets, pituitary, adrenal cortex, and the thyroid.

MEN type IIa refers to the association of phaeochromocytoma, medullary carcinoma of the thyroid, and parathyroid adenoma or hyperplasia.

MEN type IIb is the same as IIa but with a Marfanoid phenotype and intestinal and visceral ganglioneuromas.

Family members should be screened. In type I, fasting serum calcium should be measured. In type II, pentagastrin and calcium infusion tests with measurement of serum calcitonin will pick up C-cell hyperplasia. Urinary metanephrines should be measured for phaeochromocytoma.

Multiple endocrine neoplasia is a common MCQ question. MEN I is three Ps (pituitary, parathyroid, and pancreas), MEN II is two Cs [Catecholamines (i.e. phaeochromocytoma) and medullary Carcinoma of the thyroid] and parathyroid (for MEN IIa) or mucocutaneous neuromas (for MEN IIb)

- What are the initial modes of presentation for a patient with diabetes mellitus?
- How would you manage a patient with diabetic ketoacidosis?
- What are the long term complications of diabetes mellitus? How can the risk of complications be reduced?
- How would you assess whether a patient with no previous cardiovascular events should take statin therapy for an elevated serum cholesterol?
- How is osteoporosis defined?
- What are the causes of osteomalacia?
- How would you initially manage a patient with symptomatic hypercalcaemia?
- How is the diagnosis of acute gout confirmed and what is the treatment?
- If you suspected hypopituitarism what investigations would you consider?
- What are the complications of acromegaly?
- What are the physical signs of thyrotoxicosis? Which of these are specific to Grave's disease?
- What are causes of Cushing's syndrome? What investigations would help you distinguish between them?
- What are the symptoms and signs of Addison's disease?

Further reading

UKPDS Study Group. Tight blood pressure control and risk of macrovascular and microvascular complications in type 2 diabetes. *BMJ* 1998; **317:** 703–713

UKPDS Study Group. Effect of intensive blood-glucose control with metformin on complications in overweight patients with type 2 diabetes. *Lancet* 1998; **352:** 854–865

UKPDS Study Group. Intensive blood glucose control with sulphonylureas or insulin compared with conventional treatment and risk of complications in patients with type 2 diabetes. *Lancet* 1998; **352:** 837–853

The Diabetes Control and Complications Trial Research Group. The effect of intensive treatment of diabetes on the development and progression of long-term complications in insulin-dependent diabetes mellitus. *New Engl J Med* 1993; **329:** 997–986

Heart Protection Study Collaborative Group. MRC/BHF Heart Protection Study of cholesterol lowering with simvastatin in 20536 high risk individuals: a randomised placebo controlled trial. *Lancet* 2002; **360:** 7–22

Crash Course in Metabolism and Nutrition, Mosby

Turner HE and Wass JAH. Oxford Handbook of Endocrinology and Diabetes. Oxford University Press; 2002.

Tuck SP and Francis RM. Osteoporosis. *Postgrad Med J* 2002; **78:** 526–532

Million Women Study Collaborators. Breast cancer and hormone-replacement therapy in the Million Women Study. *Lancet* 2003; **362:** 419–427

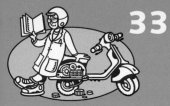

33. Musculoskeletal and Skin Disorders

Arthritis

This is common in clinical practice and examinations. Sometimes, it can affect multiple organ systems outside the joints and is responsible for considerable mortality and morbidity for patients and carers.

Rheumatoid arthritis

Rheumatoid arthritis (RA) is a systemic disease producing a symmetrical inflammatory deforming polyarthropathy with extra-articular involvement of many organs. It affects 2–3% of the population and is three times more common in women than men. The peak age of onset is between 30 and 40 years, although it can start at almost any age. There is often a family history and there is an association with HLA-DR4. The aetiology is unknown but it is thought to be autoimmune.

Clinical features

RA usually presents with an insidious onset of swollen, painful, and stiff hands and feet, progressing to involve the larger joints. Less common presentations include a relapsing and remitting monoarthritis of different large joints, a persistent monoarthritis, systemic features before joint problems are apparent, and an acute onset of widespread arthritis especially in the elderly.

General features of the disease include general malaise and fatigue; signs affecting the joints are described in Chapter 17. The metacarpophalangeal joints, proximal interphalangeal (PIP) joints, and wrists are most commonly affected (Fig. 33.1). Initially, there is joint swelling, which may progress to subluxation of joints and deformities. There is wasting of small muscles resulting from disuse atrophy, vasculitis and peripheral neuropathy. There may be tenosynovitis and bursitis; rheumatoid nodules are present in approximately 20% of patients. The feet are similarly affected.

Atlantoaxial subluxation may give rise to neurological signs, spinal cord compression and death. Other organs affected are summarised in Fig. 33.2.

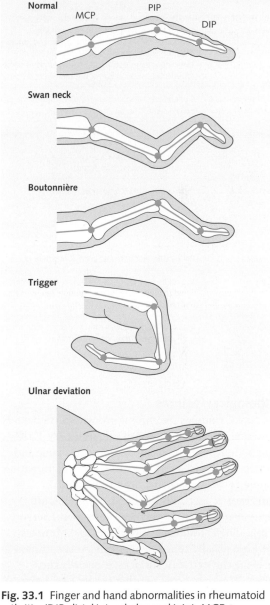

Fig. 33.1 Finger and hand abnormalities in rheumatoid arthritis. (DIP, distal interphalangeal joint; MCP, metacarpophalangeal joint; PIP, proximal interphalangeal joint.)

Organ systems affected by rheumatoid arthritis	
Organ system	**Effects**
Eyes	Sjögren's syndrome occurs in 15% of patients Scleritis causes a painful red eye, and may lead to uveitis and glaucoma Scleromalacia perforans is an uncommon complication where a rheumatoid nodule in the sclera perforates
Nervous system	Carpal tunnel syndrome (most common) Peripheral neuropathy causing glove and stocking sensory loss and occasionally motor weakness Mononeuritis multiplex due to vasculitis of vessels supplying nerves Atlantoaxial subluxation resulting in spinal cord compression
Lymphoreticular system	Generalised lymphadenopathy and splenomegaly may be present Felty's syndrome
Blood	Normochromic normocytic anaemia or iron-deficiency anaemia (see Chapter 26) ESR and CRP are raised Thrombocytosis may be found
Respiratory system	Pleural effusions (commoner in men) Rheumatoid nodules Diffuse fibrosing alveolitis Caplan's syndrome (the presence of large rheumatoid nodules and fibrosis in patients with RA exposed to various industrial dusts)
Cardiac	Pericarditis and pericardial effusions may occur
Skin	Vasculitis may produce nail-fold infarcts, ulcers, and digital gangrene Peripheral oedema may be present and is due to increased vascular permeability
Kidneys	Secondary amyloidosis may affect the kidneys leading to proteinuria, nephrotic syndrome, and renal failure

Fig. 33.2 Organ systems affected by rheumatoid arthritis. (CRP, C-reactive protein; ESR, erythrocyte sedimentation rate; RA, rheumatoid arthritis.)

Pathological features

The classic findings are chronic synovitis with pannus formation; this is composed of inflammatory T cells and polymorphs. Pannus erodes cartilage, bone and tendons. In all phases of RA, soft tissue inflammation surrounds the joint, giving rise to one of its characteristic features. Rheumatoid nodules are granulomata with a central zone of fibrinoid necrosis, surrounding palisading macrophages and fibroblasts. These are usually subcutaneous, the most common site being the extensor surfaces, especially the elbows. They can occur in other tissues (e.g. lungs, heart, and sclera). They imply being rheumatoid factor positive.

Investigations

These are discussed in Chapter 17. They should include:
- Full blood count (FBC).
- Erythrocyte sedimentation rate (ESR).
- Rheumatoid factor and other autoantibodies.

- Joint X-rays.
- Aspiration of synovial fluid, if appropriate.

Management

The aims of treatment are to control symptoms, to maintain a normal life and to modify the underlying disease process and inflammation. Physiotherapy will help to keep joints mobile, strengthen muscles, and prevent deformities. Surgery may be required to correct deformities (e.g. the repair of tendons, joint prostheses and arthrodesis). Resting the joints will relieve pain, and splints can help prevent deformities.

Drug treatment

Whilst the initial measures should include analgesia with paracetamol or preferably a non-steroidal anti-inflammatory drug (NSAID) the early use of disease-modifying antirheumatic drugs (DMARDs) is considered best practice. The aim is to slow disease progression, joint destruction and maintain function.

Drugs which modify inflammatory cytokines have recently become available. Corticosteroids remain useful and effective but have numerous long-term side effects.

Non-steroidal anti-inflammatory drugs

These drugs have both analgesic and anti-inflammatory effects; they do not alter disease progression. There are two categories. The first inhibit both forms of the enzyme cyclooxygenase (COX); examples include ibuprofen and diclofenac. This reduces the production of prostaglandins. They can have side effects, commonly gastrointestinal, including peptic ulceration and gastritis, renal impairment and fluid retention. They should be used with caution in the elderly, during pregnancy and breastfeeding, and in coagulation defects.

To reduce side effects they should be taken with food and are often combined with a proton pump inhibitor.

The second category is the selective COX-2 inhibitors (i.e. celecoxib and rofecoxib). They are effective anti-inflammatory agents with a better side effect profile, notably in reducing gastrointestinal complications. COX-2 is the inducible isoform responsible for inflammation whereas COX-1 is thought to produce the beneficial effects of prostaglandins.

Disease modifying anti-rheumatic drugs

DMARDs should now be considered early after the diagnosis of RA is made; the aim is to slow the disease process, maintaining structure and function. The most common drugs are methotrexate and sulphasalazine.

Methotrexate is a folate antagonist used in cancer chemotherapy. When taken once weekly, it has a powerful disease modifying effect on RA, often seen within 4 weeks. Its side effects include gastrointestinal, hepatic, bone marrow and pulmonary toxicity; hence, a regular full blood count and liver function tests are needed. It is contraindicated in pregnancy.

Sulphasalazine is common in the UK. It is an effective DMARD but can be limited by side effects, including rashes, gastrointestinal intolerance, bone marrow suppression and hepatitis.

Antimalarial drugs hydroxychloroquine and chloroquine can be used as DMARDs and are better tolerated. However, they are less effective against more severe RA. Retinopathy is a rare side effect.

Gold and penicillamine are now rarely used, as they can be effective agents but have marked side effects, typically bone marrow suppression, rashes and nephrotic syndrome.

Corticosteroids

Treatment with corticosteroids should be reserved for specific indications (e.g. when other anti-inflammatory drugs are unsuccessful). Low-dose prednisolone may reduce the rate of joint destruction in moderate to severe RA of less than 2 years duration. Ideally, it should only be used for short periods of time, after which treatment should be tapered off to avoid possible long-term adverse effects. Corticosteroids may also be given intra-articularly to relieve pain, increase mobility, and reduce deformity in one or a few joints.

Tumour necrosis factor inhibition

Tumour necrosis factor (TNF) is a potent proinflammatory cytokine thought to be important in RA. Two drugs are available in clinical practice. Etanercept is a TNF receptor antagonist and infliximab an antibody against TNF. They both often produce marked improvement in patients with poorly controlled disease. The main concern is infection, especially reactivation of tuberculosis. Both are expensive and current UK practice is to use them in patients with active RA not responding to at least two DMARDs, including methotrexate.

Other cytokines are being targeted and anakinra, an interleukin-1 receptor antagonist is in clinical trials.

Prognosis

RA is not just a joint disease limiting quality of life. It is a systemic disease which in its most severe form causes multiorgan dysfunction and shortens life. The life expectancy of patients whose joint disease does not remit with therapy is on average 15 years less than similar patients without RA.

Osteoarthritis

Osteoarthritis (OA) is the commonest joint condition and affects approximately half of the population by the age of 60 years. OA is a degenerative disorder affecting mainly the weight-bearing joints (e.g. the hips and knees). It is a disease of cartilage, which becomes eroded and progressively thinned as the disease proceeds. Risk factors include age, family history, obesity, male sex under age 45 years and female sex above 55 years plus systemic features (e.g. sex and growth hormones). It may also be secondary to other joint conditions and trauma.

Clinical features

Clinical signs and symptoms are described in Chapter 17. Joints commonly affected by OA are summarised in Fig. 33.3. There is pain in affected joints, which is worse with movement and towards the end of the day, superimposed on a background of pain at rest. The joints are stiff, immobile, and deformed.

On examination, there may be swelling due to bony protuberances or joint effusions, crepitus on movement, signs of inflammation, limited joint movement, and deformities. The pattern of joint involvement tends to be asymmetrical. In the hands, the most commonly affected joints are the distal interphalangeal (DIP) joints (Heberden's nodes), PIP joints (Bouchard's nodes), and first carpometacarpal joints, giving an appearance of 'square hands' (Fig. 33.4). Unlike RA, there is no systemic illness or extra-articular manifestations of the disease.

Investigations

There are no biochemical abnormalities. Diagnosis is based on clinical findings and radiological changes of loss of joint space, subchondral sclerosis, cysts, and marginal osteophytes.

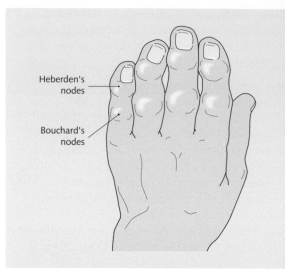

Fig. 33.4 Osteoarthritis in a hand, showing Heberden's nodes at the distal interphalangeal joints and Bouchard's nodes at the proximal interphalangeal joints.

Management

Treatment options include combinations of drugs, physical treatments (e.g. weight reduction and heat application), exercises, hydrotherapy, aids (e.g. walking sticks and special shoes), and surgery (e.g. arthrodesis, arthroplasty, joint replacement). Initially, simple analgesics (e.g. paracetamol) should be prescribed for the pain. NSAIDs are given if simple analgesia is not effective. Intra-articular corticosteroids can be used for inflammatory exacerbations. Glucosamine and chondroitin are newer medications which aim to protect cartilage and slow progression; their value is not clearly established.

Spondyloarthropathies

This term describes a group of related diseases with some common features. There is an association with HLA-B27 with familial clustering of cases. Common features include:

- Ankylosing spondylitis.
- Reiter's syndrome and reactive arthritis.
- Enteropathic arthropathies.
- Psoriatic arthritis.
- Juvenile chronic arthritis.
- Undifferentiated spondyloarthropathy.

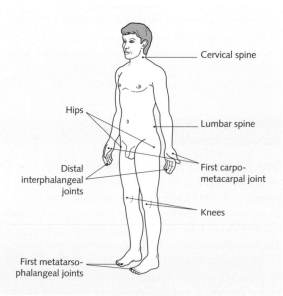

Fig. 33.3 Joints commonly affected by osteoarthritis.

Ankylosing spondylitis

This most commonly affects young men (sex ratio 2 : 1) with a prevalence of approximately 1 in 2000. HLA-B27 is present in over 90% of patients.

Clinical features

The onset is insidious with sacroiliitis causing pain in the buttocks radiating down the back of the legs. There is progressive spinal fusion with loss of movement, low back pain, and morning stiffness. Eventually the patient has a fixed kyphotic spine, hyperextended neck, spinocranial ankylosis, and a reduction in chest expansion leading to a 'question mark' posture (Fig. 33.5). Peripheral joints may be affected and tend to affect larger joints in an asymmetrical distribution. Other features include:

- General malaise.
- Uveitis: in approximately a third of cases.
- Ulcerative colitis: more common than uveitis.
- Aortic regurgitation: due to aortitis.
- Respiratory failure: secondary to kyphoscoliosis and apical fibrosis.

Investigations

The following investigations should be performed in the patient with ankylosing spondylitis:

- ESR and C-reactive protein (CRP): often raised.
- HLA-B27: provides useful supporting evidence but it is also present in the normal population.
- X-rays: sacroiliitis indicated by irregular margins and sclerosis of adjacent bone; 'bamboo' spine with squaring of the vertebrae and calcification and ossification of intervertebral ligaments.

Remember the extra articular A's complicating ankylosing spondylitis
- Apical fibrosis.
- Aortic regurgitation.
- Aortitis.
- Anterior uveitis.
- Achilles tendonitis and other enthesitides.
- Amyloidosis.

Management

Treatment includes analgesia with NSAIDs. Patients should be encouraged to exercise to prevent deformity, and to maintain movement and relieve

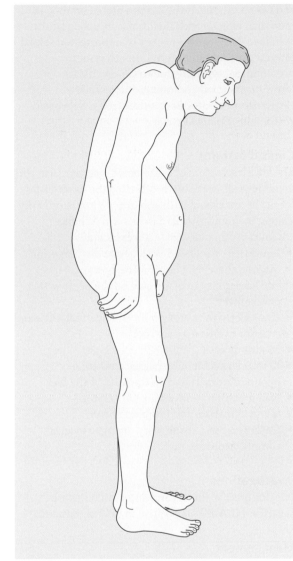

Fig. 33.5 Advancing ankylosing spondylitis. Eventually the trunk may become fixed in a fully flexed position, so that the patient cannot see directly ahead – the classic 'question mark' posture.

symptoms – sulphasalazine improves symptoms due to peripheral arthritis. TNF inhibition has been shown to be effective. Although the majority of patients will be able to maintain a normal lifestyle, the prognosis is variable. The disease may be progressive, it may remit, or there may be recurrent episodes. In extreme cases, respiratory support may be impaired due to immobility of the spine and rib cage.

Reiter's syndrome

Reiter's syndrome consists of the triad of seronegative arthritis, non-specific urethritis (NSU), and conjunctivitis. It is 20 times more common in men than women and usually affects young adults. It follows NSU with a history of unprotected sexual intercourse approximately 1 month prior to presentation, typically due to *Chlamydia* or *Urealyticum*. Less commonly, it may follow gastrointestinal infection with *Shigella*, *Salmonella*, *Yersinia*, or *Campylobacter*.

Clinical features

The arthritis is often of acute onset, polyarticular, and asymmetrical, particularly affecting the lower limbs. It may be associated with non-articular inflammatory lesions, including plantar fasciitis and Achilles tendinitis. Other clinical features include:

- Urethritis: associated with penile discharge and dysuria; there may be circinate balanitis (an erythematous circular lesion on the penis with a pale centre).
- Conjunctivitis: usually mild and bilateral; iritis and anterior uveitis may also occur.
- Mouth ulcers.
- Keratoderma blennorrhagica: a pustular hyperkeratotic lesion on the soles of the feet.
- Nail dystrophy and subungual keratosis.
- General malaise and low grade fever.
- Cardiovascular, respiratory, and neurological complications are rare.

Investigations

The diagnosis is clinical and autoantibodies are negative. HLA-B27 is positive in 60% of patients.

Management

Treatment is symptomatic with analgesia (e.g. NSAIDs) and rest of affected joints. Effusions can be aspirated. In chronic cases, sulphasalazine or azathioprine can be tried. In most cases, the acute arthritis settles within 1–2 months; approximately 50% of patients develop recurrent symptoms.

Reactive arthritis

This term describes arthritis following enteric or venereal infection as in Reiter's syndrome, but the other features of Reiter's syndrome are absent.

Psoriatic arthritis

This is a seronegative arthritis occurring in 10% of patients with psoriasis. The commonest pattern is involvement of the small joints of the hand, particularly the DIP joints, in an asymmetrical

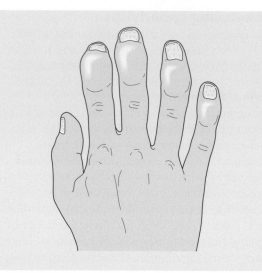

Fig. 33.6 Psoriatic arthritis involving the distal interphalangeal joints. There is 'pitting' of the nails, and there may be anycholysis.

pattern (Fig. 33.6). Other variants are described in Chapter 17. There is nail pitting and onycholysis.

Treatment is with analgesia and anti-inflammatory drugs. Immunosuppressive drugs may be effective and are used in severe cases.

Enteropathic arthropathies

This occurs in patients with inflammatory bowel disease and usually affects the knees and ankles as a monoarthritis or asymmetrical oligoarthritis. The aetiology is unknown but immune complexes in the joint may play a part. Management should be aimed at the underlying bowel disease, which will improve the arthritis. NSAIDs and joint aspiration will provide symptomatic relief.

Systemic lupus erythematosus

Systemic lupus erythematosus (SLE) is a multisystem, autoimmune connective tissue disorder. The prevalence in the UK is approximately 1 in 1000. It is nine times commoner in women, and also more common in black people. The peak age of onset is between 20 and 40 years. The aetiology is unknown but is probably multifactorial. Predisposing factors include a genetic predisposition, and environmental triggers (e.g. drugs such as hydralazine, ultraviolet light, viral infections, and immunological mechanisms).

Clinical features

The commonest early features are fever, arthralgia, malaise, tiredness, and weight loss. The following systems may be involved.

Musculoskeletal system

This is involved in over 90% of cases. There is arthralgia, the symptoms of which are clinically similar to RA although examination is often normal. There may be myalgia and myositis, and rarely there is a deforming arthropathy due to capsular laxity (Jaccoud's arthropathy). Aseptic necrosis affecting the hip or knee may rarely occur.

Skin

This is involved in approximately 80% of cases. Classically there is a 'butterfly' rash over the bridge of the nose and spreading over both cheeks (Fig. 33.7). Other features include photosensitivity, alopecia, livedo reticularis, Raynaud's phenomenon, nail-fold infarcts, purpura, urticaria, and oral ulceration.

Discoid lupus is a benign variant of SLE, with skin involvement only. There are discoid erythematous plaques on the face that progress to scarring and pigmentation. Patients with widespread skin disease may develop SLE.

Central nervous system

The central nervous system (CNS) is involved in 60% of cases. Psychiatric disturbances include depression and occasionally psychosis. Other features include:

- Seizures.
- Strokes.
- Cranial nerve lesions.
- Aseptic meningitis.
- Peripheral neuropathies.

The effects are due to arteritis and ischaemia or immune complex deposition.

Respiratory system

The respiratory system is involved in approximately 50% of cases. Pulmonary manifestations include:

- Pleurisy with pleural effusions.
- Pneumonia and atelectasis.
- Restrictive defects ('shrinking lung syndrome') with diffuse reticular-nodular shadowing on the chest X-ray.

Renal system

The renal system is involved in approximately 50% of cases. This is associated with a poor prognosis. Proteinuria and haematuria is common. There may be minimal change, and membranous or proliferative glomerulonephritis. Clinically, the patient may present with nephrotic or nephritic syndrome, hypertension or chronic renal failure.

Cardiovascular system

The cardiovascular system is involved in 40% of cases. There may be:

- Pericarditis with pericardial effusion.
- Myocarditis with consequent heart failure.
- Aortic valve lesions.
- Non-bacterial endocarditis of the mitral valve (Libman–Sachs endocarditis).

Blood and lymphatic systems

The ESR is markedly raised. There may be:

- Normochromic normocytic anaemia.
- Haemolytic anaemia.
- Leucopenia.
- Thrombocytopenia.
- Generalised lymphadenopathy.
- Hepatosplenomegaly.
- Arterial and venous thrombosis. This may be part of the antiphospholipid syndrome.

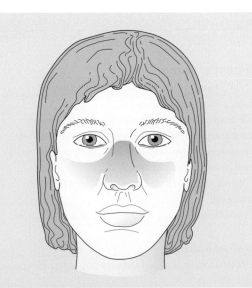

Fig. 33.7 Systemic lupus erythematosus showing the classic 'bat' or 'butterfly wing' rash.

Drug-induced lupus

Drug-induced lupus may occur with hydralazine in people who are genetically 'slow acetylators', and with procainamide, isoniazid, chlorpromazine, and anticonvulsants. It remits when the drug is stopped. Renal and CNS involvement is rare.

Investigations

The following investigations are important in patients with SLE:

- ESR: raised.
- CRP: usually normal; if raised suspect additional pathology such as infection.
- There may be anaemia, leucopenia, or thrombocytopenia.
- Antinuclear antibody: positive in almost all cases (classically homogenous staining; anti double-stranded DNA is present in about 75% of cases and is specific for SLE. The titres of anti-dsDNA rise in active disease).
- Serum complement levels: reduced in active disease; immunoglobulins raised.
- Renal biopsy: if there is involvement of the kidneys, renal biopsy shows characteristic histological changes.

Management

Patients with mild disease can be managed with aspirin or NSAIDs for joint pain. Anaemia can be corrected with transfusion, and sun block will protect from photosensitivity. For acute exacerbations, steroids are given in high doses and gradually tailed off depending on symptoms, signs, and changes in ESR.

Immunosuppressive drugs are used for patients with more serious disease (e.g. if there is renal or CNS involvement) as they have a steroid-sparing effect. Drugs used include azathioprine, chlorambucil and cyclophosphamide.

In some patients in whom NSAIDs are ineffective in controlling joint pain, or in whom skin manifestations predominate, the antimalarial drug hydroxychloroquine may be useful. It can cause retinal degeneration so vision should be formally assessed at regular intervals.

Antiphospholipid syndrome

This condition manifests as an increased risk of arterial and venous thromboses and miscarriage. It is associated with two antibodies against phospholipid. The first is the anticardiolipin antibody and the second is called the lupus anticoagulant. It causes a prolonged activated partial thromboplastin time, hence its name, but *in vivo* it is procoagulant.

Whilst first described in SLE patients this syndrome can be 'primary' (i.e. in the absence of SLE).

Treatment is specialist and often requires high levels of anticoagulation.

Polymyalgia rheumatica

Polymyalgia rheumatica (PMR) is a clinical syndrome characterised by proximal muscle pain and stiffness. The incidence increases with age and the prevalence is as much as 2% in patients aged over 60 years. It is two to three times commoner in women than men, more common in Northern Europe than Southern Europe, and is rare in non-Whites. PMR and giant cell arteritis (see p. 265) are closely linked, but either can occur in isolation.

Clinical features

Discriminating characteristics for PMR include:

- Bilateral shoulder pain with or without stiffness.
- Bilateral upper arm tenderness.
- Illness of less than 2 weeks duration.
- Morning stiffness that lasts for more than 1 hour.
- Depression with or without weight loss.
- Age greater than 65 years.
- An initial ESR of at least 40 mm/hour.

The distribution tends to be symmetrical, and systemic features such as sweating and malaise are common. True weakness does not occur, although power and range of movement may be limited by pain.

Differential diagnosis

The differential diagnosis of PMR includes:

- Late-onset RA.
- Musculoskeletal: OA, rotator cuff disease, non-specific back pain, trochanteric bursitis.
- Other neuromuscular conditions, polymyositis, and proximal myopathy.
- Occult malignancy if systemic features are marked.
- Hypothyroidism: due to myalgia and malaise.

Investigations

The following investigations are important in patients with PMR:

- ESR: usually over 40 mm per hour; very high values can occur.

- Acute phase proteins: increased (e.g. CRP).
- Alkaline phosphatase: raised in approximately 30% of patients.
- A mild normochromic normocytic anaemia is common and platelets tend to be increased.
- Temporal artery biopsy: rarely helpful.
- Tests to exclude conditions capable of mimicking PMR: rheumatoid factor, thyroid function tests, creatine kinase if muscle weakness is suspected and autoantibodies if there are features suggesting connective tissue disease.

Management

Eighty percent of symptoms improve within a few days with corticosteroids. The ESR falls to normal within 2–3 weeks and the CRP becomes normal within 1 week. An initial daily dose of 15–20 mg of prednisolone is usually adequate to control symptoms. The dose should be continued for 1 month and slowly reduced over the following month to approximately 10 mg daily.

There is no indication for prophylactic high-dose steroids to prevent blindness as with giant cell arteritis. However, patients should be warned to look out for additional symptoms such as headache or blurred vision. Steroids should be reduced slowly over the subsequent months.

Approximately 50% of patients manage to discontinue steroids within 2 years. Management should be based on the clinical response, although a rise in ESR should prompt review. Relapses are most common in the first year but the incidence falls thereafter, and are often associated with a reduction in steroid dose. Adding a NSAID to cover ache and stiffness may be of help.

In patients who are developing the side effects of steroids, a 'steroid-sparing' immunosuppressant (e.g. azathioprine) should be considered under expert supervision. Prophylaxis against osteoporosis is usually indicated. In a few patients, it is impossible to withdraw steroids altogether and so it is acceptable to maintain them indefinitely on prednisolone 2–3 mg/day.

Prognosis

The prognosis is good provided the steroid dosage is not excessive. Most patients can be reassured that treatment can usually be discontinued after 2–4 years with a low rate of recurrence thereafter.

Other connective tissue disorders

Systemic sclerosis

Systemic sclerosis is a multisystem disease that mainly occurs in middle-aged women. It presents with Raynaud's phenomenon in more than three quarters of cases. The aetiology is unknown. Familial cases occur with HLA-B8 and HLA-DR3 at increased frequency. There are abnormalities of both humoral and cellular immunity. Early in the disease, the skin is oedematous and the blood vessels show arteritis and thickening. There is an increase in collagen and progressive fibrosis of viscera.

Clinical features

There is general malaise, lassitude, fever, and weight loss. The following systems may be involved.

Skin

Systemic sclerosis is also termed scleroderma, reflecting the thickening and hardening of the skin associated with increased collagen content. Patients classically have a beaked nose, facial telangiectasia, and tight skin around the mouth causing difficulty in opening the mouth wide (Fig. 33.8). The skin becomes smooth and waxy, and atrophic with pigmentation or depigmentation. There is sclerodactyly and the fingers are 'sausage shaped'. Raynaud's phenomenon is common. There may also be subcutaneous calcification.

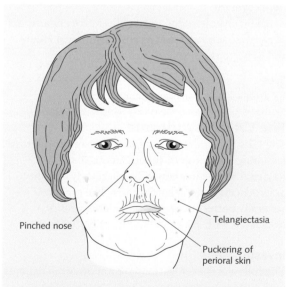

Fig. 33.8 Systemic sclerosis, showing pinched nose, multiple telangiectasia, and tightening of the skin around the mouth. The skin may also be waxy and shiny.

323

Morphoea or localised scleroderma is a relatively benign condition affecting only the skin, especially on the trunk and limbs. Plaques evolve to produce waxy, thickened skin and induration. These may enlarge or new lesions may appear over time. Resolution is associated with hyperpigmentation. Only rarely does morphoea proceed to systemic sclerosis.

Gastrointestinal system
Oesophageal involvement is very common. There is delayed peristalsis, dilatation or stricture formation leading to dysphagia or heartburn in about half of affected patients. Dilatation and atony of the small bowel may lead to bacterial overgrowth, and hence malabsorption and steatorrhoea.

Respiratory system
There is interstitial fibrosis, which predominantly affects the lower lobes of the lungs or can be diffuse. This may cause a restrictive lung defect and may progress to respiratory failure. There may be aspiration pneumonia and pulmonary hypertension.

Musculoskeletal system
There may be polyarthralgia and flexion deformities due to fibrosis of tendons. Myopathy and polymyositis can occur.

Cardiovascular system
Myocardial fibrosis can cause arrhythmias and conduction defects. Pericardial effusions can occur and right heart failure secondary to lung disease is seen.

Renal system
Renal involvement due to an obliterative endarteritis of renal vessels can lead to progressive renal failure and hypertension, which may be fatal.

Eyes
Sjögren's syndrome may occur.

The CREST syndrome
The CREST syndrome is a form of systemic sclerosis including Calcinosis of subcutaneous tissues, Raynaud's phenomenon, oEsophageal dysmotility, Sclerodactyly, and Telangiectasia. The prognosis is generally better than systemic sclerosis *per se*. It is associated with anticentromere antibodies.

Investigations
The following investigations are important in patients with systemic sclerosis:
- Antinuclear antibodies: present in 80% of patients (nucleolar pattern in scleroderma; rheumatoid factor is positive in 30%).
- ESR: often raised.
- FBC: may show a normochromic normocytic anaemia or a haemolytic anaemia.
- Hand X-rays: may show calcinosis.
- Barium swallow or oesophageal manometry: motility problems.

Management
Treatment is symptomatic (e.g. nifedipine or electrically heated gloves may help with Raynaud's phenomenon). Antacids, H_2 receptor-antagonists, or proton pump inhibitors will help relieve heartburn. Physiotherapy may help when joints are affected, and NSAIDs can be given for joint pain. Hypertensive renal crises are emergencies and should be treated aggressively with angiotensin-converting enzyme inhibitors and optimal supportive critical care.

Prognosis
The course of the disease is variable but is usually slowly progressive. Death usually occurs from lung, renal or cardiac complications. The overall mean 5-year survival is approximately 70%.

Polymyositis and dermatomyositis
Polymyositis is a disorder of muscle and is of unknown aetiology. Immunological and viral factors have been suggested. Pathologically there is necrosis of muscle fibres with regeneration and inflammation. When accompanied by a rash, it is known as dermatomyositis. It can occur at any age, with a peak incidence at around 50 years old, with women twice as likely to be affected as men. Approximately 10% of cases are associated with an underlying malignancy of bronchus, breast, stomach, or ovary. The incidence of malignancy increases with age and is more common in men.

Clinical features
The clinical features of polymyositis and dermatomyositis include the following:
- Muscle weakness and proximal muscle wasting.
- Onset: acute or chronic with progressive weakness.
- Muscle pain and tenderness: about 50% of patients.
- Fibrosis: flexion deformities of the limbs.
- Arthralgia and arthritis: about 50% of patients.
- Skin involvement: purple 'heliotrope' colour around the eyes, and sometimes the rest of the face; violaceous, oedematous lesions over the

knuckles (Gottron's papules); telangiectasia, nail-fold infarcts.
- Muscle involvement: can affect the oesophagus leading to dysphagia.
- Raynaud's phenomenon.
- Lung fibrosis.
- Respiratory muscle weakness may require ventilatory support.
- Sjögren's syndrome.

Investigations

- Creatine kinase is raised and can be used to follow the course of the disease. A raised CKMB or troponin can be seen but rarely causes clinically significant myocarditis.
- Characteristic electromyographic changes— fibrillation potentials.
- Muscle biopsy: necrosis of muscle fibres with swelling and disruption of muscle cells; fibrosis, thickening of blood vessels, and inflammatory changes.
- ESR: usually raised and there may be a normochromic normocytic anaemia; antinuclear antibodies and Jo-1 antibodies may be positive.
- Investigations for underlying malignancy.

Management

High-dose steroids should be prescribed in the acute phase. These can be gradually tailed off. Immunosuppressive drugs (e.g. methotrexate or azathioprine) may be required if there is a poor response to steroids. Physiotherapy may help to restore muscle power.

Prognosis

Adults fare better than children unless there is an underlying malignancy. The disease may be progressive, or may wax and wane. Death usually occurs from respiratory or cardiac failure.

Sjögren's syndrome

This is a chronic autoimmune disease leading to destruction of epithelial exocrine glands resulting in keratoconjunctivitis sicca (dry eyes) or xerostomia (dry mouth). It can be primary or secondary if associated with a connective tissue disorder (commonly RA). There is an association with HLA-B8 and HLA-DR3. Other exocrine glands may be involved. Systemic manifestations include:
- Arthralgia and polyarthritis.
- Raynaud's phenomenon.

- Renal involvement in 20% of patients.
- Pulmonary: fibrotic lung disease.
- Parotid gland enlargement in one third.
- Vasculitis.

There is an increased incidence of lymphoma. It is associated with other organ-specific, autoimmune diseases (e.g. thyroid disease, vitiligo, pernicious anaemia, primary biliary cirrhosis and chronic active hepatitis).

Pathologically there is a lymphocytic and plasma cell infiltrate of the secretory glands.

Investigations

The following investigations are important in patients with Sjögrens syndrome:
- Anti-Ro and anti-La antibody titres: high levels.
- Immunoglobulins: raised.
- Rheumatoid factor: always present.
- Schirmer's test: this is a method of quantifying conjunctival dryness. A strip of filter paper is put under the lower eyelid and the distance along the paper that tears are absorbed is measured. This should be more than 10 mm in 5 minutes.

Treatment

The mainstay of therapy is conservative measures to protect the eye and relieve the oral symptoms. Attempts to modify the progression of the disease have shown little reward. Hydoxychloroquine appears to be the most promising agent in studies.

Mixed connective tissue disease

This is a term used when the symptoms and signs do not fit neatly into one of the well-defined syndromes. It affects women more than men, and presents in young adults. ANA is often positive in a speckled pattern and there are high titres of antibody to an extractable nuclear antigen such as ribonucleoprotein. The condition may respond to steroids. Immunological tests for this disorder and others are summarised in Fig. 33.9.

Polyarteritis nodosa

Polyarteritis nodosa is a necrotising vasculitis which causes aneurysms of medium-sized arteries. It is rare in the UK, is more common in men than women, and the peak incidence is between the ages of 20 and 50 years. There is an association with hepatitis B surface antigen.

Immunological tests	
Test	**Associated disorder**
Antinuclear factor (ANA)	SLE: Rheumatoid arthritis Sjögren's syndrome: MCTD, systemic sclerosis
Anti double-stranded DNA antibodies	SLE
Rheumatoid factor	Rheumatoid arthritis; SLE, MCTD, Sjögren's syndrome
Anti-Ro (SSA), anti-La (SSB) antibodies	Sjögren's syndrome
Antiphospholipid antibodies (e.g. anticardiolipin)	Antiphospholipid syndrome
Anti ribonucleoprotein antibodies	MCTD
Jo-1 antibodies	Polymyositis, dermatomyositis
Antineutrophil cytoplasmic antibodies (ANCA)	pANCA (peripheral): polyarteritis nodosa cANCA (classical): Wegener's granulomatosis
Antiacetylcholine receptor antibodies	Myasthenia gravis
Anti-GM1 antibodies	Multifocal motor neuropathy, Guillain–Barré syndrome
Anti-GAD antibodies	Stiff-man syndrome

Fig. 33.9 Immunological tests. (ANA, antinuclear antibody; GAD, glutamate decarboxylase; MCTD, mixed connective tissue disease; SLE, systemic lupus erythematosus.)

Clinical features
Clinical features include the following:
- General: fever, malaise, weight loss, myalgia.
- Renal: the main cause of death. Patients may present with hypertension, proteinuria, an acute nephritic syndrome, nephrotic syndrome, or renal failure.
- Cardiac: this is the second commonest cause of death. Coronary arteritis may lead to angina and myocardial infarction. There may be pericarditis.

Other complications include mononeuritis multiplex, pulmonary infiltrates and late-onset asthma, arthralgia and visceral infarction.

Investigations
Investigations include:
- ESR and CRP: usually raised; normochromic normocytic anaemia, leucocytosis, and eosinophilia in 30% of cases.
- ANCA: 10% are pANCA positive.
- Biopsy: affected organs may demonstrate fibrinoid necrosis and cellular infiltration in the arteries.
- Angiography: demonstrates microaneurysms in affected viscera.

Management
Treatment is symptomatic, and with steroids and immunosuppressive agents. The course of the disease may be rapidly or slowly progressive. Renal failure is the main cause of death. The overall 5-year survival is 70% if appropriately treated.

Primary skin diseases

Psoriasis
Psoriasis is a usually benign inflammatory skin disease that affects 2% of the population. Pathologically there is the proliferation of keratinocytes causing acanthosis (thickening of the skin). It may present at any age with a peak incidence in the late-20s. Triggers include stress, trauma, infection, and drugs (e.g. lithium, chloroquine and β-blockers).

The most common lesion in psoriasis is a salmon-pink plaque topped by a silvery scale, most frequently found over the extensor surfaces of the limbs (e.g. elbows and knees). Involvement of the scalp with a thickened hyperkeratotic scale is also common. Plaques may be round or 'guttate' (like rain drops), geographical or circinate (ring like). Guttate psoriasis occurs conventionally after streptococcal pharyngitis. Removal of the scales leaves pinpoint bleeding sites (Auspitz's sign). Psoriasis exhibits the Koebner phenomena (i.e. it can arise at sites of trauma).

In flexural psoriasis, lesions have a pinkish glazed appearance, are clearly demarcated, and are non-scaly. The commonest sites of involvement are the groin, perianal and genital regions, and inframammary folds.

Pustular psoriasis affects the palms or soles with well-demarcated scaling and erythema. The pustules are white, yellow, green, or brown when dried.

Extradermal manifestations include nail pitting and some form of arthropathy in 10% of patients.

Management

For mild conditions, treatment other than reassurance and an emollient may be unnecessary. In more troublesome cases topical therapy can be highly effective. Systemic therapy is used only if topical treatments are inadequate.

Topical therapy

Salicylic acid enhances the rate of loss of surface scale. Side effects include irritation or toxicity when large areas are treated. Coal tar has both anti-inflammatory and antiscaling properties but its use is limited by its unpleasant appearance and odour, and it may not be used on the face. However, when the lesions are extensive, coal tar baths are useful. Dithranol is very effective in psoriasis. It can cause severe skin irritation, and should therefore be started at low concentrations and gradually built up. Calcipotriol is a vitamin D derivative that can be applied topically for mild-to-moderate psoriasis. It does not have an unpleasant odour; hypercalcaemia is a recognised complication. Corticosteroids applied topically are highly effective but rarely induce long-term remission and lead to skin atrophy. Tazarotene is a topical retinoid useful in mild-to-moderate plaque psoriasis; it can be used with steroids and is clean and convenient. Many of these drugs are formulated as shampoos for scalp psoriasis.

Systemic therapy

Ultraviolet B radiation therapy alone is helpful in mild-to-moderate, guttate or chronic plaque psoriasis. If unsuccessful, then photochemotherapy using psoralens with long-wave ultraviolet irradiation (PUVA) is effective in some patients. Special lamps are required, and short-term side effects include burning; long term, there may be cataract formation, accelerated ageing of the skin (solar elastosis), and the development of skin cancer. Acitretin is a retinoid (vitamin A derivative) given orally for severe resistant or complicated psoriasis. Side effects include dry and chapped lips, mild transient increase in the rate of hair fall, pruritus, paronychia, and nose bleeds. It is teratogenic. Cytotoxic drugs (e.g. methotrexate and cyclosporin) can be used for severe resistant psoriasis. They are for use only by specialists.

Eczema

The terms eczema and dermatitis are often used interchangeably. It affects 10% of the population. Clinically, lesions are often vesicular, rupturing to leave a raw weeping surface. They may be diffuse, irritating, and sometimes painful. There may be itching and secondary infection. Lesions can be chronic and scaling with lichenification.

Atopic eczema

This often starts in infancy with the vast majority growing out of it by the age of 12 years. Breastfeeding may help prevent atopic eczema. Clinically, there is itching and inflammation. In adults, pruritic exudative lesions are seen on the face, trunk, wrists, antecubital and popliteal fossa. Investigations include prick tests to common allergens, and raised serum immunoglobulin (Ig)E. It may be associated with asthma and hayfever.

Irritant contact dermatitis

The hands are often affected by erythema, vesiculation, and fissuring. Irritants include detergents, bleaches, soaps, etc. It may be a problem in certain occupations (e.g. hairdressers and engineers).

Allergic contact dermatitis

This requires previous sensitisation. Patch testing produces a marked, prolonged response even to dilute quantities of the allergen. The pattern of eczema depends on the site of contact. There is often a sharp cut-off where contact ends although spread to other sites may occur (autosensitisation). Thin, moist skin is the most vulnerable. Common allergens include:
- Dyes.
- Nickel: buttons and zips.

- Chromates: cement and leather.
- Lanolin: cosmetics.
- Rubber.
- Resins: glues.
- Plants.
- Topical antibiotics.
- Antiseptics.

Seborrhoeic dermatitis

This is a scaly, crusty, red, itchy eruption appearing on oily areas of the skin [e.g. the face, flexures, and scalp (dandruff)].

Management

Where possible, the cause should be established and removed. A patient with suspected contact dermatitis should be patch tested to establish the diagnosis. Atopic eczema usually requires the regular application of an emollient with short courses of a mild-to-moderate topical corticosteroid, the least potent that is effective. In more severe eczema, more potent steroids may be needed, and if itching is a major problem consideration should be given to the administration of antihistamines and possibly antibiotics to prevent secondary bacterial infection.

For dry, fissured, scaly lesions, treatment is with emollients, and emulsifying ointment as soap substitutes. For weeping eczema, treatment is with topical corticosteroids, wet dressings of potassium permanganate, and topical antibacterials. Coal tar is used occasionally in chronic atopic eczema. Cyclosporin may be used for severe resistant atopic dermatitis.

Acne vulgaris

This is a papulopustular inflammatory condition, usually affecting the face and trunk, which affects approximately 90% of adolescents. Whilst usually mild and short lived, it can persist into adulthood and/or be severely disfiguring and psychologically damaging. Overproduction of sebum leads to blockage of the sebaceous duct producing the primary lesion (the comedo or 'blackhead'). Colonisation by *Propionibacterium* acnes is probably an important factor. Healing may leave residual scarring.

Management

A sympathetic approach is needed. Dispel myths that the patient is dirty or that acne is caused by eating chocolate or greasy food. Advise on washing the face with soap and water frequently to degrease the skin. Both comedones and inflamed lesions respond well to benzoyl peroxide or azelaic acid.

Lichen planus is summed up by four Ps: peripheral, pruritis, polygonal, and purple

Topical antibiotics are used for mild-to-moderate acne and include erythromycin, tetracycline, and clindamycin. Prolonged periods of oral antibiotics (e.g. for 6 months) are also effective. Isotretinoin is a retinoid used for severe acne unresponsive to systemic antibiotics. It acts primarily by reducing sebum secretion. The drug is teratogenic. Hormone manipulation via antiandrogens and ethinyloestradiol can be highly effective.

Herpes simplex

More than 80% of adults have serologic evidence of prior herpes simplex type 1 (HSV 1) infection, usually from childhood. It is the cause of the coldsore 'herpes labialis'. HSV-2 is more commonly associated with genital herpes. Reactivation following systemic illness causes a burning, stinging neuralgia which accompanies or precedes attacks. The subsequent lesions are small groups of vesicles with an erythematous base in orolabial and genital areas. Diagnosis is clinical but vesicular fluid or scrapings can show HSV. Treatment is with topical, oral or i.v. aciclovir or oral valaciclovir. Herpes simplex may cause an encephalitis with a predilection for the temporal lobes. It presents with non specific symptoms, headaches, speech and behavioural changes. Analysis of the cerebrospinal fluid for HSV DNA is the best diagnostic tool. Untreated it can cause death and survivors are left with neurologic sequelae. Treatment is with i.v. aciclovir. Disseminated HSV may occur with immunosuppression (e.g. HIV).

Herpes (Varicella) Zoster

The primary lesion is chickenpox (varicella) usually in childhood; if occurring in adulthood it may be severe. The infection then lies dormant in the dorsal root ganglia until immunosuppression or illness causes reactivation termed shingles (Zoster). Typically dermatomal pain and paraesthesia preceeds the appearance of maculopapular then vesicular lesions within that dermatome. It is usually thoracic or in the ophthalmic division of the trigeminal nerve. Diagnosis is clinical though analysis of vesicular fluid or scrapings can demonstrate herpes zoster. If ophthalmic, or immunosuppressed, then treatment with i.v. aciclovir is indicated. Disseminated herpes can cause shingles in a non-dermatomal distribution. Corticosteroids may reduce post herpetic neuralgia. Otherwise this is best treated with carbamazepine, gabapentin or capsaicin. It may prove difficult to control and specialist advice should be sought. The patient may be isolated until non infectious and certain groups such as the immunocompromised, pregnant women or healthcare workers without previous infection should avoid contact.

Lichen planus

Lesions are purple, polygonal, and planar or flat-topped papules. The cause is unknown but may be related to disturbances of immune function. Lichen planus-like reactions occur with certain drugs, such as sulphonamides, sulphonylureas, methyldopa, thiazides, β-blockers, and drugs that alter immune function (e.g. antimalarials, gold salts, penicillamine).

The distribution of lesions is mainly peripheral and symmetrical. Scarring occurs with chronic disease. Linear lesions may follow trauma or scratching (Koebner's phenomenon). Lesions may occur on the buccal mucosa or in the nails. The presence of Wickham's striae helps to distinguish the disease. These are fine white lacy lines coursing over the papule. Postinflammatory hyperpigmentation is also a useful diagnostic sign.

The lesions usually last for 12–18 months if untreated. Systemic steroids may be required to suppress intractable itching. Less acute disease can be managed with topical corticosteroids with an antihistamine at night to control the itching.

Skin manifestations of systemic disease

There are many causes and presentations of specific systemic disease; they range from the life threatening purpuric rash of meningococcal septicaemia which must not be missed, to providing clues to chronic medical conditions. The following is a small selection, and many other diseases have skin signs which have been highlighted in the relevant chapters (e.g. chronic liver disease).

Erythema nodosum

These are painful, nodular lesions usually on the anterior shins which go through similar colour changes to a bruise. New crops of lesions emerge while earlier lesions are fading. It is five times more common in women, with a peak incidence between 20 and 50 years.

Causes of erythema nodosum
- Sarcoidosis.
- Drugs (e.g. sulphonamides, oral contraceptive pill, dapsone).
- Bacterial infections (e.g. streptococcus, tuberculosis, leprosy).
- Crohn's disease and ulcerative colitis.
- Behçet's disease.
- Leptospirosis.
- Viral and fungal infections.

Erythema multiforme

These are 'target' lesions, or circular lesions in a symmetrical distribution with central blistering. It usually occurs on the limbs. The lesions may be preceded by a prodrome of fever, sore throat, headache, arthralgia, and gastroenteritis.

In Stevens–Johnson syndrome, there is systemic illness, and lesions are present in the mouth, eye, and genital regions.

Causes of erythema multiforme
- Drugs (e.g. barbiturates, sulphonamides, penicillin, salicylates).
- Systemic infections, especially viral (e.g. mycoplasma, herpes simplex).
- Vitamin deficiency, especially niacin, and vitamins A and C.
- Collagen disorders.

Erythema marginatum

This is associated with rheumatic fever. There are pink rings on the trunk which come and go.

Pyoderma gangrenosum

This presents with violaceous nodules, which then ulcerate to produce an ulcer with an overhanging edge. They heal leaving a scar. Causes include inflammatory bowel disease, neoplasia, Wegener's granulomatosis and myeloma. Systemic steroids and cyclosporin are the first line treatment.

Vitiligo

This is characteristically well demarcated areas of depigmentation. It is associated with organ-specific autoimmune disease (e.g. Addison's, pernicious anaemia, alopecia, Hashimoto's thyroiditis). These are all associated with the HLA B8 DR3 genotype.

Specific diseases with skin manifestations

Inflammatory bowel disease

Both ulcerative colitis and Crohn's disease are causes of erythema nodosum and pyoderma gangrenosum. Crohn's is associated with aphthous ulceration and perianal skin tags, fistulae or abscesses.

Diabetes mellitus

Skin manifestations include recurrent infections, ulcers, necrobiosis lipoidica diabeticorum (shiny area on the shins with a yellowish colour and telangiecstasia), granuloma annulare (purplish annular lesions with the skin surface remaining intact), and fat necrosis at the site of injections.

Coeliac disease

Coeliac disease is associated with dermatitis herpetiformis. There are pruritic symmetrical clusters of urticarial lesions, particularly in the gluteal region and extensor aspects of the elbows and knees. They progress to vesicles and bullae. Direct immunofluorescence show granular deposits of IgA along the dermal papillae. There may be secondary bacterial infection. Treatment is with dapsone.

Hyperthyroidism

Pretibial myxoedema is red oedematous plaques on the shins due to mucin deposition.

Neoplasia

Features may include the following:
- Acanthosis nigricans (especially with gastric carcinoma): areas of pigmented rough thickening of the skin in the axillae or groin with warty lesions.
- Dermatomyositis (see p. 326).
- Erythema gyratum repens: a rare 'wood grain' erythema associated with lung cancer.
- Secondary skin metastases.
- Acquired ichthyosis: dry, scaly skin (vaguely resembling that of a fish), associated with lymphoma.
- Thrombophlebitis migrans (especially with pancreatic carcinoma): successive crops of tender nodules affecting blood vessels throughout the body.

Sarcoidosis

Erythema nodosum and lupus pernio may be present (i.e. a diffuse bluish plaque with small papules within the swelling) affecting the nose.

Neurofibromatosis

This condition is autosomal dominant and may include the following features:
- Café-au-lait spots (light brown macules).
- Axillary freckling.
- Violaceous dermal neurofibromata.
- Subcutaneous nodules.

Lyme disease

Cutaneous signs are erythema chronicum migrans. This starts off as a small red papule which gradually enlarges to form a ring with a raised border. It lasts for 2 days to 3 months. Lyme disease is caused by *Borrelia burgdorferi*, a spirochete spread by ticks from deer. Within the UK, it is most common in the New Forest. Other features include:
- Malaise.
- Migratory arthralgia.
- Neck stiffness.
- Lymphadenopathy.
- CNS abnormalities (e.g. meningitis and peripheral neuropathies).
- Cardiac disease including conduction disturbances and myocarditis.

Treatment is with tetracycline, penicillin, or third generation cephalosporin (e.g. cefotaxime).

Xanthomatosis

Tendon xanthomata are associated with familial hypercholesterolaemia (see p. 290). Eruptive xanthomata occur with greatly elevated serum lipid concentrations. Xanthelasmata are yellow plaques commonly found on the eyelids. They may indicate hyperlipidaemia.

Behçet's disease

This is a recurrent progressive systemic disease of unknown aetiology with painful ulceration of the oral and genital regions. Other features of Behçet's disease may include:
- Iritis, keratitis and hypopyon.
- Retinal vein occlusion.
- Seronegative arthritis.
- CNS complications (e.g. meningoencephalitis and cranial nerve palsies).

Treatment is with steroids for ulcers and systemic features. In resistant cases colchicine or cytotoxic drugs (e.g. azathioprine, may be needed).

Malignant skin tumours

Basal cell carcinoma

This is the commonest skin tumour and is frequently seen in elderly, fair-skinned people. Lesions mainly occur on the face, especially at the side of the nose or periorbital skin. They may be flesh-coloured papules or plaques with superficial dilated blood vessels over the surface. There may be central necrosis with ulceration or crusting and a pearly rolled edge. They may also be pigmented or cystic. They tend to be locally invasive (hence the alternative name rodent ulcer) but metastases are rare. Treatment is by surgical excision, cryotherapy, or radiotherapy.

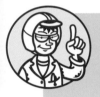

Sites of malignant melanoma with a poor prognosis are BANS: back of the arm, neck, and scalp

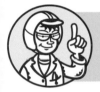

Beware of the man with a big liver and a glass eye-think of metastatic ocular melanoma

Squamous cell carcinoma

This tumour arises from the epidermis or skin appendages, and is most commonly seen on damaged or chronically irritated skin. It is invasive and can metastasise though this is rare. Viral disease (e.g. human papilloma virus) may be a predisposing factor. Tumours are hyperkeratotic, crusted and indurated, and may ulcerate. Treatment is by excision or radiotherapy. Carcinoma may develop in long standing venous ulceration; when this occurs it is termed a Marjolin's ulcer.

Malignant melanoma

This tumour is increasing in incidence and occurs particularly in fair-skinned people with exposure to sunlight. It is a major cause of cancer in young people. Some melanomas arise in pre-existing moles. Malignancy should be suspected if a pigmented lesion shows the following:

- Rapid enlargement.
- Bleeding.
- Increasing variegated pigmentation, particularly blue–black or grey.
- Ulceration.
- An indistinct border.
- Persistent itching.
- Small 'satellite' lesions around the principal lesion.

The prognosis is related to the depth of the tumour assessed histologically (Breslow thickness). The 5-year survival for patients with a tumour less than 1 mm thick is greater than 90%. If the thickness is greater than 3.5 mm, the 5-year survival rate is less than 35%.

Patients with lesions on the limbs have a better prognosis than those with truncal lesions who, in turn, have a better prognosis than those with facial lesions. Metastasis is common. Interferon may slow progression of metastases.

Management

People should avoid exposure to direct sunlight and should use sunscreen lotions. Self-examination should be practised, and people should be aware of the warning signs and symptoms listed above. Treatment is by excision with skin grafting if necessary.

- How does an inflammatory arthritis differ from osteoarthritis?
- What non joint problems are encountered with rheumatoid arthritis?
- What is the rationale behind modern therapy for rheumatoid arthritis?
- Describe the classic presentation of ankylosing spondylitis?
- Differentiate between polymyalgia rheumatica and polymyositis?
- List the organ symptoms affected by systemic lupus erythematosus and an example in each category?
- How does the appearance and distribution of psoriasis and eczema differ?
- What is the Koebner phenomenon?
- List five conditions associated with erythema nodosum?
- What is Marjolin's ulcer?

Further reading

The British Association of Dermatologists publishes guidelines and reviews of all aspects of skin disease. They are available on its website *www.bad.org.uk*.

The British Society for Rheumatology publishes guidelines and reviews of all aspects of rheumatology. They are available on its website *www.rheumatology.org.uk*.

Choy E H S and Panayi G S 2001 Mechanisms of disease: cytokine pathways and joint inflammation in rheumatoid arthritis. *N Engl J Med* **344**; 907–916

Cook and Haslam 2004 *Crash Course in Rheumatology and Orthopaedics*. Mosby

Graham-Brown R and Bourke J F 1998 *Colour Atlas and Text of Dermatology*. Mosby

Morehead K and Sack K E 2003 Osteoarthritis- What therapies for this disease of many causes? *Postgrad Med* **114**;11–17

Ruiz-Irastorza G, Khamashta M A, Hughes G R V 2001 Systemic lupus erythematosus. *Lancet* **357**; 1027–1032

Savage C O S, Harper L, Cockwell P et al 2000 Vasculitis. ABC of arterial and vascular disease. *BMJ* **320**; 1325–1328

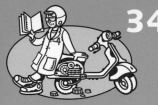

34. Haematological Disorders

Anaemia

Anaemia is a common clinical problem as it is the end result of many different pathological processes. The aetiology, clinical evaluation, complications, and investigation policy have been considered in Chapter 26. The general approach to management is outlined first, and then specific conditions are discussed in detail.

General approach to management
Discover the underlying cause
Remember that there may be more than one cause of anaemia in any one patient and this can catch out the unwary! For example, folate and iron deficiency may both be present in coeliac disease.

Fig. 34.1 shows possible causes of anaemia in rheumatoid arthritis.

Treat the underlying cause
The anaemia will recur if the underlying problem persists (e.g. peptic ulceration or colonic neoplasm).

Correct the anaemia
The method of correction will depend on the type of anaemia and presence of complications. In general, iron, vitamin B_{12}, and folate should only be prescribed when the patient has been appropriately investigated and shown to have a deficiency.

Iron replacement
Oral iron replacement therapy (e.g. ferrous sulphate should be continued for 3 months after the

haemoglobin returns to normal to replace iron stores). Side effects include nausea, change in bowel habit, and abdominal pain. (The stool colour may become very dark or black.) If side effects occur, reduce the dose to once or twice daily. Intramuscular or intravenous iron can be given but only if there is poor patient compliance with oral therapy, severe gastrointestinal disturbance with oral therapy, or malabsorption.

Vitamin B_{12} replacement
Most causes of vitamin B_{12} deficiency are due to malabsorption and so vitamin B_{12} is given by intramuscular injection. Stores are replaced by giving hydroxycobalamin. Maintenance therapy is every 3 months, which needs to be lifelong in most patients.

Folate replacement
Oral folic acid corrects anaemia and replaces folate stores (a higher dose may be needed in malabsorption states). Lower dose oral folic acid should be given as prophylaxis against neural tube defects to women prior to conception and throughout the first 12 weeks of pregnancy.

It should not be given in malignancy unless essential, as some tumours are dependent on folate, and it should not be given alone in megaloblastic anaemia unless vitamin B_{12} status has been shown to be normal, as it can precipitate the neurological complications of vitamin B_{12} deficiency (subacute combined degeneration of the cord).

Causes of anaemia in rheumatoid arthritis

- Anaemia of chronic disease
- Hypersplenism due to splenomegaly (Felty's syndrome if also neutropenic)
- Chronic blood loss from peptic ulceration due to steroid and NSAID administration
- Bone marrow suppression by disease modifying drugs such as gold and penicillamine
- Folate deficiency (increased utilisation of folate)

Fig. 34.1 Causes of anaemia in rheumatoid arthritis. (NSAID, non-steroidal anti-inflammatory drug.)

Always measure haematinics prior to blood transfusion

Blood transfusion
Whole blood should only be administered when there is hypovolaemia in addition to anaemia, as occurs in massive acute haemorrhage. In an emergency, where time does not allow crossmatching, O Rhesus-negative blood can be given

safely. In chronic symptomatic anaemia, which cannot be corrected by folate, vitamin B_{12} or iron therapy, matched packed red blood cells (RBCs) may be given. Fig. 34.2 summarises the complications of transfusion.

Splenectomy

Splenectomy is useful in hereditary spherocytosis and autoimmune haemolytic anaemia that is refractory to steroids or immunosuppressive therapy. Other indications for splenectomy include trauma, refractory idiopathic thrombocytopenic purpura, and symptomatic splenomegaly (e.g. myelofibrosis, lymphoma and leukaemia). Complications of splenectomy include thrombocytosis and increased susceptibility to infection with encapsulated bacteria (e.g. pneumococcus and Haemophilus influenzae type B). Patients should be immunised with vaccines against these two organisms. Dental treatment should be covered by antibiotic prophylaxis and any febrile episode treated quickly. Prophylactic penicillin may be indicated, either lifelong or until adulthood.

Erythropoietin

Recombinant erythropoietin (EPO) has revolutionised the management of the anaemia associated with chronic renal failure. It is given up to three times a week as subcutaneous or intravenous injections. Adequate iron stores are needed and it is less effective in inflammatory states. It is being investigated for use in other settings at present.

Complications include hypertension and the observation of a rare pure red cell aplasia associated with anti-EPO antibodies. This has not been shown with the newer novel erythropoiesis-stimulating proteins.

Anaemia of chronic disease
Aetiology and pathology

Many infective, inflammatory or malignant processes are associated with anaemia. For the aetiologies see Fig. 26.2. The pathology is multifactorial, with inappropriate utilisation of adequate iron stores, possible decrease in erythropoietin production and reduced RBC survival.

Complications of blood transfusion	
Complication	**Cause**
Haemolytic reaction	ABO incompatibility (severe), extravascular haemolysis (mild/clinically silent)
Anaphylaxis	Hypersensitivity to plasma proteins
Febrile reaction	Antibodies to white cells
Volume overload	Particularly the elderly and in megaloblastic anaemia
Coagulopathies	Platelets and clotting factors are reduced by a dilutional effect in massive transfusion
Infection	Virus (HIV, hepatitis B and C, EBV, CMV) Gram-negative bacteria (uncommon)
Haemosiderosis	With repeated transfusions
Alloimmunisation	Antibodies may develop to red cells, leukocytes, platelets and plasma proteins despite receiving compatible blood; this may cause problems the next time the patient receives a transfusion
Graft versus host disease	Uncommon: preventable by using irradiated blood (important in transplant recipients)
Air embolism	Particularly if given via central lines
Thrombophlebitis	At cannula site
TRALI (Transfusion associated lung injury)	Unpredictable, non cardiogenic pulmonary oedema

Fig. 34.2 Complications of blood transfusion. (CMV, cytomegalovirus; EBV, Epstein–Barr virus; HIV, human immunodeficiency virus.)

Presentation and complications

Presentation is with the symptoms and signs of anaemia (see p. 151), and of the primary disease. The complications are those of anaemia (see p. 152) and the underlying disease.

Investigations

Characteristic findings are:

- Normochromic normocytic anaemia (may be hypochromic, microcytic).
- Serum iron low.
- Serum ferritin high (can be normal).
- Increased iron stores in bone marrow.
- A raised erythrocyte sedimentation rate (ESR), neutrophil leucocytosis, and thrombocytosis, in addition to the anaemia constitutes a 'reactive' blood picture reflecting the primary pathology.

Treatment

- Treat the underlying disease.
- If mild and asymptomatic no treatment is necessary.
- If symptomatic, consider transfusion and rarely recombinant erythropoietin therapy.

The anaemia associated with chronic renal failure has a different pathogenesis and treatment.

Sideroblastic anaemia
Aetiology

Sideroblastic anaemia can be congenital or acquired:

- Congenital: X-linked.
- Acquired: primary – refractory anaemia with ring sideroblasts (this is a subgroup of myelodysplasia); secondary – drugs (e.g. isoniazid, pyrazinamide), alcohol, lead poisoning, myeloproliferative disease, connective tissue disease.

Pathology

- Haem cannot be incorporated into protoporphyrin to form haemoglobin.
- Erythropoiesis becomes disordered.
- Iron accumulates in the marrow.

Presentation

- Symptoms and signs of anaemia.
- No specific clinical features.

Complications

- Primary refractory anaemia with ring sideroblasts may progress to acute myeloid leukaemia (AML).
- Haemosiderosis if recurrent transfusions are given.

Investigations

- Dimorphic RBCs on blood film of normochromic and hypochromic cells.
- Mean corpuscular volume: low, normal, or slightly raised.
- Ferritin is raised.
- Ring sideroblasts in the bone marrow (these are erythroblasts where haem has accumulated in the mitochondria, causing granules which stain with Prussian blue and are situated in a perinuclear ring).

Treatment

- Withdraw any possible causative agents, such as drugs, as the anaemia may resolve.
- Folate orally may also help.
- Blood transfusion.

Lead poisoning
Aetiology

- In adults, usually due to industrial exposure or unwitting chronic lead ingestion.
- Exposure in children was typically from old toys (as toy paints used to contain lead).

Pathology

- Absorbed from the lungs or gastrointestinal tract.
- Most profound effects on bone marrow, nervous system, and kidneys.
- Also deposited in bones, teeth, nails, and hair.

Presentation

This may be non specific and chronic if lead exposure is not considered.

- Nausea, vomiting, and colicky abdominal pain.
- Altered conscious level, irritability, and seizures if encephalopathic (more common in children).
- Foot drop or wrist drop (usually adults).
- Burton's line (blue line on the gums).

Complications

- Peripheral motor neuropathy.
- Encephalopathy.
- Sideroblastic and haemolytic anaemia.
- Fanconi's syndrome (lead nephropathy).

Investigations

- Blood lead levels.
- Lead lines on X-ray: dense metaphyseal lines in children (wrists and knees) due to lead and calcium deposition.

- Hypochromic anaemia with basophilic stippling of RBCs (RNA deposition).
- Ring sideroblasts may be present in bone marrow.
- Free RBC protoporphyrin is raised.

Treatment
- Discuss with poisons information services.
- Treat with sodium calcium edetate (drug of choice), dimercaprol or penicillamine.

Hereditary spherocytosis
Hereditary spherocytosis is an inherited disease (autosomal dominant), with an incidence of 1 in 5000.

Pathology
- Deficiency or defect of spectrin, a RBC protein responsible for membrane stability.
- The normally biconcave RBCs become spherical as the membrane is more permeable.
- The cells are no longer deformable and become trapped in the spleen where they are haemolysed.
- Severity is variable.

Presentation
- Jaundice can develop at any age depending on severity.
- Splenomegaly is usually present.
- Signs of complications may also be present.

Complications
- Gallstones (pigmented) due to increased unconjugated bilirubin in the bile.
- Aplastic crises due to parvovirus infection.
- Megaloblastic anaemia due to increased folate utilisation, particularly during pregnancy (see Fig. 26.4).

Investigations
- Anaemia, which may not be present if bone marrow compensates for haemolysis.
- Spherocytosis and reticulocytosis (polychromasia) on blood film.
- Mean corpuscular haemoglobin concentration often increased.
- Erythroid hyperplasia in bone marrow (to compensate for increased breakdown).
- Increased unconjugated bilirubin and urinary urobilinogen with reduced haptoglobin levels.
- Increased lactate dehydrogenase (LDH).
- Increased osmotic fragility.

Treatment
- No treatment if the haemolysis is mild or if the patient is very young.
- Splenectomy in moderate to severe disease. 'Curative' as it eliminates haemolysis but not the membrane defect.
- Folate supplementation.
- Screen family members.

Hereditary elliptocytosis is an autosomal dominant condition with a similar but milder presentation to that of hereditary spherocytosis. The RBCs are elliptical on the blood film. Most cases require no treatment but the severity is variable, and severe forms may also require splenectomy and folate supplementation.

Glucose-6-phosphate dehydrogenase deficiency
Glucose-6-phosphate dehydrogenase (G6PD) deficiency occurs in 200 million people worldwide. It is an inherited (X-linked recessive) condition.

Pathology
- G6PD is an important enzyme in maintaining glutathione in a reduced state which provides protection against oxidative stress.
- If erythrocytes deficient in G6PD are exposed to oxidative stress, haemoglobin becomes oxidised, and forms precipitates called Heinz bodies which stick to the RBC membrane. The cells lose deformability and become trapped and destroyed in the spleen.

Presentation
- The disease affects males in the Middle East, South-East Asia, West Africa, the Mediterranean, and Southern Europe.
- The severity of disease varies, being most severe in the Mediterranean type.
- Acute episodes of intravascular haemolysis are precipitated by intercurrent illness (particularly infection), drugs (e.g. antimalarials, sulphonamides), and the ingestion of fava beans (favism).
- The patient is usually completely well in between episodes.
- In severe deficiency, chronic haemolysis with splenomegaly may occur.
- Female heterozygotes have improved resistance to falciparum malaria.

Investigations
- Between episodes: G6PD assays (concentration or activity) show deficiency; other tests are normal.
- During acute episode; the blood film shows 'bite' cells, 'blister' cells, Heinz bodies, and reticulocytosis. Features of haemolysis will be present: increased unconjugated bilirubin, reduced haptoglobin, and increased urinary urobilinogen.

Treatment
- Avoiding or stopping precipitating drugs.
- Treat any underlying infection.
- Transfusion for severe, symptomatic anaemia.
- Considering exchange transfusion and phototherapy in icterus neonatorum.

Pyruvate kinase deficiency
This is an inherited condition (autosomal recessive).

Pathology
- Pyruvate kinase is an important enzyme in the glycolytic (Embden–Meyerhof) pathway.
- In deficiency, ATP production is reduced.
- Abnormal erythrocytes are removed by the spleen.
- 2,3-DPG increases, shifting the oxygen dissociation curve to the right, resulting in better toleration of anaemia.

Presentation
This condition presents with symptoms of anaemia, jaundice and gallstones; splenomegaly is common. Severity is variable.

Complications
Complications include anaemia and gallstones.

Investigations
- Blood film: poikilocytosis (with 'prickle' cells) and reticulocytosis.
- Anaemia.
- Pyruvate kinase: assay demonstrates deficiency.

Treatment
Treatment is by blood transfusion for severe anaemia; consider splenectomy if requiring multiple transfusions.

Sickle cell anaemia

Do not deny sickle cell patients adequate analgesia during a crisis for misplaced fear of drug dependency

Sickle cell anaemia is an inherited (autosomal recessive) condition which most commonly affects Afro-Caribbeans but is also found in the Middle East and Mediterranean. The condition provides advantage in infection with falciparum malaria.

Pathology
- A single base mutation in the DNA on chromosome 11 causes substitution of glutamic acid for valine at position 6 in the β-haemoglobin chain (HbS).
- When HbS becomes deoxygenated it aggregates in an organised fashion forming polymers within the RBCs which are less soluble and less deformable.
- As a result the erythrocyte shape becomes distorted and changes from a biconcave disc to a 'sickle' shape.
- The sickle cells cannot readily pass through the microcirculation and become trapped in small vessels (causing infarction) and in the spleen (where they are destroyed – haemolysed).

Presentation
In the homozygote, severity is variable, and the disease may present from the third month onwards (as haemoglobin F levels fall). There is chronic haemolysis with intermittent crises and complications.

Types of sickle cell anaemia crisis
There are four types of sickle cell anaemia crisis:
- Aplastic: due to parvovirus B19 infection of RBC precursors. Profound anaemia and reticulocytopenia. Self-limiting but transfusion may be required.
- Sequestration: sequestration may occur in the spleen, liver, and lungs. The haemoglobin drops rapidly with a compensatory increase in reticulocytes. Splenic sequestration is seen only in children as the spleen is usually infarcted by 6 years old. Exchange transfusion may be required.

- Haemolytic: may be precipitated by infection. Seen particularly in cases with coexistent G6PD deficiency. The haemoglobin drops rapidly with a compensatory increase in reticulocytes.
- Painful: due to vascular occlusion. Can be precipitated by dehydration, hypoxia, infections, and cold exposure. Almost any organ can be affected. Small bones of the hands and feet most often affected in childhood ('hand–foot syndrome'). In older patients, the lungs, hips, shoulders, and spine are more commonly involved.

Complications
- Anaemia.
- Infection: pneumonia (*Staphylococcus pneumoniae*, *Haemophilus influenzae*), osteomyelitis (*Salmonella*).
- Vessel occlusion: splenic infarction (resulting in predisposition to infection), renal papillary necrosis, priapism, aseptic necrosis of the femoral head, transient ischaemic attacks, strokes, placental infarction, and spontaneous abortion.
- Gallstones.
- Leg ulceration.

Investigations
- Normochromic normocytic anaemia.
- Reticulocytosis, sickle cells, and target cells on film (features of hyposplenism may also be present following splenic infarction; Fig. 26.7).
- Haemoglobin electrophoresis demonstrates HbS.
- Leucocyte and platelet counts may also be raised.
- Prenatal diagnosis can be made using polymerase chain reaction techniques on chorionic villous samples.

Treatment
There are no effective treatments for the underlying disease; treatment is symptomatic.
- Long term folate (increased folate utilisation because of haemolysis).
- Immunisation against pneumococcus and *H. influenzae* (increased risk of these because of hyposplenism secondary to splenic infarction).
- Prophylactic penicillin in children.
- Supportive care during crises. Blood transfusion. Adequate analgesia and hydration plus vigorous treatment of hypoxia and infection.
- Exchange transfusions if recurrent crises or significant organ damage.

Prognosis
There is a 5% mortality in the first 10 years of life.

Note that in the sickle cell trait (a heterozygous carrier state) the disease is much milder with little or no anaemia and a normal blood film. Crises may be caused in extreme conditions. The most common complication is renal disease.

Thalassaemia
Normal haemoglobin synthesis is summarised in Fig. 34.3.

Prevalence and aetiology
The prevalence of thalassaemia is 2.5–15% in the 'thalassaemia belt' (see below). It is an inherited condition. The alpha globin gene is on chromosome 16 and the beta gene on chromosome 11.

Pathology
- Reduced production of one or more of the haemoglobin chains (most importantly α or β), which results in a relative excess and

---

Normal haemoglobin synthesis

- Normal haemoglobin is composed of four polypeptide chains (tetramer)
- At various stages of development, different polypeptide chains are produced (ζ, ε, α, γ, δ and β)
- In the embryo (first 8 weeks' gestation), three different haemoglobins are produced by the yolk sac, Hb Gower-1 (ζ_2, ε_2), Hb Gower-2 (α_2, ε_2) and Hb Portland (ζ_2, γ_2)
- Fetal haemoglobin (HbF) is composed of two α chains and two γ chains (α_2, γ_2) and is the major haemoglobin of intrauterine life. It declines rapidly around birth and constitutes less than 1% haemoglobin by 6 months of age. HbF is produced predominantly made by the liver until 30 weeks, after which the bone marrow takes over. It has an avid affinity for oxygen
- Production of β chains increases rapidly at 36 weeks' gestation; 96% adult haemoglobin is HbA (α_2, β_2), 3.5% is HbA$_2$ (α_2, δ_2) with the remainder being HbF
- The genes for the globin chains α and ζ are found clustered on chromosome 16. The genes for the remaining chains are located in a cluster on chromosome 11
- Each person has four α genes (two on each chromosome 16) and two β genes (one on each chromosome 11)

Fig. 34.3 Normal haemoglobin synthesis.

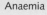

accumulation of the other chain (called 'imbalanced globin chain synthesis').

- The unstable haemoglobin precipitates, causing ineffective erythropoiesis and haemolysis.
- There is deficiency of α chains in α-thalassaemia and of β chains in β-thalassaemia.

Presentation

- α-Thalassaemia is found in populations in the Mediterranean, Africa, the Middle East and South-East Asia.
- β-Thalassaemia affects those in China, the Mediterranean, the Middle East and India.
- The clinical presentation is dependent on the underlying defect as shown in Figs 34.4 and 34.5.
- Thalassaemia provides an advantage in infection with falciparum malaria.

Microcytic anaemia is the abnormality on a blood film in β-thalassaemia trait. Differentiation from iron deficiency requires ferritin levels and clinical suspicion.

Treatment

- Transfusion to maintain an adequate haemoglobin (>10 g/dL) during childhood to ensure normal growth and development.
- Iron chelation to prevent haemosiderosis using desferrioxamine.
- Splenectomy can reduce transfusion requirements but should be avoided where possible because of the increased susceptibility to infection.
- Long term folate supplementation in severe disease (β-thalassaemia major).
- Bone marrow transplantation may be curative in some patients with β-thalassaemia major.
- Current research emphasis is on the prospect of using gene therapy techniques.
- Prenatal diagnosis and genetic counselling should be available.

Pernicious anaemia
Incidence and aetiology

This is an autoimmune condition and has an incidence of 2 per 10 000.

Pathology

- Immunoglobulin G (IgG) autoantibodies are produced against gastric parietal cells and intrinsic factor.
- This causes gastric mucosal atrophy with loss of parietal cells and achlorhydria.
- Intrinsic factor, necessary for vitamin B_{12} absorption, is not produced.

Presentation

- The onset is usually insidious and is more common after the age of 50 years, affecting females more than men.
- Higher prevalence in Scandinavian populations (fair hair and blue eyes).
- Strong association with other autoimmune diseases and blood group A.

Characteristic features of the α-thalassaemias				
Subtype	Silent carrier	α-Thalassaemia trait	HbH disease	Hydrops fetalis
Genetic abnormality	One α gene deleted	Two α genes deleted	Three α genes deleted	Four α genes deleted
Clinical features	Asymptomatic	Usually asymptomatic	Haemolytic anaemia Splenomegaly Bone changes	Hepatosplenomegaly Gross oedema Hypoalbuminaemia Extramedullary haemopoiesis
Haematological findings	No abnormality	Hypochromia microcytosis	Hypochromia Microcytosis Reticulocytosis HbH (β_4) on electrophoresis Inclusion bodies with cresyl blue	Hypochromia Microcytosis Reticulocytosis Target cells Nucleated red cells Hb Bart's (γ_4) on electrophoresis
Survival	Normal	Normal	Variable	Stillborn or death shortly after birth

Fig. 34.4 Characteristic features of the α-thalassaemias. (HbH, haemoglobin H.)

Characteristic features of the β-thalassaemias			
Subtype	β-Thalassaemia minor	β-Thalassaemia intermedia	β-Thalassaemia major
Genetic abnormality	Heterozygous abnormality in β globin gene	Homozygous or mixed heterozygous Abnormality in β globin gene	Homozygous abnormality in β globin gene
Clinical features	Usually asymptomatic	Variable Extramedullary haematopoiesis hepatosplenomegaly Skeletal deformity Gallstones Leg ulcers	Failure to thrive (3–6 months) Jaundice Extramedullary haematopoiesis hepatosplenomegaly Skeletal deformity Haemosiderosis Recurrent infections Cardiac failure Gallstones Leg ulcers
Haematological findings	Mild anaemia Microcytosis Hypochromia Target cells Poikilocytosis HbA$_2$ high HbF may be raised	Moderate anaemia but not transfusion dependent Microcytosis Hypochromia Target cells Poikilocytosis	Transfusion-dependent severe anaemia Microcytosis Hypochromia Target cells Anisopoikilocytosis Reticulocytosis Nucleated RBCs Basophilic stippling Inclusion bodies on supravital staining with methyl violet HbA absent or very low HbF high
Survival	Normal	Survive to adulthood even without treatment	Death in childhood without treatment; bone marrow transplantation may be curative

Fig. 34.5 Characteristic features of the β-thalassaemias. (Hb, haemoglobin; RBC, red blood cell.)

- Symptoms include those of anaemia and the neurological complications of vitamin B$_{12}$ deficiency.
- Examination may reveal anaemia, glossitis, lemon tint (increased bilirubin due to haemolysis), low-grade pyrexia, mild splenomegaly, and neurological signs.

Complications
- Complications of anaemia (see Chapter 26).
- Neurological abnormalities from vitamin B$_{12}$ deficiency (dementia, optic atrophy, peripheral neuropathy, subacute combined degeneration of the cord).
- Gastric carcinoma.

Investigation
- Macrocytic anaemia with typical blood film (see Fig. 26.7).
- White cell and platelet counts: may be low.
- Serum vitamin B$_{12}$: low, with abnormal Schilling test (now rarely performed).

- Megaloblastic bone marrow.
- Bilirubin: increased.
- LDH: increased (also due to breakdown of abnormal RBCs).
- Parietal cell antibody in 90% (can be seen in normal elderly).
- Intrinsic factor antibody in 50%.
- Gastroscopy should be considered to exclude gastric carcinoma.

Treatment
- Lifelong vitamin B$_{12}$ replacement (see p. 335).
- Initial response to treatment can be demonstrated by an increase in reticulocyte count.

It is often said that you should never transfuse patients with B$_{12}$ deficiency due to risk of heart failure. Response to B$_{12}$ is often rapid and routine transfusion can be avoided; however, if the patient is haemodynamically compromised or demonstrating ischaemic stress, then limited transfusion is needed.

Leukaemias

The leukaemias are a group of conditions characterised by the malignant proliferation of leucocytes in the bone marrow. The cells spill out into the blood stream and may infiltrate other organs.

In the acute leukaemias, there is a proliferation of early lymphoid and myeloid precursors (called blasts) which do not mature. The clinical course is very aggressive and rapidly fatal without treatment.

The chronic leukaemias have a more indolent course and are characterised by the proliferation of lymphoid and myeloid cells which reach maturity (lymphocytes and neutrophils respectively).

All leukaemias are best managed by specialists and chemotherapy is a huge rapidly-changing field. Most patients are in clinical trials and only the principles need be understood by students and junior doctors.

Acute lymphoblastic leukaemia
Epidemiology and aetiology
Acute lymphoblastic leukaemia (ALL) is the most common malignancy in children under 15 years. Its aetiology is unknown but is probably multifactorial. Risks include:
- Genetic predisposition: concordance in twins, Down's syndrome and ataxia telangiectasia.

Pathology
- Lymphoblasts accumulate in the bone marrow, and can cause bone marrow failure.
- Lymphoblasts circulate in the blood stream and can infiltrate the lymph nodes, liver, spleen, kidneys, testicles, and central nervous system (CNS).
- Classified according to the French–American–British system (Fig. 34.6).

FAB classification of ALL

- L1: small cells, homogenous, small or absent nucleoli, scanty cytoplasm
- L2: large cells, heterogeneous, occasional large nucleoli, more cytoplasm
- L3: large cells, homogenous, prominent nucleoli, abundant cytoplasm

---

Fig. 34.6 The French–American–British (FAB) classification of acute lymphoblastic leukaemia (ALL). Note that ALL may also be classified according to phenotype (B cell, T cell, common, null).

Presentation
- Peak incidences at age 5 years and over 65 years.
- The history is usually short as the disease is so aggressive (days to a few weeks).
- Symptoms are due to rapidly expanding tumour cells in the bone marrow causing bone pain or bone marrow failure (Fig. 34.7).
- There is fever, lymphadenopathy, and hepatosplenomegaly on examination.
- Main sites of relapse are bone marrow, CNS, and testes.

Investigations
- Normochromic normocytic anaemia with low reticulocyte count.
- High white cell count due to lymphoblasts; neutropenia may be present.
- Thrombocytopenia.
- Bone marrow is hypercellular and dominated by lymphoblasts (usually >50%).
- Cytogenetic abnormalities may be present (e.g. hyperdiploidy or the Philadelphia chromosome).
- Urate and LDH high.
- Mediastinal mass on chest X-ray in T cell-ALL.
- Cerebrospinal fluid examination may show lymphoblasts, increased pressure, and increased protein.

Treatment
All chemotherapy requires careful supportive care with hydration, prophylactic antibiotics, antiviral and antifungal drugs, septic surveillance, blood products to support pancytopenia, bone marrow colony-stimulating factors such as granulocyte colony-stimulating factor, monitoring of coagulation and allopurinol to prevent tumour lysis syndrome and gout from the increased purine metabolism.

Treatment should be managed in a specialised unit and include:
- Cytotoxic chemotherapy (induction of remission then consolidation followed by maintenance).
- CNS prophylaxis: cranial irradiation, intrathecal methotrexate.
- Testes: no prophylaxis but often a site of relapse.
- Treat with radiotherapy if relapse occurs.
- Bone marrow transplantation (allogeneic or autologous) can be curative; it is used in poor risk patients.

Features of bone marrow failure		
Cells affected	**Result**	**Manifestation**
Red cell precursors	Anaemia	Lethargy, dyspnoea, pallor
White cell precursors	Neutropenia	Recurrent infections, fever
Platelet precursors	Thrombocytopenia	Bleeding, bruising, purpura

Fig. 34.7 General features of bone marrow failure.

Prognosis

- Children: 60% 5-year survival.
- Adults: 30% 5-year survival.
- Poor prognostic indicators include increasing age, increasing white cell count, null cell or T cell phenotype, male sex, and the presence of the Philadelphia chromosome.

Acute myeloid leukaemia and acute non-lymphocytic leukaemia

Epidemiology

Acute non-lymphocytic leukaemia and AML account for 20% of all leukaemias, and 85% of adult acute leukaemias.

Aetiology

Most cases arise with no clear cause, though many risks are recognised.

- Ionizing radiation: survivors of Hiroshima.
- Chemical exposure: leather and rubber workers (benzene).
- Previous chemotherapy: alkylating agents.
- Predisposing diseases: myeloproliferative diseases, multiple myeloma, aplastic anaemia and myelodysplasia which can transform to acute leukaemia (often the cause of death).

Pathology

- Accumulation of immature haemopoietic blast cells in the bone marrow, which can cause bone marrow failure.
- Blasts can infiltrate the gums, liver, spleen, skin, and less commonly the CNS.
- Traditionally classified as shown in Fig. 34.8. As with many haematological malignancies immunohistochemistry and cytogenetics are replacing morphological factors for classification and prognosis.

Presentation

- More frequent with increasing age (median age at presentation is 50 years).
- Symptoms are due to marrow failure (Fig. 34.7, particularly skin infections) or infiltration by leukaemic cells.

French–American–British (FAB) classification of AML		
FAB subtype	**Name (predominant cell type)**	**Specific clinical features**
M1	Undifferentiated myeloblastic	–
M2	Myeloblastic	Most common
M3	Promyelocytic	DIC may cause fatal bleeding
M4	Myelomonocytic	Gingival, skin and meningeal infiltration
M5	Monocytic	Gingival, skin and meningeal infiltration Lymphadenopathy and DIC may occur
M6	Erythroleukaemia	Particularly older patients
M7	Megakaryocytic	–

Fig. 34.8 The French–American–British (FAB) classification of acute myeloid leukaemia (AML). (DIC, disseminated intravascular coagulation.)

- Bone pain, joint pain, and malaise may be prominent symptoms.
- Hepatomegaly and moderate splenomegaly are common.
- Disseminated intravascular coagulopathy has a recognised association with the M3 subtype.
- Lymphadenopathy is rare except in subtype M5.
- Gingival hypertrophy and skin lesions are features of subtypes M4 and M5.
- When the circulating white cell count is very high, leucostasis may occur, resulting in hyperviscosity symptoms.

Investigations
- Normochromic normocytic anaemia with low reticulocyte count.
- High white cell count due to circulating blasts; neutropenia may be present.
- Blasts may contain Auer rods (diagnostic of AML).
- Thrombocytopenia.
- Bone marrow is hypercellular and normal marrow is replaced by blast cells.
- Cytogenetic abnormalities may be present in around 50% of patients. For example, an 8 : 21 translocation is associated with a favourable outcome whereas monosomy of chromosome 5 is a poor marker.
- Urate and LDH high.
- Calcium and phosphate may also be raised.

Treatment
Treatment should be managed in a specialised unit and include:
- Supportive care as for all leukaemias (see ALL).
- Intensive cytotoxic chemotherapy (induction of remission, consolidation and maintenance). The exact regimen is determined by the subtype and most patients are in a clinical trial.
- Bone marrow transplantation in some patients.
- Immunotherapy is a growth area and gemtuzumab, an immunotoxin shows promise against AML in which CD33 is expressed.

Prognosis
- In most patients, cure/complete remission should be the aim, most patients enter remission and further therapy produces up to 25% long-term survivors.
- Poor prognostic factors include increasing age, very high white cell count, secondary leukaemia (e.g. previous myelodysplasia), certain cytogenetic

abnormalities, and the presence of disseminated intravascular coagulation (DIC).

Chronic lymphocytic leukaemia
Epidemiology and aetiology
Chronic lymphocytic leukaemia (CLL) is the most common leukaemia in the developed world (30% of all leukaemias). Its aetiology is unknown.

Pathology
- Proliferation of small lymphocytes in bone marrow, blood, and lymphoid tissues.
- These are morphologically mature but functionally abnormal.
- 95–98% of CLL patients have B cell phenotype (remainder are T cells).

Incidence and presentation
- The most common type of leukaemia in the developed world.
- Increasing incidence with age (90% of cases >50 years) and in males.
- Some patients are asymptomatic; others may describe malaise, weight loss, night sweats, recurrent infections, bleeding, or symptoms of anaemia.
- Lymphadenopathy is usually found (60%).
- Hepatosplenomegaly may also be present.

Investigations
- Monoclonal lymphocytosis with 'smear' or 'smudge' cells seen on film.
- Anaemia may be due to marrow infiltration or autoimmune haemolysis (Coombs' positive).
- Thrombocytopenia may be due to marrow infiltration or autoimmune destruction.
- Bone marrow shows accumulation of mature lymphocytes.
- Cytogenetic and immunological analysis will offer diagnostic and prognostic information.
- Hypogammaglobulinaemia in 50%.

Treatment
CLL usually follows an indolent course and traditionally watchful waiting has been the mainstay of therapy. Future more tailored therapy is likely as the molecular nature of CLL is elucidated.
- Observe only if asymptomatic mild disease.
- The oral alkylating agent chlorambucil is well tolerated especially in older patients.
- Intravenous fludarabine, an antimetabolite, is now the preferred agent.

- Autoimmune phenomena are responsive to oral prednisolone.
- Radiotherapy may be beneficial in symptomatic, localised disease.
- Splenectomy is sometimes used in refractory hypersplenism.

Prognosis

- Dependent on extent of disease (survival ranges from 1.5 years to over 12 years).
- In around 10% of CLL, Richter transformation to high-grade lymphoma occurs as a terminal event.

Chronic myeloid leukaemia

Incidence

CML accounts for 20% of all leukaemias. It can be considered as a myeloproliferative disease.

Pathology

A malignant proliferation of myeloid cells of unknown aetiology. There is a characteristic chromosome 9 : 22 reciprocal translocation—the 'Philadelphia chromosome'. The resulting fusion gene *bcr/abl* possesses tyrosine kinase activity and is believed to be pathogenic in CML.

Presentation

- Presents in middle age, most commonly between 40 and 60 years, with a male preponderance.
- Symptoms include lethargy, weight loss, sweats, and left hypochondrial discomfort (enlarging spleen).
- Symptoms of anaemia or thrombocytopenia may be present.
- On examination there is splenomegaly, which may be massive.
- Hepatomegaly is present in 50% of cases but lymphadenopathy is uncommon.
- The natural history is characterised by a chronic phase lasting several years, followed by an acute, aggressive phase similar to acute leukaemia.
- Leucostasis may occur in the acute phase.

Investigations

- High white cell count (often very high) with full range of immature and mature myeloid cells.
- Anaemia may be due to marrow infiltration or hypersplenism.
- Thrombocytosis is common.
- Bone marrow demonstrates accumulation of myeloid cells.

- 95% of patients have the Philadelphia chromosome on light microscopy. The other 5% demonstrate the fusion protein through molecular studies.
- Neutrophil alkaline phosphatase is low.
- Urate and LDH are high.
- Serum vitamin B_{12} is high.

Treatment

- Good supportive therapy as needed.
- Imatinib, a specific inhibitor of the tyrosine kinase activity of the Philadelphia chromosome has revolutionised treatment of CML. It is well tolerated and produces clinical and cytogenetic response in the majority of cases.
- Cytotoxic chemotherapy: hydroxyurea was the previous drug of choice.
- α-Interferon achieves good haematological control and reduction in the presence of the Philadelphia chromosome. It has unpleasant side effects and its role is unclear with the development of imatinib.
- Allogeneic bone marrow transplantation may be curative and should be considered in young patients with a human leucocyte antigen-matched sibling.
- Leucophoresis will reduce the white count quickly in leucostasis.

Prognosis

- Chronic phase: median time 2–6 years.
- Acute phase: median survival 3 months.
- Transformation is to AML in two thirds of patients and to ALL in the remainder.

The long term results of imatinib are unknown at present.

Multiple myeloma

The three principal features of multiple myeloma are:
- Skeletal abnormalities.
- Production of a monoclonal protein.
- Accumulation of plasma cells in the bone marrow.

Incidence and aetiology

The incidence of multiple myeloma is 5 per 100 000 (1% of all malignancies, 10–15% of all haematological malignancies).

Pathology

- Neoplastic proliferation of a single clone of plasma cells (a plasma cell is a terminally differentiated B cell).
- The malignant cells secrete a monoclonal immunoglobulin or light chain and normal immunoglobulin production is suppressed. The plasma cells can form tumours called plasmacytomas.
- Osteoclast activity is increased resulting in bone reabsorption.
- AL (systemic) amyloidosis affects 10% of cases.

Presentation

- Disease mainly of the elderly with a peak incidence in the seventh decade.
- Bone pain due to osteolytic lesions and pathological fractures affect two thirds of patients.
- Recurrent infections result from impaired antibody response and hypogammaglobulinaemia.
- Symptoms of anaemia may be present.
- Examination usually reveals pallor alone.
- Splenomegaly and peripheral neuropathy can occur with amyloidosis.
- Spinal cord compression and radiculopathy can result from compression by tumour or vertebral collapse.
- Polymerisation of the monoclonal antibody occasionally results in hyperviscosity syndrome.

Investigations

- Normochromic normocytic anaemia.
- Rouleaux (RBCs sticking together) and background immunoglobulin staining may be seen on the blood film.
- ESR: usually high.
- Serum protein electrophoresis demonstrates a monoclonal paraprotein. In 60% it is IgG and 25% IgA. 15% have no serum paraprotein.
- Bence-Jones protein may be found in the urine. It is immunoglobulin light chain and accounts for the 15% of myeloma with no serum paraprotein.
- Skeletal survey reveals generalised osteopenia, 'punched-out' lytic lesions ('pepperpot skull'), and pathological fractures. A radionuclide bone

scan is not helpful as it detects osteoblastic activity.
- Bone marrow aspirate shows over 10% of bone marrow cells are plasma cells. Cytogenetic analysis is increasingly helpful for prognosis.
- Calcium high (increased osteoclastic activity), alkaline phosphatase is usually normal.
- Urate high.
- Renal failure may result from a number of factors (Fig. 34.9).
- β_2-microglobulin level usually high.

Treatment

- Observation only in asymptomatic, uncomplicated disease.
- Supportive treatment with antibiotics, blood products, analgesics, and correction of hypercalcaemia where necessary.
- Vincristine, adriamycin and dexamethasone is the chemotherapy of choice in younger patients. Melphalan and prednisolone usually control symptoms and reduce tumour burden.
- Other combination cytotoxic chemotherapy can be used in refractory disease.
- High-dose chemotherapy with autologous stem cell rescue can lead to durable remission though not cure.
- Allogeneic transplantation may be curable but has a high mortality. It is an option for younger patients after proper discussion of the risks.
- Radiotherapy may be useful where there is localised disease causing bony pain.
- Interferon, thalidomide and other immunotherapy may be used by specialists in certain cases.

Prognosis

- Median survival is 3 years.
- Poor prognostic factors include high β_2-microglobulin levels (most accurate), high

Causes of renal failure in multiple myeloma
• Hypercalcaemia
• Hyperuricaemia
• Precipitated light chains
• Amyloidosis
• NSAIDs prescribed for bone pain

Fig. 34.9 Causes of renal failure in multiple myeloma. (NSAID, non-steroidal anti-inflammatory drug.)

paraprotein levels, high urea, low haemoglobin, increasing age, and low albumin.

Note that a monoclonal gammopathy may be present in the absence of myeloma in monoclonal gammopathy of uncertain significance. These patients should be monitored under long-term review as progression to malignant disease may occur.

Malignant lymphomas

Malignant lymphomas are neoplastic proliferations of lymphocytes which form solid tumours within lymphoid tissue. They are split into two broad categories on the basis of histological findings: Hodgkin's disease [Reed–Sternberg (RS) cells present] and non-Hodgkin's lymphoma (all others).

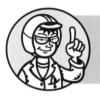

Pel-Ebstein fever is a periodic pyrexia associated with Hodgkin's lymphoma

Hodgkin's disease
Incidence and aetiology
The incidence of Hodgkin's disease (HD) is 5 per 100 000 (one of the most common malignancies in young adults). Its aetiology is unknown but there is a definite if unclear link with Epstein–Barr virus (EBV).

Pathology
- Characteristic RS cells in a background of inflammatory infiltrate.
- RS cells are large bi- or multinucleated cells with prominent 'owl-eyed' nucleoli.
- HD is divided using the Rye classification into four histological subgroups (Fig. 34.10).

Presentation
- Bimodal age at presentation with peaks at 20–29 years and above 50 years with a male preponderance in childhood HD.
- Principally affects white populations and is more common in higher socioeconomic groups.
- Symptoms are due to painless lymph node enlargement (particularly cervical, axillary, and mediastinal) and/or 'B symptoms' (Fig. 34.11).

The Rye classification of Hodgkin's disease		
Subtype	**Percentage**	**Prognosis**
Lymphocyte predominant	10	Excellent
Mixed cellularity	30	Intermediate
Lymphocyte depleted	< 5	Poor
Nodular sclerosis	60	Variable

Fig. 34.10 The Rye classification of Hodgkin's disease.

- Lymphadenopathy is supradiaphragmatic in 90% of patients and mediastinal disease may cause dry cough and exertional dyspnoea.
- Some patients describe pruritus and alcohol-induced lymph node pain.
- Affected lymph nodes feel rubbery and are non tender.
- Pallor and hepatosplenomegaly may also be found on examination.

Investigations
- The diagnosis is usually made on lymph node biopsy; staging of disease is then performed to determine the extent of disease and is central to planning appropriate treatment (Fig. 34.12).
- Normochromic normocytic anaemia, neutrophilia, eosinophilia, and thrombocytosis.
- Alkaline phosphatase raised (serum Ca^{2+} may be high).
- LDH raised in bulky disease (prognostic indicator and marker of disease activity).
- Urate high.
- ESR may be raised.
- Chest X-ray: mediastinal lymphadenopathy.
- Computed tomography (CT) scan of the thorax, abdomen and pelvis to stage the extent of the disease.
- Bone marrow examination in some patients usually shows reactive marrow only. If HD present

'B symptoms'
• Weight loss >10% of initial weight over previous 6 months • Drenching night sweats • Fever >38°C

Fig. 34.11 'B symptoms'.

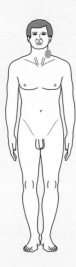

Stage I
One lymph node site only

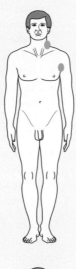

Stage II
Two lymph node sites, but on the same side of the diaphragm

Stage III
Lymph node involvement on both sides of the diaphragm

Stage IV
Disseminated disease involving one or more extralymphatic organs

Fig. 34.12 Ann Arbor staging of malignant lymphomas. Diagram shows stages I to IV. When you stage a patient you give a number (I–IV) and a letter (A or B). The letter A denotes the absence of B symptoms and B denotes the presence of B symptoms. For example, patients at stage IIA have stage II lymphoma without B symptoms.

in bone marrow then it demonstrates stage IV disease automatically.

- Staging laparotomy with splenectomy, formerly performed for early stage disease, is now almost never necessary.

Treatment

- Localised disease (stage IA–IIA): radiotherapy often with chemotherapy.
- Stage IIB–IIIA: treatment is uncertain (i.e how best to combine radiotherapy and chemotherapy).
- Extensive disease (stage IIIB–IVB): chemotherapy with ABVD (doxorubicin, bleomycin, vincristine and daunorubicin) is the accepted standard, having replaced MOPP (mustine, oncovin, procarbazine, and prednisolone).

- Relapse after radiotherapy: chemotherapy as above.
- Relapse after chemotherapy: alternative chemotherapy regimen, high-dose chemotherapy with autologous bone marrow or stem cell transplant in selected patients.

Prognosis

The outlook for the predominantly young patients is good and a positive outcome should be expected.

- Overall 5-year survival is 75% but this is greatly affected by histological type and stage of disease at presentation. Treated stage IA and IIA disease has a 10-year survival of over 80%. Even advanced disease has 5-year survival rates of 50%.

- Poor prognostic indicators include B symptoms, high stage, lymphocyte depleted histology, increasing age, high ESR, and high LDH.

Non-Hodgkin's lymphomas
Incidence and aetiology
Non-Hodgkin's lymphomas (NHL) account for 4% of all cancers, and the incidence is increasing for reasons which are unknown. Incidence increases with age (uncommon before 40 years, median age is 50 years) and the condition is more common in males. The aetiology is probably multifactorial including:

- Genetic predisposition.
- Immunosuppression (e.g. HIV infection, transplant recipients).
- Viruses (e.g. EBV, particularly Burkitt's lymphoma).
- Ionising radiation (e.g. survivors of the atomic bomb).

Pathology
- Neoplastic proliferation of B (usually) or T lymphocytes within the lymphoid system forming solid tumours which do not have RS cells.
- Heterogeneous group of conditions with many different subtypes.
- A number of different classification schemes have been developed in an attempt to identify groups of patients with similar clinical, histological, and genetic features. The most recent scheme is called the REAL (Revised European American Lymphoma) classification.
- In practical terms, NHL can be broadly divided into two groups: B or T cell lymphomas or low-grade NHL and high-grade NHL.

Presentation
- Usually presents with painless lymphadenopathy or 'B' symptoms.
- May also involve extranodal sites including skin, lung, bowel, CNS, and bone.
- Low-grade NHL has an indolent course but is not curable; high-grade NHL presents aggressively but may be cured in up to 40% of patients.
- Lymphadenopathy, hepatosplenomegaly, pallor, and involvement of extranodal sites should be looked for on examination.

Investigations
- The diagnosis is usually made on lymph node biopsy; staging investigations should then be performed to determine the extent of disease using the Ann Arbor system (Fig. 34.12).
- Circulating lymphoma cells are sometimes seen on the peripheral film.
- LDH high in bulk disease.
- Urate high.
- Paraproteinaemia and immunoparesis may be found.
- Bone marrow may be infiltrated by lymphoma cells and may cause bone marrow failure.
- Lumbar puncture as central nervous system involvement can occur.
- CT scan of the thorax, abdomen and pelvis: will determine the stage of the disease.

Cytogenetic analysis for chromosomal rearrangement and immunohistochemistry is becoming more important to provide information on both classification and also prognosis.

Treatment
Low-grade NHL
- Asymptomatic: observation only.
- Localised disease: radiotherapy.
- Symptomatic or progressive disease: oral chemotherapy (chlorambucil or cyclophosphamide).
- Combination chemotherapy can be given in refractory disease.

High-grade NHL
- Localised lesion: radiotherapy.
- Most patients require cytotoxic chemotherapy; CHOP (cyclophosphamide, doxorubicin, vincristine and prednisolone) is the gold standard.
- High-dose chemotherapy with autologous bone marrow transplantation should be considered in young, fit patients.

Rituximab is a monoclonal antibody against the B cell surface antigen CD20. It has proved highly effective against B cell NHL and its use is likely to increase and the list of indications widen.

Prognosis
- Low-grade NHL: median survival is around 8–10 years.
- High-grade NHL: 40% 5-year survival.
- Poor prognostic factors include increasing age, high LDH, extensive disease, T cell phenotype, certain extranodal sites, poor performance status, and low-grade NHL that has transformed into high-grade NHL.

Bleeding disorders

An increased tendency to bleeding can result from abnormalities of platelets, the coagulation pathway, or of blood vessels. The differential diagnosis, clinical findings, and investigation of these disorders are discussed in detail in Chapter 24. Specific conditions and their management are considered here.

Haemophilia A

Incidence and aetiology

Haemophilia A affects 1 in 8000 males. As an X-linked recessive inherited condition it affects only males.

Pathology

Decreased plasma factor VIII activity. It is classified as mild, moderate and severe depending on plasma levels (i.e. <1%, from 1–5% or >5%, respectively).

Presentation

- Severity of bleeding correlates with level of factor VIII activity (lower levels correspond to more severe symptoms).
- Bleeding may be spontaneous or secondary to trauma.
- Recurrent haemarthroses and intramuscular haematomas cause long-term disability due to arthopathy and contractures.
- Haematuria and intracranial bleeding may also occur.
- Bleeding from small cuts is usually minor (due to normal platelet function) but easy bruising occurs and bleeding following surgery may be fatal.
- After trauma, bleeding may be delayed as initial haemostasis is maintained by platelets.
- Gastrointestinal bleeding is uncommon.

Investigations

- APTT: prolonged.
- PTT: normal.
- TT: normal.
- Bleeding time: normal.
- Factor VIII assay: low.

Treatment

- Usually managed in specialised haemophilia centres.
- When there is bleeding or the patient requires surgery, factor VIII levels can be increased in two ways – mild haemophilia with desmopressin (DDAVP); moderate or severe haemophilia with recombinant factor VIII concentrates.
- Other aspects of management include analgesia (avoiding aspirin), joint replacement, synovectomy for arthropathy, regular dental care, and psychosocial and genetic support.

Prognosis

Life expectancy should be normal with current therapies.

Complications

Previously the complications of receiving factor VIII concentrates included exposure to HIV, hepatitis B and C as it was derived from donated blood. This is much reduced with recombinant factor VIII. The development of inhibitors to infused factor VIII results in a much worse prognosis.

Haemophilia B (Christmas disease)

Incidence and aetiology

Incidence is 1 per 30 000. It is also an X-linked recessive inherited condition.

Pathology

Decreased plasma factor IX activity.

Presentation

Identical to haemophilia A.

Investigations

- APTT: prolonged.
- PTT: normal.
- TT: normal.
- Bleeding time: normal.
- Factor IX assay: low.

Treatment

Treatment is with factor IX concentrates (DDAVP has no effect on factor IX levels). Otherwise treatment is the same as for haemophilia A.

Prognosis

With current therapies life expectancy should be normal.

Von Willebrand's disease

Incidence and aetiology

Von Willebrand's disease (VWD) occurs in 1% of the general population. It is an inherited (autosomal dominant) condition.

Pathology

- Deficiency of von Willebrand's factor (VWF).
- VWF is a plasma protein that acts as a cofactor in platelet adherence to the subendothelium. Platelet aggregation is normal as it involves fibrinogen and different receptors. It is also binds and stabilises factor VIII.

Presentation

- Both sexes equally affected.
- Severity of disease is variable.
- Most patients present with mucosal bleeding (epistaxis, bleeding gums, gastrointestinal bleeding). This may be worse with aspirin.
- Menorrhagia and bleeding following surgery, dental extractions, trauma, and delivery are common.
- Haemarthroses and intramuscular haematomas are rare.

Investigations

- Platelets: normal in number and structure.
- APTT: prolonged (may be normal).
- PTT: normal.
- TT: normal.
- Bleeding time: prolonged.
- VWF assays: low.
- Ristocetin platelet aggregation: abnormal.

Treatment

Aspirin should be avoided. Treatment is with DDAVP, tranexamic acid or concentrates (usually cryoprecipitate or factor VIII) in haemorrhage or perioperatively.

Prognosis

Usually normal life expectancy.

Disseminated intravascular coagulation

This is a syndrome characterised by a specific haematological response to a wide range of insults.

Aetiology

DIC may be caused by:
- Malignancy: mucus-secreting adenocarcinomas, prostate, pancreatic carcinoma, acute promyelocytic leukaemia (AML–M3).
- Infection: Gram-negative septicaemia, meningococcal septicaemia, toxic shock syndrome.
- Obstetric: amniotic fluid embolism, placental abruption, eclampsia, septic abortion.
- Tissue damage: rhabdomyolysis, fat embolism, severe trauma, burns.
- Immunological: incompatible blood transfusion, drug reaction, anaphylaxis.
- Liver disease: acute fatty liver of pregnancy, fulminant liver failure.
- Others: snake bites, acute pancreatitis.

Pathology

- Initially intravascular coagulation is precipitated by release of tissue factor or procoagulant substances into the circulation from injured cells, malignant cells, or damaged endothelium.
- Microthrombi form throughout the microcirculation causing ischaemia and infarction.
- Platelets, fibrin, and clotting factors are consumed by the thrombotic process and the fibrinolytic system becomes activated; these two processes result in a tendency to bleed, and haemorrhage may be significant.

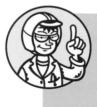

Modulation of the clotting pathway with activated protein C has shown great promise in the management of severe sepsis

Presentation

- DIC may be mild and chronic, or severe and life-threatening.
- Thrombosis can cause ischaemia or infarction in the lungs, kidneys, liver, heart, brain, or skin.
- Bleeding is often into the skin or recent venepuncture sites.
- Gastrointestinal and pulmonary haemorrhage may also occur.

Investigations

- Platelet count: low.
- PTT: prolonged.
- APTT: prolonged.
- TT: prolonged.
- Fibrinogen: low (may be normal as acute phase reactant).
- D-dimers (fibrin degradation products): high.
- Blood film: fragmented RBCs due to microangiopathic haemolysis.

Treatment

- Treatment of the underlying disease is the first priority and may resolve the DIC.
- Meticulous supportive care (e.g. fluids, antibiotics, debridement of gangrene).
- Replacement of platelets and clotting factors (using fresh frozen plasma or cryoprecipitate) may be used if there is haemorrhage or risk of haemorrhage (e.g. in surgery).
- Pharmacological inhibitors of coagulation or fibrinolysis (e.g. heparin or tranexamic acid) may be beneficial in certain circumstances but their use is controversial.

Prognosis

Mortality is 80% in severe DIC and is usually due to the underlying disease.

Thrombotic disorders

The causes of thromboembolism can be broken down by Virchow's triad:
- Changes in the vessel wall.
- Changes in the blood flow.
- Changes in the composition of the blood.

Disorders resulting in increased thrombus formation in both arteries and veins are of recent public interest with the reports of increased incidence of deep vein thrombosis after air flights, the 'economy class' syndrome.

Aetiology

Risk factors for venous thromboembolism (VTE) are outlined in Fig. 34.13.

Pathology

- Venous thrombosis can be caused by abnormal vessel walls, venous stasis, or hypercoagulable blood.
- Thrombosis may be precipitated by a specific provoking event such as surgery or a physiological state such as pregnancy.
- The lower limbs are the most common site of thrombosis.

- Small clots may break off and cause pulmonary embolus or, very rarely, cerebral infarction by paradoxical embolus in patients with a patent foramen ovale.

Presentation

- Deep vein thrombosis (DVT) causes local pain and swelling.
- The diagnosis can be difficult to make on clinical grounds.
- Pulmonary embolus (PE) causes sudden onset of pleuritic chest pain, dyspnoea, and haemoptysis.
- Inherited hypercoagulable states may present with venous thromboses without obvious precipitants, in unusual places (e.g. Budd–Chiari syndrome), at an early age or in spontaneous abortions.
- Antiphospholipid syndrome and hyperhomocysteinaemia may cause arterial as well as venous thromboses.

Investigations

- Acutely every effort should be made to confirm the diagnosis of venous thrombosis. The first step is to evaluate the pretest probability of VTE preferably via a scoring system e.g. the Well's criteria. The next is to measure the d-dimer. The third step is to perform the appropriate imaging test on the at-risk patients. This may be ultrasound, ventilation-perfusion scanning, angiography or in future magnetic resonance direct thrombus imaging.
- Careful clinical examination should be performed looking for an underlying cause such as malignancy and investigated as appropriate.
- A baseline, platelet count and clotting screen should always be performed.
- If the patient is young, ask if there have been recurrent episodes, recurrent spontaneous abortions, or a family history of thromboembolism, and consider hereditary thrombophilia. Assays are available to detect these abnormalities.

Treatment if thrombosis is proven

- Anticoagulation with low molecular weight heparin should be started. It is licensed for both DVT and PE. The lack of need for monitoring has allowed the treatment of DVT as an outpatient. The indications for unfractionated heparin are decreasing; amongst them is renal failure or mechanical heart valves.

Risk factors for venous thromboembolism		
Aetiology	Risk factor	
Inherited	Factor V Leiden mutation (Activated protein C resistance) Prothrombin 20210A mutation Antithrombin III deficiency Protein C deficiency Protein S deficency Hyperhomocysteinaemia Dysfibrinogenaemia Paroxysmal noctural Haemoglobinuria	
Acquired	Physiological	Pregnancy Childbirth Obesity Elderly
	Initiating events	Surgery Trauma Long distance travel
	Pathological	Immobility Malignancy Venous trauma Oestrogens Nephrotic syndrome Antiphospholipid syndrome Hyperviscosity syndromes

Fig. 34.13 Risk factors for venous thrombosis.

- Oral warfarin should be given simultaneously and monitored using the international normalised ratio (INR) which should be maintained between 2 and 3.
- Heparin should be continued until the INR is therapeutic. If heparin is contraindicated the hirudins (derived from leeches) may be used.

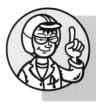 Warfarin alone is initially PROcoagulant due to its more rapid inhibition of protein C and S

In the future, ximelagatran, an oral direct thrombin inhibitor which does not require level monitoring may replace warfarin.

Treatment period
The length of time a patient should be anticoagulated is controversial and always under review, but as a general rule:
- Below knee DVT: warfarin for 3–6 months.
- Above knee DVT and PE: warfarin for 6 months.

Above knee DVTs are at increased risk of propagating along the venous system and embolising to the lungs.
- Two or more unprovoked and documented thromboses: lifelong warfarin.

Thrombotic thrombocytopenic purpura

Thrombotic thrombocytopenic purpura (TTP) is a rare disease, most common in young adults. It is a combination of signs, symptoms and characteristic blood film appearance.

Presentation
- Symptoms and signs of anaemia and bleeding.
- Neurological signs and symptoms such as lethargy, headache, confusion, seizures and hemiparesis.
- Pyrexia which is not caused by infection.

Renal impairment is rare compared with haemolytic uraemic syndrome in which renal failure is common and neurological problems rare.

Investigations

- Blood film: anaemia, reticulocytosis, thrombocytopenia and fragmented red cells (schistocytes).
- Bilirubin: increased due to haemolysis.
- LDH: elevated.
- Clotting: usually normal unless DIC.

Differential diagnosis

The differential diagnosis of microangiopathic haemolytic anaemia includes

- Haemolytic uraemic syndrome.
- TTP.
- Vasculitis.
- DIC.

Prognosis and treatment.

Plasmapheresis is the mainstay of treatment. It has vastly improved the prognosis and most people achieve a lasting response. Immunosuppression is also used.

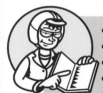

- What are 'haematinics'?
- Classify the different types of sickle cell crisis.
- What other conditions are associated with pernicious anaemia?
- How are acute and chronic leukaemias different?
- What is the prognosis from chronic lymphocytic leukaemia?
- What is the Philadelphia chromosome?
- What changes are seen on the full blood count and biochemistry in multiple myeloma?
- What is meant by 'B symptoms'?
- How does the pattern of bleeding in haemophilia differ from that in von Willebrands' disease?
- Describe five inherited conditions associated with an increased risk of venous thromboembolism?

Further reading

Bockenstedt P 2003 D-dimer in venous thromboembolism. *N Engl J Med* **349**; 1203–1204

The British Society for Haematology publishes guidelines and reviews of all aspects of haematology. They are available on its website *www.b-s-h.org.uk*.

Comprehensive but accessible review series in *Lancet* 2000 on all aspects of haematology. Vol 355 published weekly starting April 1st

Evans L S and Hancock B W 2003 Non-Hodgkin lymphoma. *Lancet* **362**; 139–146

Goldman J M and Melo J V 2003 Chronic myeloid leukemia – advances in biology and new approaches to treatment. *N Eng J Med* **349**; 1451–1464

Griffin, Arif and Mufti 2003 *Crash Course in Immunology and Haematology*, 2nd edn. Mosby

Howard M and Hamilton P 2002 *Haematology – An illustrated colour text*. Mosby

Sirohi B and Powles R 2004 Multiple myeloma. *Lancet* **363**; 875–887

Toh C H and Dennis M 2003 Disseminated intravascular coagulation: old disease, new hope. *BMJ* **327**; 924–927

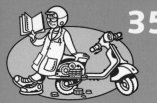

35. Infectious Diseases

Introduction

Infections affecting specific systems have been discussed in the appropriate chapters. This chapter considers three important and very different infections, human immunodeficiency virus (HIV), malaria and methicillin resistant staphylococcus aureus (MRSA).

HIV and AIDS

Epidemiology

The Department of Health states that an estimated 41 200 adults in the UK are infected with HIV, of whom 30% are unaware of the diagnosis. The World Health Organization estimates that over 40 million people worldwide are infected with HIV, more than three quarters of whom live in sub-Saharan Africa. In some countries, such as Botswana, the prevalence of HIV is approaching 40% and it is threatening the very stability of the society. The provision of drugs to these countries has become a politically contentious topic.

Aetiology

HIV-1 was first identified in 1983; it is found throughout the world and is the main cause of disease in humans.

HIV-2 is uncommon except in West Africa. The beginnings of the virus are unknown but it may have originated in central Africa. It is similar to the simian immunodeficiency virus and hence cross-species transfer has gained widespread acceptance as its origin in humans. HIV can be transmitted by sexual, parenteral, or vertical routes (Fig. 35.1).

Pathology

HIV is a lentivirus, which is a subgroup of the human retroviruses. Its genetic information is stored in a single strand of ribonucleic acid (RNA). Three specific genes produce proteins essential for HIV survival (Fig. 35.2). The virus can infect any cells expressing $CD4^+$, notably T helper cells, lymphocytes central to the immune response plus macrophages and monocytes. $CD4^+$ acts as a receptor for glycoprotein (gp120) on the virus envelope allowing the virus to enter the cell. Co-receptors such as CXCR4 and CCR5 are recognised as important and potential therapeutic targets.

The enzyme reverse transcriptase makes DNA copies of the virus RNA, which become integrated into the host cell's genome resulting in constant production of more viruses. The normal function of the infected cells is disrupted and the host cells are eventually destroyed.

Because the principal cells affected are those of the immune system, HIV infection is characterised by diseases resulting from immunodeficiency (e.g. infections and malignancies).

Presentation

There are four recognised phases of HIV infection (Fig. 35.3).

Seroconversion

Seroconversion usually occurs after 6–8 weeks incubation and severity varies significantly.

Routes of HIV transmission	
Route	**Examples**
Sexual	Vaginal intercourse, anal intercourse
Parenteral	Intravenous drug abuse, blood transfusion, needlestick injury
Vertical (i.e. from mother to fetus)	During gestation or delivery, via breast milk

Fig. 35.1 Routes of HIV transmission.

Fig. 35.2 HIV genes and the proteins they encode.

HIV genes and the proteins they encode	
Gene	Protein
Pol	Reverse transcriptase (makes DNA copies of the viral RNA) and integrase (for insertion into host DNA)
Gag	Core protein p24
Env	Encodes gp41, a transmembrane protein, and gp120, an external glycoprotein (for fusion with host cell)

Symptoms include mild 'glandular fever-type' illness, arthralgia, fever, headaches, rash, generalised lymphadenopathy, and neurological abnormalities. The illness is self-limiting and usually resolves within 8 weeks.

Asymptomatic phase

Fifty percent of untreated patients will develop the acquired immune deficiency syndrome (AIDS) after 10 years, although some will remain asymptomatic without treatment.

Generalised lymphadenopathy

Rubbery, mobile lymphadenopathy develops in multiple sites for at least 3 months prior to the onset of symptomatic disease. Biopsy shows non-specific reactive histiocytosis.

Symptomatic infection

This stage is characterised by constitutional symptoms (weight loss, diarrhoea, and fever), recurrent infections, malignancies, and neurological abnormalities (Fig. 35.4). Specific criteria (differing between the USA and Europe) for the diagnosis of AIDS exist based on CD4+ counts and the development of certain indicator diseases. Malignancies seen with increased frequency in HIV

infection are often associated with specific viral infections (Fig. 35.5).

Investigations

All investigations for HIV infection should be performed under the strictest of confidentiality. The diagnosis has immense social, financial, health, and psychological implications; counselling prior to testing is very important.

The presence of HIV infection can be assessed by the measurement of viral antigens, HIV RNA detection, the immune response to the infection (anti-HIV antibodies) or the effects of the infection (CD4+ count). Figure 35.6 summarises the findings at the different stages.

In practice, the diagnosis is usually made using HIV antibody tests. Several different methods of detection are now commercially available. If a result is positive, the test should be repeated using a different method. If that is also positive, a further serum sample should be taken and the tests repeated before the diagnosis is confirmed. In this way, false positive results are reduced to a minimum.

Note that HIV antibodies may be undetectable for up to 3 months after infection and that this is a window for false negative results.

Once the diagnosis is reached the disease activity should be assessed. This is done by quantifying both HIV RNA viral load and CD4+ cell count. The higher the viral load and the lower the CD4+ count, the worse the prognosis as the more rapid is the likely progression from HIV to AIDS. These two indicators are also used to follow the response to drug therapy.

Anaemia, thrombocytopenia, and raised β_2-microglobulin levels also correlate with disease progression.

Treatment

The treatment of HIV has changed hugely in the last ten years. HIV is not curable but the advent of highly

Phases of HIV infection	
Phase	Features
I	Seroconversion
II	Asymptomatic phase
III	Persistent generalised lymphadenopathy
IV	Symptomatic infection including AIDS

Fig. 35.3 Phases of HIV infection.

	Features of symptomatic HIV infection	
Organ/System	**Feature**	**Example**
Mouth	Infection	Candida, abscesses, gingivitis
	Premalignant	Oral hairy leukoplakia
	Malignant	**Kaposi's sarcoma**
	Others	Aphthous ulceration
Gastro-intestinal	Infection	Oesophagitis (**candida, herpes simplex (HSV), cytomegalovirus (CMV)**) Liver disease (mycobacteria, hepatitis B, CMV, microsporidia). Biliary disease (CMV, cryptosporidium, microsporidia) Colitis (Campylobacter, Salmonella, Shigella, Cryptosporidium, Giardia, CMV)
	Malignancy	**Kaposi's sarcoma**, lymphoma
	HIV - related	Enteropathy, gastropathy, malabsorption, diarrhoea **HIV wasting syndrome "Slim disease"**
Cardiovascular	HIV - related	Pericardial effusions, conduction abnormalities, dilated cardiomyopathy, pulmonary hypertension.
	Infection	Marantic endocarditis.
Respiratory	Infection	**Pneumocystis carinii pneumonia** Bacterial pneumonia **(recurrent)** Mycobacterium tuberculosis **(disseminated)** Mycobacterium avium intracellulare Fungal pneumonia (Aspergillus, Histoplasmosis **(disseminated)**)
	Malignancy	**Kaposi's sarcoma**, lymphoma
Neurological	Infection	**Toxoplasmosis** (abscess and encephalitis) **Cryptococcal meningitis** **CMV** (encephalitis, transverse myelitis) Herpes simplex(HSV), varicella zoster abscesses (VZV) and tuberculosis
	Malignancy	**Cerebral lymphoma**
	HIV-related	**Encephalopathy (HIV dementia)** **Progressive multifocal leukoencephalopathy** meningitis, myelopathy, peripheral neuropathy, inflammatory demyelinating polyneuropathy
Renal	HIV-related	HIV associated nephropathy (HIVAN) -more common in black people, males and intravenous drug users -severe nephrotic syndrome with characteristic FSGS
Haematological	Infection	Recurrent bacteraemia
	Malignancy	**Non-Hodgkin's lymphoma**
	HIV-related	Anaemia, leucopenia, thrombocytopenia.
Dermatological	Infection	Viral (HSV (severe),VZV (causing shingles molluscum contagiosum) Bacterial Fungal (candida, tinea) Scabies - contagious Norwegian scabies
	Malignancy	**Kaposi's sarcoma** Basal cell carcinoma Squamous cell carcinoma
	Others	Seborrhoeic dermatitis Psoriasis
Eyes	Infection	Retinitis (**CMV**, herpes, toxoplasma).
Musculoskeletal	HIV-related	Arthropathy

Fig. 35.4 Features of symptomatic HIV infection. AIDS defining illnesses are shown in bold.

Malignancies seen with increased frequency and associated viruses

Tumour	Associated virus
Kaposi's sarcoma	Human herpesvirus 8
Cerebral lymphoma	Epstein–Barr virus
Non-Hodgkin's lymphoma	Epstein–Barr virus
Hodgkin's disease	Not determined
Cervical carcinoma	Human papillomavirus
Anal carcinoma	Human papillomavirus

Fig. 35.5 Malignancies seen with increased frequency and associated viruses.

active anti-retroviral therapy (HAART) has changed the disease from one to die from, to one to live with. Many patients with AIDS have made remarkable recoveries in their health. The aim is to reduce viral load to as low as possible and raise $CD4^+$ counts. HAART involves the use of several drugs from different classes in order to reduce the development of resistant viral strains and to maximise the treatment response. In contrast to the pre HAART era, drug therapy is begun early in the disease process. The three common classes are:

- Nucleoside analogue reverse transcriptase inhibitors (e.g. zidovudine and didanosine).
- Non-nucleoside analogue reverse transcriptase inhibitors (e.g. efavirenz and nevirapine).
- Protease inhibitors (e.g. indinavir and saquinavir).

Treatment should be under HIV specialists and the exact regime varies from person to person. The legion of potential side effects and interactions from these drugs provides another reason for specialist care.

Figure 35.7 shows the sites of action of the HIV drugs. Two new treatment targets are integrase inhibitors and fusion inhibitors of which enfuvirtide is a recently launched example.

Because HIV treatment has improved so the management of HIV associated infections and malignancy has diminished and changed. Infections seen in HIV are shown in Fig. 35.8. HIV is partly responsible for the slight increase in notification of tuberculosis in the UK since 1990. The most well known HIV malignancy is Kaposi's sarcoma. Treatment includes HAART, local chemotherapy, interferon or cryotherapy. Systemic therapy is with liposomal doxorubicin.

Prevention

Despite HAART, there is no 'cure' for HIV infection; therefore, preventative measures must remain the highest priority. Such measures include education, the provision of clean needles for intravenous drug abusers, the use of condoms, the screening of blood products and organs donated for transplantation, and avoidance of breastfeeding in HIV-positive mothers. At present, a vaccine is not likely in the near future.

Prognosis

This is strongly related to viral load and $CD4^+$ count. Untreated patients with a $CD4^+$ count <50 per µl have a 90% three year mortality whilst it is only 25% if the count is >250 per µl. The long-term prognosis in people who respond well to HAART with high $CD4^+$ counts and unrecordable viral loads is not known but many are asymptomatic and living normal lives more than 10–15 years post diagnosis.

Investigation at different stages of HIV infection

Phase	Viral replication	p24	HIV antibodies	$CD4^+$ count
Seroconversion	High	Detectable until HIV antibodies appear	Detectable 3 weeks to 3 months after exposure	Transient fall due to high viral load, but returns to normal when HIV antibodies appear
Asymptomatic phase	Low	Undetectable as antibody in excess to antigen	Detectable	Normal
Symptomatic phase	High	Detectable	Detectable	Falls; when $<200 \times 10^6$/L risk of infection is very high and development of AIDS is likely

Fig. 35.6 Investigation at different stages of HIV infection.

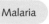

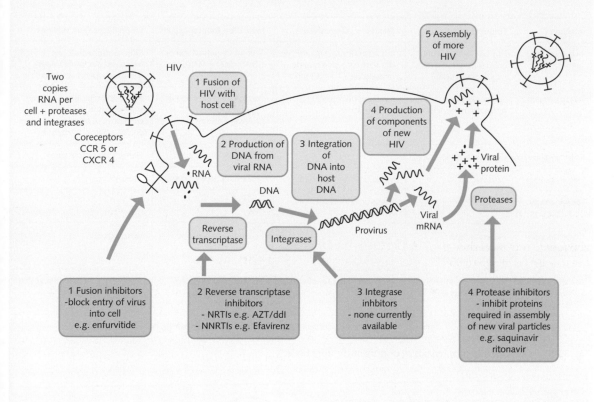

Fig. 35.7 Site of action of HIV drugs. (NRTIs, nucleoside reverse transcriptase inhibitors; NNRTIs, non-nucleoside reverse transcriptase inhibitors; AZT, zidovudine; ddI, didanosine.)

Malaria

Epidemiology

Worldwide, malaria affects over 200 million people and causes 2 million deaths each year. It is endemic in the tropics and subtropics. It is seen in temperate zones when imported by people who have visited or come from endemic areas. In the UK, approximately 2000 cases are notified each year.

Aetiology

The disease is caused by protozoal infection with one of the species of the genus *Plasmodium* (*P. vivax*, *P. ovale*, *P. malariae*, or *P. falciparum*).

Pathology

Malaria is spread from an infected person to a non-infected person by sporozoites from the bite of a female Anopheles mosquito. The sporozoites multiply in hepatocytes leading to thousands of merozoites that then invade red blood cells. At schizogony, the red blood cell bursts, releasing malaria parasites, malaria antigen, haemoglobin, cytokines, especially tumour necrosis factor and other constituents of the red blood cells, into the blood stream causing the typical clinical picture.

This occurs every 72 hours in *P. malariae* (quartan malaria), every 48–72 hours in *P. vivax* and *P. ovale* (tertian malaria) and every 48 hours in *P. falciparum* (subtertian malaria). *Plasmodium vivax*, *P. ovale*, and *P. malariae* invade up to 2% of the circulating red blood cells. *Plasmodium falciparum* may affect over 10% of cells, producing a potentially life-threatening illness.

Fig. 35.9 demonstrates the life cycle of malaria.

Presentation

Malaria is characterised by periodic high fevers, sweating, and rigors, which coincide with schizogony. Suspect it in all people returning from a malarial

Treatment and prophylaxis of opportunistic infections				
Infection	Treatment	Treatment alternatives	Indication for prophylaxis	Prophylactic drug regimes
Pneumocystis carinii	High-dose intravenous cotrimoxazole. Steroids may be beneficial	Intravenous pentamidine, or clindamycin + primaquine, or dapsone + trimethoprim	Secondary prevention or CD4+ <200 × 10⁶/L	Oral cotrimoxazole, or nebulized pentamidine, or dapsone + pyrimethamine
Toxoplasmosis	Sulphadiazine + pyrimethamine + folate	Clindamycin replacing sulphadiazine	Secondary prevention or CD4+ <200 × 10⁶/L positive serology	Pyrimethamine + sulphadiazine, or clindamycin, or cotrimoxazole, or dapsone
Cytomegalovirus	Ganciclovir or foscarnet	—	Secondary prevention	Ganciclovir or foscarnet
Herpes simplex	Aciclovir	Valaciclovir or foscarnet	Secondary prevention	Aciclovir
Herpes zoster	Aciclovir	Valaciclovir or foscarnet or famciclovir	—	—
Cryptococcal meningitis	Fluconazole or amphotericin B and/ or flucytosine	—	Secondary prevention	Fluconazole
Mycobacterium avium-intracellulare	Rifampicin + ethambutol + clarithromycin	Rifabutin replacing rifampicin	Secondary prevention	Azithromycin or clarithromycin
Candida	Fluconazole	Ketoconazole or itraconazole	Secondary prevention	Fluconazole

Fig. 35.8 Treatment and prophylaxis of opportunistic infections.

area. Nausea, vomiting, abdominal pain, headache, cough, and arthralgia may also be present. Splenomegaly is commonly found but mild icterus and massive hepatomegaly may also be present. Fig. 35.10 summarises the complications of *P. falciparum* malaria.

Malaria prophylaxis does not offer 100% protection

Investigations
- Thin and thick blood films : thick films allow parasites to be identified, thin films are useful in species identification. Degree of parasitaemia is important. Repeat films may be needed.
- Anaemia and leucocytosis may occur. Thrombocytopenia is common.
- Urea and electrolytes: renal failure.
- C reactive protein: normally raised.
- Coagulopathy: may be a feature of *P. falciparum* infection.
- Liver function tests: including raised bilirubin (from haemolysis) often become abnormal.
- Hyponatraemia: *P. falciparum*.
- Hypoglycaemia may be seen in severe cases.

Treatment
The treatment of malaria is under constant review as resistant strains develop. Up-to-date information

regarding prophylaxis and treatment of malaria should be obtained from local infectious disease centres.

Acute therapy
Management of the acute episode includes:
- Supportive care as appropriate; severe cases should be managed in a critical care setting.
- Chloroquine for *P. vivax, P. ovale*, and *P. malaria*.
- Quinine (intravenous if severe) and fansidar for *P. falciparum* as most cases are chloroquine resistant; mefloquine (lariam), proguanil/ atovaquone (malarone) or halofantrine can also be used.
- Exchange transfusion may be useful when there is a high level of parasitaemia.

Eradication therapy
The eradication of liver parasites to prevent future relapse:

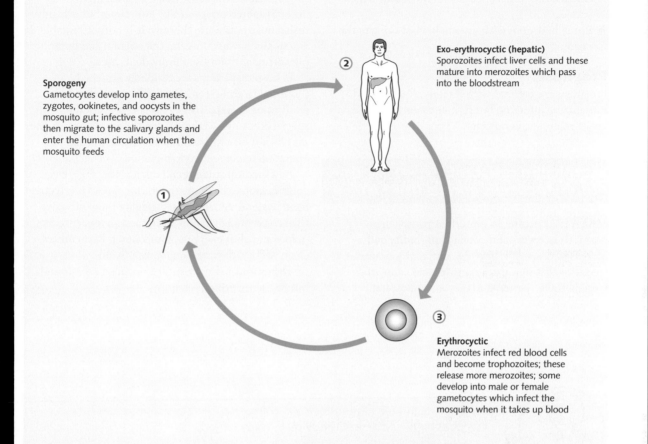

Sporogeny
Gametocytes develop into gametes, zygotes, ookinetes, and oocysts in the mosquito gut; infective sporozoites then migrate to the salivary glands and enter the human circulation when the mosquito feeds

Exo-erythrocyctic (hepatic)
Sporozoites infect liver cells and these mature into merozoites which pass into the bloodstream

Erythrocyctic
Merozoites infect red blood cells and become trophozoites; these release more merozoites; some develop into male or female gametocytes which infect the mosquito when it takes up blood

Fig. 35.9 The malaria transmission cycle.

- Is necessary in *P. ovale* and *P. vivax*.
- Primaquine is used. Consider testing for glucose-6-phosphate dehydrogenase deficiency prior to commencing treatment.

Complications of infection by *Plasmodium falciparum*

- Cerebral malaria (hyperpyrexia, coma, death)
- Hypoglycaemia
- Acute respiratory distress syndrome
- Seizures
- Severe intravascular haemolysis with haemoglobinuria ('blackwater fever')
- Acute renal failure
- Hepatic necrosis
- Jaundice
- Haemolytic anaemia
- Lactic acidosis
- Coagulopathy (including DIC)

Fig. 35.10 Complications of infection with *Plasmodium falciparum*.

Prevention

With the emergence of resistant organisms, the avoidance of mosquito bites and mosquito control take on greater importance.

Chemoprophylaxis

For chemoprophylaxis, refer to up-to-date information (e.g. the British National Formulary or the London School of Hygiene and Tropical Medicine). It should be started 1 week prior to travel and continued for at least 4 weeks after return.

Medications used include chloroquine, malarone, mefloquine and doxycycline. All have side effects and the risks and benefits should be made available to patients.

Avoidance of mosquito bites

- Mosquito nets and repellents.
- Wear appropriate clothing, particularly long-sleeves and trousers around dawn and dusk, which

is when the female Anopheles mosquito is most active.

- Spray bedroom with insecticide last thing in the evening.

Prognosis

Prognosis is excellent with *P. vivax*, *P. ovale*, and *P. malariae* infection but *P. falciparum* is still a life-threatening condition.

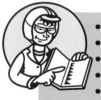

Methicillin resistant *Staphylococcus aureus* (MRSA)

MRSA has become an important pathogen in hospitals in terms of mortality, morbidity and increased costs. It is also the source of sometimes sensationalist newspaper articles and cause of trepidation to patients as they enter hospital.

It results in the same range of presentations as other *Staphylococcus aureus* infections but is highly resistant to antibiotic therapy. It is not untreatable. It is sensitive to vancomycin, teicoplanin and linezolid plus other antibiotics in individual cases.

In hospital patients are routinely screened (nose/axilla/groin) for MRSA. Those positive have eradication therapy, barrier nursing if needed and special precautions taken in certain situations (e.g. they may be last on a theatre list so it can be cleaned post operation to prevent contamination of other patients).

As a medical student and doctor, the single biggest contribution to be made to limiting spread is effective hand hygiene. Alcohol based gels are more effective than conventional handwashing and are easier to use before and after every patient contact. Remember to clean your stethoscope regularly as well!

Other multi-drug resistant organisms are found but the same principles apply.

- How does the human immunodeficiency virus cause disease in humans?
- What does highly active antiretroviral therapy mean?
- In malaria what may the full blood count and blood film show?
- What methods of prevention should you advise in a malarial area?
- Name two antibiotics to which MRSA is sensitive?

Further reading

The British HIV Association publishes guidelines and reviews on HIV. They are available on its website *www.bhiva.org*.

The British Society for Antimicrobial Chemotherapy has information about MRSA and other bacterial infections encountered. It can be viewed on its website *www.bsac.org.uk*.

Girou E, Loyeau S, Legrand P et al 2002 Efficacy of handrubbing with alcohol based solution versus standard handwashing with antiseptic soap: randomised clinical trial. *BMJ* **325**: 362–366

Information on tropical medicine can be obtained from the London School of Hygiene and Tropical Medicine at its website www.lshtm.ac.uk.

Kilby J M and Eron J J 2003 Novel therapies based on mechanisms of HIV-1 cell entry – Review article. *N Engl J Med* **348**: 2228–2238

Murray H W, Pepin J, Nutman T B et al 2000 Recent advances in tropical medicine. *BMJ* **320**: 490–94

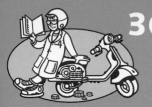

36. Drug Overdose

Epidemiology

Drug overdose results in 10% of all acute hospital admissions and 4.7% of all hospital admissions in 12–20-year-olds.

Aetiology

Overdose may be due to the following:
- Accidental: particularly in children.
- Deliberate: self-administration in suicide or parasuicide, homicide, or child abuse (e.g. Munchausen's by proxy).
- Iatrogenic: uncommon (e.g. interacting drugs).

Presentation

History

Drug overdose in many patients may result in a mild illness requiring little intervention. However, some patients take many tablets or cocktails of drugs causing a life-threatening state requiring intensive care and may be fatal. Around 80% of patients are conscious and able to provide a history. In all patients, particularly the unconscious, make every effort to talk to family, friends, and the ambulance staff. Always consider overdose in any unconscious patient. Where possible, try to establish the following facts.

What drugs were taken and when?

It is very common for more than one drug to be taken, and alcohol is often also used. Try to establish which tablets were taken, how many and how long ago to establish the likely ongoing risk. However, it is good policy to treat the patient and not the history as this may be unreliable.

Try to assess the suicidal risk

Have they taken an overdose before? What events led to the overdose? Did the patient intend suicide at the time or was it a reaction to acute stress such as an argument? Was the act premeditated (e.g. were tablets collected over a period of time, was a suicide note left, were the tablets taken when the patient expected to be alone for a while)? What did they do after taking the tablets—did they ring for their partner or ambulance immediately? Does the patient feel suicidal now? Would they do it again?

Figure 36.1 summarises features indicating a high suicidal risk.

Examination

The examination should be in three stages: assess how ill the patient is, look for evidence to suggest the likely drug(s) involved, and look for complications of overdose.

How ill is the patient?

The first priority is ABC—ensure the patient has an adequate Airway, Breathing (respiration) and Circulation. Assessment of coma scale, pulse, blood pressure, temperature, and BM (glucose estimation) should then be made.

Is there any evidence to suggest underlying cause?

Relatives or ambulance staff may have brought bottles from the scene. Look for evidence on the patient such as diabetic cards or hospital appointment cards (e.g. it may be an insulin overdose). Also look for:
- Pinpoint pupils: opiates, organophosphates.
- Dilated pupils: tricyclic antidepressants, amphetamines, cocaine.
- Nystagmus: phenytoin, alcohol.
- Papilloedema: carbon monoxide.
- Burns around the mouth: corrosives.
- Hyperventilation: aspirin.

Features indicating a high suicide risk
• Elderly
• Male
• Previous suicide attempts
• Unemployed
• Socially isolated (single, living alone)
• Chronic debilitating illness (psychiatric or physical)
• Drug or alcohol abuse

Fig. 36.1   Features indicating a high suicide risk.

- Hypothermia: chlorpromazine.
- Needle marks: opiates, benzodiazepines, stimulants.

Have any complications occurred?
Figure 36.2 summarises complications of drug overdose. Note that a low-reading thermometer can be used to detect hypothermia.

Investigations

- Paracetamol and salicylate levels should be measured in all patients.
- Urea and electrolytes, blood glucose, serum osmolarity.
- Baseline clotting and liver function tests in paracetamol overdose.
- Drug levels can be measured in the blood, gastric contents, and urine, but this is not necessary in the majority of patients.
- Electrocardiogram: if clinically indicated (e.g. arrhythmia).
- Chest X-ray: if evidence of aspiration.

Management

The management of drug overdose can be divided into three parts: general measures for all patients, specific measures according to the drug taken, and psychiatric assessment and social input when the patient recovers physically.

General approach
Supportive care
- If unconscious, clear airway and give oxygen via a face-mask.
- If no gag reflex, call anaesthetist as the patient may need endotracheal intubation.

Complications of drug overdose
• Coma
• Respiratory depression
• Hypotension or hypertension
• Arrhythmias
• Seizures
• Head injury
• Hypothermia or hyperthermia
• Aspiration pneumonia
• Rhabdomyolysis
• Gastric stress ulceration

Fig. 36.2 Complications of drug overdose.

- Some patients may require assisted ventilation.
- Gain intravenous access, keep patient with head downwards, and give i.v. fluids for hypotension unless there is cardiogenic shock (central venous pressure monitoring may be necessary).
- Nurse semiprone and measure observations regularly – some patients who walk into A&E may deteriorate rapidly.
- Attach cardiac monitor if arrhythmia is suspected or the patient is known to have taken tricyclic antidepressants.
- In arrhythmia, correct hypoxia, acidosis or electrolyte balance; antiarrhythmic agents should be used with caution as they can exacerbate the arrhythmia.
- Convulsions should be treated with intravenous benzodiazepines.
- Prevent gastrointestinal absorption.

Gastrointestinal absorption may be prevented by either emptying the stomach or preventing bowel absorption.

Emptying stomach
- Indications: consider gastric emptying within 4 hours for most drugs; within 6 hours after opiates and anticholinergics; within 12 hours after tricyclic antidepressants, salicylates, and aminophylline.
- Contraindications: ingestion of caustic, corrosive, or petroleum derivatives.

There are two methods of gastric emptying: induced emesis (vomiting) or gastric lavage:
- Induced emesis – syrup of ipecacuanha; particularly useful in children; should not be given if the patient is drowsy or likely to become drowsy because of the risks of aspiration; is of limited value in preventing absorption.
- Gastric lavage – used where induced emesis is refused, contraindicated, or unsuccessful (usually in the unconscious patient whose airway is protected by a cuffed endotracheal tube).

Preventing absorption in the bowel
- Activated charcoal binds poisons in the stomach preventing absorption.
- More effective the sooner it is given.
- Doses may be given every 4 hours to increase the elimination of certain drugs (aspirin, carbamazepine, phenobarbitone, quinine).
- Contraindicated in drowsy patients (risk of aspiration).

- Ineffective for iron, lithium, potassium, alcohol, and cyanide.

Increase elimination of drug

Elimination of drugs can be increased using forced alkaline diuresis or dialysis.

Forced alkaline diuresis

- Increases renal drug excretion.
- Used in severe salicylate, phenobarbitone, and amphetamine overdose.
- Can cause fatal fluid overload, electrolyte disturbance, or acid-base disturbance, and should be monitored very carefully.

Dialysis

Dialysis should be used in severe overdose when other methods are contraindicated or unsuccessful. The techniques include peritoneal or haemodialysis and haemoperfusion.

Specific antidotes

Advice for overdose of any drug or ingestion of any poisons can be obtained 24 hours a day from a number of poisons information centres. Each A&E department and hospital switchboard will have a list of national numbers.

Figure 36.3 summarises the specific management of overdose of some of the more common drugs.

Psychiatric and social assessment

Once the acute event and medical management is completed, an assessment of the patient's psychiatric state (ongoing suicidal risk) and social circumstances should be made, however trivial the overdose may have appeared. Where appropriate, psychiatrists and social care workers should be involved.

Specific measures in the management of drug overdose		
Drug	Toxic side effects	Specific management
Opiates	Respiratory depression, drowsiness or coma, pinpoint pupils, hypotension, bradycardia, hypothermia, pulmonary oedema	Naloxone 0.8–2 mg intravenously (may need to be repeated every 2–3 minutes to a maximum of 10 mg due to its short half-life); can be administered by continuous intravenous infusion
Benzodiazepines	Drowsiness, dysarthria, nystagmus, ataxia, coma, respiratory depression; fairly safe if taken alone but potentiate the effects of other sedative drugs which are often taken at the same time	Flumazenil 200 µg over 15 seconds, then 100 µg every 60 seconds until response (maximum dose 1 mg); should be used cautiously
Paracetamol	Nausea and vomiting in the first 24 hours; acute hepatocellular necrosis may develop after 3 days ith as few as 20 tablets causing jaundice, encephalopathy, hypoglycaemia and abdominal pain; renal tubular necrosis may also occur	Monitor blood pressure, prothrombin time, glucose, creatinine, pH, and for signs of encephalopathy: these parameters determine the need for specialist referral; check paracetamol levels from 4 hours onwards (treatment may begin before result is available if significant overdose suspected); use nomogram to determine whether antidote should be given if less than 24 hours since tablets were taken Give acetylcysteine (Parvolex) by intravenous infusion Oral methionine may be given instead if overdose less than 12 hours before
Aspirin	Nausea, vomiting, tinnitus, deafness, sweating, hyperventilation, tachycardia, delirium, seizures, coma, impaired clotting, hypokalaemia, hypoglycaemia, metabolic acidosis (respiratory alkalosis initially)	Correct dehydration, hypokalaemia and hypoglycaemia If plasma salicylate levels >500 mg/L (3.6 mmol/L), the patient should have forced alkaline diuresis under close supervision In severe poisoning (>700 mg/L or 5.1 mmol/L), haemodialysis may be life-saving
Iron	Usually accidental affecting children causes haemorrhagic enteritis (corrosion) with nausea, vomiting, abdominal pain, haematemesis, bloody diarrhoea, acute hepatocellular necrosis, metabolic acidosis, peritonitis, hypotension, coma	Desferrioxame by intravenous or intramuscular injection
Digoxin	Nausea, vomiting, diarrhoea, hyperkalaemia, bradyarrhythmias, tachyarrhythmias, altered colour vision, delirium	Correct electrolyte disturbance Temporary ventricular pacing in atrioventricular Block digoxin-specific antibody fragments (Digibind) in severe overdose
β-blockers	Bradycardia, hypotension, cardiac failure, convulsions, coma, asystole	Atropine intravenously for bradycardia Glucagon intravenously in severe overdose
Heparin	Haemorrhage	Intravenous protamine sulphate
Warfarin	Haemorrhage	Intravenous vitamin K, intravenous infusion of concentrates of factors II, VII, IX, and X, or fresh frozen plasma

Fig. 36.3 Specific measures in the management of drug overdose with certain of the more common drugs. (U&Es, urea and electrolytes.)

- What is the specific therapy of choice for a significant paracetamol overdose? Which parameters should be closely monitored to assess the need for transfer to a specialist unit?

Further reading
Crash Course in Pharmacology

Vale A and Bateman D N. Poisoning. *Medicine* 2003; **31:** 1–76

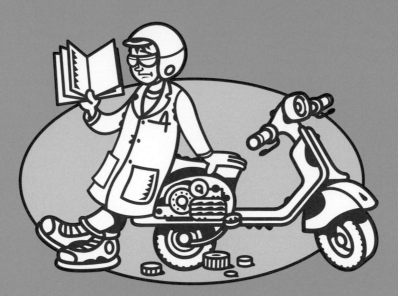

HISTORY, EXAMINATION AND COMMON INVESTIGATIONS

37. Taking a History   369

38. Examination of the Patient   379

39. The Clerking   405

40. Common Investigations   409

37. Taking a History

General principles: the bedside manner

Despite the constant progress in medical knowledge and diagnostic techniques, the history as taken from the patient remains the cornerstone of practice. From the first meeting, a patient decides whether or not they think the doctor is competent and trustworthy, based on the doctor's general manner and attitude. Mutual trust is the foundation of the good doctor–patient relationship.

There is no easy recipe for developing a good bedside manner but courtesy, patience, and letting the patient express their ideas, concerns, and expectations are essential ingredients.

Whenever you meet a patient, introduce yourself politely and do not forget relatives or friends who might also be present. Try to put the patient at ease, as visiting the doctor is very stressful for most people, particularly if they think that they have a serious illness. If you cannot speak the same language, try to get an interpreter. If a patient has hearing difficulties, sit closer, write things down or speak louder!

The aims of the history are as follows:
- To establish rapport with the patient.
- To obtain an accurate, sequential account of the patient's symptoms and create a differential diagnosis.
- To ask specific questions to focus on the most likely diagnoses.
- To determine risk factors for these possible diagnoses.
- To assess whether complications have occurred on the basis of associated symptoms.
- To put this problem or problems into the context of the patient's life.

We have outlined a standard approach to obtaining the history. However, the important thing is that you develop an approach with which you are comfortable and then practise it again and again. In this way you will not miss things out and you will be able to concentrate more on what the patient is telling you rather than what comes next.

Watch the patient closely, as facial expression and body posture can sometimes tell you more than the words themselves. If you are looking up, they will also feel that you are genuinely listening to what they are saying. It is important to strike a good balance between recording the history accurately and maintaining eye contact.

As a general principle, start the consultation by asking very open-ended questions, such as 'How are you?', 'How can I help?' or 'What symptoms have made you come to the clinic today?' This gives the patient the opportunity to say what they want. Then ask more specific questions to clarify important aspects.

As a rule, it is preferable to take the history and then write it down afterwards; it enables you to listen and appear to be listening without distraction plus you can organise your thoughts before committing them to paper. However, when you are learning it may be easier to make notes as you go along; you can also have prompts on your paper to enable you to fill in all sections. As you gain experience, you will find it easier to memorise the patient's history and write it down later.

The history

At the start of every history you should always:
- Document the date, time, and place of consultation. (Remember that the clerking is a legal document.)
- Record the age, sex, and occupation of the patient.
- Document who referred the patient and if they were seen as an emergency.

Presenting complaint

This is a sentence or short list explaining the reason the patient has seen you today. It is always written in the patient's own words: medical jargon comes later. Resist the temptation to write the entire history in this section, particularly when there are multiple symptoms; however, mentioning an obvious background condition can be helpful (e.g. 'One week increasing shortness of breath and productive cough. Known 10-year history of COPD').

History of the presenting complaint

This is where the presenting complaint is explored in great detail. It is impossible to describe a system that will work for all complaints in every situation. You will need to develop your own techniques and quirks.

- Aim to obtain a coherent, sequential chronological description of the events leading to the consultation.
- Ask the relevant questions to the symptoms e.g. for pain, where is it? What is its character?
- Keep the differential diagnoses for a symptom in your mind and seek evidence to confirm or refute them.
- Use the review of symptoms questions for the system you suspect to fill in extra detail (e.g. if the complaint is a cough, ask about dyspnoea, pain, sputum, etc., and record it in the presenting complaint).
- Ask about the relevant risk factors (e.g. if pulmonary embolus is suspected ask about immobility, travel, etc.).
- Recapitulate the history back to the patient, as this helps cement the story in your mind and reassures them you are listening.
- If the history is long, or vague, using the opening question 'So when did you last feel well?' gives a platform to begin from.
- Seek collateral history from witnesses, friends or family where necessary (e.g. after a seizure).
- With chronic complaints, it is vital to ask about how the symptoms are affecting the patient's life.

Finally, ask if they have any thoughts or worries as to what the diagnosis may be; this can be very enlightening and will help you build a good working relationship as you will be addressing their concerns. What the doctor is interested in and what the patient is interested in can be diametrically opposed.

The first section of this book 'A patient presents with' gives an idea of the variety of potential histories. The way to become skilled in history taking for both clinical practice and examinations is to try and clerk as many patients as you can with the range of listed presentations. It is important to write these up with a list of diagnoses and a plan, then practise

At the end of the history ask two questions:
- 'Is there anything else you are worried about or want to tell me?' It is possible that the patient may now feel ready to tell you about their main concern.
- 'Is there anything that you are worried this might be?' There is often visible relief when this question is asked and it enables you to address the patient's real feelings about his or her illness.

presenting to other people. Then ask yourself how you could do it better next time.

Past medical history

Ask the patient if they have had any previous operations or medical problems. It is prudent to probe a little about each illness and how the diagnosis was made. Remain sceptical about diagnoses that the patient is labelled with. Lists of past history are commonly and sometimes wrongly carried forward from one hospital visit to the next. Record the history in chronological order and, where possible, record the year, hospital and consultant involved for each episode. Many patients may forget past illnesses, particularly if anxious, and it is worth developing a routine to ask them specifically about diabetes, hypertension, angina or heart disease, rheumatic fever, tuberculosis, epilepsy, asthma/emphysema/bronchitis, jaundice, stroke, or transient ischaemic attacks.

Medications

Record which medications the patient is currently taking, how often and at what dose. If the prescribed medications are not being taken ask why. Ask if there have been any recent changes in medication. Always ask what drugs the patient has taken in the past. For example, a patient with pulmonary fibrosis as a consequence of amiodarone may well have stopped taking it years before! Finally, ask about any non prescription medications that may be obtained from a chemist or health food shop.

Allergies

Does the patient have any allergies to any medications or anything else at all, no matter how trivial? If yes, what was the exact nature of the reaction? It is worth asking about penicillin directly as many patients state they have a penicillin allergy but, on closer questioning, they may describe a non-specific symptom and a beta-lactam antibiotic can be given safely if the need is there.

If the patient says they have no allergies it is traditional to write 'no known drug allergies'.

Family history

Do any diseases 'run' in the patient's family? Record illnesses in close relatives, including age of death where relevant. Drawing a family tree can be helpful in some patients.

Social history

The importance of this part of the history is to establish how the illness affects the patient's life and how they are coping at home. Ask about:
- Who is at home? If they have a partner, are they fit and well?
- Do they have dependent children? Who is looking after them at the moment?
- What is the home like? If the patient is elderly, is there a warden?
- If the patient is disabled, have appropriate modifications been made?
- Do they need help with daily tasks, such as washing, dressing, feeding, cleaning, or shopping?
- Is there a nearby relative who helps, or does the patient have meals-on-wheels, a home help, or a district nurse?
- What is their occupation? Details of their past and present occupation can be important (e.g. industrial lung disease).
- Are they still able to work despite the current problem?
- Some diagnoses can be particularly important in relation to work, such as heavy goods vehicle drivers and epilepsy.
- Do they smoke? Smoking is a significant cause of many diseases.
- Alcohol past and present. Record as units per week (Fig. 37.1).
- Do they use 'recreational' drugs? These have health, social, and financial implications.

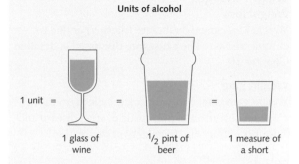

Units of alcohol

1 unit = 1 glass of wine = 1/2 pint of beer = 1 measure of a short

Fig. 37.1 Units of alcohol. These refer to standard pub measures of wine and spirits and standard strength beer.

- Have they recently been abroad? They may have been exposed to different infective agents.
- Do they have pets (particularly budgerigars, pigeons, and parrots)?
- Sexual history is not appropriate in every history but may be important (e.g. for hepatitis or HIV).

Systems review

Patients occasionally focus on one minor symptom while omitting to tell you of another more significant symptom. In fact, this can be a deliberate act, asking the doctor to deal with a simple problem (e.g. sore throat) while deciding whether to ask for help with the real worry such as impotence or chest pain. Performing a quick systems review will prevent you from missing other important diseases.

Alternatively, if the symptoms are multiple and non-specific, a review of systems can shine light on the consultation and aid a differential diagnosis.

The symptoms to ask about in each system are outlined below. This list cannot be exhaustive and some symptoms are repeated as they cross organ systems though with different emphasis.

General symptoms
Fatigue
This is a non-specific symptom which can accompany many organic as well as psychiatric diseases. Look particularly for evidence of anaemia or hypothyroidism.

Appetite
Anorexia is a feature of many diseases, again organic and psychiatric; increased appetite despite weight loss is seen in hyperthyroidism.

Weight changes
Weight loss
Weight loss can be deliberate (dieting) or due to chronic disease. The causes are discussed in detail in Chapter 10.

Weight gain
Weight gain is seen in pregnancy, hypothyroidism, Cushing's syndrome, polycystic ovarian disease and 'comfort eating' due to anxiety or depression.

Sweats
Drenching sweats occurring at night are seen in lymphoma, chronic leukaemia, and tuberculosis.

Pruritus (itching)
Pruritus can be due to local skin disease or systemic disease as shown in Fig. 37.2.

Sleep pattern
If there is difficulty in sleeping, ask if the problem is in going to sleep or in waking early. Difficulty in getting off to sleep is often due to worry or anxiety, whereas early morning wakening is a feature of depression. Sleep apnoea is common and can be debilitating as hypersomnolence limits daytime function.

Cardiovascular symptoms
Chest pain
Establish the site, radiation, character, exacerbating and relieving factors, and severity; discussed in detail in Chapter 1.

Dyspnoea
Exertional dyspnoea can be due to poor left ventricular function, pulmonary oedema, arrhythmia, or valvular disease.

Orthopnoea is breathlessness on lying flat, usually from increased pulmonary venous congestion. This symptom can be present in diaphragm palsy and even in chronic obstructive pulmonary disease, as diaphragmatic input to ventilation is less efficient when the patient is lying flat.

Paroxysmal nocturnal dyspnoea is waking during the night due to severe breathlessness (pulmonary oedema).

Sudden onset of breathlessness, irrespective of body position or exercise, is often due to arrhythmia (see Chapter 2).

Syncope
Syncope is the transient loss of consciousness and motor tone, which may be due to arrhythmia, valvular heart disease, postural hypotension, or vertebrobasilar insufficiency (Chapter 19).

Palpitations
Palpitations mean different things to different people and they should be explored carefully as they may be insignificant or they may be life threatening (see Chapter 3).

Ankle swelling
This can be due to right ventricular failure, low plasma oncotic pressure (e.g. decreased albumin levels), drugs (e.g. calcium channel blockers), or it can be gravitational.

Calf swelling
This can be due to:
- Deep vein thrombosis: recent travel, immobility or surgery, pregnancy, combined oral contraceptive pill, family history, malignancy.
- Ruptured Baker's cyst: in the elderly, secondary to osteoarthritis of the knee.
- Muscle trauma.
- Cellulitis.
- Tumour: sarcoma (rare).

Claudication
Intermittent claudication due to peripheral vascular disease causes calf, thigh, or buttock pain on exercise. The amount of exercise required to cause pain tends to be consistent although it often deteriorates slowly. It is relieved within a predictable period of time on rest.

Causes of pruritus	
Cause	**Examples**
Skin disease	Scabies, eczema, lichen planus, urticaria, dry skin (elderly, hypothyroidism)
Systemic disease	Hepatic (biliary obstruction, pregnancy) Malignancy (particularly lymphoma) Haematological (polycythaemia, iron deficiency) Chronic renal failure Drugs (sensitivity, opiates) Endocrine (diabetes mellitus, hyper/hypothyroidism, carcinoid syndrome) Parasitic (trichinosis) Neurological (multiple sclerosis) Psychogenic

Fig. 37.2 Causes of pruritus.

Spinal claudication due to spinal stenosis also causes calf, thigh, or buttock pain on exertion, possibly by causing occlusion of the spinal arteries. However, the claudication distance tends to be variable. The pain can also be brought on by prolonged standing and is also often bilateral. The pain improves with rest (though improvement takes longer with ischaemic pain) or with lumbar spine flexion (less pain on climbing hills than going downhill).

Respiratory symptoms
Dyspnoea
Clarify the degree of dyspnoea and its consequences; try and separate respiratory dyspnoea from cardiac causes though there is much overlap (see Chapter 2).

Cough
This can be a minefield for the doctor. However there are no short cuts in its evaluation (see Chapter 5).

Sputum
How much sputum is produced? There is often little sputum in bronchial carcinoma but copious amounts in bronchiectasis. Ask about its colour, texture and time course;
- Yellow: infection, acute asthma (due to eosinophils).
- Green: infection.
- Frothy: pulmonary oedema.
- Rusty: lobar pneumonia (pneumococcal).
- Blood: see Chapter 5.
- Taste: foul in bronchiectasis and abscess.
- Smell: foul in bronchiectasis.

Chest pain
Chest pain is usually pleuritic in chest disease (Chapter 1), and is often due to pneumonia, pneumothorax, and pulmonary embolus.

Wheeze
Patients with airways obstruction sometimes notice an audible expiratory wheeze.

Hoarse voice
This may be caused, for example, by recurrent laryngeal nerve palsy in bronchial carcinoma.

Sleep disordered breathing
Sleep disorders are common and cause personal and professional problems to the patient. Poor sleep causes daytime somnolence which can be disabling or potentially lethal if you fall asleep driving. The most common is obstructive sleep apnoea. Ask about snoring, whether sleep is refreshing, morning headaches and restless leg movements. The patient's partner is often the best source of information.

Gastrointestinal disease
Abdominal pain
Establish the site, radiation, character, exacerbating and relieving factors, and severity. This is discussed in detail in Chapter 12.

Dysphagia
Dysphagia means difficulty in swallowing. Ask about:
- Where do things get stuck? This may give a clue as to the site of the lesion.
- Is there difficulty with solids, fluids or both? Neuromuscular disorders tend to present with dysphagia for fluids at onset, whereas mechanical obstruction results in dysphagia for solids at onset.

The causes of dysphagia are outlined in Fig. 37.3.

Vomiting
What does the vomitus look like?
- Yellow-green: upper gastrointestinal (GI) contents plus bile.
- Brown (faeculent): lower small bowel contents.
- Bright-red blood: active upper GI bleeding (Chapter 8).
- Coffee grounds': 'old' upper GI bleeding.

How 'violent' was the vomiting? Projectile vomiting indicates pyloric stenosis, most commonly seen in infants, but may arise as a consequence of duodenal ulceration in adults.

Indigestion
'Heartburn' or 'dyspepsia' is due to reflux of the gastric contents into the oesophagus.

Bowel habit
Has there been a change? Ask about diarrhoea and constipation, or the presence of one alternating with the other. (For more on this see Chapter 9).

Rectal bleeding
Is the bleeding with or without mucus? The causes of rectal bleeding are summarised in Fig. 37.4. Anal and rectal lesions result in fresh blood on the outside of the stool, on the paper on wiping, or in the pan. Higher lesions result in blood intermixed with the

Fig. 37.3 Causes of dysphagia.

Causes of dysphagia	
Disorder	**Examples**
Oropharyngeal lesions	Stomatitis, pharyngitis, quinsy, lymphoma
Intrinsic oesophageal and gastric lesions	Peptic stricture Carcinoma of oesophagus or gastric fundus Foreign body Oesophageal web (Paterson–Brown–Kelly or plummer–Vinson syndrome) Infection (*Candida albicans*) Pharyngeal pouch Schatzki's ring (oesophagogastric junction in hiatus hernia) leiomyoma of oesophageal muscle
Extrinsic oesophageal compression	Goitre with retrosternal extension Intrathoracic tumours (lymphoma, bronchial carcinoma) Enlarged left atrium
Neuromuscular disorders	Achalasia Scleroderma Diffuse oesophageal spasm Diabetes mellitus Myasthenia gravis Myotonia dystrophica Bulbar or pseudobulbar palsy e.g. motor neurone disease or troke Diphtheria
Psychological	Globus hystericus

stool. Melaena implies upper GI bleeding and the passage of altered blood.

Tenesmus

Tenesmus is the painful desire to defecate when there is no stool in the rectum. This is due to a lesion in the lumen or wall of the rectum mimicking faeces.

Genitourinary symptoms
Dysuria

This is discomfort during or after micturition due to urinary tract infection or recent urethral instrumentation (catheter or cystoscope).

Causes of rectal bleeding
• Haemorrhoids • Anal fissure • Carcinoma (anus, rectum, or colon) • Polyps • Diverticulitis (including Meckel's diverticulum) but not diverticulosis • Colitis (infective, ulcerative, Crohn's, ischaemic) • Angiodysplasia

Fig. 37.4 Causes of rectal bleeding.

Urine

What does the urine look like?
- Cloudy: infection, precipitated urates or phosphates.
- Frothy: proteinuria.
- Orange: very concentrated urine, bilirubin, rifampicin.
- Red: haematuria, haemoglobinuria, myoglobinuria, rifampicin.
- Black: 'blackwater fever' due to *Plasmodium falciparum*.
- Dark on standing: porphyria.
- Green: drugs containing methylene blue (commercial analgesics).

See Chapter 14 for the causes of haematuria and proteinuria.

Frequency

Increased frequency of micturition can be due to:
- Bladder irritation: infection, stones, tumour.
- Outflow obstruction: prostatic hypertrophy, urethral stricture.
- Neurological: multiple sclerosis.

Note that, in polyuria, there is an increased volume of urine as well as frequency of micturition.

Nocturia
This can be due to any of the causes of polyuria (see Chapter 13) and increased frequency.

Hesitancy
Hesitancy, followed by a poor stream with terminal dribbling, are features of prostatic enlargement.

Loin pain
This can be associated with renal disease (Chapter 12).

Incontinence
This can be either urge incontinence (e.g. detrusor instability) or stress incontinence (e.g. weak pelvic musculature following childbirth). It can be functional as people with mobility problem may not be able to get to the loo quick enough.

Menstruation
Determine the pattern of the normal cycle. Then ask about flow (heavy or light), intermenstrual bleeding, post coital bleeding, or dysmenorrhoea.

Discharge
Vaginal or penile discharge can indicate infection.

Neurological symptoms
Headache
This is another problem symptom for the doctor with the diagnosis ranging from the trivial to the fatal. Stay alert for warning symptoms (see Chapter 16).

Dizziness
This can also be unsteadiness (Chapters 19 and 23).

Limb weakness, paraesthesiae and sensory loss
These are covered in detail in Chapter 23.

Syncope
See Chapter 19.

Disturbed vision
Vision can be affected by lesions of the optic pathway or of the nerves controlling eye movements (third, fourth, sixth), or conjugate gaze.

Disturbed hearing
Ask about deafness, tinnitus, and vertigo (Chapter 25).

Disturbed smell
Anosmia can result from head injury, nasal polyps, following viral upper respiratory tract infections or frontal lobe tumours.

Altered speech
There are three types of disordered speech:
- Dysarthria: difficulty in articulating speech, but language content is completely normal.
- Dysphonia: difficulty in voice production.
- Dysphasia: difficulty in understanding or expressing language; caused by lesions affecting the dominant cerebral hemisphere (usually the left).

Fig. 37.5 shows the characteristic speech abnormalities that result from lesions at specific anatomical sites.

Metabolic and endocrine symptoms
Most symptoms will have been described in previous chapters. In particular, look for a history suggestive of hyper- or hypothyroidism (Fig. 37.6) and diabetes mellitus (Fig. 37.7).

Musculoskeletal symptoms
Weakness
This is covered in detail in Chapter 21.

Pain
Pain can arise in the muscles (Chapter 21), joints (Chapter 17), or bones (Fig. 37.8).

Stiffness
Stiffness, particularly after inactivity (e.g. early morning stiffness), is a feature of inflammation.

Joint swelling
This can be caused by infection, inflammation, blood (haemarthrosis), or crystal deposition.

Disability
How do the symptoms affect lifestyle? This is extremely important in patients with rheumatological diseases.

Skin symptoms
Rash
The distribution may be very helpful in determining the diagnosis (Chapter 18).

Pruritus
For the causes of pruritus, see Fig. 37.2.

	Causes and features of abnormalities of speech	
Site of lesion	**Causes**	**Features of speech**
Dysarthria Mouth	Ulcers, macroglossia	Slurred
Lower cranial nerve lesions (9th to 12th)	Bulbar palsy (stroke, poliomyelitis, motor neuron disease, syringobulbia, malignancy)	Nasal quality, slurred Associated features such as dysphagia
Upper cranial nerve lesions (9th to 12th)	Pseudobulbar palsy (stroke, motor neuron disease, multiple sclerosis)	Spastic speech, like 'Donald duck' Associated features like dysphagia and emotional lability
Cerebellum	Multiple sclerosis, stroke, tumour, hereditary ataxias, alcohol, hypothyroidism	Scanning ('staccato') speech Flow is broken Syllables explosive
Extrapyramidal	Parkinsonism	Difficulty initiating speech Monotonous and slightly slurred
Toxic	Acute alcohol intoxication	Slurred
Dysphonia Neuromuscular junction	Myasthenia gravis	Weak, nasal speech Deteriorates on repetition
Vocal cord disease	Tumour, viral laryngitis, tuberculosis, syphilis	Weak volume, husky quality
Vocal cord paralysis	Recurrent laryngeal nerve palsy (mediastinal carcinoma, intrathoracic surgery or trauma, aortic aneurysm)	Weak volume, husky quality
Dysphasia Broca's area (inferior frontal gyrus)	Infarction, bleeding, space-occupying lesion	Expressive dysphasia Comprehension intact Difficulty in finding appropriate words and so speech non-fluent
Wernicke's area (superior temporal gyrus)	Infarction, bleeding, space-occupying lesion	Receptive dysphasia Fluent speech but words are disorganised or unintelligible Comprehension impaired
Frontotemporoparietal lesion	Infarction (left middle cerebral artery), bleeding, space-occupying lesion	Global dysphasia Marked receptive and expressive dysphasia
Posterior part of superior temporal/inferior parietal lobe	Infarction, bleeding, space-occupying lesion and raised intracranial pressure, dementia	Nominal aphasia Unable to name specific objects Other aspects of speech preserved

Fig. 37.5 Causes and features of abnormalities of speech arising from lesions at specific anatomical sites.

Precipitants

Has there been any recent change in detergents, soap, shampoo, etc?

Haematological symptoms

These can be summarised as follows:

- Symptoms of anaemia: low haemoglobin (Chapter 26).
- Recurrent infections: low white cell count.
- Bleeding or bruising: low platelets (Chapter 24).
- Any recent glandular swelling?

Good history taking is not easily taught or learnt the night before an examination. It is acquired through experience, lots of it!

Differences in the history between hyperthyroidism and hypothyroidism		
Symptom	Hyperthyroidism	Hypothyroidism
Temperature intolerance	Heat	Cold
Weight	Decreased	Increased
Appetite	Increased	Decreased
Bowel habit	Diarrhoea	Constipation
Psychiatric	Anxiety, irritability	Poor memory, depression
Menstruation	Oligomenorrhoea	Menorrhagia
Others	Palpitations, sweating, eye changes, pretibial myxoedema, acropachy	Dry skin, brittle hair, arthralgia, myalgia

Fig. 37.6 Differences in the history between hyperthyroidism and hypothyroidism.

Symptoms of diabetes mellitus	
Mechanism	Symptoms
Due to hyperglycaemia	Polyuria Polydipsia Fatigue Blurred vision Recurrent infections, e.g. *Candida* Weight loss (type I)
Due to complications	Peripheral neuropathy Retinopathy Vascular disease

Fig. 37.6 Symptoms of diabetes mellitus.

To start with, learn and follow a system. As you improve you will begin to adapt it to respond to the patients' replies

Causes of bone pain	
Cause	Example
Tumour	Primary tumour (benign or malignant), metastases
Infection	Osteomyelitis (*Staphylococcus, Haemophilus influenzae, Salmonella*, tuberculosis)
Fracture	Traumatic, pathological
Metabolic	Paget's disease, osteomalacia

Fig. 37.8 Causes of bone pain.

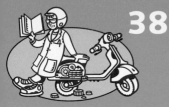

38. Examination of the Patient

Introduction

When it comes to examining patients, practice really does make perfect. Examiners will be able to tell whether you have examined many patients or not within the first 2–3 minutes of seeing you in action! Therefore, take every opportunity you have to rehearse your technique. Let others watch you examine and comment. These could be your teachers or fellow students. The more you do it, the more comfortable you will be with the patient, you will use the right words to get the patient to do what you need and, as in history taking, you will stop worrying about what comes next and start thinking about which physical signs are absent or present and their interpretation.

First things first

There are three essential things you must do whenever you see a patient:

- Introduce yourself, shake hands, and explain to the patient what you would like to do and why, thereby obtaining their consent for the examination.
- Ask the patient to move into the position required for the system you are looking at, expose the area concerned, and then make sure that the patient is comfortable and that their privacy is respected and modesty maintained.
- From the moment you first see the patient, try to decide whether they look well or ill. There is plenty of time while an examiner introduces you to the patient, and while the patient undresses and gets on to the couch, for you to gain a lot of information. Can the patient walk? Can they undo buttons? Are they breathless? Are they in pain? Can they see? Are they deaf? Are there any handy clues around the bed (diabetic drinks, wheelchair, nebulizer, catheter)? Taking time to do this has several advantages: it will help you with the diagnosis, it helps to prioritise your approach as a practising clinician, and it will calm your nerves in clinical examinations.

You will probably find that all clinical teachers will show you a slightly different format for examination technique. The important thing is to develop an approach that you are comfortable with and then keep practising it until it becomes second nature.

In examinations you will almost always be asked to examine a particular system: 'examine this gentleman's chest', 'what do you notice about this lady's face?' This chapter describes the technique for each system and how to interpret the clinical signs you will find. When, as a doctor, you see a patient you will need to be able to examine the whole patient and focus your attention on relevant areas.

General inspection

It is medical etiquette that all clinical examinations are performed from the right hand side of the patient. The most important thing is to decide is how well or ill the patient is, as described above. Other specific abnormalities should then be looked for.

Cyanosis

This is a bluish discoloration which is seen when the concentration of reduced (deoxygenated) haemoglobin in the blood rises above 1.5 g/dL. Central cyanosis is seen best in the tongue and lips. It is caused by underlying respiratory or cardiovascular disease. Peripheral cyanosis can be due to either central cyanosis or reduced peripheral circulation, as poorly perfused peripheral tissue will take up oxygen more readily. Reduced peripheral circulation is seen in shock, cold weather, and vascular abnormalities. Cyanosis is seen rarely in anaemia but occurs more readily in polycythaemia.

Very rarely, other forms of reduced haemoglobin, such as methaemoglobin or sulphaemoglobin, can cause cyanosis.

Jaundice

Jaundice is the yellow discoloration of the skin, sclera, and mucous membranes due to serum bilirubin concentrations greater than 30 μmol/L, which becomes more obvious at concentrations greater than 50 μmol/L. Jaundice can be due to

Causes of hypothermia	
Cause	**Examples**
Exposure	At home in patients who are immobile On treks or after prolonged water immersion in the young
Infection	Septicaemia from any cause
Endocrine	Hypothyroidism, hypopituitarism
Toxic	Alcohol abuse, drug overdose
Drugs	Hypnotics, e.g. benzodiazepines
Hypothalamic damage	Failure of thermoregulation

Fig. 38.1 Causes of hypothermia.

increased bilirubin production, abnormal bilirubin metabolism in the liver, or reduced bilirubin excretion (see Chapter 11).

Yellow skin (particularly palms and soles) with normal sclera can be due to carotenaemia (excessive consumption of carrots, or hypothyroidism).

Pallor

Generalised pallor can be racial, inherited (albinism), or due to anaemia, shock, myxoedema, or hypopituitarism. Localised pallor is seen in disruption of the arterial supply, as in Raynaud's phenomenon.

Hydration

Signs of dehydration include dry mucous membranes, tachycardia, postural hypotension, decreased skin turgor, and altered consciousness level if severe. If the patient is in hospital, hydration status should be monitored more accurately using weight, fluid balance charts, and central venous pressure (if very ill).

Overhydration can sometimes result from the overenthusiastic administration of intravenous fluids, particularly in the elderly. Clinical signs include raised jugular venous pressure (JVP), pulmonary oedema, a third heart sound and peripheral oedema.

Temperature

Fever can accompany numerous infectious, inflammatory, and malignant diseases. If associated with an acute infection, the patient often looks flushed, sweaty, and unwell. A swinging pyrexia may be a feature in the presence of an abscess. An intermittent fever may occur in lymphoma or in malaria, where it recurs every few days. For more on this, see Chapter 6.

Hypothermia is a particular problem of the elderly, alcoholics, and patients with dementia. A patient becomes hypothermic when the core temperature falls below 35 °C. The causes are summarised in Fig. 38.1.

Pigmentation

Generalised pigmentation is usually of racial origin but may also arise in haemochromatosis (greyish–bronze), occupational exposure (slate-grey appearance with argyria in silver workers), and with some drugs (slate-grey with amiodarone).

Adrenocorticotrophic hormone (ACTH) can mimic the action of melanocyte-stimulating hormone, and therefore when its levels are raised, pigmentation increases e.g. Addison's disease (particularly in skin creases, pressure areas, buccal mucosa, scars), Cushing's disease (ACTH-secreting pituitary tumour), ectopic ACTH production and Nelson's syndrome (following bilateral adrenalectomy for Cushing's disease).

Chronic illness may be associated with pigmentation, common examples being chronic liver disease and chronic uraemia.

As well as Addison's disease, local areas of pigmentation may be seen in Peutz–Jeghers' syndrome (brown lesions around the lips) and neurofibromatosis (café-au-lait patches).

Localised areas of depigmentation, particularly affecting the back of the hand and neck, are seen in vitiligo, an autoimmune disease of the skin affecting melanocytes. It may be associated with other autoimmune diseases.

Breast examination

Breast examination should be performed in women who have symptoms of breast disease or when an underlying malignancy is suspected. Do not forget that breast tissue extends into the axillae. Breast examination must be approached sensitively with a full explanation. Male students and doctors should have a female chaperone to help put the patient at ease (and to protect themselves from accusations of inappropriate behaviour).

Lymphadenopathy

Examine all lymph node sites (Fig. 38.2). Always examine the cervical lymph nodes standing behind the patient. The causes for generalised and localised lymphadenopathy are discussed in Chapter 22.

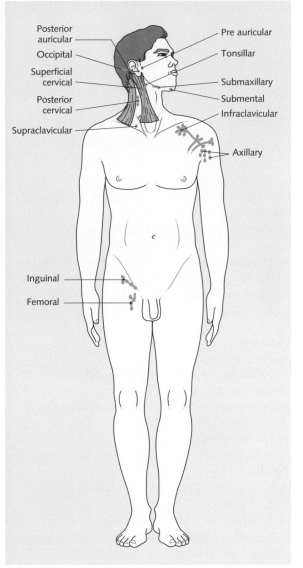

Fig. 38.2 Examination of lymph node sites.

If lymphadenopathy is present, pay special attention to examination of the spleen and liver.

The face and body habitus

Examiners will often take you to a patient and simply ask 'what is the diagnosis in this patient?' or 'what do you notice about this gentleman's face?' The conditions in Fig. 38.3 are often known as 'spot diagnoses'—they have characteristic physical features and often come up in examinations.

Common 'spot diagnoses'	
Disease	**Examples**
Endocrine	Hypothyroidism, hyperthyroidism, acromegaly, Cushing's syndrome, Addison's disease
Metabolic	Paget's disease, chronic liver disease, uraemia / stigmata of dialysis
Neuromuscular	Parkinson's disease, myotonia dystrophica, facial nerve palsy, Horner's syndrome, ptosis, choreoathetosis
Connective tissue	SLE, scleroderma, Marfan's syndrome, ankylosing spondylitis
Hereditary	Turner's syndrome, Down's syndrome Klinefelter's syndrome, achondroplasia
Cardiovascular	Mitral facies Cyanotic congenital heart disease
Physiological	Chloasma of pregnancy
Haematological	Thalassaemia
Infection	Congenital syphilis
Dermatology	Pigmentation, purpura, psoriasis, neurofibromatosis, Osler-Weber-Rendu (hereditary haemorrhagic telangiectasia) herpes zoster, pemphigoid/pemphigus, necrobiosis lipoidica diabeticorum.

Fig. 38.3 Common 'spot diagnoses'—all have characteristic physical signs.

The neck

When asked to examine the neck, there will usually be a thyroid mass or lymphadenopathy. However, do not forget the salivary glands, branchial cyst, pharyngeal pouch, cervical rib, carotid body tumour, and cystic hygroma. Causes of lymphadenopathy are described in Chapter 22. Figure 38.4 lists the causes of thyroid enlargement.

 If you find no abnormality in the neck, examine the jugular venous pressure, listen to the carotid artery for bruits, and re-examine for cervical rib

First, look very carefully at the neck, lifting the hair out of the way if necessary. Look for obvious

Causes of thyroid gland enlargement	
Form of enlargement	**Causes**
Diffuse enlargement (goitre)	• Idiopathic • Physiological—puberty, pregnancy • Autoimmune—Hashimoto's and Graves' diseases • Iodine deficiency—endemic, e.g. Derbyshire neck • Thyroiditis—de Quervain's (viral), Riedel's (autoimmune) • Drugs—carbimazole, lithium, sulphonylureas • Genetic—dyshormonogenesis (Pendred's syndrome)
Solitary nodule	• Thyroglossal cyst • Prominent nodule in multinodular goitre • Adenoma • Cyst • Carcinoma (papillary, follicular, anaplastic, medullary) • Lymphoma

Fig. 38.4 Causes of thyroid gland enlargement.

masses, scars, skin changes, or deformity. If there is a mass in the region of the thyroid gland, ask the patient to take a sip of water into their mouth and then swallow—a goitre will move upwards on swallowing. In addition, ask the patient to open the mouth and then watch as they protrude the tongue forward—a thyroglossal cyst will move upwards. If a mass is present, determine the properties shown in Fig. 38.5. Percussion is useful to determine retrosternal extension of a goitre. Bruits may be audible in the thyroid gland (thyrotoxicosis) or carotid artery (atheroma). If you find a thyroid mass, you should go on to assess thyroid status as shown in Fig. 38.6.

The hands

The hands can provide a wealth of information for the alert clinician. When you are asked to examine the hands, consider the normal structures present and examine them in turn. Where appropriate, go on to examine the functional use of the hand

Features of any mass
• Site • Shape • Size including upper, lower and lateral limits • Consistency • Tenderness • Fluctuance • Fixation to underlying or overlying structures • Transillumination (where appropriate) • Local lymph node involvement • Bruit

Fig. 38.5 Features to determine for any mass.

(e.g. undoing a button or picking up a pen). This is particularly important in neurological abnormalities and destructive arthritides, (e.g. rheumatoid arthritis, RA).

Hands
- Blue: peripheral cyanosis.
- Pallor: anaemia (skin creases) and Raynaud's phenomenon.
- Pigmentation: Addison's disease (skin creases).
- Depigmentation: vitiligo.
- Palmar erythema (Fig. 38.7).

Nails
- Koilonychia: spoon-shaped nails seen in iron deficiency.
- Leuconychia: white nails due to hypoalbuminaemia (Fig. 38.8).
- Clubbing: an increase in angle between nail-plate and fold to over 180°. The causes are shown in Fig. 38.9.
- Splinter haemorrhages: terminal lesions usually due to trauma, proximal lesions found in infective endocarditis, and vasculitis.
- Quincke's sign: capillary pulsation in the nail-bed due to aortic regurgitation.
- Beau's lines: horizontal grooves in the nails caused by temporary arrest of nail growth due to acute severe illness.
- Onycholysis: separation of the nail from the nail-bed due to psoriasis, trauma, fungal infections, and hyperthyroidism.
- Yellow nails: yellow nail syndrome with lymphatic hypoplasia (peripheral oedema and pleural effusions).

Examination of thyroid status		
	Hyperthyroidism	**Hypothyroidism**
Mood	Irritability, anxiety	Depression, slowness
Weight	Thinness	Overweight
Hands	Fine tremor, palmar erythema, sweaty palms, *acropachy	Puffiness, anaemia, Tinel's sign (carpal tunnel syndrome)
Pulse	Tachycardia, atrial fibrillation	Bradycardia
Face	Lid lag, lid retraction, *exophthalmos, *ophthalmoplegia, *chemosis	Loss of outer third of eyebrow, puffy eyes, 'toad-like' facies, xanthelasmata
Skin	*Pretibial myxoedema (shins)	Dry, thin hair
Neuromuscular	Proximal myopathy	Slow relaxing ankle jerks, cerebellar signs

Fig. 38.6 Examination of thyroid status. *Denotes features that are specific to Grave's disease.

- Half-and-half nails where the proximal nail is white and the distal nail is brown or red due to chronic renal failure.

Tendons
- Xanthomata: hypercholesterolaemia.
- Dupuytren's contractures (thickening of the palmar fascia): associated with alcoholic liver disease, epileptics treated with phenytoin, vibrating tools, and familial and idiopathic causes.

Joints
- Destructive arthropathy: RA, psoriasis, gout.
- Heberden's nodes: osteophytes of the distal interphalangeal joints.
- Bouchard's nodes: osteophytes of the proximal interphalangeal joints.

Neuromuscular
- Localised wasting: ulnar or median nerve lesions.
- Generalised wasting: C8/T1 anterior horn cell, nerve root or brachial plexus damage, combined median and ulnar nerve damage, disuse atrophy in severe arthritis, profound cachexia.
- Myotonia: failure to relax after voluntary contraction seen in myotonia dystrophica.

Other signs
- Sclerodactyly (tightening of the skin causing tapering of the fingers): look also for Calcinosis, Raynaud's phenomenon, Oesophageal dysmotility (ask the patient if they have difficulty on swallowing), and Telangiectasia—hence CREST syndrome (where the S stands for sclerodactyly).
- Spade hands: acromegaly.
- Asterixis: a coarse flapping tremor seen when the hand is oustretched with the wrist extended and fingers apart. It is caused by metabolic encephalopathy (e.g. liver failure, carbon dioxide retention, uraemia).

Causes of palmar erythema	
Causes	**Examples**
Physiological	Pregnancy Puberty Familial
Pathological	Chronic liver disease Rheumatoid arthritis Thyrotoxicosis Oral contraceptive pill Polycythaemia

Fig. 38.7 Causes of palmar erythema.

Causes of hypoalbuminaemia	
Causes	**Examples**
Reduced intake	Malnutrition
Reduced synthesis	Liver disease
Increased utilisation	Chronic illness
Increased loss	Nephrotic syndrome (kidneys) Protein-losing enteropathy (gut) Severe burns (skin)

Fig. 38.8 Causes of hypoalbuminaemia.

Causes of clubbing	
Causes	**Examples**
Respiratory	Tumour: bronchial carcinoma, mesothelioma Chronic suppuration: abscess, bronchiectasis, empyema Fibrosis: from any cause Vascular: arteriovenous malformation
Cardiovascular	Congenital cyanotic heart disease Subacute bacterial endocarditis Atrial myxoma
Gastrointestinal	Inflammatory bowel disease Lymphoma Cirrhosis
Endocrine	Thyrotoxicosis (acropachy)
Familial	Autosomal dominant

Fig. 38.9 Causes of clubbing.

- Action tremor: this is rapid and fine in amplitude. It is worsened by holding the hands in a particular posture (e.g. hands outstretched) or by movement. It is characteristic of benign essential tremor, thyrotoxicosis and excessive caffeine intake and is an exaggeration of physiological tremor.
- Resting tremor: the thumb moves across the tips of the fingers. This 'pill-rolling' tremor is worst at rest and is characteristic of parkinsonism.
- Intention tremor: this is absent at rest, present on maintaining a posture, and exaggerated by movement. It is characteristic of disorders of the cerebellum and its connections.

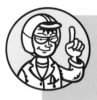

When examining the hands, always look at the elbows for a psoriatic rash, rheumatoid nodules, or gouty tophi

The cardiovascular system

General inspection
- Does the patient look well or ill?
- Are they lying flat?
- Are they cachectic (cardiac cachexia)?
- Do they have Marfan's syndrome (aortic regurgitation, mitral regurgitation), Down's

syndrome (atrial septal defect), or Turner's syndrome (aortic coarctation, ventricular septal defect, less often—atrial septal defect, aortic stenosis)?

Position
Help the patient to adopt a comfortable position at 45° with the chest exposed. In women, cover the chest until ready to examine the praecordium.

Hands
- Clubbing: subacute bacterial endocarditis (SBE) and congenital cyanotic heart disease.
- Cyanosis: peripheral vasoconstriction, pulmonary oedema, and right-to-left shunt.
- Splinter haemorrhages: SBE.
- Janeway's lesions: non-tender macules in the palms due to SBE.
- Osler's nodes: painful nodules on the pulps of the fingers due to SBE.
- Quincke's sign: aortic regurgitation.
- Xanthomata: hypercholesterolaemia-vascular disease.

Radial pulse
- Rate: normally between 60 and 100 b.p.m. (see Chapter 3).
- Rhythm: regular or irregular (see Chapter 3).
- Radioradial delay: dissecting thoracic aortic aneurysm.
- Radiofemoral delay: coarctation of the aorta.
- Character: best determined by palpation of a larger artery (e.g. brachial or carotid arteries).

Blood pressure
- Level: hypertension is a risk factor for vascular disease.
- Lying and standing: postural hypotension.
- Right and left: left may be lower than right in aortic dissection.
- Wide pulse pressure: in the elderly and aortic regurgitation.
- Narrow pulse pressure: aortic stenosis.
- Pulsus paradoxus: exaggerated fall in pulse pressure during inspiration resulting in a faint or absent pulse in inspiration; caused by severe asthma or cardiac tamponade.

Brachial and carotid artery
- Character: collapsing (Fig. 38.10), slow-rising (aortic stenosis), bisferiens (mixed aortic valve

Causes of a collapsing pulse	
Causes	**Examples**
Physiological	Elderly Pregnancy Exercise
Pathological	Aortic regurgitation Patent ductus arteriosus Fever Thyrotoxicosis Anaemia Arteriovenous shunts

Fig. 38.10 Causes of a collapsing pulse.

If the JVP is not visible at 45°, try sitting the patient upright, laying the patient flat and eliciting the hepatojugular reflux as it may be either too high or too low to be seen

disease), alternans (severe left ventricular failure), and jerky (hypertrophic obstructive cardiomyopathy).

- Corrigan's sign: prominent carotid pulsation due to aortic regurgitation.

Jugular venous pressure

When assessing JVP, the patient should be at 45° with their head rested on a pillow (this relaxes the sternocleidomastoid muscles). Pulsation should be up to 3 cm above the sternal angle (8 cm above right atrium). Differences between JVP and carotid pulsation in normal subjects are shown in Fig. 38.11. JVP acts as a manometer for right atrial pressure and is raised when right atrial pressure is raised (Fig. 38.12). Abnormalities in the waveform result from specific underlying pathologies (Fig. 38.13).

Restrictive cardiomyopathy, constrictive pericarditis and pericardial tamponade are all associated with Kussmaul's sign (JVP rises during inspiration) and Friedrich's sign (steep y descent due to sudden collapse in diastole of high atrial pressure and its subsequent rapid ascent due to failure of ventricular relaxation).

Face

- Central cyanosis: pulmonary oedema and right-to-left shunt.
- Anaemia: possible high output cardiac failure.
- Malar flush: pulmonary hypertension due to mitral valve disease.
- Jaundice: haemolysis due to mechanical valves.
- Xanthelasmata: hypercholesterolaemia (vascular disease).
- Teeth: source in bacterial endocarditis.
- Mouth: high-arched palate in Marfan's syndrome.
- De Musset's sign: head nodding due to aortic regurgitation.
- Roth's spots in the retina: bacterial endocarditis.

Praecordium

Look for scars and deformities, including:

- Sternotomy scar: arterial bypass grafts and valve replacements.

Differences between JVP and carotid pulsation		
Feature	**Carotid pulsation**	**JVP**
Palpable	Yes	No
Number of visible peaks	One	Two
Occlusion by gentle pressure	No	Yes (fills from above)
Sitting upright	No change	Height falls
Lying flat	No change	Height rises
Gentle pressure on liver	No change	Height rises (hepatojugular reflux)
Deep inspiration	No change	Height falls

Fig. 38.11 Differences between jugulovenous pulsation (JVP) and carotid pulsation.

Causes of a raised JVP

- Right ventricular failure
- Volume overload (overenthusiastic intravenous fluids)
- Superior vena caval obstruction (JVP is non-pulsatile)
- Tricuspid valve disease (stenosis and regurgitation)
- Pericardial effusion causing tamponade
- Constrictive pericarditis

Fig. 38.12 Causes of a raised jugulovenous pressure (JVP).

- Mitral valvotomy scar under the left breast: always look for it as it indicates a previously closed mitral valvotomy.
- Skeletal deformities—can cause an ejection systolic flow murmur.

Apex beat

The apex beat should be at the mid-clavicular line in the fifth left intercostal space.

- Lateral displacement: left or severe right ventricular dilatation. Lung pathology may also cause displacement.

- Impalpable: obesity, pleural effusion, pericardial effusion, chronic obstructive airways disease, and dextrocardia (palpable on the right!).
- Tapping: mitral stenosis (palpable first heart sound).
- Heaving: 'pressure overload' in aortic stenosis, or hypertension.
- Thrusting: 'volume overload' in aortic regurgitation, mitral regurgitation (ventricle usually markedly displaced).
- Diffuse: left ventricular dilatation.
- Double impulse: left ventricular aneurysm or hypertrophic cardiomyopathy.

Palpation

Parasternal heave is caused by the enlargement or hypertrophy of the right ventricle.

A thrill is a palpable murmur and indicates significant valve disease; it can be systolic or diastolic and therefore its position in the cardiac cycle should be assessed by timing its relation to a central pulse. Palpate in all valve areas (Fig. 38.14).

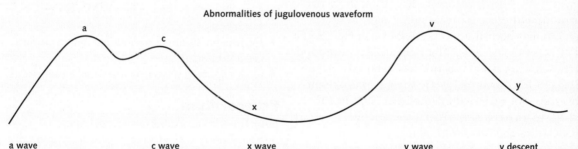

Abnormalities of jugulovenous waveform

a wave	c wave	x wave	v wave	y descent
Atrial systole	Increasing RV pressure before TV closes	Atrial relaxation during ventricular systole	Atrial filling at end of ventricular systole	Tricuspid valve opens prior to atrial contraction
Absent a wave: • Atrial fibrillation Large a waves: • Tricuspid stenosis • Right ventricular hypertrophy due to pulmonary hypertension or pulmonary stenosis Giant a waves: • 'Cannon waves' due to atrial contraction against closed TV due to VT, complete heart block, nodal tachycardia		Absent x descent: • Atrial fibrillation Steep x descent: • Constrictive pericarditis • Pericardial tamponade	Large v waves: • Tricuspid regurgitation	Slow y descent: • Tricuspid stenosis Steep y descent: • Constrictive pericarditis • Restrictive cardiomyopathy • Pericardial tamponade • Tricuspid regurgitation

Fig. 38.13 Abnormalities of jugulovenous waveform. (VT, ventricular tachycardia; TV, tricuspid valve.)

Aortic (second intercostal space, right sternal edge)

Pulmonary area (second intercostal space, left sternal edge)

Tricuspid area (left sternal edge)

Mitral area (fifth intercostal space)

Fig. 38.14 Positions of auscultation of the cardiac valves.

Auscultation

- Listen in all four areas with the bell and diaphragm (Fig. 38.14).
- Roll the patient to the left hand side to listen with the bell at the axilla for mitral stenosis.
- Sit the patient forward to listen with the diaphragm at the left sternal edge in expiration for aortic regurgitation.
- Listen to the first and second sounds, then for third and fourth sounds.
- Are there any murmurs? (see Chapter 4.)
- Listen for additional sounds including opening snap, ejection click, pericardial knock or rub, and mechanical valves.
- Time any abnormalities against the carotid pulsation.
- Listen to the carotid arteries for bruits (atheroma) or radiation of aortic stenotic murmur.

Evidence of cardiac failure

- Examine lung bases for pulmonary oedema and pleural effusions indicating left ventricular failure.
- Sacral oedema occurs in right ventricular failure.

- Hepatomegaly occurs in right ventricular failure; it will be pulsatile if there is tricuspid regurgitation.
- Pitting oedema occurs in right ventricular failure and is almost always bilateral.

Peripheral pulses

Pulses in the legs may be diminished in peripheral vascular disease. Systolic and diastolic murmurs may be heard in the femoral arteries due to aortic regurgitation (pistol shots and Duroziez's sign).

The respiratory system

General inspection

- Does the patient look well or ill? Is the patient alert?
- Cachexia: underlying malignancy.
- Sputum pot: examine.
- Nebulizer: bronchospasm.
- Distress: breathless at rest and moving around in the bed.
- Pursed lip breathing: chronic small airways obstruction.
- Voice: hoarse in bronchial carcinoma (recurrent laryngeal nerve palsy).
- Lymphadenopathy: supraclavicular, cervical, and axillary.
- Respiratory rate: normally around 12–16 breaths per minute.

Position

Help the patient to adopt a comfortable position at 45° with the chest exposed. In women, cover the chest until you are ready to examine it.

Hands

- Clubbing: malignancy, fibrosis, and chronic suppuration. Bronchial carcinoma (especially squamous cell) associated with clubbing may also cause hypertrophic pulmonary osteoarthropathy—swelling and pain, particularly in the wrists and ankles, with subperiosteal new bone formation on X-ray.
- Cyanosis: peripheral vasoconstriction and respiratory failure.
- Wasting of small muscles: infiltration of T_1 by bronchial neoplasm (Pancoast's tumour).
- Tar-stained fingers: increased likelihood of malignancy and obstructive airways disease.
- Asterixis: carbon dioxide retention.

- Evidence of conditions with may involve the lungs (e.g. systemic sclerosis, rheumatoid arthritis) (see Chapter 33).

Pulse
- Tachycardia: severe respiratory disease (e.g. acute asthma or pneumonia).
- Bounding: carbon dioxide retention.
- Atrial fibrillation: malignancy and pneumonia.

Blood pressure
Pulsus paradoxus is seen in severe acute asthma.

JVP
- Right ventricular failure: chronic respiratory disease with pulmonary hypertension.
- Superior vena caval obstruction: bronchial carcinoma.
- Large a waves: cor pulmonale.

Face
- Central cyanosis: respiratory failure.
- Anaemia: chronic respiratory disease, particularly malignancy.
- Horner's syndrome: apical carcinoma (Pancoast's tumour) involving cervical sympathetic nerves (see Chapter 31).
- Fine tremor: β-agonists.
- Plethoric facies: polycythaemia.

Trachea
Warn the patient before you palpate the trachea! Note the following:
- Tracheal deviation reflects pathology in the upper mediastinum (Fig. 38.15).
- Check the position of the apex beat to confirm lower mediastinal shift.
- Feel for tracheal tug in acute respiratory distress.

Causes of tracheal deviation	
Towards lesion	**Away from lesion**
Collapse	Tension pneumothorax
Apical fibrosis	Massive pleural effusion
Pneumonectomy	Large mass (e.g. thyroid)

Fig. 38.15 Causes of tracheal deviation.

- The distance from the cricoid cartilage to the suprasternal notch should be three to four finger breadths – this distance reduces in hyperinflation.

Inspection
Perform inspection, palpation, percussion, and auscultation on the front of the chest first. Then sit the patient forward, palpate for lymphadenopathy, and then repeat the examination on the back of the chest. Typical patterns of respiratory abnormalities are shown in Fig. 38.16.

On inspecting the chest assess the following:
- Respiration: use of accessory muscles (respiratory distress).
- Recession: intercostal and subcostal (respiratory distress).
- Scars: including previous surgery and chest drains.
- Deformity: in particular, Harrison's sulci (indrawn costal margins) and pectus carinatum due to severe childhood asthma; barrel chest is seen in long-standing airways obstruction due to hyperinflation.
- Radiotherapy: markings or skin changes indicate previous treatment for underlying malignancy.

Expansion
- Ask the patient to take a deep breath in and out and watch closely.
- Place your hand firmly on the chest laterally with fingers apart and thumbs lifted off the chest wall touching each other.
- The chest should expand by at least 5 cm on deep inspiration.
- Any significant pulmonary disease will reduce expansion.
- In unilateral disease, the affected side will move less than the other.
- Note any chest wall tenderness, which is usually caused by musculoskeletal abnormalities.

Vocal fremitus
Ask the patient to say '99' and palpate with the ulnar border of the hand. Increased vocal fremitus indicates consolidation (sometimes fibrosis and above pleural effusion); decreased indicates pleural effusion or collapse.

Percussion
Compare one side with the other and remember the axillae. The following signs are important:
- Hyper-resonant: pneumothorax.

Findings on clinical examination of common respiratory diseases						
Pathology	General signs	Tracheal deviation	Palpation	Percussion note	Breath sounds	Causes
Pneumothorax	Tachycardia and hypotension in tension pnueumothorax	Away from affected side if tension	Reduced expansion, reduced TVF	Normal or hyper-resonant	Reduced or absent	Spontaneous (particularly tall healthy males and Marfan's syndrome), trauma, airways obstruction, cystic fibrosis, pulmonary abscess
Consolidation	Pyrexia, tachycardia	None	Reduced expansion, increased TVF	Dull	Increased vocal resonance whispering pectoriloquy, bronchial breath sounds	Pneumococcus, *Haemophilus influenzae*, *Staphylococcus aureus*, *Klebsiella*, *Pseudomonas*, *Mycoplasma*, *Legionella*, *Influenza type A*, *Aspergillus*
Pleural effusion		Away from affected side if large	Reduced expansion, reduced TVF	Stony dull	Absent	Transudate (<30g/L protein): cardiac failure, liver failure, nephrotic syndrome, Meigs' syndrome, myxoedema Exudate (>30g/L protein): malignancy, pneumonia, pulmonary embolus, rheumatoid arthritis, SLE, subphrenic abscess, pancreatitis, trauma, Dressler's syndrome
Collapse		Towards affected side	Reduced expansion, reduced TVF	Dull	Reduced or absent	Foreign body or mucus plugs (asthma, aspergillosis) within the bronchial lumen, bronchial carcinoma arising from the bronchus itself, extrinsic compression by enlarged lymph nodes (malignancy, tuberculosis)
Fibrosis	Clubbing	Towards affected side if apical disease	Reduced expansion, increased TVF	Normal or dull	Fine inspiratory crepitations	Cryptogenic fibrosing alveolitis, sarcoidosis, drugs (amiodarone, bleomycin), radiation, inhalation of dusts (asbestos, coal), extrinsic allergic alveolitis, ankylosing spondylitis, rheumatoid arthritis, systemic sclerosis, tuberculosis
Bronchiectasis	Clubbing, purulent sputum	Normal	Normal or reduced expansion, normal or increased TVF	Normal or dull	Coarse inspiratory crepitations, occasional polyphonic wheeze	Congenital (cystic fibrosis, Kartagener's syndrome, hypogammoglobulinaemia), idiopathic, bronchial obstruction (foreign body, carcinoma, lymphadenopathy), infection (childhood measles or whooping cough, tuberculosis, aspergillosis, postpneumonia)
Bronchospasm	Hyperexpanded chest, tremor (if on β-agonist), Harrison's sulci, pectus carinatum	Normal	Reduced expansion, normal TVF	Normal, hyper resonant over bullae, reduced liver dullness	Polyphonic wheeze, crepitations in chronic obstructive airways disease	Anaphylaxis

Fig. 38.16 Findings on clinical examination of common respiratory diseases. (TVF, tactile vocal fremitus.)

389

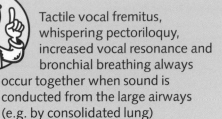

Tactile vocal fremitus, whispering pectoriloquy, increased vocal resonance and bronchial breathing always occur together when sound is conducted from the large airways (e.g. by consolidated lung)

- Dull: solid organ (liver or heart), consolidation, collapse, pleural thickening, peripheral tumours, and fibrosis.
- Stony dull: pleural effusion.

Auscultation
- Vesicular breath sounds: these are normal.
- Bronchial breathing, whispering pectoriloquy, increased vocal resonance: consolidation (sometimes fibrosis and above pleural effusion).
- Wheeze: small airways obstruction (polyphonic or generalised), large airway obstruction (e.g. bronchial carcinoma (monophonic or localised), and cardiac failure).
- Fine crackles: pulmonary fibrosis.
- Medium crackles: cardiac failure.
- Coarse crackles: infection.
- Early crackles: chronic obstructive pulmonary disease.
- Absent breath sounds: pleural effusion.
- Pleural rub: pleural irritation due to pneumonia or pulmonary embolus.
- Click: during systole this is occasionally heard in a small left pneumothorax (Hamman's sign).

Other signs
- The liver may be palpable if it is pushed down by hyperexpanded lungs, enlarged due to right ventricular failure, or if there are metastases from a bronchial carcinoma.
- Pitting oedema indicates right ventricular failure.
- Peak flow should be assessed if airflow obstruction is suspected.

The upper border of the liver is normally at the sixth rib in the right midclavicular line. If the percussion note remains resonant below this, the lungs are hyperinflated

The abdomen

General inspection
- Appearance: does the patient look well or ill?
- Pain.
- Patient's position: think of peritonism if very still, appendicitis (psoas irritation) if right knee flexed, and renal colic if rolling around in agony.
- Cachexia: chronic disease, particularly malignancy.
- Drowsy: encephalopathy (hepatic or uraemia).
- Hydration (see p. 382).

Hands
- Clubbing: cirrhosis, inflammatory bowel disease and gastrointestinal lymphoma.
- Leuconychia: liver failure, nephrotic syndrome, protein-losing enteropathy.
- Koilonychia: chronic iron deficiency, consider occult neoplasm particularly in the stomach and caecum.
- Palmar erythema: cirrhosis.
- Asterixis: hepatic encephalopathy and uraemia.
- Dupuytren's contracture: alcoholic liver disease.
- Half-and-half nails: renal failure.
- Bullae (blisters): porphyria cutanea tarda due to alcoholic liver disease.

Arms
- Scratch marks: obstructive jaundice (particularly primary biliary cirrhosis) and lymphoma.
- Muscle wasting: proximal myopathy due to alcohol, steroid excess, or underlying malignancy (paraneoplastic).
- Bruising: hepatic impairment.

Face
- Jaundice: prehepatic, hepatic, or posthepatic (see Chapter 11).
- Anaemia: from any cause (see Chapter 26).
- Xanthelasmata: hypercholesterolaemia (primary biliary cirrhosis or nephrotic syndrome).
- Kayser–Fleischer rings: Wilson's disease (best seen by slit-lamp examination).

Mouth
- Hydration.
- Glossitis: iron deficiency and megaloblastic anaemia.
- Pigmentation: Addison's disease, chronic liver disease, chronic renal failure and Peutz-Jeghers' syndrome (see p. 382).

- Telangiectasia: hereditary haemorrhagic telangiectasia (Osler–Weber–Rendu syndrome).
- Crohn's disease: lip swelling and mucosal ulceration.
- Gingival hypertrophy (Fig. 38.17).

Neck

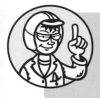 Always palpate the neck from behind the patient with the neck slightly flexed to relax the sternocleidomastoid muscles

Look for left supraclavicular lymphadenopathy – caused by metastasis from underlying gastrointestinal carcinoma (Virchow's node or Troisier's sign).

Trunk

Spider naevi arise in the distribution of the superior vena cava – five or more suggest underlying chronic liver disease, pregnancy, or hyperthyroidism.

Gynaecomastia and sexual hair loss indicate chronic liver disease.

Position

Ask the patient if they are comfortable lying flat. If so, help the patient to do this with the head on one pillow and arms relaxed by the sides. Expose from below the breasts (in women) or the nipples (in men) down to the symphysis pubis.

Inspection

Observe closely looking for the following:

- Scars: previous surgery or trauma.
- Distension (Fig. 38.18).
- Obvious mass: including movement with respiration.

- Bruising: Cullen's (para-umbilical) and Grey Turner's (flanks) signs in acute pancreatitis.
- Dilated veins: inferior vena cava obstruction (venous flow is upwards).
- Caput medusae: portal hypertension (venous flow is away from the umbilicus).
- Pulsation: abdominal aortic aneurysm.
- Striae: pregnancy or Cushing's syndrome.
- Node: umbilical nodule (Sister Mary Joseph's nodule) is a metastasis from intra-abdominal malignancy.
- Peristalsis: if visible this indicates an obstruction, though it may be normal in a thin or elderly patient.

Palpation

 Always look at the patient's face when palpating the abdomen—it will often tell you a lot!

Before you touch the patient, ask if they are tender anywhere and start palpation away from that area. Feel gently in each of the four quadrants, noting tenderness or masses. Then feel more deeply in each quadrant to determine the characteristics of any mass found (Fig. 38.5).

If a mass is present, consider what structures normally lie at that site and what disease processes might affect that structure (see Chapter 12). Next, palpate for hepatomegaly and splenomegaly starting in the right iliac fossa. Examine for renal masses by bimanual palpation. If hepatomegaly or splenomegaly are present, comment on consistency (smooth or irregular) and size in centimetres (not finger

Causes of gingival hypertrophy	
Cause	**Examples**
Acute myeloid leukaemia	Monocytic, myelomonocytic
Drugs	Cyclosporin, phenytoin, nifedipine
Infection	Gingivitis
Scurvy	See p. 117
Physiological	Pregnancy

Fig. 38.17 Causes of gingival hypertrophy.

Causes of generalised abdominal swelling	
Cause	**Aetiology**
Fluid	Ascites
Faeces	Constipation
Fetus	Pregnancy
Flatus	Bowel obstruction
Fat	Obesity
Fibroids	And any other tumour or organomegaly

Fig. 38.18 Causes of generalised abdominal swelling.

Causes of hepatomegaly	
Cause	**Examples**
Cirrhosis	Any cause*, particularly primary biliary cirrhosis and haemochromatosis
Tumour	Benign, malignant, primary (hepatocellular carcinoma), and metastases
Venous congestion	Right ventricular failure, Budd–Chiari syndrome, tricuspid disease
Infection	Viral hepatitis*, abscess, syphilis, Weil's* disease, hydatid disease, brucellosis
Cysts	Polycystic disease
Haematological	Lymphoproliferative disease*, myeloproliferative disease*
Metabolic	Storage diseases*, amyloidosis*
Inflammatory	Sarcoidosis*

Fig. 38.19 Causes of hepatomegaly. Remember the 'Cs' for common causes: cirrhosis, carcinoma, and cardiac failure. Note that the liver may appear large in the absence of true hepatomegaly when it is pushed down by a hyperinflated lung (as in acute asthma or chronic obstructive airways disease) and when a Riedel's lobe is present (normal anatomical variation of the right hepatic lobe). *Denotes the causes of hepatosplenomegaly.

breadths) beneath the costal margin (the causes of hepatomegaly are shown in Fig. 38.19); the causes of splenomegaly are discussed in detail in Chapter 22. A palpable liver must also be assessed for pulsatility (tricuspid regurgitation), tenderness and bruits.

Do not forget the distinguishing features of the spleen and kidney (see Fig. 22.2); the causes of a renal mass are summarised in Fig. 38.20.

Finally, palpate for abdominal aortic aneurysm and examine the groins for lymphadenopathy and hernias.

Causes of unilateral and bilateral palpable kidneys	
Type	**Cause**
Unilateral	Tumour (hypernephroma, nephroblastoma) Hydronephrosis, pyonephrosis Hypertrophy of single functioning kidney, perinephric abscess or haematoma, polycystic disease (only one kidney palpable)
Bilateral	Polycystic kidneys (autosomal dominant in adults, autosomal recessive in children) Amyloidosis Bilateral hydronephrosis

Fig. 38.20 Causes of unilateral and bilateral palpable kidneys.

Percussion

Always percuss from resonance to dullness. Use percussion to determine the size of the liver and spleen starting at the chest, moving inferiorly. Percuss over any masses to determine their consistency. Always assess for ascites by looking for a fluid thrill and shifting dullness. Fig. 38.21 summarises the causes of ascites.

Auscultation

- Bowel sounds may be normal, increased, or decreased: increased in bowel obstruction (high-pitched and tinkling) and absent in the ileus (functional motor paralysis of the bowel) due to any cause (Fig. 38.22).
- Arterial bruits: may be heard over stenosed vessels such as renal arteries.
- Venous hum in the epigastrium: portal hypertension.
- Friction rubs: may rarely be heard over the liver (infarction, tumour, or gonococcal perihepatitis) or spleen (infarction).
- Succussion splash: any cause of gastric outlet obstruction e.g. pyloric stenosis. It can only be assessed more than 2 hours after a meal or may be falsely positive.

Other signs

- Look at the legs for pitting oedema (Fig. 38.23).
- In the clinical examinations, if you say that you would also like to examine the genitalia and perform a rectal examination, you will usually be taken to the next case. When seeing patients as a

Causes of ascites	
Type	**Cause**
Transudate (protein <25 g/L)	Cardiac failure Liver failure Hypoproteinaemia Meigs' syndrome Myxoedema Constrictive pericarditis (rare) Cirrhosis with portal hypertension
Exudate (protein >25 g/L)	Intra-abdominal malignancy Infection (tuberculosis, perforation, spontaneous) Pancreatitis Budd–Chiari syndrome Lymphatic obstruction (chylous)

Fig. 38.21 Causes of ascites.

Causes of ileus
• Following intra-abdominal surgery where the gut has been handled • Peritonitis • Pancreatitis • Hypokalaemia • Uraemia • Diabetic ketoacidosis • Intra-abdominal haemorrhage • Retroperitoneal haematoma • Retroperitoneal trauma, e.g. surgery for aortic aneurysm • Anticholinergic drugs

Fig. 38.22 Causes of ileus.

practising clinician, always consider whether these examinations are appropriate. In some circumstances, they are essential, such as rectal bleeding, iron deficiency, or change in bowel habit.
• If there is hepatosplenomegaly, go on to examine all lymph node sites, bearing in mind myeloproliferative and lymphoproliferative disorders, sarcoidosis, viruses such as Epstein–Barr virus, and liver disease complicated by portal hypertension.

The nervous system

All medical short case examinations will involve at least one neurology case—this usually fills medical

Causes of lower limb oedema	
Cause	**Examples**
Pitting	Unilateral: Deep venous thrombosis Unilateral compression of veins (nodes, tumour) Bilateral: Right ventricular failure Tricuspid stenosis Constrictive pericarditis Hepatic failure Nephrotic syndrome Protein-losing enteropathy Inferior vena cava obstruction (thrombosis, nodes, tumour) Immobility Kwashiorkor
Lymphatic (non-pitting)	Obstruction by nodes, tumour or infection (filariasis) Congenital hypoplasia (Milroy's disease) Myxoedema

Fig. 38.23 Causes of lower limb oedema.

students and membership candidates with fear and dread!

Although it is true that neuroanatomy is complicated and many different diseases can affect each part, the end result is a limited repertoire of patterns of signs. The best approach is to identify which signs are present using a well-rehearsed technique and consider where the lesion is likely to be. You can then think of which diseases affect that part of the nervous system and look for additional evidence to support the diagnosis.

The clinical signs and common diseases associated with different parts of the nervous system are discussed in detail in Chapter 23. This section covers a practical approach to the examination technique itself. It is particularly important to practise this routine over and over again as it is the most difficult to perform competently and will be all the more impressive if you can do it well!

General inspection
• Appearance: does the patient look well or ill?
• Level of consciousness: is the patient conscious or unconscious?
• Age: a young patient is more likely to have multiple sclerosis or an inherited disease; an elderly patient is more likely to have had a stroke.
• General clues: is there a wheelchair (the problem also affects the legs) or diabetic drinks (peripheral neuropathy or stroke)?
• Posture: how is the patient sitting? Is the patient leaning towards one side (hemiparesis)? Is there a tremor at rest (parkinsonism)?
• Speech: when the patient speaks does the speech sound normal? (see Fig. 37.5)

Cranial nerves
Features and examinations of the cranial nerves include the following.

First cranial nerve (olfactory)
• Sensory only.
• This is not routinely tested, but ask the patient if they have noticed anything abnormal about their sense of smell.
• Sense of smell can be tested using bottles containing essences, though this test is rarely performed. (Note that ammonia should not be used as it also stimulates the trigeminal nerve.)
• Anosmia can result from head injury (fracture of the cribriform plate), upper respiratory tract

393

infection, tumour (olfactory groove meningioma or glioma), or Kallmann's syndrome (anosmia with hypogonadotrophic hypogonadism).

Second cranial nerve (optic)

- Sensory only.
- Pupillary reflexes: the pupillary reactions to light and accommodation should be tested. It is essential to understand the sympathetic and parasympathetic innervation of the pupils as well as the neurological pathways involved in the light and convergence reflexes if pupillary abnormalities are to be understood (see *Crash Course in Nervous System and Special Senses*). Pupillary abnormalities in coma patients are described in Fig. 19.5. Other clinical abnormalities include:
  - Physiological anisocoria—slight difference in size.
  - Senile miosis—small, irregular pupils in old age.
  - Afferent pupillary defect (complete lesion of optic nerve). If the left eye is affected, shining light in it fails to cause constriction in either eye—absent direct and consensual reflexes. However, if light is shone in the right eye the left eye dilates (i.e. the right eye consensual reflex is intact).
  - Relative afferent pupillary defect (RAPD; Marcus–Gunn pupil). This occurs if there is incomplete damage to the afferent pathway (e.g. previous retrobulbar neuritis due to multiple sclerosis). The swinging light test is performed (i.e. the light is moved from one eye to the other alternately). If the left eye has a RAPD, there will be delayed conduction along its afferent pathway. Therefore, if the light is initially shone in the left eye, both pupils will constrict; on moving the light to the right eye, bilateral constriction occurs again; when the light returns to the left eye, the pupil dilates initially due to its delayed afferent conduction. This is diagnostic of a RAPD.

- Horner's syndrome—see Miscellaneous Neurological Disorders.
- Argyll Robertson pupil—a small irregular pupil that 'accommodates but does not react' (i.e. fixed to light but constricts on convergence). Almost diagnostic of neurosyphilis (occasionally occurs in diabetes mellitus).
- Myotonic pupil (Holmes–Adie pupil)—a dilated pupil that reacts very slowly to light and constricts incompletely to convergence. Most common in young females and, if combined with absent tendon reflexes, this is Holmes–Adie syndrome.
- Visual acuity: ask the patient to read some print or Snellen's chart (with spectacles if normally worn). Test each eye separately. Any lesion from the cornea, lens, retina, optic nerve, optic chiasm, optic radiation, or occipital cortex can result in reduced acuity.
- Visual fields: test each eye individually. Make sure your eyes are on the same level as the patient's. Move your fingers from beyond your visual field inwards and ask the patient to tell you when they can see them. Check each quadrant. Use a red hat pin to determine the blind spot. Typical field defects are shown in Fig. 38.24. Vision can be formally assessed using perimetry. If the visual

Visual field defects		
Defect	Site of lesion	Causes
Tunnel vision	Retina	Glaucoma, retinitis pigmentosa, laser therapy for diabetic retinopathy
Enlarged blind spot	Optic nerve	Papilloedema (due to any cause)
Central scotoma	Macula, optic nerve	Optic atrophy, optic neuritis, retinal disease affecting macula
Monocular visual loss	Eye, optic nerve	Extrinsic compression, toxic optic neuropathy
Bitemporal hemianopia	Optic chiasm	Pituitary tumour, craniopharyngioma, sella meningioma
Quadrantic hemianopia	Temporal lobe (superior) Parietal lobe (inferior)	Stroke, tumour
Homonymous hemianopia	Occipital cortex, optic tract	Stroke, tumour

Fig. 38.24 Visual field defects.

fields are intact look for inattention by simultaneously stimulating both the left and right.

- Fundoscopy: common abnormalities on fundoscopy are papilloedema (Fig. 38.25), optic atrophy (Fig. 38.26), diabetic retinopathy (Fig. 38.27), hypertensive retinopathy (Fig. 27.23), and retinitis pigmentosa—a familial condition. Pigmentary retinal degeneration may also occur in other conditions such as Refsum's disease and Laurence–Moon–Biedl syndrome.

Third, fourth, and sixth cranial nerves

- Control the eye's movements.
- Ask the patient to follow your finger with their eyes and tell you if they 'see double'.
- Look for nystagmus. This is involuntary rhythmic eye oscillation. It occurs physiologically at the extremes of lateral gaze and >2 beats are required for it to be significant. Cerebellar lesions cause nystagmus on lateral gaze that is more coarse on the ipsilateral side. Lesions of the vestibular apparatus and its connections can cause nystagmus (see p. 147). Brainstem lesions may cause unusual patterns of nystagmus. Congenital causes and early loss of central vision (e.g. albinism) may cause pendular nystagmus.
- Assess conjugate gaze by asking the patient to look at your hand and then to a finger on your other hand, and then from one to the other as quickly as possible. If there is an internuclear ophthalmoplegia (a lesion in the medial longitudinal fasciculus), there will be slow

Causes of optic atrophy	
Cause	**Examples**
Pressure on optic nerve	Tumour, glaucoma, aneurysm, Paget's disease
Demyelination	Multiple sclerosis
Vascular	Central retinal artery occlusion
Metabolic	Diabetes mellitus, vitamin B_{12} deficiency
Toxins	Methyl alcohol, tobacco, lead, quinine
Trauma	Including surgery
Consecutive	Due to extensive retinal disease such as choroidoretinitis
Hereditary prolonged papilloedema	Friedreich's ataxia, Leber's optic atrophy

Fig. 38.26 Causes of optic atrophy.

movement in the adducting eye and nystagmus in the abducting eye. If one eye is covered, or if convergence is attempted, adduction is normal as this is a disorder of conjugate gaze. Internuclear ophthalmoplegia is usually caused by multiple sclerosis but may occasionally result from vascular lesions.

Stages of diabetic retinopathy	
Stage	**Features**
Background	Dot haemorrhages (microaneurysms), blot haemorrhages, hard exudates
Preproliferative	All of the above, plus multiple soft exudates (cotton wool spots), flame haemorrhages, venous beading and loops, IRMAs
Proliferative	All of the above, plus new vessel formation on retina or iris (rubeosis iridis), retinal detachment, preretinal or vitreous haemorrhage, glaucoma (with rubeosis iridis)
Maculopathy	Hard exudates (possibly in a ring – 'circinate') within a disc width of the macula; decreased acuity not correcting with a pinhole suggestive of macular oedema (therefore must check acuity)

Fig. 38.27 Stages of diabetic retinopathy. Note that cataracts are also more common in diabetes, and that retinopathy may have been treated by laser photocoagulation (burns around the periphery of the retina, destroying ischaemic tissue and thus reducing the drive for new vessel formation). (IRMA, intraretinal microvascular abnormality.)

Causes of papilloedema	
Cause	**Examples**
Raised intracranial pressure	Tumour, abscess, hydrocephalus, haematoma, benign intracranial hypertension, cerebral oedema (trauma)
Venous occlusion	Central retinal vein thrombosis, cavernous sinus thrombosis
Malignant hypertension	Grade IV hypertensive retinopathy
Acute optic neuritis	Multiple sclerosis, sarcoidosis
Metabolic	Hypercapnia, hypoparathyroidism
Haematological (rare)	Severe anaemia, acute leukaemia

Fig. 38.25 Causes of papilloedema.

- Diplopia in all directions of gaze may result from myasthenia gravis, ocular myopathy or disease in the surrounding tissue of eye, such as Graves' disease, tumour, or orbital cellulitis.

Third cranial nerve (oculomotor)

- Motor supply to levator palpebrae superioris, all orbital muscles except the superior oblique and lateral rectus muscles, and parasympathetic tone to pupillary reflex.
- Controls pupillary reflexes, in addition to the second cranial nerve. Test the reaction to light and accommodation (as above).
- Lesion of this nerve results in ptosis and a dilated pupil with no reaction to light or accommodation. The eye looks 'down and out' at rest and is unable to look upwards or inwards.
- Causes of third cranial nerve lesions are infarction, posterior communicating artery aneurysm (which is painful), mononeuritis multiplex (see p. 132), demyelination, tumour, and neurosyphilis. Medical, as opposed to mechanical compressive, causes of third nerve palsy often spare the parasympathetic nerve fibres (i.e. there is 'pupillary sparing'). Conversely, compressive lesions are associated with relatively less ophthalmoplegia. This is because the parasympathetic fibres run on the surface of the nerve.

Fourth cranial nerve (trochlear)

- Motor supply to the superior oblique muscle.
- Patient may have the head tilted away from the lesion.
- Diplopia on looking down and away from the lesion with one image at an angle to the other.
- Fourth cranial nerve lesions are usually associated with third cranial nerve lesions and have a similar aetiology.

Patients with a fourth cranial nerve palsy have difficulty with vision when walking downstairs or reading a book

Sixth cranial nerve (abducens)

- Motor supply to the lateral rectus.
- There is diplopia on abduction of the affected eye with two images side by side.
- Sixth cranial nerve lesions are caused by mononeuritis multiplex, diabetes mellitus, demyelination, tumour, infarction, thiamine deficiency (Wernicke's encephalopathy), raised intracranial pressure (false localising sign), and neurosyphilis.

Fifth cranial nerve (trigeminal)

- Sensation to the face (ophthalmic, maxillary, and mandibular branches).
- Motor supply to the muscles of mastication (temporalis, masseter, and pterygoid muscles).
- Test sensation in the distribution of each division comparing one side with the other.
- Remember the corneal reflex, which requires intact motor function of the seventh cranial nerve for blinking.
- Ask the patient to clench the teeth.
- Ask them to hold the mouth open while you try to push it shut.
- Test jaw jerk, which is increased in pseudobulbar palsy, and reduced or absent in bulbar palsy.
- The causes of fifth cranial nerve lesions are shown in Fig. 38.28.

Fig. 38.28 Causes of a trigeminal nerve lesion.

Causes of a trigeminal nerve lesion	
Cause	**Examples**
Brainstem	Tumour, infarction, demyelination, syringobulbia
Cerebellopontine angle	Acoustic neuroma, meningioma
Petrous temporal bone	Trauma, tumour, middle ear disease, herpes zoster
Cavernous sinus	Tumour, thrombosis, aneurysm of internal carotid artery
Peripheral	Meningeal tuberculosis, syphilis, lymphoma, carcinoma, sarcoid

Seventh cranial nerve (facial)

- Sensation of taste from the floor of the mouth, the soft palate, and anterior two thirds of the tongue.
- Motor supply to the muscles of facial expression and the stapedius muscle.
- Parasympathetic supply to the salivary and lacrimal glands.
- Ask the patient to wrinkle the forehead, screw the eyes tightly shut, show the teeth, and blow the cheeks out.
- In lower motor neurone lesions all the muscles are affected.
- In upper motor neurone lesions, the upper half of the face and emotional expressions are spared (e.g. normal eye closure and wrinkling of the forehead).
- Taste is not usually examined formally but ask if the patient has noticed any recent change. Involvement of the nerve to stapedius causes hyperacusis (increased sensitivity to high pitched or loud sounds).
- Fig. 38.29 summarises the causes of facial nerve palsies.

Whenever you see a lower motor neurone lesion of the facial nerve, look around the ear for a herpes zoster rash (Ramsay Hunt syndrome)

Eighth cranial nerve (vestibulocochlear)

- Sensory to the utricle, saccule, and semicircular canals (vestibular), and to the organ of Corti (cochlea).

- Ask if the patient has noticed any difficulty with hearing.
- Assess the ability of the patient to hear whispered numbers with the other ear covered.
- Rinne's test: place a vibrating tuning fork on the mastoid process and then at the external auditory meatus—the test is positive if the sound is louder when the fork is held at the external auditory meatus (i.e. air conduction) than when placed on the mastoid process (i.e. bone conduction). This is normal. An abnormal test (Rinne negative) indicates conductive deafness.
- Weber's test: place a vibrating tuning fork at the centre of the forehead; the sound will be heard towards the normal ear in sensorineural deafness or towards the affected ear in conductive deafness.
- The causes of vestibular disease are shown in Fig. 25.3.
- The causes of conductive and sensorineural deafness are described in Fig. 38.30.

Ninth and tenth cranial nerves

- Look at palatal movement (ask the patient to say 'Aah').
- No palatal elevation on the affected side, with the uvula pulled towards the normal side.
- Check the gag reflex (ninth, sensory; tenth, motor).
- Fig. 38.31 summarises diseases affecting these nerves.

Ninth cranial nerve (glossopharyngeal)

- Sensory to pharynx and carotid sinus and taste to the posterior third of the tongue.
- Motor supply to the stylopharyngeus muscle.
- Parasympathetic to the parotid gland.

Fig. 38.29 Causes of facial nerve palsies.

Causes of facial nerve palsies	
Cause	Examples
Upper motor neuron central	Stroke, tumour
Lower motor neuron pons	Stroke, tumour, demyelination, motor neurone disease
Cerebellopontine angle	Acoustic neuroma, meningioma
Petrous temporal bone	Bell's palsy, herpes zoster (Ramsay-Hunt)
Middle ear disease	Infection, tumour
Peripheral	Trauma, parotid disease, mononeuritis multiplex, sarcoid, Guillain-Barré syndrome

Fig. 38.30 Causes of deafness.

Causes of deafness	
Cause	Examples
Conductive	Wax, foreign body, otitis externa, injury to tympanic membrane, otitis media, ofosclerosis (e.g. Paget's disease), middle ear tumour (e.g. cholesteatoma)
Sensorineural	Presbycusis (due to old age), noise induced, drugs (aminoglycosides, aspirin overdose), infection (meningitis, syphilis, measles), congenital (maternal rubella, cytomegalovirus, toxoplasmosis), Ménière's disease, acoustic neuroma, trauma, Paget's disease

Tenth cranial nerve (vagus)
- Sensory to the larynx.
- Motor supply to the cricothyroid and the muscles of the pharynx and larynx.
- Parasympathetic to the bronchi, heart, and gastrointestinal tract.

Eleventh cranial nerve (accessory)
- Cranial root provides the motor supply to some muscles of the soft palate and larynx.
- Spinal root provides the motor supply to the trapezius and sternocleidomastoid muscles.
- Ask the patient to shrug the shoulders and test against resistance.
- Ask the patient to turn his or her head against your resisting hand and test the sternocleidomastoid muscle bulk.

Twelth cranial nerve (hypoglossal)
- Provides the motor supply to the styloglossus, hyoglossus, and all intrinsic muscles of the tongue.
- Ask the patient to open the mouth. Look for wasting and fasciculation, indicating a lower motor neurone lesion of the tongue.
- Then ask the patient to protrude the tongue. If there is a unilateral lesion the tongue will deviate towards the side of the lesion.
- Upper motor neurone lesions are due to stroke, tumour, or motor neurone disease.

- Lower motor neurone lesions are due to diseases in the posterior fossa, skull base, and the neck, including tumour, motor neurone disease, syringobulbia, trauma, and poliomyelitis.

The upper limbs
Inspection
- Wasting: lower motor neurone lesion, muscle disease, and disuse.
- Fasciculation: lower motor neurone lesion.
- Scars: particularly from surgery.
- Deformity: may cause mononeuropathy by entrapment, and contractures may be the result of neurological disease.
- Tremor (Fig. 38.32).

 Do not confuse the asterixis of metabolic encephalopathy with a tremor

Pronator drift
- Ask the patient to hold his or her arms outstretched before them with the palms facing upwards.
- Marked weakness due to any cause will become immediately apparent.

Fig. 38.31 Causes of glossopharyngeal, vagus, and accessory nerve palsies.

Causes of glossopharyngeal, vagus and accessory nerve palsies	
Cause	Examples
Central (brainstem)	Tumour, infarction, syringobulbia, motor neuron disease
Peripheral	Tumour or aneurysm near the jugular foramen, trauma of skull base, Guillain–Barré syndrome, poliomyelitis

Fig. 38.32 Causes of tremor.

Causes of tremor		
Type	**Features**	**Causes**
Resting	Seen when patients relaxed with hands at rest	Parkinsonism
Postural	Seen when hands held outstretched	Benign essential tremor Anxiety Thyrotoxicosis β_2-agonists
Intention	Seen when patients try to touch examiner's finger with their own finger	Cerebellar disease

- Ask the patient to keep their arms still and close their eyes.
- If there is an upper motor neurone lesion (affecting the parietal lobe), the arm will drift downwards and the palm will turn downwards.

Tone
Reduced tone is a feature of a lower motor neurone lesion or cerebellar lesion. Hypertonia may manifest as either spasticity or rigidity. Spasticity describes the sudden build up of increased tone during the first few degrees of passive movement. The resistance lessens as the movement is continued and this is characteristic of upper motor neurone lesions. This is often described as the 'clasp-knife' phenomenon. Rigidity describes the sustained resistance to passive movement seen in extrapyramidal conditions (e.g. parkinsonism). This may be described as 'lead pipe' rigidity and when associated with a tremor gives rise to 'cogwheel' rigidity.

Power
All muscle groups should be tested and scored (Fig. 38.33). You will need to learn the root value for each movement (Fig. 38.34). Remember to compare muscle power of one side to the other for each group.

Coordination
Ask the patient to alternately touch their nose and your finger. In cerebellar disease, there will be an intention tremor and past pointing (i.e. the patient overshoots the examining clinician's finger consistently towards the side of the lesion). Ask the patient to tap one palm with alternating sides of the other hand as quickly as possible (demonstrate to the patient what you would like them to do). In cerebellar disease, this will be slow, poorly coordinated, and the action of the moving hand has a high amplitude—this is dysdiadochokinesis.

Reflexes
Practise as often as you can. Learn the root value of each reflex—these are clinically useful as well as helpful in examinations! (Fig. 38.35). Reflexes can be reduced, normal or increased. They will be reduced or absent in lower motor neurone lesions, sensory neuropathy, and severe muscle disease (disruption of reflex arc), and will be exaggerated in upper motor neurone lesions.

Sensation
Test each dermatome (Fig. 38.36) for the sensation of light touch, pinprick (and temperature). Then, starting distally, check vibration and joint position sense. Remember the different pathways these senses take (Fig. 38.37).

The lower limbs
Inspection
- Wasting: lower motor neurone lesion, muscle disease, and disuse.
- Fasciculation: lower motor neurone lesion.
- Scars: particularly from surgery.

Grading muscle power	
Grade	**Features**
0	No movement at all
1	Flicker of movement only
2	Movement only when gravity excluded
3	Movement against gravity only
4	Movement against gravity and some additional resistance
5	Normal power

Fig. 38.33 Grading muscle power.

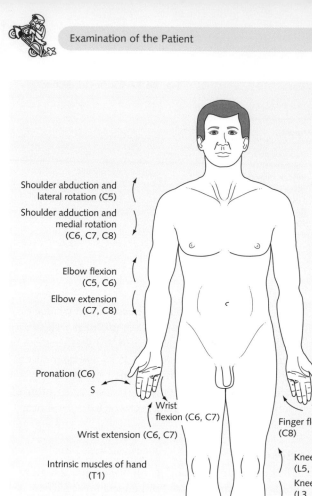

Fig. 38.34 Nerve roots for each muscle group movement.

Shoulder abduction and lateral rotation (C5)

Shoulder adduction and medial rotation (C6, C7, C8)

Elbow flexion (C5, C6)

Elbow extension (C7, C8)

Pronation (C6)

Wrist flexion (C6, C7)

Wrist extension (C6, C7)

Intrinsic muscles of hand (T1)

Hip flexion (L2, L3)

Hip extension (L4, L5)

Finger extension (C7)

Finger flexion (C8)

Knee flexion (L5, S1)

Knee extension (L3, L4)

Dorsi flexion (L4, L5)

Plantar flexion (S1, S2)

Inversion (L4)   Eversion (S1)

- Deformity: may cause mononeuropathy by entrapment, and contractures may be the result of neurological disease.
- Pes cavus: Charcot–Marie–Tooth disease, Refsum's disease.
- Catheter: neurogenic urinary incontinence.
- Walking aids: wheelchair and stick indicating degree of disability.

Gait
- Ask the patient to walk for 2–3 metres, turn and walk back, then walk heel to toe (cerebellar

ataxia), and finally stand on toes and on heels (any muscle weakness will now manifest itself).
- Make sure you walk with the patient so you can catch them if they fall.
- An immense amount of information can be gained by careful study of these aspects of gait (Fig. 23.3).

Tone
Reduced tone is a feature of a lower motor neurone lesion or cerebellar lesion. Tone may be increased in an upper motor neurone lesion or

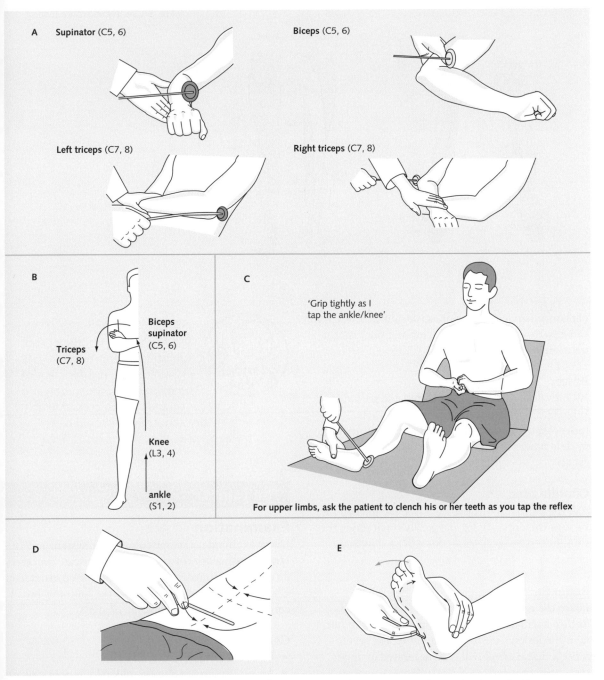

Fig. 38.35 Eliciting reflexes. (A) Upper limb tendon reflexes. (B) A simple way to remember root values of reflexes. (C) Testing ankle jerk with reinforcement. (D) Abdominal reflexes: test in four quadrants shown. (E) The normal response is a downgoing hallux. In an upper motor neurone lesion, the hallux dorsiflexes and other toes fan out (the Babinski response).

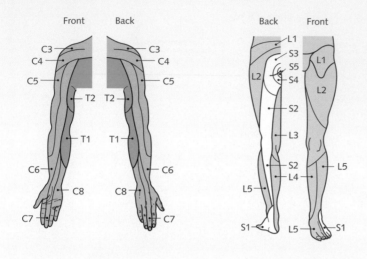

Fig. 38.36 Dermatome testing.

parkinsonism. Test for clonus (usually at ankle, but can also do at patella), signifying an upper motor neurone lesion.

Power

All muscle groups should be tested and scored (Fig. 38.33). Learn the nerve roots for each movement (Fig. 38.34). Remember to compare muscle power of one side to the other for each group.

Coordination

Ask the patient to lift the leg, place the heel on the knee of the opposite leg and gently run it down the shin. In cerebellar disease, this will be slow and clumsy.

Reflexes

Learn the root value of each reflex (Fig. 38.35). Reflexes will be reduced or absent in lower motor neurone lesions, sensory neuropathy, and severe muscle disease, and will be exaggerated in upper motor neurone lesions. Check plantar response, which is normally downgoing but will be upgoing in upper motor neurone lesions.

Sensation

Test each dermatome (Fig. 38.36) for sensation of light touch, pinprick (and temperature). Then, starting distally, check vibration and joint position sense. Check specifically for peripheral neurology—'stocking' distribution.

The sensory pathways are shown in Fig. 38.37.

Sensory testing is difficult and subjective. A thorough inspection and examination of tone, power, coordination and reflexes should help to predict which sensory abnormality should be expected

The joints

Examination

Diseases affecting the musculoskeletal system and how to distinguish between different disease processes on clinical examination have been discussed in detail in Chapter 17. However, remember the following broad components to the examination of joints.

General

- Does the patient look well or ill?
- Anaemia: chronic disease, blood loss (peptic ulcer due to non-steroidal use), bone marrow suppression (immunosuppressive therapy), haemolysis (autoimmune associated with systemic lupus erythematosus), and hypersplenism (Felty's syndrome in RA).
- Face: scleroderma, systemic lupus erythematosus, cushingoid facies (long-term steroid therapy).
- Stooped: ankylosing spondylitis and osteoporosis.

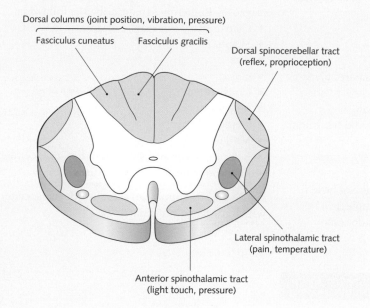

Dorsal columns (joint position, vibration, pressure)

Fasciculus cuneatus   Fasciculus gracilis

Dorsal spinocerebellar tract
(reflex, proprioception)

Lateral spinothalamic tract
(pain, temperature)

Anterior spinothalamic tract
(light touch, pressure)

Sensory pathways			
Sensation	Tested using	Pathway	Level of decussation
Pain	Neurotip	Lateral spinothalamic tract	At level of sensory root within one spinal segment
Temperature	Tuning fork for cold	Lateral spinothalamic tract	At level of sensory root within one spinal segment
Light touch	Cotton wool	Anterior spinothalamic tract	At level of sensory root within several spinal segments
Vibration	Tuning fork	Posterior columns (fasciculus gracilis and fasciculus cuneatus)	Medulla oblongata
Joint position sense	Move fixed joints	Posterior columns (fasciculus gracilis and fasciculus cuneatus)	Medulla oblongata
Two-point discrimination	Orange stick	Posterior columns (fasciculus gracilis and fasciculus cuneatus)	Medulla oblongata

Fig. 38.37 (A) Anatomy of sensory pathways within the spinal cord. (B) Tests for different sensory modalities.

Look

- Deformity.
- Scars: previous surgery.
- Erythema: acute inflammation or infection.
- Swelling: osteophytes, synovial hypertrophy, and acute inflammation.
- Muscle wasting: disuse, nerve entrapment, mononeuritis multiplex, or long-term steroid therapy.

Feel

- Increased temperature: acute inflammation or infection.
- Tenderness.
- Effusions.
- Crepitus on movement.

Move

- Active and passive movement.

- Is pain associated with movement?
- Is the joint stable? Are there intact ligaments and supporting musculature?

What is the underlying cause?

- Psoriatic rash.
- Subcutaneous rheumatoid nodules:particularly at the elbow.
- Gouty tophi: on the pinna and elbow.
- Look for evidence of long-term steroid treatment (Fig. 32.15).

Disability

It is very important to get an impression of how limiting the joint problem is. for example, in a patient with RA, ask the patient to undo some buttons or write their name with a pen.

look at a rash, you will be awarded marks for giving a good description, even if you are unable to make a diagnosis. Remember to describe the following:

- Distribution: this can be diagnostic in itself.
- Shape.
- Size.
- Colour.
- Consistency.
- Temperature.
- Tenderness.
- Margins.
- Relation to the surface: raised, flat, or ulcerated.
- Fixation to underlying structures.

Figure 38.38 summarises skin disorders associated with underlying systemic disease.

The skin

The clinical approach to skin rashes has been discussed in detail in Chapter 18. When asked to

Skin disorders associated with underlying systemic disease	
Disease	**Skin manifestation**
Diabetes mellitus	Necrobiosis lipoidica diabeticorum, granuloma annulare, acanthosis nigricans
Sarcoidosis	Lupus pernio, scar infiltration, erythema nodosum
Malignancy	Dermatomyositis, acanthosis nigricans, necrolytic migratory erythema (glucagonoma), erythema gyratum repens (usually bronchial carcinoma), thrombophlebitis migrans (pancreatic carcinoma)
Liver disease	Spider naevi, palmar erythema, leukonychia, porphyria cutanea tarda, pigmentation
Renal disease	Uraemic frost (rare), pale yellow pigmentation, half-and-half nails
Hyperlipidaemia	Xanthelasmata, tendon xanthomata, eruptive xanthomata
Neurofibromatosis	*Café-au-lait* patches, axillary freckling, neurofibromas, plexiform neuromas

Fig. 38.38 Skin disorders associated with underlying systemic disease.

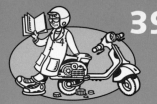

39. The Clerking

Introduction

The doctor's 'clerking' is a written summary of the patient's history and examination. It is a legal document and should be precise, complete, and legible. Avoid using abbreviations – although the meaning may be obvious to you, they may be interpreted very differently in a different speciality or hospital. However, in real life, abbreviations litter the medical notes and you ought to be familiar with the most common ones.

The 'history of presenting complaint' section is a useful place to document the most relevant positive and negative historical points. Less relevant details can be recorded in their appropriate sub-section. For example, in the case below, the relevant negative historical points have been included in the 'history of presenting complaint' rather than elsewhere in the clerking.

At the end of the clerking, the salient points should be emphasised in a summary statement. You should then, always, compile a 'problem list'. This is often forgotten by students and junior doctors alike, but is invaluable in planning appropriate investigations and management. In some patients, it will not be appropriate, or even possible, to take a full history and perform a full clinical examination (e.g. in an emergency situation). We have outlined a clinical example.

As a student, it is good practice to be very thorough as it helps you to learn the relevant questions and to avoid missing anything important. However, with practice, you will learn to tailor carefully the clinical approach to each patient based on their individual, and often very different, needs.

Medical sample clerking

Hospital No. X349282

BLOGGS, Joe DOB 29/4/46
58 year old man

01/01/04 07.20   Referred by General practitioner

PC   Shortness of breath

> 1. Presenting complaint should be brief, but it is helpful to mention relevant background information.

HPC   4-day history of worsening dyspnoea. Gradual onset over hours.
            Initially noted while climbing stairs at home. Over the last 12 hours
            has become short of breath at rest. No periods of relief since onset.
            Relieving/exacerbating factors:
            Relieved by rest. Exacerbated by exertion.
            Associated symptoms:
            Cough productive of green sputum for 3 days.
            Sharp left sided posterior chest pain worsened by coughing and inspiration.
            Feels 'feverish'.
            Relevant direct questions:
            Usually unlimited exercise tolerance
            Lifelong non-smoker
            No asthma, tuberculosis exposure, occupational exposure to
            chemicals or asbestos.
            No pets or travel abroad
            No haemoptysis, worsening of chest pain on exertion, ankle swelling, calf pain
            palpitations, trauma to chest wall, orthopnoea or paroxysmal nocturnal dyspnoea.

> 2. Mention only the relevant negatives.

> 3. A useful way of recording important negatives on one line.

PMH   1963   appendectomy
            1972   duodenal ulcer (no symptoms since)

            No diabetes, hypertension, rheumatic heart disease, epilepsy, jaundice, cerebrovascular disease

S/E   General - fatigue lately, appetite unchanged, weight stable, no sweats or pruritus
            CVS - as above
            RS - As above
            GIT - No current indigestion. No symptoms like previous duodenal ulcer.
                        No vomiting/dyspnoea/abdominal pain
            GUS - No urinary symptoms
            NS - No headache/syncope. No dizziness/limb weakness/sensory loss. No disturbed vision/
                        hearing/smell/speech
            MS - No joint pain/stiffness/swelling. No disability
            Skin - No rash/pruritus/bruising

DH   No regular or over the counter medication.
            Penicillin allergy - facial swelling and
            rash as young child

> 4. Always record the dose and frequency of any drugs – remember you'll be writing the drug chart later! Always document that you have asked about drug allergies

Fam Hx   Father died of 'heart attack' aged 52
            Mother died of 'old age' at 88

Social Hx   Lives with wife who is fit and well
            Own house. Stairs
            Completely independent
            Never smoked
            Alcohol: 24 units per week
            Sexual history: not appropriate
            No recent overseas travel
            No pets
            Occupation: hotel porter

O/E   General: unwell, short of breath. Can complete sentences. Not
using accessory muscles of inspiration. Sweaty.
No cyanosis or clubbing. No pallor
Temperature: 38.5 C

> **5.** Record your initial observations – they are important. 'Alert and chatty' or 'Distressed and looks unwell' tell you a lot about the patient.

CVS   Pulse 104 bpm regular, normal character
BP 110/70 mmHg (right)
JVP normal
No praecordial scars/chest deformities
Apex beat normal position and character
No parasternal heave/thrills
Auscultation; heart sounds normal. No added sounds. No oedema.
Peripheral pulses palpable.

hs ———+——————||————————+——

              1   2   1

> **6.** You can use diagrams to clarify your examination findings

Dull percussion note
↑vocal fremitus
Bronchial breath sounds
↑vocal resonance
Whispering Pectoriloquy
No pleural rub

RS   Trachea central
Respiratory rate is 28/min
Expansion symmetrical and normal
Vocal fremitus increased at left base posteriorly
Dull percussion note at left base posteriorly
Bronchial breath sounds at left base with increased vocal resonance and whispering pectorilquy

Abdomen   Appendectomy scar right iliac fossa. No veins/distension
Palpation: soft and non-tender. No palpable masses or organomegaly
Percussion note normal
Auscultation bowel sounds normal
Genitalia not examined
Rectal examination: not performed

soft + non-tender
° masses
o organomegaly
Bowel sounds normal

NS   Higher function normal
Cranial nerves: I: normal
II: PERLA (pupils equal in reaction to light and accommodation)
normal fundi and visual fields
III, IV, VI: no diplopia/nystagmus
V, VII, VIII, IX, X, XI, XII: normal
Upper and lower limbs: power, tone, coordination, sensation all normal

Reflexes		Right	Left
	Biceps	++	++
	Supinator	++	++
	Triceps	++	++
	Knee	++	++
	Ankle	+	+
	Plantar	↓	↓

Joints and skin   Normal

Summary   58 year old male non-smoker presents with a 4 day history of worsening exertional dyspnoea associated with a productive cough, pleuritic left sided chest pain and symptoms of fever. On examination he is short of breath and tachypnoeic. He has a pyrexia and signs of consolidation at the left base. The most likely diagnosis is left-sided community acquired pneumonia.

Problem list   Dyspnoea? Left basal pneumonia.
Penicillin allergy.

7. Sign your notes, including printed surname and bleep number

PARKER, 552

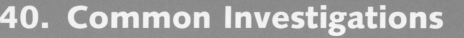
Introduction

By the time it comes to organising investigations, the good clinician will already have a fairly clear idea of what he or she is likely to find. The investigation plan should be well structured, starting with simple non-invasive tests designed to answer specific questions. Remember two important rules:

- Do not request a test if you do not know why you are doing it. There is nothing worse than getting an abnormal result and wondering whether it is important or not!
- If a test is worth requesting, always make sure you see the result—it may be the clue you need.

If you are given an investigation to comment on in any examination, always describe what the investigation is, the patient's name, and the date it was performed. This is a good habit to get into, as the name will usually tell you what sex the patient is, their age and possibly their ethnic background. As a practising clinician, it is also important as patients' results occasionally find their way into the wrong set of notes.

The cardiovascular system

Cardiac enzymes

The traditional method of diagnosing myocardial necrosis is to measure the change in levels of several enzymes released by damaged myocardium over subsequent days (Fig. 40.1). These include creatine kinase (CK) and its cardiac isoform CK-MB, aspartate aminotransferase (AST) and lactate dehydrogenase (LDH). CK remains valuable but their value has changed with the use of Troponin I and T measurements. Troponins are specific to heart muscle and are involved in the myocyte contraction generated by actin and myosin filaments. A normal subject will have negligible levels of serum troponin. Therefore any increase in the troponin level indicates myocardial damage. After cardiac chest pain, a single measurement is performed at 6–12 hours and, if positive, need not be repeated.

It is raised by any myocardial damage and will be elevated with myocarditis. There is debate concerning the level at which it should be considered significant in renal failure as it is excreted by the kidneys.

Electrocardiogram

The 12-lead electrocardiogram (ECG) is an assessment of the electrical activity of the heart. Ten electrodes are attached to the patient giving 12 different 'views' of the heart (Fig. 40.3). Diagnostic information is obtained by considering the different components of the ECG. When starting to interpret ECGs, always be systematic to avoid missing abnormalities.

Rate

Divide 300 by the number of large squares between two QRS complexes to give the number of b.p.m. (each large square represents 0.2 seconds). Normal

Elevation of cardiac enzymes post myocardial infarction (CK, AST, LDH)			
	Begins to size (hours)	Peak (hours)	Returns to normal (days)
Enzyme			
CK-MB	1-6	12-24	1-2
CK	6	24	2-3
AST	12	24-48	3-5
LDH	24	48-72	10-14
Troponin	6	12-24	14

Fig. 40.1 Elevation of cardiac enzymes and troponin post myocardial infarction. (CK, creatine kinase; AST, aspartate aminotransferase; LDH, lactate dehydrogenase.)

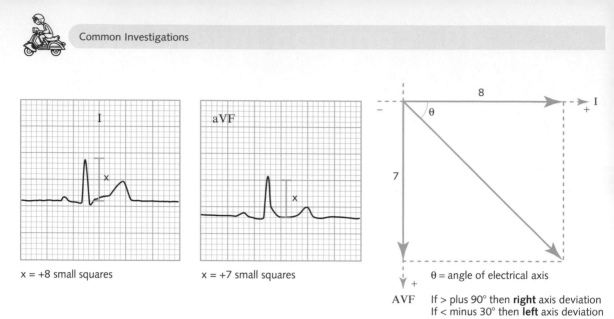

x = +8 small squares | x = +7 small squares | θ = angle of electrical axis

AVF   If > plus 90° then **right** axis deviation
If < minus 30° then **left** axis deviation

Fig. 40.2 The position of the anterior electrodes for a 12-lead electrocardiogram.

rate is 60–100 b.p.m. Causes of sinus tachycardia and bradycardia are shown in Fig. 40.4.

Rhythm

Are the QRS complexes regular? If irregular is it irregularly irregular and is each QRS preceded by a P wave (Chapter 3)?

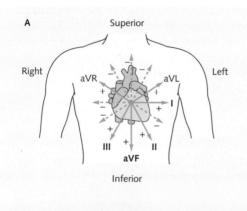

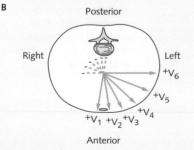

Fig. 40.3 The 12 different views of the heart given by a 12-lead electrocardiogram. (A) Superior perspective. (B) Posterior perspective.

Causes of sinus tachycardia and sinus bradycardia	
Sinus tachycardia	**Sinus bradycardia**
Anxiety	Physical fitness
Exercise	Sinoatrial node disease
Anaemia	Hypothermia
Shock	Hypothyroidism
Fever	Cholestatic jaundice
Pregnancy	Raised intracranial pressure
Thyrotoxicosis	Postmyocardial infarction
Pulmonary embolus	Drugs, e.g. β-blockers
Cardiac failure	
Drugs, e.g. β-agonists	

Fig. 40.4 Causes of sinus tachycardia and sinus bradycardia.

In tachycardia

In sinus tachycardia, a P wave precedes each QRS complex and the rhythm is regular. If there are no P waves and the rhythm is irregular, consider atrial fibrillation, atrial flutter with variable block, and frequent ectopic beats.

If no P waves are present and the rhythm is regular, consider atrial tachycardia, atrial flutter with 2 : 1 block, and ventricular tachycardia.

In bradycardia

If P waves are small or absent, check for hyperkalaemia. In sinus bradycardia, P waves are present and the rhythm is regular.

In first-degree heart block, P waves are present with a regular rhythm, but the PR interval is prolonged >200 ms.

In second-degree heart block, two or more P waves are present between each QRS (2 : 1 or 3 : 1 heart block). In Mobitz I (second-degree,

Wenckebach heart block), the PR interval gradually lengthens until one P wave is not conducted. In Mobitz II, the PR interval is constant with dropped beats.

In third-degree heart block, P waves are present but are completely independent of regular QRS complexes caused by an escape ectopic pacemaker.

 Check whether the complexes are regular by marking five QRS complexes on a piece of paper. Move it along by one complex and your marks should coincide exactly

Axis

The axis is the average direction of spread of electrical activity through the ventricles. The normal axis lies between −30° and +90° (Fig. 40.5). There are several ways of working out the axis, some more quantitative than others. The most accurate is to measure the size of the net deflection in leads I and AVF and create a right angled triangle, the hypotenuse of which is the electrical axis. The axis

can then be calculated accurately. This is illustrated in Fig. 40.2.

P wave

The P wave represents electrical activity of the right and left atria.

It is tall with P pulmonale (i.e. >2.5 mm), which is caused by hypertrophy of the right atrium, as in tricuspid stenosis or pulmonary hypertension. The P wave is bifid and widened (like an 'm') with P mitrale, which is caused by hypertrophy of the left atrium as in mitral stenosis.

PR interval

The PR interval represents the time for electrical activity to pass from the sinoatrial node to the atrioventricular (AV) node—it should be 0.12–0.2 seconds (three to five small squares).

It is prolonged in heart block (see above) and shortened in Wolff–Parkinson–White and Lown–Ganong–Levine syndrome due to accessory pathways connecting the atria and ventricles. In Wolff–Parkinson–White syndrome there is also a slurred upstroke of the R wave, which is called a delta wave.

QRS complex

The QRS complex represents ventricular depolarisation; its different morphology in the different leads represents the different views of the heart in each lead; it should last less than 0.12 seconds (three small squares).

It is broad if depolarisation has spread through an abnormal route, either due to disruption of the pathway, as in bundle branch block, or because it has started somewhere other than the AV node, as in ventricular ectopic beats or ventricular tachycardia.

Q waves should be less than 0.04 seconds (one small square) and less than two small squares deep. Abnormally wide and deep 'pathological' Q waves are permanent features of previous myocardial infarction (MI).

The height of the R wave in V_5 and V_6 should be less than 25 mm. The R wave may be abnormally tall in left ventricular hypertrophy (Fig. 40.6); the QRS complexes may be abnormally small in pericardial effusion, obesity and chronic obstructive pulmonary disease (COPD).

ST segment

The ST segment should not be greater than 1 mm above or below the isoelectric line. (Causes of ST elevation are shown on p. 6). ST depression is an

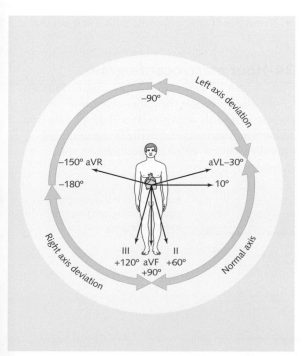

Fig. 40.5 Axis determination on electrocardiogram.

Features of left ventricular hypertrophy
• S wave in V_1 and R wave in V_5 or $V_6 \geq 35$ mm • R wave in $V_{5-6} > 27$ mm • S wave in $V_{1-3} > 30$ mm • ST depression in I, aV1, V_{4-6} • T wave inversion in I, aV1, V_{4-6} • Left axis deviation

Fig. 40.6 Features of left ventricular hypertrophy.

indication of myocardial ischaemia. Down-sloping depression with inverted T waves can be evidence of digoxin usage.

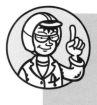

To make a definite diagnosis of left ventricular hypertrophy, voltage criteria in addition to repolarisation abnormalities must be present

T wave
The T wave represents ventricular repolarisation and should be less than 10 mm in height. Peaked T waves are seen in acute MI and hyperkalaemia. Small, flattened T waves may be seen in hypokalaemia. Inverted T waves are a feature of myocardial ischaemia, infarction, and 'strain' pattern with ventricular hypertrophy.

QT interval
The QT interval is the time from ventricular depolarisation (start of QRS) to complete ventricular repolarisation (end of T wave). It should be less than 0.44 seconds (which is two large squares). The QT interval varies inversely with heart rate (i.e. shortens in tachycardia). It can be corrected for rate by calculating $QT/_{R-R}$.

The QT interval is increased in hypocalcaemia, hypomagnesaemia, drugs (amiodarone, β-blockers, tricyclic anti-depressants), Jervell–Lange–Neilsen and Romano–Ward syndromes or severe myocardial disease, when the variability in QT can be wide from beat to beat (QTc dispersion) reflecting disordered electrical conduction.

U wave
The U wave is often a normal variant but is more prominent in hypokalaemia.

Exercise electrocardiogram
This is still the first-line investigation in the diagnosis of coronary artery disease in most centres. It has a sensitivity of 70% and specificity of 80% compared to angiography. It is safe provided the exclusion criteria are followed (Fig. 40.7). The resting ECG is taken. The patient then performs exercise until symptoms develop or the protocol is complete. Regular pulse, blood pressure, and ECGs are recorded. Evidence of myocardial ischaemia (ST depression and T wave inversion) and rate-induced arrhythmias are looked for.

The test is useful for the following:
• Assessment of severity of ischaemic heart disease.
• Prognosis following MI.
• Exercise-induced palpitations.
• Diagnosis of atypical chest pain – is it angina or not?

24-Hour electrocardiogram
The 24-hour ECG records cardiac rhythm over a 24-hour period while the patient continues with their normal daily activities. It will detect transient arrhythmias and is useful in the investigation of episodic syncope, palpitations, dizziness, and dyspnoea.

Fig. 40.7 Contraindications to electrocardiogram treadmill exercise testing.

Contraindications to ECG treadmill exercise testing
• Acute myocardial infarction within 2 days • Acute coronary syndrome • Severe aortic stenosis • Uncontrolled arrhythmia • Blood pressure >200/120 mm Hg • Left bundle branch block - difficult to interpret ECG changes • Patient physically unable to adequately stress their heart

Chest X-ray

Chest radiography (CXR) can give much information regarding both the underlying diagnosis, as well as subsequent complications. This is summarised in Fig. 40.8. Pulmonary oedema is described in Fig. 40.9.

Echocardiography

Echocardiography is an ultrasound technique that can be performed via a transthoracic or transoesophageal (TOE) approach. It gives structural information of the heart. TOE gives better images especially with suspected endocarditis or aortic dissection and larger patients.

Colour doppler can be used to look at blood flow and pressure gradients across valves. It is useful in the diagnosis of the following:

- Pericardium: effusion.
- Myocardium: left ventricular hypertrophy, left ventricular dysfunction, cardiomyopathies.
- Endocardium: atrial myxoma, vegetations, thrombus.
- Valves: stenosis and regurgitation with estimation of pressure across valves.
- Congenital heart disease: including atrial and ventricular septal defects.
- Aorta: aneurysm and dissection.

The use of dobutamine allows the assessment of hibernating myocardium in the same manner as stress thallium testing.

Thallium perfusion scan

Thallium perfusion scan monitors cardiac uptake of radioactive thallium in a similar manner to potassium. Areas with a poor coronary blood supply are identified as 'cold spots'. The response to a stressor, either adenosine or dobutamine, can be used to assess for potentially reversible ischaemia and hence those people who would benefit from revascularisation. This test can be used in patients unable to use a treadmill, such as those with osteoarthritis affecting the lower limbs.

Cardiac catheterisation

The right side of the heart is catheterised via the femoral vein (usually the right). The left side of the heart and coronary arteries are catheterised via the femoral artery. It provides the following information:

- Pressure in different chambers of the heart and the great vessels.
- Pressure gradient across the valves.
- Anatomy of the coronary arteries: following injection of radio-opaque dye.
- Assessment of blood flow: valvular regurgitation or across septal defects.
- Oxygen concentrations: in different heart chambers in assessment of shunts.

Therapeutic measures include:
- Angioplasty
- Valvotomy.
- Arterial stent insertion.

Underlying diagnoses and complications in the cardiovascular system detectable on chest X-ray		
Region	Diagnosis	X-ray findings
Pericardium	Tuberculosis or constrictive pericarditis	Calcification
Myocardium	Effusion Left ventricular dilatation Right ventricular dilatation Left atrium Left ventricular aneurysm	Globular cardiomegaly Cardiomegaly with left ventricle displaced inferolaterally Cardiomegaly Double right heart border; splaying of carina Calcified mural thrombus
Endocardium	Rheumatic heart disease	Calcification
Valves	Valve replacement Mitral stenosis Atheroma	Sternal wires; metallic valves; surgical clips Widened carina, calcified valve, straight left heart border Calcification
Aorta	Coarctation Dissection	Rib notching Widened mediastinum
Lungs	Pulmonary oedema	Fig. 40.9

Fig. 40.8 Underlying diagnoses and complications in the cardiovascular system detectable on chest X-ray.

Chest X-ray features of pulmonary oedema
• Upper lobe veins dilatation • Kerley B lines • Bat's wing shadowing (perihilar oedema) • Fluid in the horizontal fissure • Pleural effusion (usually bilateral but can be unilateral)

Fig. 40.9 Chest X-ray features of pulmonary oedema.

The respiratory system

Chest X-ray

You should develop your own routine for looking at a CXR so as not to miss important features, particularly when there is a glaring abnormality that immediately distracts attention. This should include the trachea, mediastinum (nodes, vessels), cardiac outline, diaphragms (including the costo- and cardiophrenic angles), lung fields themselves, bones, and soft tissues. The radiological findings for common respiratory diseases are outlined in Fig. 40.10.

Peak expiratory flow rate

Peak expiratory flow rate (PEFR) is obtained using a simple hand held device and measures the maximal flow rate in L/min. It is reduced in airflow obstruction. However, as an absolute value PEFR is not very useful; they can be easily performed by patients at home or in hospital and are good for monitoring disease control in an asthmatic patient.

Lung function tests

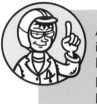

ALWAYS look at a chest X-ray in a systematic manner. The heart size is best assessed on a posterior-anterior (PA) projection

Radiological findings associated with common respiratory diseases	
Abnormality	**Radiological findings**
Airways obstruction (asthma, emphysema, chronic bronchitis)	Lungs hyperexpanded with flat hemidiaphragms allowing visualisation of anterior aspects of sixth ribs; apical bullae may be seen in emphysema; look specifically for pneumothorax which may complicate bronchospasm or for evidence of infection which may have caused it
Pneumonia	Hazy opacification, often limited to one lobe or segment but may be diffuse; bronchi remain patent and may form air bronchograms; sometimes associated with collapse or pleural effusion
Pulmonary embolus	Often no abnormality; elevated hemidiaphragm, local oligaemia, wedge atelectasis, and pleural effusions may be seen
Tumour	Localised opacification; look for small rounded opacifications or hilar lymphadenopathy suggesting metastases
Pleural effusion	Dense opacity in the lower zone with edges curved upwards (meniscus); hemidiaphragm and heart border not visible; mediastinum may shift if effusion massive; look for causes of effusion such as tumour; need at least 500 ml of fluid before detectable on chest X-ray
Fibrosis	Diffuse 'ground glass', nodular or reticular shadowing may progress to honeycomb lung if severe; mediastinum may shift towards disease due to loss of lung volume
Pneumothorax	Increased translucency due to absence of vascular shadowing and visible visceral pleura; mediastinum will shift only if pneumothorax massive or under tension; look for underlying pathology such as airways obstruction
Tuberculosis	Apical mass with hilar lymphadenopathy with or without pleural effusion; may become calcified; apical fibrosis and miliary mottling indicate postprimary disease
Bronchiectasis	May be normal; thickened bronchi may be visible as tramline or ring shadows; look for dextrocardia (Kartagener's syndrome)
Pulmonary oedema	See Fig. 40.9

Fig. 40.10 Radiological findings associated with common respiratory diseases.

Spirometry

Measurements of airflow rates and forced vital capacity are obtained using a spirometer (hand held spirometers are available). The patient breathes in to maximum inspiration (total lung capacity, TLC) and then exhales into the spirometer as quickly and for as long as possible i.e to residual volume (RV). The volume expelled is plotted against time. The flow rate is calculated from the gradient at any point of the volume–time graph. When flow rate is plotted against volume you obtain the 'flow–volume loop'. The pattern of this gives clues to underlying pathology.

The FEV_1 (forced expiratory volume in 1 second) is the volume exhaled in the first second of the test. The FVC (forced vital capacity) is the total volume exhaled. Both measurements are related to age, sex, and height, and nomograms are used to provide predicted or 'normal' parameters. The FEV_1 can be expressed as a percentage of the FVC and is 70–80% in normal subjects.

Where there is obstruction to airflow, as in bronchospasm, the FEV_1 is very much reduced. Although the total lung volume is increased, the FVC will also be slightly reduced due to air trapping as the small airways collapse. However, the reduction in FEV_1 is much greater than that for FVC and the FEV_1/FVC ratio is reduced (Fig. 40.11).

A repeat test should be performed after the administration of bronchodilators to determine if there is a reversible element present.

Restrictive defects, e.g. due to pulmonary fibrosis, are characterised by reduced lung volumes and reduced FVC. The FEV_1 will be normal or slightly reduced. The FEV_1/FVC ratio is therefore normal or increased (Fig. 40.11).

Lung volumes

The values of TLC, RV and other volumes are calculated when functional residual capacity is measured using either a helium dilution technique or whole body plethysmography. Emphysema characteristically has large lung volumes and fibrotic lung disease small volumes.

Transfer factor

Transfer factor (TLCO) is a measurement of the ease with which the alveoli permit diffusion of carbon monoxide from alveolus to blood. The diffusion is across the alveolar–capillary membrane (i.e. movement from the alveolus to the blood) and is dependent on three conditions:

- An adequate blood supply to the areas of lung ventilated (i.e. ventilation-perfusion, V/Q) matching.
- Efficient diffusion across the alveolar–capillary membrane.
- Adequate amounts of normal haemoglobin.

TLCO should be corrected for the haemoglobin concentration. If it remains abnormal, it indicates that the pathology present is at the alveolar level.

TLCO will be low when any of the three above steps are affected, as in emphysema or pulmonary fibrosis. It will be raised in polycythaemia, left-to-right shunts, and pulmonary haemorrhage.

Pleural fluid

A sample should be aspirated if:

- The effusion is not clearly explained (e.g. by cardiac failure).
- It is unilateral.
- Pneumonia is suspected.
- Systemic symptoms are present.

It should be checked for protein and LDH concentration with simultaneous blood levels to classify it as an exudate or transudate (use Light's criteria), cytology if malignancy is suspected and microscopy, Gram stain and culture for infection. pH measured on a blood gas machine is now recommended as <7.2 suggests infection. Other tests (e.g. amylase, rheumatoid factor, adenosine

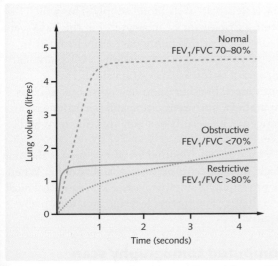

Fig. 40.11 Spirometry in normal patients, and those with obstructive and restrictive pulmonary defects.

deaminase) should only be performed if the clinical situation dictates.

Arterial oxygen saturation

This is measured indirectly via a finger probe; it reflects the percentage of oxygenated haemoglobin in arterial blood. It is useful in assessing patients in both emergency and clinic situations but has several drawbacks. It gives no measure of pCO_2 or acid–base balance and can be distorted by peripheral hypoperfusion or the presence of abnormal haemoglobin such as carboxyhaemoglobinaemia.

Arterial blood gases

Arterial blood gases are key to assessing the type and severity of respiratory conditions and disturbances of acid–base balance. It is usually taken from the radial artery. The important variables measured or derived are the partial pressures of oxygen and carbon dioxide (pO_2 and pCO_2), pH plus bicarbonate concentration and base excess.

When looking at blood gas results, remember these three tips:
- Look at the pH—normal, acidosis or alkalosis?
- Look at the pCO_2—does it correlate to the change in pH? Respiratory or compensatory?
- Look at the bicarbonate–base excess—does it correlate to change in pH? Metabolic or compensatory?

- pO_2 : This is related to the partial pressure of oxygen in the inspired air and then the ease with which it diffuses into the blood.
- pCO_2 : This is related to ventilation, i.e. the product of tidal volume and respiratory rate. High pCO_2 indicates hypoventilation and vice versa. Carbon dioxide can be thought of as an 'acidic' gas and hence high pCO_2 causes a respiratory acidosis.
- pH : This is the measure of the acid–base balance of the blood. It is tightly regulated between 7.35–7.45 in normal subjects. It is a logarithmic scale of hydrogen ion concentration, so small changes of pH reflect larger changes in the ion concentration.

- Bicarbonate : this should be considered an alkaline ion; it is increased in a metabolic alkalosis and decreased in metabolic acidosis.
- Base excess : The normal value is −2 to +2. It reflects the amount of 'base' (alkali) that is in excess of that needed for normal pH. That means a *positive base excess* is a consequence of a metabolic alkalosis ('an excess of base'). A *negative base excess* is a consequence of metabolic acidoses (i.e. you need to add base to restore the pH to normal).

If an acid/base disturbance persists for long enough the body compensates, either via bicarbonate homeostasis in the kidneys or respiratory changes in pCO_2. Therefore if the pCO_2 is chronically raised as in COPD, the kidneys compensate by retaining bicarbonate ions. This is a 'compensated respiratory acidosis'. Persisting metabolic acidosis will lead to hyperventilation, lowering the pCO_2 normalising the pH, a 'compensated metabolic acidosis'.

Arterial blood gas analysis may seem difficult at first; it requires practice and the application of simple rules on which to build.

Ventilation–perfusion scan

Technetium-99m-(^{99m}Tc)-labelled albumin is injected intravenously and detected in the lungs by a gamma camera – this is the perfusion scan. Areas not perfused are identified as 'cold spots'.

Pulmonary ventilation is demonstrated by the inhalation of xenon-133 (^{133}Xe), which is also detected by a gamma camera.

In pulmonary emboli, an area of well-ventilated lung is deprived of its blood supply. This will create a discrepancy ('mismatch') in the V/Q scans that is diagnostic of pulmonary embolism (PE). Where a V/Q scan is not possible, a CT pulmonary angiogram or formal angiogram should be considered. In other pulmonary diseases, such as pneumonia, both ventilation and perfusion are reduced. This results in a non-specific 'matched' defect.

V/Q scans are reported in most centres as showing a high, intermediate, or low probability of PE. When the probability is intermediate or low, careful clinical re-evaluation and further investigations are usually required.

Computed tomography scan

Most lung pathology can be detected by a standard CXR. However, computed tomography (CT) scanning provides more detailed information. It has two modes, the 'lung windows' for assessment of the lung parenchyma and conventional views of the mediastinum and pleura. High resolution CT (HRCT) provides much thinner cross sectional images and is now the optimal non invasive investigation of parenchymal lung disease. CT is indicated in several situations including:

- Demonstration and staging of bronchogenic carcinoma / metastases or mediastinal masses.
- Demonstration of parenchymal and pleural disease.

Spiral CT allows the acquisition in one breath of the whole thorax. It has allowed CT pulmonary angiography to become a highly effective technique to show pulmonary emboli without invasive angiography instead of V/Q scanning especially in those with pre existing lung disease.

Bronchoscopy

Fibre-optic bronchoscopy is performed under local anaesthetic and allows direct visualisation of the vocal cords and bronchial tree. It is important in the diagnosis and sometimes treatment of pulmonary disease.

Central tumours can be visualised and biopsied. Transbronchial biopsy of the lung will provide diagnostic tissue in interstitial lung disease.

Bronchoalveolar lavage is important in the diagnosis of some infections (tuberculosis, *Pneumocystis pneumonia*), peripheral tumours, and some unusual diseases (e.g. histiocytosis X).

Lung biopsy

Biopsy may be necessary in the diagnosis of tumours, interstitial lung disease, and infections when other techniques have failed to provide adequate information. The tissue can be obtained by transthoracic needle biopsy under ultrasound or CT guidance, mediastinoscopy, mediastinotomy, video assisted thoracoscopy, and open biopsy at thoracotomy.

The gastrointestinal system

Liver function tests

Liver function tests (LFTs) comprise two distinct groups. The first measure hepatocyte function and damage. These include alanine and aspartate aminotransferases (ALT and AST) that are released by damaged hepatocytes (e.g. hepatitis), albumin and prothrombin time, which both reflect hepatocyte synthetic function.

The second group indicate obstructive liver and biliary tree disease. These include alkaline phosphatase (ALP) and gamma glutamyl transpeptidase, They tend to be more raised than ALT in biliary tree pathology. However, there is much overlap.

Bilirubin is produced by red cell destruction and then conjugated by the liver to enable excretion. It is raised in many liver disorders giving the clinical sign of jaundice. It can be useful to know if the hyperbilirubinaemia is predominantly conjugated or unconjugated.

Serum amylase

Amylase is produced by the salivary glands and the exocrine pancreas. It is used as an indicator of acute pancreatitis though can be raised in other conditions (Fig. 40.12).

Ascitic Fluid

Ascites is present in many gastrointestinal (GI) and liver pathologies. A sample can be aspirated simply and analysed for protein content, infection (white cell count, Gram stain and culture) and malignancy (cytology).

Plain abdominal X-ray

Plain X-rays are of limited use in GI disease. Erect chest X-ray is often done at the same time to assess for acute perforation of an abdominal viscus. Fig. 40.13 shows radiological changes that may be found in specific diseases.

Causes of a raised serum amylase
• Acute pancreatitis
• Perforated peptic ulcer
• Ruptured ectopic pregnancy
• Acute cholecystitis
• Diabetic ketoacidosis
• Severe glomerular disease
• Myocardial infarction
• Mumps
• Salivary calculi

Fig. 40.12 Causes of a raised serum amylase.

Radiological abdominal abnormalities associated with gastrointestinal diseases	
Diagnosis	**Radiological abnormality**
Intestinal obstruction	Proximal bowel distension; absent bowel gas distally; air–fluid levels on the erect film
Perforation of a viscus	Subdiaphragmatic free gas on the erect film
Sigmoid volvulus	Grossly distended loop of sigmoid colon often extending from the pelvis to the xiphisternum (looks like a coffee bean)
Acute pancreatitis	'Sentinel loop' of dilated adynamic small bowel; 'ground glass' appearance if ascites present
Chronic pancreatitis	Pancreatic calcification
Calculi	90% of urinary tract stones and 10% of gallstones are radio-opaque
Abdominal aortic aneurysm	Calcified aneurysmal abdominal aorta

Fig. 40.13 Radiological abdominal abnormalities associated with gastrointestinal diseases.

Ultrasound scan, CT scan, and magnetic resonance imaging

These are useful in defining intra-abdominal anatomical abnormalities and pathologies such as fluid (ascites, abscess), tumour and stones (biliary, urinary tract). Ultrasound is cheaper, more accessible and, is often used as the first-line investigation. CT and magnetic resonance imaging (MRI) are particularly helpful in examining the deeper structures that are not always adequately visualised on ultrasound, which include the pancreas and retroperitoneum. Contrast can be given to improve information obtained and computer software has allowed the reconstruction of two-dimensional images to give three-dimensional pictures as in CT colonoscopy.

Barium swallow

The progress of swallowed barium is recorded. This procedure is used in the investigation of dysphagia. It should be performed prior to endoscopy in patients to demonstrate oesophageal anatomy and prevent perforation by the endoscope. It will demonstrate anatomical lesions in the oesophagus including strictures, carcinoma, web, or pharyngeal pouch, and motility abnormalities such as achalasia.

Barium meal

Barium is taken with effervescent tablets producing a double-contrast image of the stomach and proximal duodenum. This will demonstrate anatomical abnormalities including ulcers and polyps. However, most patients with gastric pathology will need a histological diagnosis and endoscopy with the option of biopsy is the investigation of choice.

Small bowel contrast studies

Barium can be introduced into the small bowel in two ways—in a small bowel follow-through, barium is swallowed and its journey to the terminal ileum is recorded; and in a small bowel enema, barium is delivered to the distal duodenum via a nasojejunal tube. It is useful in the diagnosis of small bowel polyposis, Crohn's disease, and malignancies, such as lymphoma.

Barium enema

A double-contrast picture of the colon and terminal ileum is produced by introducing barium and air into the rectum. The rectum is poorly visualised and should be examined by sigmoidoscopy. Typical abnormalities will be seen in polyps, malignancy, ulcerative colitis, and Crohn's disease.

Endoscopy

Various 'scopes' are now available, enabling direct visualisation of the whole GI tract with the exception of the third part of the duodenum to the terminal ileum (Fig. 40.14).

As well as visualising pathology, biopsies can be taken for histological diagnosis. Contrast can also be injected into the pancreatic and biliary tree (endoscopic retrograde cholangiopancreatogram).

Endoscopy is also important in treatment for the following reasons:

- Strictures can be dilated.
- Stents and prosthetic tubes can be placed through malignant lesions causing obstruction.
- Varices can be banded or injected with sclerosing agents.

'Scopes' used to examine the gastrointestinal tract	
'Scope'	**Bowel visualised**
Gastroscope	Oesophagus, stomach, first two parts of duodenum
Colonoscope	Rectum, entire colon, terminal ileum
Flexible sigmoidoscope	Rectum, descending colon
Rigid sigmoidoscope	Rectum, lower sigmoid colon
Proctoscope	Anus, lower rectum

Fig. 40.14 'Scopes' used to examine the gastrointestinal tract.

- Polyps can be removed.
- Bleeding lesions can be injected with adrenaline or cauterised.

Liver biopsy

Percutaneous liver biopsy is often indicated to establish histological diagnosis. It is not without risk, especially of bleeding. If the risk is considered high then a transjugular approach is safer.

The urinary system

Urine

Urine should be collected by taking a midstream specimen which minimises contamination by skin commensals.

The urine should have a dipstick test which gives an indication of urinary pH, specific gravity, protein, glucose, ketones, and blood. Some dipsticks offer nitrite and leucocyte detection which are useful in diagnosing urinary tract infection. Causes of proteinuria and haematuria are discussed in detail in Chapter 14. Glycosuria is usually due to high plasma glucose concentration (diabetes mellitus).

Heavy ketonuria is a feature of diabetic ketoacidosis, although ketones will become present in the urine on fasting for several hours.

Microscopy is performed to determine the number of red blood cells (RBCs) and white blood cells (WBCs), and the presence of bacteria or casts. A urinary tract abnormality is likely to be present if there are more than two RBC or five WBCs per high-powered field, RBC or WBC casts, or a large number of bacteria ($>1 \times 10^5$/mL). The urine can be cultured to confirm a urinary tract infection and to determine sensitivities to available antibiotics. If tuberculosis is suspected, three early morning specimens should be examined.

Urea and creatinine

Urea is produced by the liver from amino acids, while creatinine is a product of tissue breakdown; both are excreted by the kidneys. Levels of both in the plasma are dependent on a balance between production and excretion. Creatinine is freely filtered by the glomerulus with a small amount of tubular secretion and no reabsorption; as such it is used as a simple marker of glomerular filtration rate (GFR). It is not linearly related to GFR. This can be shown using calculated GFR via the Cockcroft–Gault equation. For a 50-year-old man weighing 70 kg, a rise in creatinine from 100 to 200 μmol/L reduces GFR from 80 to 40 mL/min. A rise from 400 to 800 μmol/L (which would worry most students and doctors) reduces GFR from just 20 to 10 mL/min. This can also show that 'normal range creatinine does not equal normal renal function'.

Normal range creatinine DOES NOT always mean normal renal function

In renal failure, urea and creatinine will be raised proportionally. In an upper GI bleed, urea will be raised but creatinine remains normal (high protein intake: blood absorbed by the small intestine). The urea : creatinine ratio is also raised in dehydration. A low ratio occurs in chronic liver disease, low-protein diet, and haemodialysis. Creatinine may also be low in those with reduced muscle bulk.

Plain X-ray

A plain X-ray ('KUB' film) is most useful in the diagnosis of renal stones, of which 90% are radio-opaque. It also demonstrates renal size, shape, and position.

Renal ultrasound

Renal ultrasound is good at detecting renal size, cysts, stones, tumours, and urinary outflow obstruction (hydronephrosis), but gives little information regarding the pelvicalyceal system and is a poor predictor of renal artery stenosis. It provides no information about renal function.

Intravenous urography

Renally excreted contrast is injected intravenously and a series of X-rays are taken at specific time intervals. Information regarding anatomy and excretion is gained by following the movement of contrast from the renal parenchyma, through the pelvicalyceal system, to the ureters and bladder. It detects renal scarring due to chronic parenchymal disease, pelvicalyceal pathology and the location of calculi.

CT scan

CT scan provides detailed anatomical information. It is important in staging malignancy and the examination of regions poorly visualised by other techniques, such as the retroperitoneal and perinephric areas.

Radioisotope studies

Renal scintigraphy can provide information about gross renal anatomy, obstruction, the relative contribution of each kidney to overall renal function, and features suggestive of renal artery stenosis. Its accuracy is increased by the coadministration of captopril—the 'captopril renogram'.

Renal angiography

Contrast is injected directly into the renal arteries via a catheter introduced into the femoral artery. This is the gold standard test for the diagnosis of renovascular disease. It also allows therapeutic stenting of stenoses. Magnetic resonance angiography is an excellent non invasive alternative.

Cystoscopy

Cystoscopy allows the direct visualisation of the bladder mucosa. It is useful in the diagnosis and sometimes treatment of bladder carcinoma.

Renal biopsy

Renal biopsy is performed transcutaneously under ultrasound guidance. It is essential in the assessment of suspected renal parenchymal disease and of transplanted kidneys. It may be complicated by frank retroperitoneal haemorrhage, haematuria, pain, and, in the long term, arteriovenous malformation. Biopsy material should be evaluated

by light microscopy, electron microscopy, and immunofluorescence.

The nervous system

Tests useful in the diagnosis of neurological disease have been described in Chapter 23.

Metabolic and endocrine disorders

Diabetes mellitus

Diabetes mellitus (DM) is characterised by chronic hyperglycaemia. It can be primary, as in type 1 (insulin-dependent DM, IDDM) and type 2 (non-insulin-dependent DM, NIDDM), or secondary to pancreatic disease (chronic pancreatitis, haemochromatosis, cystic fibrosis), endocrine disease (Cushing's syndrome, acromegaly), pregnancy, or drugs (steroids).

Diagnosis

Glycosuria is very non-specific but may prompt further investigation. This is performed by asking the patient to fast overnight and then measuring the blood glucose next morning: 'fasting glucose'. It may be diagnostic of diabetes. If further tests are needed then an oral glucose tolerance test is carried out. With this the patient fasts overnight, a blood glucose is measured and then they drink 75 g of glucose. Blood glucose is then measured at 1 and 2 hours. From these, diabetes or one of the impaired glucose metabolism states may be diagnosed. See Chapter 32 for the most recent guidelines for interpretation of these results.

Monitoring response to diet or treatment

Glycated haemoglobin (HBA1c) gives a measurement of overall glycaemic control over the previous 2–3 months. Fructosamine gives a measurement of overall glycaemic control over the previous 1–3 weeks.

Hypothalamus-pituitary-adrenal axis

Figure 40.15 summarises the normal control of cortisol. Excess circulating cortisol causes the clinical picture of Cushing's syndrome. It may result from increased release of adrenocorticotrophic hormone (ACTH), excess cortisol production in the adrenal glands, or by the

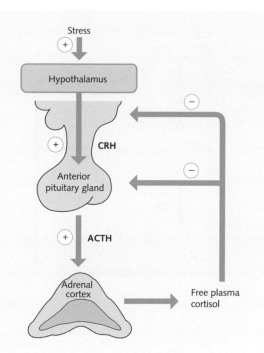

Fig. 40.15 Hypothalamus–pituitary–adrenal axis. (ACTH, adrenocorticotrophic hormone; CRH, corticotrophin-releasing hormone.)

oral administration of corticosteroids. Pseudo-Cushing's syndrome may arise in alcohol abuse and endogenous depression.

Reduced circulating cortisol results from reduced pituitary ACTH production, or reduced adrenal cortisol production.

Tests useful for determining the site of the lesion in cortisol excess and deficiency are given in Fig. 40.16.

Plasma cortisol

Plasma cortisol will vary throughout the day in normal individuals and should be measured at 09.00 hours and midnight. Normal circadian rhythm will be lost and levels raised in Cushing's syndrome. Very low or absent cortisol levels at a time of suspected Addisonian crisis confirms inadequate production of cortisol.

Tests for cortisol excess
Urinary cortisol

A 24-hour estimation of urinary free cortisol is a better predictor of Cushing's syndrome than plasma cortisol.

	Investigations in abnormalities of the hypothalamus–pituitary–adrenal axis				
	Cushing's disease	Ectopic ACTH production	Adrenal hyperproduction of cortisol	Pituitary hypoproduction of ACTH	Adrenal hypoproduction of cortisol
Causes	Pituitary adenoma	Bronchial carcinoma, Carcinoid tumour	Adenoma, carcinoma	Tumour, infarction, corticosteroids	Addison's disease, amyloid, TB, metastases, Waterhouse–Friderichsen syndrome
Plasma cortisol	High	High	High	Low	Low
Plasma ACTH	High	Very high	Very low	Low	High
Urinary free cortisol	High	High	High	Low	Low
Overnight dexamethasone suppression test	No suppression	No suppression	No suppression	Not applicable	Not applicable
High-dose dexamethasone suppression test	Suppression	No suppression	No suppression	Not applicable	Not applicable
Short Synacthen test	Not applicable	Not applicable	Not applicable	No stimulation	No stimulation
Long Synacthen test	Not applicable	Not applicable	Not applicable	Stimulation	No stimulation

Fig. 40.16 Investigations in abnormalities of the hypothalamus–pituitary–adrenal axis. (ACTH, adrenocorticotrophic hormone.)

Plasma ACTH

This is very high in ectopic ACTH production, moderately raised in Cushing's syndrome (pituitary adenoma), and very low in adrenal adenoma or carcinoma.

Overnight dexamethasone suppression test

Here, 1 mg oral dexamethasone is taken at midnight; plasma cortisol is measured at 09.00 hours the next morning. In normal patients, ACTH and cortisol production will be suppressed by negative feedback.

In all cases of Cushing's syndrome, suppression will not occur. In patients with Cushing's disease, the feedback mechanism is less sensitive than normal as ACTH levels are chronically elevated. Ectopic ACTH production has no feedback mechanism; ACTH is always suppressed in those with an adrenal cause.

High-dose dexamethasone suppression test

Plasma cortisol is measured; 2 mg oral dexamethasone is taken every 6 hours for 2 days. After 48 hours from the first dose, plasma cortisol is remeasured. In normal individuals, the plasma cortisol should be suppressed to at least half its initial value. This dose of dexamethasone should overcome the less sensitive feedback mechanism in Cushing's disease but will not cause suppression in ectopic ACTH production and adrenal hyperfunction.

Tests for cortisol deficiency
Short Synacthen stimulation test

Plasma cortisol is measured (>150 nmol/L normally) and 0.25 mg Synacthen (which has the same biological action as ACTH) is given i.m. or i.v. Plasma cortisol is remeasured after 60 minutes. In normal patients, cortisol will rise by a minimum of 200 nmol/L to at least 500 nmol/L. The response will be poor in any case of cortisol under-production.

Long Synacthen stimulation test

Here, 1 mg Synacthen is given by intramuscular injection daily for 3 days. Adrenal glands suppressed by the prolonged administration of corticosteroids show a response to this level of stimulation. No response will be seen in adrenal hypofunction.

The hypothalamus–pituitary–thyroid axis

Figure 40.17 summarises the normal control of thyroid hormones. Thyroid status can now be easily

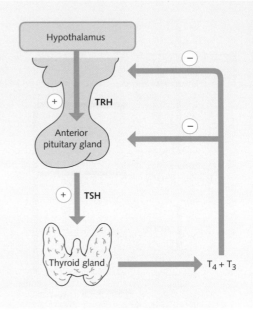

Fig. 40.17 Hypothalamus–pituitary–thyroid axis. (TRH, thyrotropin-releasing hormone; TSH, thyroid-stimulating hormone.)

assessed by the measurement of thyroid-stimulating hormone (TSH), total thyroxine (T_4) and total tri-iodothyronine (T_3) (Fig. 40.18). Approximately 99% of circulating T_4 and T_3 is bound to protein (mostly thyroxine-binding globulin). It is the free T_4 and T_3 that is physiologically active and can be measured separately.

Pituitary function tests

If suspected, initial blood tests should include TSH, T4, T3 prolactin, growth hormone and insulin-like growth factor-1, luteinising and follicle stimulating hormones, testosterone and cortisol. Pituitary fossa imaging is then undertaken (e.g. CT/MRI or lateral skull X-ray).

Calcium metabolism

Calcium homoeostasis is dependent on the normal availability of calcium and vitamin D and normal functioning of the parathyroid glands, kidneys, and gut (Fig. 40.19).

Plasma calcium

Total plasma calcium is measured and should be adjusted for albumin concentration (half is protein bound but it is the unbound that is physiologically active). The most accurate measurement is in the fasted patient with a sample taken without a cuff.

Biochemical abnormalities in thyroid disease					
	Primary thyrotoxicosis	Secondary thyrotoxicosis	Primary hypothyroidism	Secondary hypothyroidism	Sick euthyroid syndrome
Causes	Thyroiditis, toxic adenoma, multinodular goitre, carcinoma, amiodarone	Pituitary adenoma	Thyroiditis, iodine deficiency, dyshormonogenesis, antithyroid drugs, post irradiation/^{131}I therapy	Hypopituitarism, isolated TSH deficiency	Acute severe illness
TSH	Low	High	High	Low	Normal or low
Total or free T_4 and T_3	T_3 high (first) then T_4 high	T_3 high (first) then T_4 high	T_4 low (first) then T_3 low	T_4 low (first) then T_3 low	T_4 and T_3 low

Fig. 40.18 Biochemical abnormalities in thyroid disease. (T_3, tri-iodothyronine; T_4, thyroxine; TSH, thyroid-stimulating hormone.)

Fig. 40.19 Calcium homeostasis. (PTH, parathyroid hormone.)

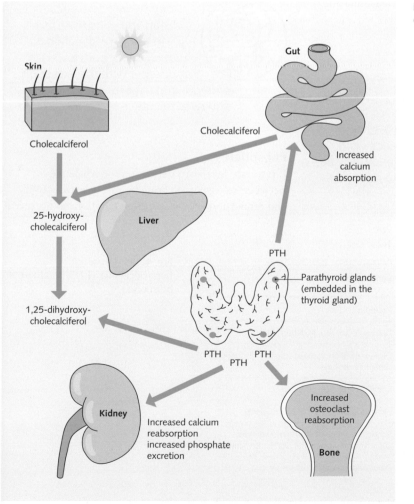

Causes of hypercalcaemia	
Mechanism	**Example**
Increased calcium intake	Milk–alkali syndrome
Increased vitamin D intake	Self-administered, iatrogenic
Increased activity of vitamin D	Sarcoidosis, lymphoma, Addison's disease
Increased production of PTH	Primary hyperparathyroidism (adenoma, hyperplasia, carcinoma), tertiary hyperparathyroidism (hyperplasia)
Production of PTH-related peptide	Squamous carcinoma, renal cell carcinoma
Increased osteoclastic activity	Osteolytic metastases, multiple myeloma
Increased bone turnover	Hyperthyroidism
Increased renal tubular calcium reabsorption	Familial hypocalciuric hypercalcaemia (autosomal dominant)

Fig. 40.20 Causes of hypercalcaemia. (PTH, parathyroid hormone.)

Causes of hypercalcaemia and hypocalcaemia are shown in Figs 40.20 and 40.21.

Calcium and phosphate levels vary in the same direction (i.e. both higher or both lower) in all diseases with the exception of hypo- and hyperparathyroidism, and renal failure

In hypocalcaemia always check magnesium.
Hypomagnesaemia often follows hypocalcaemia and magnesium supplementation may be needed for the calcium to respond to treatment

Phosphate
Phosphate levels are dependent on a balance between release from bone by osteoclastic activity, and renal tubular reabsorption. Parathyroid hormone

Fig. 40.21 Causes of hypocalcaemia. (PTH, parathyroid hormone.)

Causes of hypocalcaemia	
Mechanism	**Example**
Reduced calcium intake	Dietary deficiency, malabsorption
Reduced vitamin D intake/production	Dietary deficiency, malabsorption, reduced sunlight exposure
Reduced activation of vitamin D	Renal disease, liver disease
Increased inactivation of vitamin D	Enzyme induction by anticonvulsants
Reduced production of PTH	Surgical removal of parathyroid glands, autoimmune, congenital (DiGeorge syndrome)
Resistance to PTH	Pseudohypoparathyroidism
Hypoalbuminaemia	Shock

(PTH) increases phosphate release from bone but reduces renal reabsorption, with the overall effect of lowering phosphate concentrations.

Alkaline phosphatase

Alkaline phosphatase is found in osteoblasts, liver, and the placenta. Isoenzymes can be measured to determine the origin of high levels. Alkaline phosphatase concentrations will be increased in bone disease if there is an increase in the number or activity of osteoblasts, as in Paget's disease, osteomalacia, metastases, healing fractures, and hyperparathyroidism.

Parathyroid hormone

PTH concentration can be measured by radioimmunoassay. It is elevated in hyperparathyroidism and pseudohypoparathyroidism, and low or undetectable in primary hypoparathyroidism.

The overall pattern of abnormalities in these investigations is typical, as shown in Fig. 40.22.

Musculoskeletal and skin disease

Muscle disease is investigated by measuring muscle enzymes, electromyography, and muscle biopsy, as described in Chapter 23. The investigation of joint and connective tissue diseases is described in Chapter 17, and characteristic findings on investigation of skin pathology are discussed in Chapter 18.

Haematological disorders

Full blood count
Haemoglobin

Haemoglobin is needed for oxygen carriage to the tissues. Insufficient quantities result in the signs and symptoms of anaemia. Remember, it is not a diagnosis and should be investigated as in Chapter 26. In general, men have higher levels than women until menstruation has ceased. A typical reference value is 13.5–17.5 g/dL in men and 11.5–15.5 g/dL in women.

In polycythaemia, haemoglobin levels are above the normal range. It may be true where the total RBC volume is increased, or relative where the total RBC volume is normal but the plasma volume is decreased (Fig. 40.23).

Mean corpuscular volume

This index is invaluable in evaluating the cause of anaemia. Typical reference range is 80–95 fL. The causes of a raised and low mean corpuscular volume are described in Chapter 26. The red cell distribution width will help to demonstrate the presence of dimorphic cell populations.

Pattern of biochemical abnormalities in bone disease				
Disease	Calcium	Phosphate	Alkaline phosphatase	PTH
Osteoporosis	N	N	N	N
Osteomalacia	↓	↓	↑	N or ↑
Paget's disease	N	N	↑↑	N
Metastases	↑	↑	↑	PTH-rp may be ↑
Renal failure	↓	↑	N or ↑	N or ↑
Primary hyperparathyroidism	↑	↓	N (slightly ↑)	↑
Primary hypoparathyroisism	↓	↑	N	↓
Pseudo-hypoparathyroidism	↓	↑	N	↑

Fig. 40.22 Pattern of biochemical abnormalities in bone disease. (N, normal; PTH-rp, parathyroid hormone related peptide.)

Causes of polycythaemia		
Primary polycythaemia (myeloproliferative disorder)	Secondary polycythaemia ($\uparrow$ erythropoietin production)	Relative ($\downarrow$ plasma volume)
Polycythaemia rubra vera	Chronic hypoxia: pulmonary disease, cyanotic heart disease, high altitudes, obesity (pickwickian syndrome), methaemoglobinaemia Inappropriate erythropoietin: renal disease, cerebellar haemangioblastoma, hepatocellular carcinoma, uterine myomata, phaeochromocytoma	Stress Polycythaemia Dehydration Plasma loss (burns)

Fig. 40.23 Causes of polycythaemia.

Reticulocytes

Reticulocytes normally comprise 0.5–20% of the RBCs; they are immature RBCs that still contain ribosomal RNA. They are present in the peripheral blood for up to 2 days after leaving the bone marrow before they become mature RBCs. The number of reticulocytes present in the peripheral blood will increase when the bone marrow is producing large numbers of RBCs. This is seen 2–3 days after acute blood loss and in haemolysis.

White cell count

A standard reference for total white cell count is $4.0–11.0 \times 10^9/L$. The total count comprises neutrophils, lymphocytes, monocytes, eosinophils, and basophils (Fig. 40.23).

Platelet count

A typical reference range for platelet count is $150–400 \times 10^9/L$. The causes of thrombocytopenia are discussed in Chapter 24, and the causes of thrombocytosis are shown in Fig. 40.25.

Causes of abnormalities of the white cell count			
White cell	Normal value ($\times 10^9/L$)	Increased	Decreased
Neutrophils	2.5–7.5	Bacterial infections, uraemia, inflammation, malignancy, steroids, acute haemorrhage, myeloproliferative disorders	Bone marrow failure, hypersplenism, infections (HIV, typhoid), racial, drugs (phenytoin, tolbutamide), connective tissue disease (SLE, rheumatoid arthritis)
Lymphocytes	1.5–3.5	Infections (viral, TB, brucellosis), CLL, ALL, non-Hodgkin's lymphoma, thyrotoxicosis	Bone marrow failure, HIV, drugs (cytotoxics)
Monocytes	0.2–0.8	Infection (TB, brucellosis), inflammation (UC, Crohn's disease), connective tissue disease (SLE, rheumatoid arthritis), AML, malignancy	Bone marrow failure
Eosinophils	0.04–0.44	Allergy (urticaria, drugs), parasite infection (filariasis, amoebiasis), skin disease (psoriasis, dermatitis herpetiformis), polyarteritis nodosa, Hodgkin's disease, pulmonary eosinophilia, eosinophilic leukaemia	Bone marrow failure
Basophils	0.01–0.1	Infection (varicella), hypothyroidism, myeloproliferative disorders	Bone marrow failure

Fig. 40.24 Causes of abnormalities of the white cell count. (ALL, acute lymphoblastic leukaemia; AML, acute myeloid leukaemia; CLL, chronic lymphocytic leukaemia; HIV, human immunodeficiency virus; SLE, systemic lupus erythematosus; TB, tuberculosis; UC, ulcerative colitis.)

Causes of thrombocytosis	
Primary	Essential thrombocythaemia
Secondary	Inflammation Malignancy Chronic infection Post splenectomy Haemorrhage Surgery or trauma

Fig. 40.25 Causes of thrombocytosis.

A 'reactive' blood picture consists of a normochromic normocytic anaemia, neutrophilia, thrombocytosis and raised erythrocyte sedimentation rate. It suggests underlying inflammation, infection or malignancy

If you cannot see any abnormality, look specifically at the apices for a small pneumothorax, TB or cervical rib, behind the heart for a hiatus hernia (air-fluid level), left hemidiaphragm for lower lobe pathology, at the soft tissues for unilateral mastectomy, and below the diaphragms for free gas

Erythrocyte sedimentation rate

The erythrocyte sedimentation rate is a measure of the rate of RBC sedimentation over 1 hour. The normal range varies between laboratories, increases with age, anaemia and is higher in women. It is a non-specific indicator of inflammation, infection, and malignancy.

Haematinics

These comprise ferritin, vitamin B_{12} and folate; they are the building blocks for red cell production. They should be measured in anaemic patients especially

prior to blood transfusion. Iron study interpretation is shown in Chapter 26.

Blood film

A peripheral blood film is non-invasive and provides information on a whole range of haematological conditions.

Bone marrow examination

Aspirate and trephine are usually taken from the posterior iliac crest under local anaesthesia (aspirate may also be obtained from the sternum). A smear of bone marrow cells is made from the aspirate, allowing a detailed examination of the proportion and differentiation of different cell lines in the bone marrow. Infiltration by other cells (carcinoma) and iron reserves can also be assessed (Perl's stain). Cytogenetic analysis of the aspirate may give diagnostic and prognostic information. The trephine consists of a core of bone containing marrow cells, and is important in determining marrow cellularity and infiltration.

Coagulation assessment

Rudimentary coagulation is assessed by measurement of the prothrombin time, activated partial thromboplastin time, thrombin time, and bleeding time (Chapter 24).

D-dimers

These are fibrin degradation products and are elevated in any thrombotic condition. They are sensitive but not very specific for a given condition. Due to their high negative predictive value, they are commonly measured in suspected venous thromboembolism. In this situation, a negative result is the most useful as it provides strong evidence against deep vein thombosis/PE.

Miscellaneous tests

C-Reactive Protein

This is an acute phase protein produced by the liver in response to inflammation and infection. It responds quickly to changes in disease state and hence is very useful to monitor response to treatment (e.g. antibiotics).

Tumour markers

These are commonly raised in certain malignancies but also in other pathologies. They are useful in following

427

response to therapy in diagnosed cancer. However their role in screening and 'diagnostic trawling' is debated due to inadequate sensitivity and specificity.

The widest debate is that surrounding prostate specific antigen (Fig. 40.26).

Common tumour markers		
Tumour marker	Malignancy	Also elevated in the following
Prostate Specific Antigen (PSA)	Prostate	Benign prostatic hypertrophy
Alpha fetoprotein AFP	Hepatocellular carcinoma	Hepatitis, cirrhosis
Carcinoembryonic antigen CEA	Gastrointestinal carcinoma	Cirrhosis, pancreatitis
CA 125	Ovary, breast	Cirrhosis, peritonitis
CA 19-9	Pancreatitis	Cholestasis
CA 153	Breast	Benign breast disease.

Fig. 40.26 Common tumour markers.

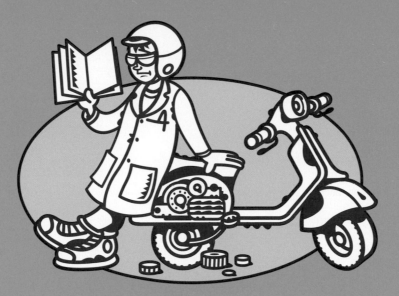

SELF ASSESSMENT

Multiple-choice Questions	431	MCQ Answers	451
Short-answer Questions	441	SAQ Answers	461
Extended-matching Questions	443	EMQ Answers	465
Patient-management Problems	449		

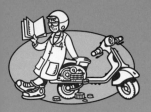

Multiple-choice Questions

Gastroenterology

1. Gastroesophageal reflux disease:

(a) Is becoming decreasingly common
(b) Can be exacerbated by smoking
(c) Can be excluded by oesophagogastroduodenoscopy (OGD)
(d) Is treated surgically in the first instance
(e) Causes pre-malignant ulceration of the oesophagus

2. Peptic ulcer disease:

(a) *Helicobacter pylori* infection is more commonly associated with duodenal ulcers than gastric ulcers
(b) May occur following non-steroidal anti-inflammatory drug use
(c) All gastric ulcers must be biopsied
(d) Gastric ulceration can be reliably distinguished from duodenal ulceration on history alone
(e) *Helicobacter pylori* eradication should be performed for all duodenal ulcers

3. Upper gastrointestinal haemorrhage:

(a) A detailed history and examination is a priority
(b) A large bleed causes an immediate decrease in haemoglobin concentration
(c) Causes an increase in urea concentration
(d) The investigation of choice is oesophagogastroduodenoscopy
(e) Re-bleeding carries a higher mortality

4. The following are features of ulcerative colitis:

(a) Transmural inflammation
(b) Pseudopolyps
(d) Skip lesions
(e) Less common in smokers

5. Colorectal cancer:

(a) The majority occur in patients with a strong family history
(b) Inflammatory bowel disease involving the colon is a risk factor
(c) Right-sided tumours usually present earlier
(d) May present with an iron deficiency anaemia alone
(e) Only a minority of tumours can be resected surgically

6. Pseudomembranous colitis:

(a) Is caused by *Clostridium difficile* itself
(b) Almost always follows antibiotic therapy
(c) Is diagnosed by demonstrating an erythematous, ulcerated mucosa covered by a membrane on sigmoidoscopy
(d) May be complicated by toxic dilation of the colon
(e) Is treated with intravenous metronidazole

7. Irritable bowel syndrome:

(a) Is rare
(b) Is more common in males
(c) May present with rectal bleeding
(d) Is a diagnosis of exclusion
(e) Is usually treated with 100% success

8. The following can be said of gallstones:

(a) Most are radio-opaque
(b) They are often asymptomatic
(c) Their incidence increases with age
(d) They are associated with haemolytic anaemia
(e) They may cause bowel obstruction

9. Acute pancreatitis:

(a) Is commonly caused by excess alcohol
(b) Often presents with mild abdominal discomfort
(c) May cause peri-umbilical bruising
(d) Is diagnosed by characteristic abdominal X-ray findings
(e) xxxxx

10. The following may be said of viral hepatitis:

(a) Hepatitis A may cause chronic hepatitis
(b) Hepatitis B is transmitted via the faecal–oral route
(c) Chronic hepatitis B infection may be complicated by hepatocellular carcinoma
(d) Hepatitis C causes acute hepatic failure
(e) Hepatitis E is transmitted via the faecal–oral route

Genitourinary Disorders

1. Glomerular pathology may present in the following ways:

(a) Proteinuria
(b) Haematuria
(c) Hypertension
(d) Renal failure
(e) Nephritic syndrome

2. Nephrotic syndrome:

(a) Haematuria is a key feature
(b) Is always due to a primary glomerulonephritis
(c) May cause frothy urine
(d) Is associated with hypercholesterolaemia
(e) Is associated with an increased risk of venous thromboembolism

3. If glomerular disease is suspected the following investigations should be performed:

(a) 24-hour urine collection
(b) Urine microscopy
(c) Complement levels
(d) Serum and urine immunoelectrophoresis
(e) Anti-neutrophil cytoplasmic antibody and anti-glomerular basement membrane antibody

4. The following can be said of acute renal failure:

(a) The urine output always decreases
(b) Hypovolaemia is a common cause
(c) The mortality is low
(d) Few survivors regain normal renal function
(e) An early ultrasound scan is important

5. The following complications of acute renal failure require urgent dialysis therapy:

(a) Pulmonary oedema
(c) Serum creatinine >500 µmol/L
(d) Resistant hyperkalaemia
(e) Uraemic pericarditis

6. Severe hyperkalaemia:

(a) Can cause life-threatening arrhythmias
(b) 10 mL of 10% calcium gluconate intravenously helps reduce potassium levels rapidly
(c) Salbutamol nebulisers reduce serum potassium
(d) Correction of acidosis reduces serum potassium
(e) Insulin/dextrose infusions caused potassium excretion

7. The following can be said of chronic renal failure:

(a) Chronic glomerulonephritis is a rare cause
(b) All cases require a kidney biopsy for diagnosis
(c) Tight blood pressure control is very important
(d) Dietary modifications focus on increased calorie intake to avoid malnutrition
(e) Macrocytic anaemia is a feature

8. Urinary tract infections:

(a) Are more commonly seen in females
(b) Affect 5% of the female population at least once
(c) Are always symptomatic
(d) Are less common in patients with urinary catheters
(e) Never ascend to involve the kidneys

9. The following are causes of hyponatraemia:

(a) Chronic congestive cardiac failure
(b) Conn's syndrome
(c) Diabetes insipidus
(d) Diuretic therapy
(e) Severe hyperlipidaemia

10. The following ECG changes may be seen in hypokalaemia:

(a) Tall, tented T waves
(b) U waves
(c) Widened QRS complex
(d) Prolonged PR interval
(e) Elevated ST segment

Neurology

1. Stroke:

(a) The majority are caused by cerebral haemorrhage
(b) In supratentorial strokes with homonymous hemianopia, patients can see on the hemiplegic side
(c) A CT scan is essential to diagnose a stroke
(d) Affected patients can be managed on any ward
(e) Aggressive early lowering of blood pressure reduces the risk of recurrence

2. Giant cell arteritis:

(a) Has a peak incidence at age 40 years
(b) May cause pain while eating
(c) The erythrocyte sedimentation rate is always elevated
(d) Treatment should be delayed until the diagnosis is confirmed as steroids can themselves be toxic
(e) Temporal artery biopsy is always diagnostic

3. Migraine:

(a) Affects approximately 2% of the population
(b) May cause hemiplegia
(c) Is a risk factor for stroke
(d) Acute attacks may be treated with β-blockers
(e) 5-HT antagonists, such as sumatriptan, should be taken regularly

4. Parkinson's disease:

(a) Is more common in males
(b) The tremor is characteristically made worse by movement
(c) The neurological signs are always symmetrical
(d) Depression is a commonly associated problem
(e) Long-term levodopa replacement therapy is associated with significant side-effects

5. Multiple sclerosis:

(a) Is a recognised sequela of bacterial meningitis
(b) Is most common in patients over 50 years
(c) Demyelinating lesions characteristically occur at a particular site in any given patient
(d) Symptoms may worsen following exercise or a hot bath
(e) Steroid therapy improves the prognosis

6. Bacterial meningitis:

(a) May spread at institutions
(b) A non-blanching petechial rash suggests allergy to an antibiotic
(c) Investigations must be completed before commencing therapy
(d) Lumbar puncture should be deferred if there is evidence of raised intracranial pressure
(e) Oral antibiotic therapy is appropriate unless the patient is too ill to swallow

7. Epilepsy:

(a) Is the only cause of generalised tonic-clonic seizures
(b) Epilepsy cannot be diagnosed without an abnormal EEG
(c) All patients must be commenced on anti-epileptic therapy after their first seizure to prevent another
(d) Sodium valproate may cause tremor
(e) Hypoglycaemia may precipitate status epilepticus

8. The following are features of raised intracranial pressure:

(a) Headache, worse with coughing and sneezing
(b) Nausea and vomiting
(c) Hiccoughs
(d) Papilloedema
(e) Lateral gaze palsy

9. Motor neurone disease:

(a) Is more common in males
(b) Has a peak incidence at age 40 years
(c) Rarely causes sensory problems
(d) May cause a combination of upper and lower motor neurone signs
(e) Treatment with riluzole can be curative

10. Bell's palsy:

(a) Affects the fifth cranial nerve
(b) Does not affect the hearing
(c) The musculature of the forehead on the affected side is spared
(d) Few patients make a full recovery
(e) High-dose prednisolone is of no benefit

Endocrine

1. The following results fulfil the WHO criteria for diagnosis of diabetes mellitus:

(a) Fasting plasma glucose 6.1 mmol/L
(b) Random plasma glucose 12.3 mmol/L with polyuria/polydipsia
(c) Fasting plasma glucose 5.3 mmol/L
(d) 2-hour oral glucose tolerance test result of 11.4 mmol/L
(e) 2-hour oral glucose tolerance test result of 8.3 mmol/L

2. Diabetes mellitus may present as follows:

(a) Weight gain
(b) Peri-anal abscess
(c) At routine eye testing
(d) With polyuria and polydipsia
(e) A life-threatening coma

3. The following can be said of therapy in diabetes mellitus:

(a) Insulin replacement is the priority in treatment of diabetic ketoacidosis
(b) Most young diabetics can be managed with dietary modification alone
(c) Tight glycaemic control reduces microvascular complications
(d) Strict blood pressure control only reduces macrovascular complications
(e) Hypoglycaemic episodes are the main obstacle to improved glycaemic control

4. Osteoporosis:

(a) Has a prevalence of 20% in white females aged 80 years or over
(b) Can be caused by hypothyroidism
(c) Can be painful
(d) Causes an elevated alkaline phosphatase
(e) The diagnosis is usually confirmed by bone biopsy

5. Hypercalcaemia:

(a) Malignancy is a rare cause
(b) May be associated with severe loin pain
(c) Parathyroid hormone levels should be normal unless hyperparathyroidism is the cause
(d) The immediate management of symptomatic hypercalcaemia is bisphosphonate therapy
(e) Frusemide is useful in therapy

6. Gout:

(a) Is commoner in men
(b) Commonly presents as an oligoarthropathy
(c) May be precipitated by diuretics
(d) A normal serum urate excludes the diagnosis
(e) Acute gout is treated with allopurinol

7. Acromegaly:

(a) Results from the excessive secretion of prolactin
(b) May be associated with homonymous hemianopia
(c) Is a secondary cause of diabetes mellitus
(d) Is diagnosed by measurement of random growth hormone levels
(e) Is always managed surgically

8. The following may be features of thyrotoxicosis of any aetiology:

(a) Atrial fibrillation
(b) Pre-tibial myxoedema
(c) Lid retraction
(d) Menorrhagia
(e) Proptosis

9. Cushing's syndrome:

(a) Is always caused by an adrenocorticotropic hormone-secreting pituitary adenoma
(b) May cause hyperkalaemia
(c) Causes weight loss
(d) 24-hour urinary free cortisol is a useful screening test
(e) Drug therapy with metyrapone is the treatment of choice for Cushing's disease

10. Addison's disease:

(a) Is associated with vitiligo
(b) May occur acutely in meningococcal septicaemia
(c) May cause hyperpigmentation
(d) Serum electrolytes usually show hyponatraemia
(e) Maintenance steroid therapy is given monthly

Respiratory disease

1. The physical signs of an uncomplicated large pneumothorax include:

(a) The trachea is deviated towards the affected side
(b) Increased percussion note over the pneumothorax
(c) Symmetrical expansion of the chest
(d) Increased breath sounds over the pneumothorax
(e) Crepitus over the upper chest

2. Asthma:

(a) Is a clinical diagnosis based on episodic wheezing, cough and dyspnoea
(b) Is excluded by normal spirometry
(c) Cough may be the only symptom
(d) Can be diagnosed by diurnal variation of peak flow rate
(e) Is declining in incidence

3. In a patient with severe asthma:

(a) The peak flow measure is unhelpful
(b) A normal pCO_2 is reassuring
(c) Intravenous magnesium is indicated
(d) Death is extremely rare
(e) Intravenous bronchodilator is much better than nebulised therapy

4. Predictors of severity of community acquired pneumonia include:

(a) Blood urea >7 mmol/L
(b) Diastolic blood pressure <80 mmHg
(c) Respiratory rate >30 per minute
(d) Confusion
(e) Age >65 years

5. Pleural effusion:

(a) A protein level of >40 g/L indicates a transudate
(b) Removal of >1.5 L fluid at a time may cause pulmonary oedema
(c) The signs include stony dullness, absent breath sounds and bronchial breathing at the upper border on the side of the effusion
(d) A blood-stained effusion is usually benign
(e) Bilateral effusions are highly sinister of malignancy

6. Pulmonary embolus:

(a) The S1Q3T3 pattern is the most common ECG abnormality
(b) Results in matched defects on V/Q scanning
(c) Is associated with undiagnosed malignancy
(d) One of the earliest signs is a resting tachycardia
(e) Requires 1 year of warfarin therapy

7. The following have shown proven benefit in chronic obstructive pulmonary disease:

(a) Smoking cessation
(b) Oxygen as needed at home
(c) Routine use of inhaled corticosteroids
(d) Non-invasive ventilation
(e) Pulmonary rehabilitation

8. Squamous cell carcinoma of the lung:

(a) Is associated with the syndrome of inappropriate antidiuretic hormone secretion
(b) Is associated with hypercalcaemia
(c) Is the most common cause of Eaton–Lambert myasthenic syndrome
(d) Chemotherapy is the mainstay of treatment
(e) Can cause adrenal metastases

9. Malignant mesothelioma:

(a) Is a tumour of the lung parenchyma
(b) Usually accompanies pulmonary asbestosis
(c) Is diagnosed by pleural plaques on chest X-ray or CT
(d) Has a good prognosis
(e) May result in compensation for patient and/or family

10. Obstructive sleep apnoea:

(a) Always occurs in overweight people
(b) Is best treated by surgery
(c) Causes excessive daytime sleepiness
(d) Is associated with non-respiratory disorders
(e) Can be the presenting feature of hypothyroidism

Infectious disease

1. Human immunodeficiency virus:

(a) Is an RNA retrovirus
(b) Cannot be transmitted from mother to child
(c) Seroconversion can be asymptomatic
(d) Commonly presents as *Pneumocystis* pneumonia
(e) Is best treated by single therapy with azidothymidine

2. The following are common causes of urinary tract infection:

(a) *Pseudomonas*
(b) *Escherichia coli*
(c) *Staphylococcus aureus*
(d) *Proteus*
(e) *Streptococcus pneumoniae*

3. The following bacteria are paired with an appropriate antibiotic for empirical therapy:

(a) *Streptococcus pneumoniae* and amoxicillin
(b) MRSA and flucloxacillin
(c) *Pseudomonas* and ciprofloxacin
(d) *Escherichia coli* and trimethoprim
(e) *Streptococcus viridans* and benzylpenicillin/gentamicin

4. Malaria:

(a) Occurs within 1 month of returning from the affected area
(b) *Plasmodium vivax* is the most serious form
(c) Is excluded by a thick film examination
(d) Hypoglycaemia can occur
(e) Chloroquine is the drug of choice in severe malaria

5. The following patients are at risk of tuberculosis:

(a) The elderly
(b) Rheumatoid arthritis
(c) Alcoholics
(d) Human immunodeficiency virus positive
(e) Sarcoidosis

History taking

1. The following are important in the patient with a chronic cough:

(a) Nocturnal symptoms
(b) Taking angiotensin II receptor blockers
(c) Change in voice character
(d) Nasal problems chronic cough if no pre-existing lung disease is present)
(e) Occupation

2. The following drugs and side effects are correctly linked:

(a) Nitrofurantoin and pulmonary fibrosis
(b) Angiotensin-converting enzyme inhibitors and angio-oedema
(c) Digoxin and visual field defects
(d) Amiodarone and photosensitive rash
(e) Ethambutol and disturbance of colour vision

3. The following are correct:

(a) 20 cigarettes per day for 20 years equals 20 pack years
(b) 30 cigarettes per day for 25 years equals 32.5 pack years
(c) A 750 mL bottle of wine contains 4 units
(d) A pint of bitter contains 2 units
(e) Alcohol problems can be initially assessed with the 'CAGE' questions

Investigations

1. When investigating suspected pulmonary embolus:

(a) The d-dimer is not useful
(b) The diagnosis is confirmed by the presence of right bundle branch block
(c) A V/Q scan is adequate if the patient has chronic obstructive pulmonary disease
(d) The troponin level will be unrecordable
(e) If the CT pulmonary angiogram is negative for pulmonary embolism then a formal angiogram should be performed to confirm the diagnosis

2. On respiratory function testing the following are true:

(a) The forced vital capacity is from total lung capacity to functional residual capacity
(b) When assessing respiratory muscle weakness (e.g. Guillain–Barré) the peak flow rate is best
(c) FEV1 of 50% predicted with FEV1/FVC ratio of 65% is consistent with obstructive lung disease
(d) The transfer factor is reduced in pulmonary fibrosis
(e) The transfer factor is increased in pulmonary haemorrhage

3. Arterial blood gas monitoring:

(a) pCO_2 can be considered an 'alkaline' gas
(b) pCO_2 is low or normal in type 1 respiratory failure ventilation is adequate)
(c) Metabolic compensation involves the retention of bicarbonate ions by the liver
(d) A raised anion gap is compatible with the presence of exogenous acid in the blood
(e) An increased base excess accompanies a rise in bicarbonate levels

4. On the electrocardiogram:

(a) The PR interval is measured from the end of the P wave to the start of the QRS complex
(b) Normal electrical axis is from −30 to +90°
(c) P mitrale is suggested by a peaked P wave taller than 2.5 mm in lead II
(d) Q waves in leads II, III and AVF indicate a previous transmural anterior myocardial infarction
(e) The normal QRS duration is 0.1 s

5. The following are causes of an increased mean corpuscular volume:

(a) Hypothyroidism
(b) Alcohol
(c) Pernicious anaemia
(d) Beta-thalassaemia trait
(e) Chronic renal failure

6. Causes of a high erythrocyte sedimentation rate include:

(a) Multiple myeloma
(b) Anaemia
(c) Polycythaemia
(d) Increasing age
(e) Giant cell arteritis

7. Causes of hypercalcaemia include:

(a) Renal cell carcinoma
(b) Milk–alkali syndrome
(c) Renal failure
(d) Sarcoidosis
(e) Pseudopseudohypoparathyroidism

8. The following are paired correctly:

(a) Increased urea to creatinine ratio with gastrointestinal bleeding
(b) High alkaline phosphatase and gamma glutamyltranspeptidase with hepatitis
(c) Positive d-dimer and venous thromboembolism
(d) High troponin and polymyositis
(e) High HBA1c and poor diabetic control

9. When performing a short Synacthen test:

(a) You are testing for excess cortisol production
(b) A flat response is a normal response
(c) It is performed overnight
(d) Synacthen is synthetic adrenocorticotropic hormone
(e) It can separate adrenal and pituitary causes of cortisol deficiency

10. The chest X-ray:

(a) Loss of the right heart border indicates consolidation in the right lower lobe
(b) Cardiomegaly is defined as a cardiothoracic ratio of >0.5 in a posteroanterior film
(c) Airspace (alveolar) shadowing could be caused by pulmonary infection
(d) Sarcoidosis may cause bilateral hilar lymphadenopathy
(e) Kerley B lines are perihilar in distribution

Haematological disorders

1. Features of iron deficiency include:

(a) Clubbing of the nails
(b) Koilonychia
(c) Low serum ferritin
(d) Gynaecomastia
(e) Rapid response to oral iron therapy

2. Which of the following are true about sickle-cell disease:

(a) It is an X-linked condition
(b) Crises may be precipitated by cold
(c) Priapism may be a feature of a crisis
(d) Streptococcal osteomyelitis is a long-term complication
(e) Patients should be regarded as 'asplenic'

3. Leukaemia:

(a) A common presenting triad is infection, bleeding and fatigue
(b) Chronic lymphocytic leukaemia (CLL) usually transforms to acute leukaemia
(c) CLL requires the Philadelphia chromosome to be present for diagnosis
(d) A platelet count of 40×10^9 should not usually be associated with bleeding
(e) Acute lymphocytic leukaemia is the most common acute leukaemia in adults

4. Disseminated intravascular coagulation:

(a) Is associated with AML-M7
(b) Can complicate severe infection
(c) Manifests as uncontrolled bleeding
(d) Has no specific therapy
(e) Fibrinogen is increased to attempt to stem bleeding

5. Haemophilia A:

(a) Is a lack of clotting factor IX
(b) Needs plasma levels to fall to 50% normal before symptoms occur
(c) Is characterised by mucosal bleeding
(d) Is associated with an increased international normalised ratio
(e) Patients are at an increased risk of HIV

6. In lymphoma the following are `B' symptoms:

(a) Painless lymphadenopathy
(b) Fever >38 °C
(c) Drenching night sweats
(d) Pruritus
(e) Abdominal pain

7. Hodgkin's lymphoma:

(a) Is separated from non-Hodgkin's lymphoma by the absence of Reed–Sternberg cells
(b) Alcohol may induce pain in the enlarged lymph nodes
(c) May be suspected from chest X-ray
(d) Has a poor prognosis
(e) Is confined to older patients

8. When dealing with a patient with suspected pernicious anaemia:

(a) A Schilling test is mandatory for diagnosis
(b) It is a condition characterised by decreased B_{12} production
(c) Low platelet and white cell count should cast doubt on the diagnosis
(d) Treatment is difficult and likely to need regular blood transfusions
(e) Addison's disease may be found

9. Anaemia of chronic disease:

(a) Has a microcytic appearance on blood film
(b) Has a low ferritin
(c) The serum iron can be low
(d) Should respond to erythropoietin
(e) Can be caused by chronic inflammatory conditions

10. The following blood film findings and diagnosis are correctly linked:

(a) Heinz bodies and G6PD deficiency
(b) Howell–Jolly bodies and splenectomy
(c) Target cells and renal failure
(d) Basophilic stipling and lead poisoning
(e) Hypersegmented polymorphs and iron deficiency

Cardiovascular disorders

1. Heart murmurs:

(a) Mitral stenosis with atrial fibrillation would give a diastolic murmur with presystolic accentuation
(b) A pansystolic murmur loudest at the apex radiating to the axilla is most likely mitral regurgitation
(c) Left-sided heart murmurs are best heard in inspiration
(d) Aortic regurgitation is best heard in the left lateral position
(e) An opening snap is heard in aortic stenosis just after the first heart sound

2. There is published evidence to support the following statements:

(a) Aspirin improves mortality in acute myocardial infarction
(b) tPA may be better than streptokinase for thrombolysis of acute anterior myocardial infarction
(c) Patients with elevated cholesterol and coronary artery disease benefit from statin therapy
(d) The mortality of patients with severe chronic heart failure is improved with therapy with bisoprolol
(e) The mortality of chronic heart failure patients is improved by low doses of spironolactone

3. After acute myocardial infarction:

(a) A positive troponin is required to initiate thrombolysis
(b) ST elevation in leads I, AVL, V5 and V6 indicates lateral myocardial infarction
(c) Aspirin should be given as soon as possible
(d) In non diabetic patients blood sugar levels need not be controlled
(e) β-blocker therapy should wait until the second day post myocardial infarction

4. Atrial fibrillation:

(a) Can cause heart failure in previously well-controlled heart disease
(b) Results in an increased risk of stroke
(c) Is usually caused by rheumatic fever
(d) Results from the irregular conduction of P waves to the ventricle
(e) May be a finding in acute pulmonary embolus

5. The following drugs should be used in non ST segment elevation myocardial infarction:

(a) Clopidogrel
(b) β-blockers
(c) Amlodipine
(d) Streptokinase
(e) Diamorphine

6. Chronic left ventricular failure:

(a) Can be classified by the New York Heart Association scale
(b) Diuretics improve survival
(c) Digoxin has no role unless in atrial fibrillation
(d) May predispose to ventricular arrhythmias
(e) All patients should try angiotensin-converting enzyme inhibitors unless contraindicated

7. The following are correct about rheumatic fever:

(a) Carditis is the most common major criterion
(b) Is classified by the Glasgow score
(c) It results in St Vitus' dance
(d) Is caused by group A β-haemolytic streptococci
(e) The aortic valve is the most likely to be chronically damaged

8. The jugulovenous pressure (JVP):

(a) Is measured from the suprasternal notch with the patient sitting at 45°
(b) Reflects right ventricular preload
(c) Cannon waves indicate complete heart block
(d) An elevated non-collapsing JVP may indicate superior venacaval obstruction
(e) Tricuspid regurgitation results in large V waves

9. The following are causes of essential hypertension:

(a) Conn's syndrome
(b) Phaeochromocytoma
(c) Coarctation of the aorta
(d) Renal artery stenosis
(e) Chronic renal failure

10. When examining the pulse:

(a) The character should be assessed centrally
(b) A slow rising pulse indicates mitral stenosis
(c) Pulsus alternans indicates poor left ventricular function
(d) Rate, rhythm, volume and character should be assessed
(e) The heart rate will decrease during inspiration in sinus arrhythmia

Musculoskeletal and skin disorders

1. The following are systemic consequences of rheumatoid arthritis:

(a) Carpal tunnel syndrome
(b) Obstructive lung disease
(c) Pericardial effusion
(d) Splenomegaly
(e) Skin ulcers

2. The following are common causes of erythema multiforme:

(a) Mycoplasma pneumonia
(b) Tuberculosis
(c) Herpes infection
(d) *Borrelia burgdorferi*
(e) Ulcerative colitis

3. Treatments for osteoarthritis include:

(a) Weight loss
(b) Non steroidal anti-inflammatory drugs
(c) TNF-α blocking drugs
(d) Joint replacement
(e) Physiotherapy

4. Gout:

(a) Commonly affects the hips and knees
(b) Crystals are positively birefringent
(c) May be precipitated by chemotherapy
(d) Allopurinol is used to treat acute attacks
(e) The serum urate is used to diagnose acute attacks

5. Ankylosing spondylitis is associated with:

(a) Aortic stenosis
(b) Apical lung fibrosis
(c) Stiffness worse in the evening after activity
(d) Low frequency of positive test for HLA-B27
(e) Amyloidosis

Examination

1. Hand signs:

(a) Clubbing may be caused by uncomplicated chronic bronchitis
(b) Koilonychia usually indicates liver disease
(c) Osler's nodes and Bouchard's nodes both occur in osteoarthritis
(d) Splinter haemorrhages are due to embolic rather than immunological phenomena
(e) Psoriatic arthropathy affects most joints in the hands but usually spares the distal interphalangeal joints

2. The following would suggest an upper rather than a lower motor neurone lesion:

(a) Fasciculation
(b) Increased tone
(c) Extensor plantar response
(d) Clonus
(e) Relatively little wasting

3. Pulsus paradoxus:

(a) The volume of the pulse increases in inspiration
(b) Can be confirmed by detecting >10 mmHg difference in systolic pressure during the breathing cycle
(c) Is a sign of severe asthma
(d) Is called pulsus paradoxus because it is the opposite of what normally happens to the pulse
(e) Can occur in cardiac tamponade

4. The following would help to distinguish between a kidney and a spleen in the left upper quadrant:

(a) Dullness to percussion
(b) A notch on the medial border
(c) Ability to 'get above' the mass
(d) Ability to ballot the mass
(e) A family history of kidney failure

5. The following are characteristic of a jugular venous, as opposed to carotid, pulsation:

(a) Palpable pulse
(b) Movement with respiration tamponade is a paradoxical rise of the JVP in inspiration).
(c) A double waveform
(d) Movement with posture
(e) No effect when pressure applied below the right costal margin

6. The physical signs of a large uncomplicated pneumothorax include:

(a) Tracheal deviation away from the pneumothorax
(b) A clicking sound synchronous with the heart sounds
(c) Symmetrical expansion of the chest
(d) Increased breath sounds over pneumothorax
(e) Increased percussion note over pneumothorax

The Clerking

1. The following can be said of a medical clerking:

(a) It is a legal document
(b) It is essential to follow a particular order
(c) The time and date are essential
(d) It should incorporate a problem list
(e) It should be completed with a signature and bleep number

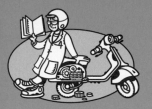

Short-answer Questions

1. What electrocardiographic changes are seen in untreated acute ST elevation myocardial infarction and what is the time course of these changes?

2. How is psoriasis distributed over the skin and what coexisting non-dermatological problems may be found?

3. What factors predispose a person to the development of venous thromboembolism?

4. How is the nephrotic syndrome defined and what are the most common causes of this syndrome?

5. What is the differential diagnosis of a young patient presenting with cervical lymphadenopathy?

6. Discuss the management of a patient with an acute stroke

7. What clinical findings would indicate the presence of severe aortic stenosis on examination?

8. Briefly describe the management of a patient with suspected giant cell (temporal) arteritis

9. How is pneumonia subclassified and how does this affect treatment?

10. What is the life expectancy of a patient newly diagnosed with HIV infection?

11. What are the physical signs of intravascular volume depletion?

12. How would you demonstrate the presence of haemolysis in the circulation?

13. Is a CT scan mandatory before performing a lumbar puncture in a patient with suspected meningitis? Justify your answer.

14. What are the cardinal physical signs of parkinsonism? Name two common causes other than idiopathic Parkinson's disease.

15. What syndromes may be caused by gallstones?

16. How would you manage a patient with acute gout who also suffers from renal failure?

17. List the findings on lumbar puncture that distinguish bacterial from viral meningitis.

18. Describe the common infections that can give rise to diarrhoea.

19. Describe the clinical features and investigations that help to distinguish ulcerative colitis from Crohn's disease.

20. How may diabetes mellitus affect the eye?

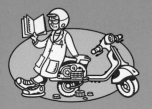

Extended-matching Questions

1. Chest pain

A. Aortic stenosis
B. Angina pectoralis
C. Inferior non ST elevation myocardial infarction
D. Anteroseptal non ST elevation myocardial infarction
E. Asthma
F. Costochondritis
G. Pulmonary embolus
H. Mitral valve prolapse
I. Hypertrophic obstructive cardiomyopathy
J. Dressler's syndrome

For each of the following patients, select the most likely diagnosis from the list of options.

1. A 56-year-old man with hypertension and known angina presents with central tight chest pain similar to his normal angina but increasing in frequency and now present at rest. ECG shows ST depression and T wave inversion in leads V1–4.

2. A 45-year-old man presents with pleuritic chest pain 6 weeks after a myocardial infarction. A friction rub can be heard on auscultation and the ECG shows ST elevation in all leads.

3. A 64-year-old woman smoker with hypertension and hypercholesterolaemia reports 4 weeks of reproducible retrosternal 'band-like' chest tightness on exertion. It is relieved by rest. ECG is normal.

4. A previously well 45-year-old woman smoker presents with left-sided pleuritic chest pain and dyspnoea on exertion. ECG shows right axis deviation and T wave inversion in leads V1–3. Resting oxygen saturations are 93% on air.

5. A 25-year-old rower presents with chest pain and dizziness on exertion. He has a pan systolic murmur at the apex and fourth heart sound on examination. ECG shows left ventricular hypertrophy. His uncle died aged 32 years from an unknown cause.

2. Haematuria

A. Benign prostatic hypertrophy
B. Goodpasture's syndrome
C. Acute pyelonephritis
D. Acute cystitis
E. Prostatic carcinoma
F. Ureteric calculi
G. Bladder carcinoma
H. Renal cell carcinoma
I. Wegener's granulomatosis
J. IgA nephropathy

For each of the following patients, select the most likely diagnosis from the list of options.

1. A 23-year-old woman presents with fever, tachycardia and tenderness in the left loin. The white cell count is raised and the urine is cloudy.

2. A 70-year-old man describes intermittent colicky left loin pain, weight loss and night sweats. He has noted testicular changes which, on examination, are a varicocele. The haematuria is macroscopic.

3. A 36-year-old woman presents with malaise, recurrent epistaxis, haemoptysis and microscopic haematuria. Examination reveals septal perforation and nodules on the chest X-ray. The serum creatinine is elevated at 307 µmol/L.

4. A 39-year-old man presents to the emergency department in high summer with severe colicky right loin pain radiating down into the scrotum. Examination is unremarkable and the dipstick shows haematuria.

5. A 78-year-old man with longstanding nocturia, poor urinary stream and terminal dribbling notices macroscopic haematuria towards the end of the urine stream. He has become more lethargic and is troubled by lower back pain.

3. Dyspnoea

A. Pulmonary tuberculosis
B. Aspergilloma
C. Diaphragmmatic palsy
D. Interstitial lung disease
E. Bronchpneumonia
F. Pneumoconiosis
G. Mesothelioma
H. Left ventricular systolic dysfunction
 I. Sarcoidosis
J. Diastolic cardiac dysfunction

For each of the following patients, select the most likely diagnosis from the list of options.

1. A 45-year-old man with two previous anterior myocardial infarctions, hypertension and diabetes describes increasing dyspnoea, especially orthopnoea. Cardiomegaly is noted on chest X-ray.

2. The above patient undergoes coronary artery bypass graft surgery involving a prolonged intensive care admission. He remains dyspnoeic but his orthopnoea is more pronounced. Chest X-ray appears to show more elevated hemidiaphragms.

3. A 51-year-old patient with dyspnoea has marked bibasal crackles on auscultation. The dyspnoea does not improve with diuretics and subsequent echocardiography is normal.

4. A 60-year-old ex-builder presents with dyspnoea and cough. Chest X-ray shows extensive pleural thickening and calcification plus a pleural effusion. This is blood stained at aspiration.

5. A 40-year-old homeless patient presents with dyspnoea, weight loss, cough and haemoptysis. The chest X-ray shows left upper lobe consolidation with cavitation. Heaf testing is strongly positive.

4. Abnormal full blood counts

A. Pernicious anaemia
B. Acute lymphoblastic leukaemia
C. Liver failure
D. Folate deficiency anaemia
E. Acute myeloid leukaemia
F. Hodgkin's lymphoma
G. Disseminated intravascular coagulopathy
H. Multiple myeloma
 I. Intravenous heparin therapy

For each of the following patients, select the most likely diagnosis from the list of options.

1. A 63-year-old woman presents with lethargy, malaise and bone pain. Investigations show a normocytic anaemia, elevated serum urea, creatinine and calcium levels. The total protein is raised though the albumin is within the normal range.

2. A 40-year-old man presents with lethargy, malaise and several recent chest infections. A full blood count result is all within the normal ranges but the blood film comments on the presence of Auer rods.

3. A 64-year-old woman with vitiligo has a full blood count measured for investigation of lethargy. She is anaemic and has a mean corpuscular volume of 120 fL. Her haematinics are abnormal and she has anti-gastric parietal cell antibodies in her serum.

4. A 34-year-old man undergoing mechanical ventilation for severe pneumonia begins to bleed from percutaneous puncture sites and mucosal surfaces. The platelet count and haemoglobin, which had been normal, begin to fall and his clotting tests including d-dimers become deranged.

5. A 24-year-old woman with lethargy, malaise and night sweats notices enlarged lymph glands in her neck. A full blood count is carried out before biopsy. An eosinophilia is the only abnormality.

5. Rheumatological

A. Rheumatoid arthritis
B. Osteoarthritis
C. Reiter's syndrome
D. CREST syndrome
E. Polymyalgia rheumatica
F. Polymyositis
G. Ankylosing spondylitis
H. Systemic lupus erythematosus
I. Antiphospholid syndrome
J. Mixed connective tissue disorder

For each of the following patients, select the most likely diagnosis from the list of options.

1. A 27-year-old man has noticed that he is finding it increasingly hard to 'get going in the mornings'. This is specifically due to backache. He feels better as the day goes on. Examination shows a decreased range of movement of the spine.

2. A 25-year-old Afro-Caribbean woman is referred for investigation of three miscarriages. She is concerned by how her skin reacts to sunlight and the development of alopecia. Her musculoskeletal symptoms are of a small joint arthralgia. Proteinuria is present on urine testing.

3. A 55-year-old man with a body mass index of greater than 35 is troubled by pain in the left hip. This is predominantly present on weight bearing and is worsened by exercise. X-ray reports loss of the joint space.

4. A 31-year-old woman reports dysuria, conjunctivitis and right knee pain. She is normally fit and well, although was off work for 10 days before presentation with diarrhoea.

5. A 44-year-old man has become weaker over the last month. He is now unable to get out of his chair without assistance. His voice has become weak and his muscles are tender. The creatine kinase is raised and he has type 2 respiratory failure on blood gas analysis.

6. Signs on chest examination

A. Bronchial breathing
B. Expiratory wheeze
C. Trachea deviated to left
D. Trachea deviated to right
E. Stridor
F. Increased percussion note
G. Whispering pectoriloquy
H. Inspiratory crackles
I. Intercostal muscle recession
J. Stony dullness

For each of the following patients, select the physical signs that best fit the clinical scenario from the list of options.

1. A patient with a large retrosternal goitre.

2. A right tension pneumothorax.

3. A patient with right upper lobe fibrosis due to sarcoidosis.

4. A patient with poorly controlled asthma.

5. A patient with a large pleural effusion.

445

7. Abdominal swellings

A. Aortic aneurysm
B. Ascites
C. Fibroid uterus
D. Polycystic kidneys
E. Ventral hernia
F. Transplanted kidney
G. Ovarian cyst
H. Hepatomegaly
 I. Splenomegaly
J. Enlarged bladder

For each of the following patients with a palpable abdominal mass, suggest the most likely cause from the list of options.

1. A 34-year-old male with Cushingoid features has a smooth mass palpable in the right iliac fossa.

2. An 81-year-old with urinary incontinence following a hernia repair and a suprapubic smooth tender mass.

3. A 35-year-old lady is admitted with a thunderclap headache and has masses in both hypochondria.

4. A 79-year-old lady complains of a swelling in the centre of her abdomen that appears when she sits up and disappears when she lies down.

5. A 38-year-old lady is admitted smelling of alcohol. She is confused with multiple spider naevi, asterixis and a tense swollen abdomen.

8. Headache

A. Meningitis
B. Encephalitis
C. Subarachnoid haemorrhage
D. Tension headache
E. Migraine
F. Cluster headache
G. Glaucoma
H. Giant cell arteritis
 I. Trigeminal neuralgia
J. Raised intra-cranial pressure

For each of the following patients, select the most likely diagnosis from the list of options.

1. A 21-year-old university student presents with a severe headache of gradual onset. He cannot tolerate the light and is febrile.

2. A 73-year-old heavy smoker is seen in clinic with a 3-month history of worsening headaches. They are most troublesome in the morning and are exacerbated by coughing. He has haemoptysis.

3. A 39-year-old businessman presents with a rapid onset of severe pain around his right eye that is associated with lacrimation and has been occurring nightly for 2 weeks.

4. A 69-year-old lady describes a worsening headache and pain in her jaw when she chews. Her vision is normal. Her erythrocyte sedimentation rate is 88 mm/hour.

5. A 28-year-old male with a family history of kidney problems presents with a sudden onset severe headache. He has neck stiffnes.

9. Altered level of consciousness

A. Brain stem infarction
B. Drug overdose
C. Hepatic failure
D. Hypoglycaemia
E. Hyponatraemia
F. Hypothermia
G. Meningitis
H. Renal failure
I. Schizophrenia
J. Subarachnoid haemorrhage

For each of the following patients, select the most likely diagnosis from the list of options.

1. A 93-year-old lady is brought in following a sudden loss of consciousness. Two days later, she remains deeply unconscious with pinpoint pupils.

2. A 42-year-old man is brought in after a sudden collapse. Sub-hyaloid haemorrhages are seen on fundoscopy.

3. A 22-year-old woman is brought in having been found in the street. She responds to painful stimuli and has pinpoint pupils.

4. A 46-year-old woman is found collapsed at home. She is unrousable, pyrexial and has a purpuric rash.

5. An elderly hypertensive lady is admitted in a post-ictal state after a witnessed tonic-clonic seizure. She has recently been commenced on a diuretic for her hypertension.

10. Endocrine tests

A. 2-hour oral glucose tolerance test
B. Dexamethasone suppression test
C. Domperidone test
D. Insulin-like growth factor 1 measurement
E. Insulin stress test
F. Prolonged fast
G. Prolonged glucose tolerance test
H. Synacthen test
I. Thyrotropin-releasing hormone test
J. Water deprivation test

For each of the following clinical scenarios, select the most appropriate investigation from the list of options.

1. A patient presents with headaches. You notice inter-dental spacing, large hands and feet, hypertension and prominent supra-orbital ridge.

2. A 39-year-old woman complains of episodic fainting, which is most likely to occur if she misses a meal.

3. A 28-year-old lady with vitiligo complains of lethargy. She is noted to have pigmented palmar creases and oral mucosa.

4. A 29-year-old man has recently been discharged following a significant head injury. He now presents with polyuria, polydipsia and hypernatraemia.

5. A 50-year-old woman is referred to clinic with hirsutism, weight gain, diabetes and hypertension.

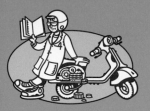

Patient-management Problems

1. A 50-year-old man presents with a chronic productive cough, weight loss and a history of tuberculosis as a child. How would you confirm your suspicion of a reactivation of tuberculosis? What therapy would you use? What are your responsibilities for public health? Could there be a different diagnosis?

2. A 34-year-old woman is referred to clinic for investigation of arthralgia, which is worse in the mornings. What features in the history, examination and investigations would support a diagnosis of rheumatoid arthritis? What is the drug treatment for rheumatoid arthritis and how has it changed?

3. A 57-year-old man describes increasing shortness of breath especially at night and decreased exercise abilities. He had a myocardial infarction 4 years before this and has been told he has 'cardiac failure'. He has heard from a friend that this is very serious and nothing can be done. How will you explain his condition to him? How would you investigate him? What therapies are available? Is it true that 'nothing can be done'?

4. A 72-year-old woman complains to you of acute low back pain. Initial investigations reveal hypercalcaemia and a high erythrocyte sedimentation rate. What is your differential diagnosis? If the hypercalcaemia requires treatment, how would it be done? What investigations are needed to establish the diagnosis?

5. A 62-year-old woman with a 50 pack-year smoking history has noticed new onset wheeze and increasing dyspnoea on exertion. Her chest is hyperexpanded on examination and chest radiography. Spirometry shows an FEV1 of 45% predicted with a FVC of 80% predicted. This is unchanged with bronchodilators. She thinks she has asthma. Is she correct? If not, what is an alternative diagnosis? What interventions have survival benefit for her? What drug and non-pharmacological therapies should be initiated?

6. A young woman aged 25 years attends your clinic because she was found to have a cholesterol level of 6.9 mmol/L at a health club membership check-up. Does she need lipid lowering therapy with a statin? The next patient is a 58-year-old diabetic man with a previous myocardial infarction and a cholesterol of 5.4 mmol/L. Should he be taking a statin? Consider the differences between primary and secondary prevention. What are the risks and benefits? What advice would you give to the first patient?

7. A previously well 41-year-old man is referred to you when a routine blood sample shows a serum creatinine level of 450 μmol/L. He says he has recently started new medications. What results and findings may require emergency treatment? What drugs are you interested in? Which investigations are required and how can you begin to separate acute from chronic renal failure on the information obtained?

8. A 56-year-old man, weighing 65 kg, with chronic renal failure and a serum creatinine of 510 mmol/L is referred to your nephrology clinic. Can you estimate his glomerular filtration rate? How would you assess and modify any elements that could preserve renal function? What are the medical consequences of chronic renal failure? He asks you if he will need dialysis – is he correct and what options are available to him?

9. A previously well 35-year-old woman attends clinic. She is feeling tired all the time and has had several respiratory tract infections in the last few months. On examination, you notice she is anaemic. Subsequent full blood count confirms anaemia and leucocytosis with numerous blast cells. She asks you what blast cells are and what that means. How do you answer her? What further investigations are needed? She thinks a bone marrow examination sounds too painful and does not want this. How would you explain its importance (think of molecular biology and cytogenetic analysis)? How is treatment becoming more focussed in haematological malignancy?

10. A 47-year-old man is referred by the emergency department with central chest pain. The ECG shows ST depression in the anterior chest leads. He has had aspirin. A medical student suggests thrombolysis is needed. Is he correct? If not, why not? What other therapies should be started? What are the alternative diagnoses? Will troponin measurement be useful in his treatment planning?

MCQ Answers

Gastroenterology

1. Gastroesophageal reflux disease:

(a) F: Frequency is increasing
(b) T: Other risk factors include obesity, caffeine, excess alcohol
(c) F: OGD may be normal whereas videofluoroscopy or 24-hour intraluminal pH monitoring may demonstrate acid reflux
(d) F: Medical treatment and lifestyle advice are the mainstay of therapy
(e) T: Barrett's oesophagus

2. Peptic ulcer disease:

(a) T: 95% versus 70%
(b) T: Very common
(c) T: Gastric cancer may present as an ulcer
(d) F: They have similar presentations
(e) T: All duodenal ulcers should receive eradication therapy as 95% of duodenal ulcers are associated with *Helicobacter pylori* infection

3. Upper gastrointestinal haemorrhage:

(a) F: Priority is given to ensuring haemodynamic stability
(b) F: A drop in haemoglobin concentration does not occur until the lost volume is replaced and haemodilution occurs
(c) T: Both by volume contraction in the circulation and therefore pre-renal impairment and because the bleed causes protein absorption which is broken down in the liver to make urea
(d) T: Should be performed within 4 hours if suspect a variceal bleed. Within 12–24 hours if patient shocked on admission or has significant co-morbidity
(e) T: Re-bleed mortality is 40% and therefore it is important to prevent rebleeds

4. The following are features of ulcerative colitis:

(a) F: This is a feature of Crohn's. Only the mucosa and submucosa are inflamed in ulcerative colitis
(b) T: Mucosal ulcers give rise to the appearance of polyps between them
(c) F: These are characteristic of Crohn's disease
(d) F: The inflammation in ulcerative colitis always involves the rectum and extends proximally in a continuous pattern
(e) T: Crohn's disease is more common in smokers

5. Colorectal cancer:

(a) F: 90% occur in those without a strong family history
(b) T: This applies to both Crohn's and ulcerative colitis
(c) F: They remain asymptomatic longer because the stool has a liquid consistency in the ascending colon and therefore obstruction occurs less readily
(d) T: A high index of suspicion is important in patients with anaemia, rectal bleeding or altered bowel habit
(e) F: Over 90% can be resected surgically

6. Pseudomembranous colitis:

(a) F: It is due to toxins produced by *Clostridium difficile*
(b) T: Most antibiotics can cause it
(c) F: The diagnosis is made by demonstration of the presence of *Clostridium difficile* toxin in a stool sample
(d) T: As with all forms of colitis
(e) F: Oral therapy is required – metronidazole or less commonly vancomycin

7. Irritable bowel syndrome:

(a) F: It is the commonest diagnosis made in gastroenterology clinics
(b) F: Commonest in young females
(c) F: This should encourage a search for other pathology
(d) T: There is no accepted definition or diagnostic test
(e) F: Therapy is rarely 100% successful

8. The following can be said of gallstones:

(a) F: 10% are, whereas 90% of renal stones are radio-opaque
(b) T: Therefore, in deciding to remove the gallbladder, it is important to ensure the patient's symptoms are from the gallbladder
(c) T: Said to be associated with the 5 'F's: fat, fertile, female, forties, fair
(d) T: Increased bile pigment from the breakdown of haemoglobin
(e) T: Gallstone ileus – a gallstone perforates through the gallbladder into the duodenum and passes on to obstruct the terminal ileum

9. Acute pancreatitis:

(a) T: The other common cause is gallstones
(b) F: There is usually severe abdominal pain
(c) T: This is Cullen's sign. Bruising in the flanks may also occur – Grey–Turner's sign. Both are due to retro-peritoneal haemorrhage
(d) F: The abdominal X-ray may show a dilated 'sentinel loop' of jejunum. The diagnostic test is a markedly raised serum amylase
(e) XXX

10. The following may be said of viral hepatitis:

(a) F: It may relapse but chronic hepatitis does not occur
(b) F: Transmission is perenteral
(c) T: This is the case also for other causes of chronic hepatitis
(d) F: The acute disease is usually asymptomatic
(e) T

Genitourinary Disorders

1. Glomerular pathology may present in the following ways:

(a) T: Up to 0.15 g/24 hours is normal
(b) T: This is usually microscopic (i.e. not visible to the naked eye)
(c) T: It is important to exclude secondary causes of hypertension particularly in young patients
(d) T: A decrease in glomerular filtration rate causes an increase in serum urea and creatinine
(e) T: Combination of proteinuria, haematuria, impaired renal function, oliguria and hypertension

2. Nephrotic syndrome:

(a) F: The key features are gross proteinuria, hypoalbuminaemia and oedema
(b) F: Other common causes include diabetic nephropathy, amyloidosis, vasculitis, infections and drugs
(c) T: Patients may report this when there is heavy proteinuria
(d) T: Cholesterol levels may be very high
(e) T: If thrombus forms in the renal veins, there may be loin pain, haematuria and an acute deterioration of renal function

3. If glomerular disease is suspected the following investigations should be performed:

(a) T: To assess creatinine clearance and 24-hour urinary protein excretion
(b) T: Red cell casts indicate glomerular disease
(c) T: May be depleted in lupus nephritis, mesangiocapillary glomerulonephritis and post-infectious glomerulonephritis
(d) T: To exclude myeloma
(e) T: Wegener's disease, microscopic polyangiitis and anti-glomerular basement membrane disease may respond well to prompt immunosuppression and therefore it is important not to miss these diagnoses

4. The following can be said of acute renal failure:

(a) F: Acute renal failure can be non-oliguric
(b) T: This is probably the most common cause seen in hospital
(c) F: Mortality is 30–70%
(d) F: Approximately 60% regain normal renal function
(e) T: To exclude obstructive uropathy which may be easily relieved thereby reversing the acute renal failure

5. The following complications of acute renal failure require urgent dialysis therapy:

(a) T: Particularly if the patient is anuric and therefore cannot be diuresed
(b) T: Sodium bicarbonate therapy may also be used
(c) F: The absolute creatinine level *per se* does not determine the need for emergency dialysis
(d) T: This problem is worse if urine output is poor
(e) T: The same would apply to other manifestations of severe uraemia (e.g. seizures)

6. Severe hyperkalaemia:

(a) T: It may therefore be fatal
(b) F: It is useful to stabilise the myocardium, but does not reduce potassium concentration
(c) T: Cause potassium to re-distribute intracellularly
(d) T: Causes potassium to re-distribute intra-cellularly
(e) F: Cause potassium to re-distribute intracellularly

7. The following can be said of chronic renal failure:

(a) F: The commonest cause of end-stage renal failure
(b) F: Usually limited to those with normal sized kidneys where the history and investigations suggest an intrinsic renal problem
(c) T: This reduces the rate of decline in renal function
(d) F: Phosphate and potassium intake are reduced as their renal secretion is impaired; sodium intake is also reduced to prevent fluid retention
(e) F: Failure of erythropoietin production by the kidneys combined with impaired utilisation of iron in erythropoiesis usually causes a normochromic normocytic anaemia

8. Urinary tract infections:

(a) T: Closer proximity of urethra to anus
(b) F: 25–35% of females have symptoms of urinary tract infection at least once
(c) F: Asymptomatic bacteriuria – no symptoms but urine yields growth of >100 000 microbes per mL on culture
(d) F: Infection is a common complication of urinary catheterisation
(e) F: Acute pyelonephritis often requires intravenous antibiotics and fluids

9. The following are causes of hyponatraemia:

(a) T: Secondary hyperaldosteronism causes sodium and water retention
(b) F: May cause hypernatraemia
(c) F: Causes hypernatraemia
(d) T: Common cause – both loop and thiazide diuretics can do this
(e) T: Pseudohyponatraemia

10. The following ECG changes may be seen in hypokalaemia:

(a) F: T waves are small or inverted
(b) T: Appear after T waves
(c) F: Feature of hyperkalaemia
(d) T
(e) F: May be depressed

Neurology

1. Stroke:

(a) F: 10–20% are caused by haemorrhage
(b) F: The visual field defect is on the hemiplegic side
(c) F: The diagnosis is clinical. CT scanning is important to distinguish haemorrhage from infarction
(d) F: Management in a specialised stroke unit has been shown to improve patient outcome
(e) F: Avoid lowering blood pressure in the acute phase. Impaired cerebral autoregulation of blood flow may result in cerebral hypoperfusion

2. Giant cell arteritis:

(a) F: Commonest in patients over 60 years
(b) T: Involvement of the vessels supplying the muscles of mastication may cause 'jaw claudication'
(c) F: It is usually elevated, but a normal erythrocyte sedimentation rate does not exclude the diagnosis
(d) F: Treatment is started promptly if there is strong clinical suspicion to avoid irreversible visual loss
(e) F: 'Skip lesions' may cause false negatives

3. Migraine:

(a) F: Approximately 10%
(b) T: This may occur during the aura. Other focal neurological deficits have been described
(c) T
(d) F: β-blockers have a role to play in prophylaxis, but not in treatment of acute attacks
(e) F: They are useful in aborting acute attacks

4. Parkinson's disease:

(a) F: Affects men and women equally
(b) F: Characteristically a resting tremor
(c) F: Commonly starts on one side
(d) T: This should be recognised and appropriate treatment and support offered
(e) T: Nausea and vomiting are common. Late side-effects include dyskinesia and other motor problems

5. Multiple sclerosis:

(a) F: There is no association
(b) F: Mean age of onset is 30 years
(c) F: The hallmark of multiple sclerosis is lesions disseminated in site and time
(d) T: Uthoff's phenomenon
(e) F: Steroids are useful for acute relapses, but do not alter the course of the disease

6. Bacterial meningitis:

(a) T: Bacterial meningitis is a notifiable disease
(b) F: This is characterisitic of meningococcal septicaemia
(c) F: Investigations should never delay prompt therapy
(d) T: In this stuation an urgent CT brain scan is required – if normal, proceed to lumbar puncture
(e) F: Parenteral antibiotics are given if bacterial meningitis is suspected

7. Epilepsy:

(a) F: Other causes must be excluded before a diagnosis of epilepsy is made
(b) F: The diagnosis is clinical. 10–15% of the population have an abnormal EEG
(c) F: Many centres reserve therapy until after a second seizure
(d) T: Other common side-effects include weight gain and hair thinning
(e) T: Unless confident that the serum glucose is normal, intravenous dextrose should be given; thiamine is given concurrently in alcoholics to avoid precipitating Wernicke's encephalopathy

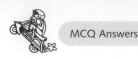

8. The following are features of raised intracranial pressure:

(a) T: Also often worse in the morning
(b) T
(c) F: This is a feature of diaphragmatic irritation
(d) T: This is a late sign
(e) T: The sixth nerve has a long intracranial course and may be affected by increased intracranial pressure – a 'false-localising sign'

9. Motor neurone disease:

(a) T: Slightly
(b) F: Peak incidence is at age 50–70 years
(c) F: Never causes sensory problems
(d) T
(e) F: It only offers a small increase in lifespan

10. Bell's palsy:

(a) F: It is an idiopathic lesion of the seventh cranial nerve
(b) F: Hyperacusis occurs when the nerve to stapedius is affected
(c) F: There is a lower motor neurone pattern of weakness
(d) F: Most patients recover fully in a few weeks
(e) F: It may reduce damage and/or speed recovery if given early

Endocrine

1. The following results fulfil the WHO criteria for diagnosis of diabetes mellitus:

(a) F: Impaired fasting glycaemia – investigate with an oral glucose tolerance test
(b) T
(c) F: Normal
(d) T
(e) F: Impaired glucose tolerance

2. Diabetes mellitus may present as follows:

(a) F: Although obesity is a common cause of type II diabetes mellitus poorly controlled undiagnosed diabetes will cause weight loss
(b) T: Diabetics are prone to infection
(c) T: A chronic complication such as diabetic retinopathy may be the mode pf presentation
(d) T: Filtered glucose exceeds renal tubular reabsorptive capacity and causes an osmotic diuresis
(e) T: This may be diabetic ketoacidosis in type I diabetes or hyperosmolar non-ketotic coma in type II diabetes

3. The following can be said of therapy in diabetes mellitus:

(a) F: Intravenous fluid replacement is the priority
(b) F: Type I diabetics all require insulin therapy
(c) T: This was demonstrated by the diabetes control and compliance test in type I diabetes and the UK Prospective Diabetes Study (UKPDS) in type II diabetes
(d) F: UKPDS also demonstrated a reduction in microvascular complications
(e) T: Reducing glucose levels increases the risk of hypoglycaemia

4. Osteoporosis:

(a) F: Prevalence is approximately 50%
(b) F: Hyperthyroidism is a secondary cause
(c) F: Osteoporosis is painless. The fractures it may cause are painful
(d) F: Blood tests, including a bone profile, are normal
(e) F: Bone densitometry is used most commonly to estimate bone mineral density

5. Hypercalcaemia:

(a) F: Primary hyperparathyroidism and malignancy are the commonest causes
(b) T: Renal stone formation may occur
(c) F: They should be suppressed
(d) F: Hydration with normal saline precedes bisphosphonate therapy
(e) F: Previously it was used to induce a calciuresis after rehydration, but it is far less effective than bisphosphonate therapy

6. Gout:

(a) T: Commoner in drinkers and higher socio-economic classes as well
(b) F: Acute gout characteristically causes a monoarthritis – often of the first metatarsophalangeal joint
(c) T: A common cause
(d) F: It is more useful for monitoring therapy, and can be normal in gout
(e) F: Allopurinol can exacerbate acute gout. Non-steroidal anti-inflammatory drugs are most commonly used to treat acute gout

7. Acromegaly:

(a) F: Most commonly due to growth hormone secreting pituitary adenoma. If this compresses the pituitary stalk, the tonic negative influence of dopamine on prolactin secretion may be lost, causing hyperprolactinaemia
(b) F: Pituitary lesions classically cause bitemporal visual field defects
(c) T: Acromegalics have an increased risk of cardiovascular disease and also suffer from hypertension and cardiomyopathy
(d) F: Growth hormone is assessed during an oral glucose tolerance test – it should normally be suppressed
(e) F: Octreotide, a somatostatin analogue, inhibits growth hormone secretion

8. The following may be features of thyrotoxicosis of any aetiology:

(a) T: Sinus tachycardia is also common
(b) F: Specific to Grave's disease
(c) T: Due to sympathetic innervation of levator palpebrae; thyrotoxicosis causes stimulation of the sympathetic nervous system
(d) F: A feature of hypothyroidism; thyrotoxicosis causes oligomenorrhoea
(e) F: Specific to Grave's disease

9. Cushing's syndrome:

(a) F: This causes Cushing's disease but is only one of the causes of Cushing's syndrome
(b) F: More likely to cause hypokalaemia and hypernatraemia
(c) F: Weight gain with a centripetal distribution of fat deposition is characteristic
(d) T: Plasma cortisol measurements are less useful
(e) F: Trans-sphenoidal surgery to resect the adenoma is the treatment of choice

10. Addison's disease:

(a) T: Autoimmune adrenal destruction causes up to 90% of cases of Addison's disease; this is associated with other autoimmune conditions
(b) T: Waterhouse–Friedrichsen syndrome results from adrenal haemorrhage/infarction
(c) T: Due to high levels of adrenocorticotropic hormone in primary adrenal failure
(d) F: Electrolytes are usually normal but, in an impending crisis, there may be hyponatraemia and/or hyperkalaemia
(e) F: Usual replacement therapy is oral hydrocortisone 20 mg in the morning and 10 mg at night – to mimic physiological diurnal variation

Respiratory disease

1. The physical signs of an uncomplicated large pneumothorax include:

(a) F: Deviated away
(b) T
(c) F: Decreased on affected side
(d) F: Decreased
(e) F: May occur with pneumomediastinum

2. Asthma:

(a) T
(b) F: Often normal between attacks, compare with chronic obstructive pulmonary disease
(c) T: A common cause of explained chronic cough
(d) T: More than 20%
(e) F: Increasing, cause unknown

3. In a patient with severe asthma:

(a) F: Values less than 33% predicted indicate a life-threatening event
(b) F: Worrying, implies the patient is becoming tired
(c) T: Bronchodilator
(d) F: Approximately 1500 deaths per year in the UK
(e) F: Little evidence for this statement

4. Predictors of severity of community acquired pneumonia include:

(a) T
(b) F: <60 mmHg or systolic blood pressure <90 mmHg
(c) T
(d) T
(e) T: The above comprise the 'CURB 65' score

5. Pleural effusion:

(a) F: Exudate – remember Light's criteria
(b) T: Rare
(c) T
(d) F: High suspicion for malignancy
(e) F: Most common cause is inadequately treated heart failure

6. Pulmonary embolus:

(a) F: Classical but uncommon
(b) F: Unmatched, ventilation normal
(c) T
(d) T: Part of clinical risk score
(e) F: 3–6 months adequate for a first event

7. The following have shown proven benefit in chronic obstructive pulmonary disease:

(a) T: Beneficial at all stages of the disease
(b) F: Only long-term oxygen therapy prolongs survival
(c) F: Only if FEV1 <50% predicted and two exacerbations in last year
(d) T: Improved survival in acute setting
(e) T: Improved symptoms and exercise tolerance

8. Squamous cell carcinoma of the lung:

(a) F: Small (Oat) cell cancer
(b) T: Increased parathyroid hormone secretion
(c) F: Small cell
(d) F: Surgery main chance of cure
(e) T: Brain, bone and liver as well

9. Malignant mesothelioma:

(a) F: Pleura
(b) F: In only approximately 15%
(c) F: Evidence of asbestos exposure only
(d) F: Little effective treatment at present
(e) T: Usually caused by industrial asbestos exposure

10. Obstructive sleep apnoea:

(a) F: Many have normal body mass index
(b) F: First-line therapy is nocturnal continuous positive-airways pressure support
(c) T: Assess with Epworth sleepiness score
(d) T: Hypertension and possibly coronary artery disease
(e) T

Infectious disease

1. Human immunodeficiency virus:

(a) T
(b) F
(c) T
(d) F: Formerly a very common mode of presentation
(e) F: Combination therapy has radically altered prognosis

2. The following are common causes of urinary tract infection:

(a) T
(b) T: The most common community organism
(c) F
(d) T
(e) F: The most common cause of community acquired pneumonia

3. The following bacteria are paired with an appropriate antibiotic for empirical therapy:

(a) T: In community acquired pneumonia
(b) F: vancomycin or teicoplanin are indicated
(c) T: Try and limit use because it is the only oral antipseudomonal antibiotic available
(d) T: Trimethoprim remains a good antibiotic for community urinary tract infection; however, resistance is increasing
(e) T: For bacterial endocarditis

4. Malaria:

(a) F: Can present many months after return
(b) F: *Plasmodium falciparum*
(c) F: Three needed by convention
(d) T: Especially in severe malaria
(e) F: Most now chloroquine resistant. Use quinine

5. The following patients are at risk of tuberculosis:

(a) T
(b) F: Treatment with TNF-α blocking drugs may allow reactivation of latent tuberculosis
(c) T
(d) T
(e) F: Can cause mediastinal lymphadenopathy and impaired cell mediated immunity can give a negative Heaf test)

History taking

1. The following are important in the patient with a chronic cough:

(a) T: May indicate asthma or gastrooesophageal reflux disease
(b) F: Angiotensin-converting enzyme inhibitors are implicated in chronic cough
(c) T: Can indicate malignancy
(d) T: With asthma and reflux, it comprises the three most common causes of chronic cough if no pre-existing lung disease is present
(e) T: Occupational exposure to irritants

2. The following drugs and side effects are correctly linked:

(a) T: If diagnosis suspected as about amiodarone and cytotoxics
(b) T: Can be years after drugs commenced
(c) F: Colour vision affected
(d) T: Can cause slate-grey skin changes
(e) T. Test before starting therapy and warn patient to monitor for signs

3. **The following are correct:**

   (a) T
   (b) F: 30 cigarettes = 1.5 packs per day multiplied by 25 years equals 37.5 pack years
   (c) F: Six units
   (d) T
   (e) T

Investigations

1. **When investigating suspected pulmonary embolus:**

   (a) F: When combined with a low clinical risk score can allow exclusion of pulmonary embolism
   (b) F: It supports the diagnosis indicating right heart strain
   (c) F: Underlying lung disease is an indication for a CT pulmonary angiogram
   (d) F: It may rise slightly as the right ventricle is stressed, not diagnostic
   (e) F: Under normal circumstances, no other tests are needed and an alternative diagnosis should be considered

2. **On respiratory function testing the following are true:**

   (a) F: From total lung capacity to residual volume
   (b) F: Vital capacity is best
   (c) T: Chronic obstructive pulmonary disease cannot be diagnosed without objective evidence of obstructive lung disease
   (d) T: Diffusion of gases is limited
   (e) T: Due to blood in the alveoli

3. **Arterial blood gas monitoring:**

   (a) F: Acid in that rising levels in the blood lower pH
   (b) T: Oxygenation is the problem, ventilation is adequate
   (c) F: The kidney
   (d) T: For example lactate, ketoacidosis
   (e) T: The two are synonymous

4. **On the electrocardiogram:**

   (a) F: From the beginning of the P wave
   (b) T
   (c) F: P pulmonale
   (d) F: Inferior
   (e) T: Increased width indicates ventricular conduction delay (i.e. bundle branch block)

5. **The following are causes of an increased mean corpuscular volume (MCV):**

   (a) T
   (b) T
   (c) T: B_{12} deficiency
   (d) F: Low MCV
   (e) F: Normal MCV

6. **Causes of a high erythrocyte sedimentation rate (ESR) include:**

   (a) T
   (b) T
   (c) F: Lowers ESR
   (d) T
   (e) T: Often key to decision making

7. **Causes of hypercalcaemia include:**

   (a) T: Other causes of lytic lesions in bone are lung, breast, thyroid and prostatic malignancy
   (b) T: Increased calcium intake
   (c) F: Hypocalcaemia
   (d) T
   (e) F: Normal biochemistry

8. **The following are paired correctly:**

   (a) T
   (b) F: Traditionally indicate obstructive biliary disease such as gallstones
   (c) F: Many things elevate the d-dimer and it is a test in which a negative result is more useful
   (d) F: Creatine kinase is increased as it is released when skeletal muscle is damaged. Troponin is cardiac specific
   (e) T: Used to monitor therapy

9. **When performing a short Synacthen test:**

   (a) F: Cortisol deficiency
   (b) F: Should rise with Synacthen in normal individuals
   (c) F: Dexamethasone suppression test is performed overnight
   (d) T
   (e) F: Need long Synacthen test or adrenocorticotropic hormone levels

10. **The chest X-ray:**

    (a) F: Right middle lobe
    (b) T
    (c) T: Other options include pulmonary haemorrhage or oedema
    (d) T: Other causes include lymphoma or tuberculosis
    (e) F: At the peripheries in pulmonary oedema

Haematological disorders

1. **Features of iron deficiency include:**

   (a) F
   (b) T: 'Spoon' shaped nails
   (c) T: The most important blood investigation though can be raised in acute illness
   (d) F
   (e) F: Several months required to replenish iron stores

2. Which of the following are true about sickle-cell disease:

(a) F: Autosomal recessive, defect on chromosome 11
(b) T: Also infection, dehydration and hypoxia
(c) T
(d) F: *Salmonella osteomyelitis*
(e) T: Has infarcted in most adults. At risk of infection as individuals are post splenectomy

3. Leukaemia:

(a) T: Affects all three main cell lines
(b) F: Often indolent requiring little active therapy
(c) F: Common in chronic myeloid leukaemia
(d) T
(e) F: Acute myeloid leukaemia

4. Disseminated intravascular coagulation:

(a) F: AML-M3
(b) T
(c) T: Although initially a pro-coagulant condition
(d) T: Treatment of the cause is the first priority
(e) F: Fibrinogen and platelets are reduced, prothrombin time and activated partial thromboplastin time are prolonged

5. Haemophilia A:

(a) F. This is haemophilia B (Factor VIII is deficient)
(b) F: Levels can fall to 5% before problems occur
(c) F: Haemarthrosis and haematomas
(d) F: Activated partial thromboplastin time
(e) F: Formerly true but safer blood products and recombinant Factor VIII have effectively eliminated this

6. In lymphoma the following are 'B' symptoms:

(a) F
(b) T
(c) T: The third 'B' symptom is weight loss more than 10% of initial body weight in 6 months
(d) F
(e) F

7. Hodgkin's lymphoma:

(a) F: The presence of Reed–Sternberg cells is required
(b) T: Reason unknown
(c) T: Results in bilateral hilar lymphadenopathy
(d) F: Most respond to therapy. In early stage disease, cure should always be the aim
(e) F: One of the most common cancers of young adults

8. When dealing with a patient with suspected pernicious anaemia:

(a) F: Now rarely performed
(b) F: Decreased absorption of B_{12} due to lack of intrinsic factor
(c) F: B_{12} deficiency is a rare cause of pancytopenia
(d) F: Responds well to B_{12} replacement
(e) T: Pernicious anaemia is associated with a wide range of other autoimmune diseases

9. Anaemia of chronic disease:

(a) F: Normocytic appearance
(b) F: Normal or high
(c) T: The problem is of iron utilisation not deficiency
(d) F: Anaemia of renal failure responds to erythropoietin
(e) T: Other causes include malignancy and chronic infection

10. The following blood film findings and diagnosis are correctly linked:

(a) T
(b) T
(c) F: Liver disease
(d) T
(e) F: B_{12} deficiency

Cardiovascular disorders

1. Heart murmurs:

(a) F: The presystolic murmur only occurs with sinus rhythm as it is the result of atrial contraction
(b) T
(c) T
(d) F: At the left sternal edge in expiration
(e) F: Opening snap occurs in mitral stenosis. Ejection click in aortic stenosis

2. There is published evidence to support the following statements:

(a) T: ISIS-2
(b) T: GUSTO
(c) T: SSSS
(d) T: CIBIS II
(e) T: RALES

3. After acute myocardial infarction:

(a) F: The decision is made on the history, electrocardiogram and absence of a contraindication
(b) T
(c) T: It is commonly given by the paramedics
(d) F: Good glycaemic control improves outcome for all. DIGAMI
(e) F: Use on day 1 improves mortality. ISIS-1

4. Atrial fibrillation:

(a) T: The loss of atrial systole impairs ventricular filling, this can tip a patient into overt heart failure
(b) T: Consider warfarin for all in long-term atrial fibrillation
(c) F: In the UK, age, hypertension and ischaemic heart disease are more common
(d) F: P waves are absent
(e) T

5. The following drugs should be used in non ST segment elevation myocardial infarction:

(a) T: The CURE study
(b) T
(c) F: The rate slowing calcium channel blockers, diltiazem or verapamil may be used if β-blockers are contraindicated
(d) F: Thrombolysis may worsen outcome
(e) T: For analgesia, consider nitrate infusion as well

6. Chronic left ventricular failure:

(a) T: 1 to 4 (most severe)
(b) F: Improve symptoms not survival
(c) F: More commonly used in USA in sinus rhythm
(d) T: Especially in dilated ventricles. Consider implantable defibrillators
(e) T: Absolutely. Improved therapy along with spironolactone and β-blockers

7. The following are correct about rheumatic fever:

(a) F: Arthritis
(b) F: This is for pancreatitis. For rheumatic fever use the revised (Duckett) Jones criteria
(c) T: Sydenham's chorea, a major criterion
(d) T
(e) F: Mitral

8. The jugulovenous pressure:

(a) F: Sternal angle
(b) T: Clinical central venous pressure
(c) T: Can be seen in patients with a VVI pacemaker
(d) T: Mediastinal mass (e.g. lung cancer or lymphoma)
(e) T: In time with the carotid pulse

9. The following are causes of essential hypertension:

(a) F
(b) F
(c) F
(d) F
(e) F: These are all causes of secondary hypertension

10. When examining the pulse:

(a) T: Carotid pulse if possible
(b) F: Aortic stenosis
(c) T
(d) T: Always, and remember to assess equality between left and right
(e) F: Increase as vagal tone is decreased

Musculoskeletal and skin disorders

1. The following are systemic consequences of rheumatoid arthritis:

(a) T
(b) F: Commonly restrictive due to pulmonary fibrosis
(c) T: Pericarditis
(d) T: May include Felty's syndrome
(e) T: A vasculitic phenomenon

2. The following are common causes of erythema multiforme:

(a) T
(b) F: Erythema nodosum
(c) T
(d) F: Erythema chronicum migrans in Lyme disease
(e) F: Pyoderma gangrenosum or erythema nodosum

3. Treatments for osteoarthritis include:

(a) T: Crucial
(b) T
(c) F: Rheumatoid arthritis
(d) T
(e) T

4. Gout:

(a) F: Small joints of feet and hands
(b) F: Negatively birefringent in gout. Positively in pseudogout
(c) T: Increased purine turnover. Ensure high fluid intake and prophylactic allopurinol
(d) F: For prevention. Non-steroidal anti-inflammatory drugs or colchicine for acute episodes
(e) F: It is a clinical diagnosis and the urate may be normal

5. Ankylosing spondylitis is associated with:

(a) F: Aortic regurgitation
(b) T: With kyphosis, can lead to chronic respiratory failure
(c) F: Remember it is an inflammatory arthritis
(d) F: >90%. The highest results for any seronegative arthropathy
(e) T

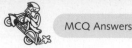

Examination

1. Hand signs:

(a) F: May be present if complicated by carcinoma
(b) F: It is a sign of iron deficiency
(c) F: Osler's nodes are a feature of endocarditis
(d) F: Caused by immune complex formation
(e) F: There are different patterns of psoriatic arthropathy. It is common for the distal interphalangeal joints to be involved

2. The following would suggest an upper rather than a lower motor neurone lesion:

(a) F: A lower motor neurone feature
(b) T: Typically with a 'clasp-knife' pattern, as opposed to the rigidity seen in extrapyramidal disease
(c) T
(d) T: May be elicited at the knee or ankle
(e) T: There may be some disuse atrophy, but significant muscle wasting is a feature of lower motor neurone lesions

3. Pulsus paradoxus:

(a) F: It decreases
(b) T: This is how pulsus paadoxus is defined
(c) T
(d) F: It is an exaggeration of the normal change in pulse volume with the respiratory cycle
(e) T: Also a feature of constrictive pericarditis

4. The following would help to distinguish between a kidney and a spleen in the left upper quadrant:

(a) T: Characteristic of a spleen
(b) T: Characteristic of a spleen
(c) T: If the mass is a kidney, you should be able to 'get above' it (i.e. palpate between the mass and costal margin)
(d) T: Kidneys are ballotable
(e) T: May suggest inherited polycystic kidney disease

5. The following are characteristic of a jugular venous, as opposed to carotid, pulsation:

(a) F: A venous pulsation cannot be felt
(b) T: Normally falls with inspiration; Kussmaul's sign in cardiac tamponade is a paradoxical rise of the jugular venous pulse (JVP)   in inspiration
(c) T: The normal JVP has an 'a' and 'v' wave
(d) T: As the patient reclines, the JVP moves higher in the neck
(e) F: The JVP rises if pressure is applied below the right costal margin – hepatojugular reflux

6. The physical signs of a large uncomplicated pneumothorax include:

(a) F: This feature suggests a tension pneumothorax requiring emergency management
(b) T: This is Hamman's sign and occurs occasionally with left-sided pneumothoraces and also in pneumomediastinum
(c) F: Reduced expansion on side of pneumothorax
(d) F: Breath sounds are reduced over pneumothorax
(e) T: It is said to be hyper-resonant

The Clerking

1. The following can be said of a medical clerking:

(a) T
(b) F: In certain cases it is better to change the order to emphasise more relevant features
(c) T
(d) T: This is useful in planning appropriate investigations and treatment
(e) F: It is also essential to print your name

SAQ Answers

1. The changes and time course are as follows:
   - Tall peaked 'hyperacute' T waves occur early after infarction.
   - The ST segment becomes elevated within minutes to hours of infarction. It is typically convex.
   - Pathological Q waves occur within 6–24 hours of infarction, usually as the ST segment settles.
   - The T waves invert after 12–48 hours.
   - Remember the pattern of infarction indicates the artery/territory damaged.
   - The persistence of ST elevation in the anterior leads can suggest the presence of an aneurysm of the left ventricle. Q waves usually remain and indicate a previous myocardial infarction on the resting ECG, even after full recovery.

2. Psoriasis is characterised by salmon-pink plaques over the extensor surfaces of the limbs, the navel, behind the ears and in the hair line. The nails may have a pitted appearance and an arthropathy exists in approximately 10% of patients. This can take one of a variety of forms.
   - Asymmetrical terminal joint involvement.
   - Rheumatoid arthritis like pattern.
   - Sacroiliitis.
   - Arthritis mutilans.

3. Many conditions are considered risk factors for venous thromboembolic (VTE) disease. They can be divided into inherited and acquired factors. Inherited factors include haematological disorders such as Factor V Leiden deficiency and prothrombin 20210A gene mutation. Acquired factors include malignancy, pregnancy, obesity, immobility and antiphospholipid syndrome. It is stated in UK guidelines that smoking is NOT an independent risk for VTE. For a full list, see Chapter 34.

4. Nephrotic syndrome is characterised by proteinuria of more than 3 g/24 hours, serum albumin of less than 20 g/dL and peripheral oedema. It is often accompanied by hyperlipidaemia and a hypercoagulable state. Its causes can be divided into primary glomerular disease or secondary to systemic disease. These include diabetes, systemic lupus erythematosus, amyloidosis, drugs such as gold or penicillamine, HIV or Hodgkin's disease.

5. Painful lymphadenopathy suggests local pyogenic infection from the territory which drain into the cervical nodes or local or systemic viral infection. Painless enlargement of glands may be a manifestation of lymphoma, sarcoidosis or HIV infection. Chronic infections presenting with cervical lymphadenopathy include tuberculosis, toxoplasma and brucellosis.

6. Aspirin should be given within the first 48 hours. This has a prognostic benefit. Ideally, this treatment is commenced after a CT scan has excluded intracranial haemorrhage but it can be given while the results of the CT scan are awaited. It is important to assess the patient's ability to swallow and, if this is impaired, administer intravenous fluids. The patient should be managed on a specialised Stroke Unit – this has been shown to improve outcome. Neurosurgical review should be considered for intracranial haemorrhages, particularly those in the posterior fossa. Supportive care is important and attention must be payed to hydration, pressure areas, nutrition, early physiotherapy and occupational therapy, as well as the needs of the family. Speech therapy may also be required. It is important not to lower blood pressure during the acute phase because disordered cerebral autoregulation of blood flow may lead to hypoperfusion and exacerbate ischaemia.

7. The pulse has a slow rising low volume character. The apex beat is heaving and undisplaced in nature. A systolic thrill maybe palpable in the aortic area. The second heart sound is quiet. An ejection click and fourth heart sound maybe heard. Remember the volume of the ejection systolic murmur is NOT correlated with severity. The blood pressure can demonstrate a narrow pulse pressure. The symptoms to ask about are dyspnoea, angina and syncopal episodes. ECG may show left ventricular hypertrophy.

8. Giant cell arteritis (GCA) is a medical emergency because it poses a significant risk of blindness if untreated. The main symptom is headache, and this can be associated with jaw claudication, a tender non-pulsatile artery on examination and systemic symptoms of a vasculitic process. The most important blood test is the erythrocyte sedimentation rate (ESR). Although a high result is non-specific, a normal ESR makes GCA less likely. Because of the risk of ischaemic optic neuritis, therapy with high-dose corticosteroids should not be withheld if the clinical suspicion is high enough. The definitive diagnosis may be made with a temporal artery biopsy. Traditionally, this should be performed within 48 hours; however, it is useful beyond this period.

9. Pneumonia can be divided into various subsets [e.g. community acquired pneumonia (typical and atypical), hospital (nosocomial) acquired pneumonia, aspiration pneumonia and pneumonia in 'at risk' groups such as the immunocompromised]. The clinical importance of this is that the microbiological agents responsible show a different distribution in each group and hence different empirical therapy is indicated. This knowledge, coupled with the use of scoring system to assess severity, will enable more effective management of patients with pneumonia.

461

10. Unknown! The development of highly active antiretroviral therapy has transformed the prognosis and the long-term survival is unknown. There is a variety of new drugs and therapeutic targets being developed. Patients are fit and well 15–20 years after diagnosis. Some patients with HIV have undergone successful organ transplantation.

11. The peripheries may be cool and poorly perfused. A tachycardia develops and the pulse pressure widens. If decompensation occurs, the blood pressure falls. A useful physical sign is the presence of a significant postural drop in blood pressure. Skin turgor is reduced and jugular venous pressure is low (may not be seen). If the urine output is recorded, this decreases. Dry mucous membranes suggest dehydration, but may simply reflect poor mouth care in a sick patient or the use of inhaled non-humidified oxygen.

12. A blood film may show fragmented red blood cells, polychromasia, macrocytosis, spherocytes or elliptocytes. The reticulocyte count increases reflecting increased marrow activity. Bilirubin levels are elevated as is lactate dehydrogenase. Haptoglobin levels fall if there is free haemoglobin in the circulation (intravascular haemolysis) and urinary urobolinogen increases.

13. No. It is safe to proceed with lumbar puncture if there are no signs of raised intracranial pressure (see Chapter 31). If a lumbar puncture is performed in a patient with raised intracranial pressure, there is a risk of herniation through the foramen magnum (i.e. coning). This is potentially fatal.

14. The cardinal physical signs are tremor, rigidity and bradykinesia. The tremor is most marked at rest and is characteristically a 'pill-rolling' tremor of index finger over thumb at 4–6 Hz. The rigidity is present throughout the range of movement. When combined with the tremor, a 'cog-wheeling' pattern of rigidity may emerge. Bradykinesia describes difficulty in initiating movements and their slowness.

Drugs with a dopamine antagonist action are common causes of parkinsonism (e.g. metoclopramide). Arteriosclerotic disease can cause parkinsonism and this responds poorly to dopamine replacement therapy. It is this poor response and the presence of vascular risk factors or cerebrovascular disease that gives the diagnosis away.

15. Gallstones are often asymptomatic but may cause acute or chronic cholecystitis, biliary colic (stone impacted in neck of gallbladder or cystic duct) or obstructive jaundice. Other presentations include cholangitis (infection of the bile ducts causing right upper quadrant pain, jaundice and fever with rigors), pancreatitis, empyema, and gallstone ileus where the gallstone perforates the gallbladder, ulcerates into the duodenum and passes on to obstruct the terminal ileum. The long-term presence of gallstones may be associated with gallbladder carcinoma.

16. Acute gout is usually managed with non-steroidal anti-inflammatory drugs (NSAIDs). Allopurinol is usually avoided until after the acute attack has settled because it may cause a flare up of acute gout. NSAIDs are contra-indicated in renal failure because they cause a deterioration in the glomerular filtration rate. Colchicine is an alternative but causes diarrhoea and vomiting and the dose needs to be adjusted in renal failure. Steroids can be useful to settle an acute attack of gout. In particular, intra-articular steroid injection can give rapid symptom relief.

17. The inflammatory response in bacterial meningitis is usually more pronounced than in viral meningitis. This leads to a higher cerebrospinal fluid (CSF) pressure, a higher protein content, and a more dense inflammatory cell infiltrate, which results in a more turbid CSF. These changes are suggestive but not diagnostic for bacterial meningitis. Stronger evidence for a bacterial cause is provided by polymorphonuclear cells on microscopy, rather than mononuclear cells, and a CSF glucose level of less than two-thirds of the blood glucose level.
Confirmatory evidence of bacterial meningitis is given by the presence of organisms on a Gram-stain (or a Ziehl-Neelsen slain for tuberculosis) and culture of the organism. (See Chapter 34, Fig. 34.7)

18. Infectious diarrhoea can be caused by many organisms by different pathological processes, which include toxin production, enteroadherence of organisms, mucosal invasion, or as part of a systemic infection. *Staphylococcus aureus, Bacillus cereus* and *Clostridium perfringens* all have a preformed toxin and give rise to food poisoning starting with vomiting and then leading to diarrhoea. Organisms that give rise to diarrhoea by enterotoxin production are enterotoxigenic *Escherichia coli* and *Vibrio cholerae,* whereas *Clostridium difficile* and *E. Coli 0157:H7* produce a cytotoxin. Enteroadherence is observed with *Cryptosporidium* and *Giardia.* Mucosal invasion is a feature of infection with viruses, e.g. *rolavirus* and *Campylobacter sp.,* *Salmonella, Shigella* and *Entamoeba histolytica.* Systemic infections that can cause diarrhoea include viral hepatitis, Legionnaire's disease, measles and toxic shock syndrome.

19. The clinical features more common in ulcerative colitis include rectal bleeding, toxic megacolon, and malignancy with long-standing disease. In Crohn's disease, palpable abdominal masses, strictures, small bowel involvement, and fistulas are more likely. The barium enema in ulcerative colitis shows: loss of the normal haustral pattern, the bowel is smooth like a 'hose pipe'. Ulcers and pseudo-polyps may be seen, and oedema of the colonic wall produces widening of the presacral space. In Crohn's disease it may show skip lesions, a coarse cobblestone appearance of the mucosa, and fibrosis producing narrowing of the intestine—'string sign'—with proximal dilatation. Biopsy of the affected mucosa via sigmoldoscopy or colonoscopy is usually the best way of distinguishing between the two. Transmural segmental involvement, with granulomas, fibrosis, fistulas, and mesenteric fat and lymph node involvement, supports Crohn's

disease. In ulcerative colitis there is continuous mucosal inflammation with neutrophillic infiltration and epithelial damage resulting in multiple ulcerations. Infiltration of the crypts by neutrophills leads to crypt microabcesses, loss of goblet cells, and submucosal aedema.

20. Diabetes mellitus may affect the eye in many ways. When examining the eye in a diabetic patient one should examine the visual acuity, which may be impaired. The iris may show rubeosis, a cataract may be present, and the retinal changes include background retinopathy (dot and blot haemorrhages, hard exudates, colton wool spots), proliferative retinopathy (new vessel formation, scars, vitreal haemorrhages, retinal detachments), macular oedema, and the laser coagulation burns of previous therapy.

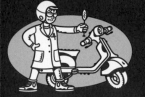

EMQ Answers

EMQ answers 1.1–1.5
(1.1) D: The ECG changes indicate anteroseptal ischaemia.
(1.2) J.
(1.3) B.
(1.4) G: Not all chest pain and ECG changes are cardiac in origin. Remember to look for underlying causes of pulmonary embolism.
(1.5) I: This is of autosomal dominant inheritance.

EMQ answers 2.1–2.5
(2.1) C.
(2.2) H: The presence of a varicocele indicates possible tumour spread to the left renal vein. Remember the venous drainage of the left testicle.
(2.3) I: The presence of upper airway symptoms and signs implies this is Wegener's rather than other 'pulmonary–renal' syndromes.
(2.4) F.
(2.5) E: The back pain is worrying as it may indicate the presence of bony metastases.

EMQ answers 3.1–3.5
(3.1) H.
(3.2) C: Cardiac failure is not the only cause of orthopnoea. Cardiac surgery, internal jugular catheterisation and prolonged ICU admission are all associated with phrenic nerve dysfunction.
(3.3) D: Not all crackles heard on ausculatation are caused by cardiac failure.
(3.4) G.
(3.5) A.

EMQ answers 4.1–4.5
(4.1) H: The elevated total protein is due to the excess immunoglobulin produced. Plasma cells maybe seen on the peripheral blood film.
(4.2) E.
(4.3) A: B_{12} deficiency may be found with other autoimmune diseases. Schilling tests are rarely carried out now.
(4.4) G.
(4.5) F: Eosinophilia – 'Hodgkins, histamine or helminths' (The three 'H's).

EMQ answers 5.1–5.5
(5.1) G.
(5.2) H: The recurrent miscarriages indicate the antiphospholipid syndrome may also be present.
(5.3) B: Compare the pattern of symptoms of osteoarthritis versus inflammatory arthritis.
(5.4) C.
(5.5) F: If severe, the respiratory muscles may be involved.

EMQ answers 6.1–6.5
(6.1) E: Stridor is an inspiratory noise resulting from tracheal compression. A thyroid goitre may displace the trachea but as it is in the midline this may be either to the left or right.
(6.2) C: The trachea is pushed away by the increasing pressure in the right hemithorax.
(6.3) D: Scarred fibrotic tissue pulls the trachea towards itself.
(6.4) B: Airflow obstruction during expiration causes a polyphonic expiratory wheeze.
(6.5) J: The fluid causes a stony dull percussion note and reduced air entry. Expansion may also be reduced.

EMQ answers 7.1–7.5
(7.1) F: This is a common place to put a transplanted kidney. His Cushing's syndrome can be explained by steroid therapy to prevent organ rejection.
(7.2) J: Elderly men may have bladder outflow obstruction due to enlarged prostate glands. These may cause urinary retention with overflow incontinence, for example, post-operatively.
(7.3) H: She has polycystic kidneys. These are associated with an increased risk of subarachnoid haemorrhage.
(7.4) E: Divarification of the recti is accentuated by sitting up.
(7.5) B: She has ascites due to decompensated alcoholic liver disease. The decompensation causes encephalopathy and may be precipitated by an alcohol binge.

EMQ answers 8.1–8.5
(8.1) A: This must be treated as suspected meningitis.
(8.2) J: He has a bronchial carcinoma with cerebral metastases.
(8.3) F: Clusters last 4–12 weeks and are followed by pain free periods of months.
(8.4) H: Prompt therapy with steroids is required to avoid permanent damage to her vision. A temporal artery biopsy may confirm the diagnosis, but may be falsely negative due to 'skip lesions'.
(8.5) C: This man has adult polycystic kidney disease and has had a subarachnoid haemorrhage. There is an increased incidence of subarachnoid haemorrhage in polycystic kidney disease.

EMQ answers 9.1–9.5

(9.1) A: The sudden onset suggests a vascular cause. Loss of consciousness is rare in strokes unless the brainstem is affected.

(9.2) J: The sudden onset again suggests a vascular cause and in this context the sub-hyaloid haemorrhages are pathognomonic of subarachnoid haemorrhage.

(9.3) B: The most likely explanation is an opiate overdose. This could be assessed by giving the patient naloxone (an opiate antagonist).

(9.4) G: This must be treated as meningitis until proven otherwise.

(9.5) E: Diuretic therapy is a common cause of hyponatraemia which in turn can cause an altered mental state and seizures.

EMQ answers 10.1–10.5

(10.1) D: The suspected diagnosis is acromegaly. A useful screening test is IGF-1 levels. An isolated measurement of growth hormone level is not useful.

(10.2) F: Investigations directed at finding an endocrine cause for suspected hypoglycaemic episodes are usually negative. However, the only way to exclude an insulinoma is to conduct a prolonged fast and measure serum glucose and C-peptide levels if symptoms occur.

(10.3) H: Autoimmune Addison's disease is suspected. Administration of an exogenous adrenocorticotropin hormone (Synacthen) will fail to produce an increase in serum cortisol.

(10.4) J: His cranial diabetes insipidus will be demonstrated by a failure to concentrate the urine during a water deprivation test as the serum osmolality rises. If desmopressin is administered the urine will concentrate within an hour as the renal tubules remain responsive to antidiuretic hormone.

(10.5) B: Cushing's syndrome is suspected and will be confirmed if the admistration of exogenous steroids fails to suppress adrenal steroid synthesis.

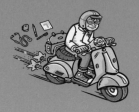

Index

A

α_1-antitrypsin deficiency 198
5-aminosalicylic acid (5-ASA) 230, 231
5-HT antagonists 266
6-mercaptopurine 231
10-point abbreviated mental test score 114, **115**
12-lead ECG 409–12
  axis 411
  different views of the heart **410**
  P wave 411
  for palpitations 18
  position of the anterior electrodes **410**
  PR interval 411
  QRS complex 411
  QT interval 412
  rate 409–10
  rhythm 410–11
  ST segment 411–12
  T wave 412
  U wave 412
^{14}C trioleate breath test 47
24-hour ambulatory blood pressure
    measurement 83
24-hour collection of urine 78, 80
24-hour ECG 18, 124, 187, 412
24-hour Holter monitoring 169
24-hour intraluminal pH monitoring 38, 221
24-hour urinary catecholamine and metanephrine
    excretion 83
24-hour urinary protein excretion and creatinine
    clearance 245, 250
30 point MMSE (mini-mental state
    examination) 114
α-blockers 183
α-interferon 344
α-thalassaemia 339
AA amyloid **127**
AAFB (acid alcohol-fast bacilli) 202
'AB/CD rule' 182
abbreviated mental test score 114, **115**
abdominal aortic aneurysm **418**
abdominal CT scan 80
abdominal distension 66
abdominal examination 390–3
  for polyuria and polydipsia 72
abdominal pain 57, 63–7
  differential diagnosis **64**

  examining the patient 65–6
  history in the patient 63, 65
  investigating the patient 66–7
  as a symptom of gastrointestinal disease 373
abdominal swelling, causes 391
abdominal ultrasound
  for abdominal pain 66
  for change in bowel habit 47
  for dyspepsia 38
  for jaundice 59
  for lymphadenopathy and splenomegaly 128
abdominal X-ray
  for abdominal pain 66
  for acute colitis 230
  for acute pancreatitis 237
  for change in bowel habit 46
  for gastrointestinal disease 417
  for haematuria and proteinuria 80
  for UTIs 253
abducens (sixth cranial nerve) 395–6
above knee DVT 352
ABPA (allergic bronchopulmonary aspergillosis)
    214–15
absence attacks 275
ABVD (doxorubicin, bleomycin, vincristine and
    daunorubicin) 347
acanthus nigricans 330
acarbose 287
accelerated hypertension 183
accessory (eleventh cranial nerve) 398
accessory nerve palsies, causes **398**
ACE inhibitors
  and coughs 30
  and renal failure 251, 252, 324
  and treatment of acute MI 166
    secondary prevention 169
  and treatment of chronic cardiac
    failure 177
  and treatment of hypertension 182–3
  and treatment of IgA nephropathy 247
  and treatment of NSTEMI 162
  and treatment of stroke patients 263
acetazolamide 268
aciclovir 279
  see also intravenous aciclovir
acid alcohol-fast bacilli (AAFB) 202
acid reflux 37, 38, 221

acidosis 167
  see also systemic acidosis
acitretin 327
acne rosacea 100
acne vulgaris 100, 328
acoustic neuroma **146**
acquired cranial diabetes insipidus 304
acquired ichthyosis 330
acquired nephrogenic diabetes insipidus 305
acromegalic gigantism 302
acromegaly 302–3
ACTH 301
  and pigmentation 380
  and the treatment of multiple sclerosis 272
  see also ectopic ACTH syndrome; plasma ACTH
ACTH-secreting tumours 301
actinic keratoses 99
action tremor in the hands 384
activated partial thromboplastin time 143
activated protein C 350
acute bacterial meningitis 272
acute cholecystitis 236
acute colitis 230
acute coronary syndromes 161
  see also acute MI; NSTEMI; unstable angina
acute diverticulitis 233
acute gastritis 222
acute GI obstruction 45
acute gout 95, 299–300
acute haemofiltration 179
acute headache 87, 265
  differential diagnosis **88**
acute heart failure 177, 179, 185
acute ischaemia of the bowel 234
acute leukaemias 341
acute lymphoblastic leukaemia (ALL) 341–2
acute MI 161, 162–9
  adverse risk factors 163
  changes induced by **163**
  complications 166–8
    subsequent inpatient management 168
  diagnosis 163–4
  management 164–6
    emergency care 164
  rehabilitation 168
  secondary prevention 168–9
acute myasthenia 131
acute myeloid leukaemia (AML) 342–3
acute myocardial infarction with ST elevation
    (STEMI) 161
acute nephritis 246

acute neurological deficit 119–24
acute non-lymphocytic leukaemia 342–3
acute pancreatitis 237–8
  radiological abdominal abnormalities **418**
acute postinfective polyneuropathy 279
acute pyelonephritis 253
  management 254
acute renal failure see ARF
acute respiratory distress syndrome (ARDS)
    211, 218
acute respiratory failure, prognosis 211
acute respiratory infections and COPD 199
acute rheumatic fever 189–90
acute thrombolysis 123
acute urethral syndromes 253
acute viral hepatitis 238–40
  clinical features 240
  investigations 240
  management 240
acute-contact allergic dermatitis 100
Addison's disease 47, 53, 311–13
adenocarcinomas 204, 222, 225
adenomatous polyps 232
adenosine 173
  see also intravenous adenosine
adrenal glands, disorders 310–13
adrenal insufficiency, symptoms 51, **312**
adrenocortical tumours 310
adrenocorticotrophic hormone see ACTH
adriamycin 345
adult polycystic kidney disease 254
adult TB 202
afferent pupillary defect 394
AFP (alpha fetoprotein) **428**
age
  and hypertension 183
  and IHD 157
AIDS
  defining illnesses **357**
  diagnosis 356
air pollution and COPD 198–9
airways obstruction
  radiological findings **414**
  see also asthma; chronic bronchitis;
      emphysema
alanine aminotransferase (ALT) 240, 417
albumin 46
alcohol 222
  effect on lymphadenopathy 128
  relationship between blood pressure and 180
  units of **371**

alcohol withdrawal 114
alcoholic hepatitis 243–4
alcoholic liver disease 243–4
aldosterone 178, 313
alfacalcidol 297, 299
alkaline phosphatase 425
ALL (acute lymphoblastic leukaemia) 341–2
allergic asthma 195
allergic bronchopulmonary aspergillosis
        (ABPA) 214–15
allergic contact dermatitis 327–8
    see also acute-contact allergic dermatitis
allergies, recording 371
allogeneic bone marrow transplantation 344, 345
allopurinol 252, 300
alopecia **103**
alpha fetoprotein (AFP) **428**
Alport's syndrome 245
ALT (alanine aminotransferase) 240, 417
alteplase 164–5
amantadine 270
amiloride 241
amine precursor: uptake and decarboxylation
        (APUD) cells 227
aminosalicylates 230
amiodarone 167, 170, 171, 173, 174, 179, 187
amitriptylline 267
AML (acute myeloid leukaemia) 342–3
amlodipine 160
amoxicillin 253
amphotericin 215
ampullary carcinoma 237
amyloidosis 187
amyotrophic lateral sclerosis 278
anaemia 141, 149–54, 333–40, 385
    correcting 333
    differential diagnosis 149–50
    examining the patient 150–1
    general approach to management 333–4
    history in the patient 150
    investigating the patient 152–4
    in RA 95, 333
    in renal failure 252
anaemia of chronic disease 334–5
    causes **149**
    changes on blood film **152**
    interpretation of iron storage results **153**
    investigations 154
anakinra 317
anal carcinoma **358**
analgesic rebound headache 89, 267

anaplastic carcinoma 204, 310
anatomical lesions, symptoms and signs **134–5**
ANCA 246
ANCA positive vasculitis 246
angina 3, **166**
    see also stable angina
angiodysplasia 153
angiography 162, 168, 234, 264, 326
    see also carotid angiography; cerebral
        angiography; coronary angiography; left
        ventricular angiography; magnetic
        resonance angiography; mesenteric
        angiography; pulmonary angiography
angioplasty 5, 7, 192
    for NSTEMI 162
    see also primary angioplasty
angioplasty and stenting 161
angiotensin II receptor blockers (ARB) 178,
        183, 251
angiotensin-converting enzyme inhibitors see
        ACE inhibitors
anion-exchange resins 291
ankle swelling 372
ankylosing spondylitis 10, 95, 97, 319
Ann Arbor staging of malignant lymphomas **347**
anorexia 371
anosmia 375, 393–4
ANP (atrial natriuretic peptide) release **70**
antacids 221, 223, 324
anti-arrhythmic drugs 173–4
anti-DNase 246
anti-dsDNA 246
anti-endomysial antibodies 226
anti-GBM (antiglomerular basement membrane)
        antibodies 246
anti-retroviral therapy (HAART) 358
anti-secretory therapy 223, 235
antiandrogens 255, 328
antibiotics 227, 230, 231
    and pseudomembranous colitis 234
    and treatment of acne vulgaris 328
    and treatment of meningitis 273
    and treatment of UTIs 253–4
    see also prophylactic antibiotics
anticholinergics 197, 201, 270, 272
    and gastric emptying 364
anticholinesterase 280
anticoagulation 184, 185, 247
    and treatment of stroke patients 263
anticonvulsants 322
antidotes for drug overdose 365

antidouble-stranded DNA antibodies 97
antiemetics 266
antiepileptic drugs 276–7
  changing 276–7
  withdrawing 277
antifibrotic agents 243
antiglomerular basement membrane (anti-GBM)
      antibodies 246
antiglomerular basement membrane disease 246
antihistamines 328
antimalarial drugs 317
antimotility drugs 235
antineutrophil cytoplasmic antibodies see ANCA
antinuclear antibodies 97, 246, 322, 324
antiphospholipid syndrome 322
antiplatelet drugs 160
antiplatelet treatment 169
antireticulin antibodies 226
antispasmodic drugs 233, 235
antistreptolysin O titre 246
antithyroid drugs 308
anxiety 1, 16
aorta, coarctation of 191–2
aortic pain 63
aortic regurgitation 22, 25–6, 186
aortic stenosis 24–5, 185–6, 192
aortography 192
apex beat 386
aplastic sickle cell anaemia crisis 337
apomorphine 270
appetite 371
APUD (amine precursor: uptake and
      decarboxylation) cells 227
ARB (angiotensin II receptor blockers) 178,
      183, 251
ARDS (acute respiratory distress syndrome) 218
ARF **70**, 247–50
  aetiology 247–8
  clinical features 248
  investigations 248–9
  management 249
  prognosis 250
Argyll Robertson pupil 394
arms and examination of the abdomen 390
arrhythmias 5, 15, 105, 169–74, 179
  causes 169
  clinical features 169
  investigations 169
arrhythmias and conduction disorders 167
arterial blood gases 109, 115, 209, 237, 416
  assessment for chest pain 7
  assessment for dyspnoea 12

arterial bruits 392
arterial oxygen saturation 12, 416
arthralgia 93
arthritis 189–90, 315
    see also chronic arthritis; OA; psoriatic arthritis;
        RA; septic arthritis; spondyloarthropathies
arthroscopy 97
artificial hearts 179
ascites 66, 240–1, 417
  causes **392**
ASD (atrial septal defect) 191
aspartate aminotransferase (AST) 163, 240,
      409, 417
aspartate transaminase 4
aspergillus clavatus 215
aspergillus fumigatus 215
aspiration 212
    see also joint aspiration
aspiration pneumonia 209
  drug choice **210**
aspirin
  management of overdose **366**
  and treatment of acute MI 165
    secondary prevention 169
  and treatment of acute rheumatic fever 190
  and treatment of atrial fibrillation 170
  and treatment of IHD 160
  and treatment of NSTEMI 162
  and treatment of pericarditis 168
  and treatment of stroke patients 262
  and treatment of transient ischaemic attacks
      (TIAs) 263
AST (aspartate aminotransferase) 163, 240,
      409, 417
asterixis 383, 387, 390
asthma 37, 195–8
  aetiology 195
  clinical features 196
    to differentiate COPD from **200**
  diagnosis 196
  differential diagnosis 196
  incidence 195
  management 196–8, **199**, 217
    chronic therapy 197
    emergency treatment 197–8, **199**
  pathophysiology 195–6
  radiological findings **414**
asymptomatic bacteriuria 253
asymptomatic phase of HIV 356
  investigation **358**
atenolol 160, 162
atherosclerosis 158–9

atopic eczema 327
  management 328
atovaquone 360
atrial fibrillation 167, 169–70, 388
  causes 169
  treatment 170
  see also fast atrial fibrillation
atrial flutter 170
atrial myxoma 190
atrial septal defect (ASD) 191
atrioventricular (AV) block 167
atrophy **103**
atropine 167, 172
atypical facial pain 267
atypical naevus 99
atypical pneumonia 209
  drug choice **210**
audiometry 147
auditory evoked potentials 137
aural symptoms of vertigo 146
auriculotemporal neuralgia 267
auscultation
  of the abdomen 392
  and the cardiovascular system 387
  and examining the patient with
      breathlessness 12
  and the respiratory system 390
Auspitz's sign 327
autoantibodies
  and investigating pericarditis 187
  and sensory and/or motor neurological
      deficits 136
  and stroke patients 124
autoantibody screens for lymphadenopathy and
      splenomegaly 128
autoimmune gastritis 222
autoimmune (Hashimoto's thyroiditis) 305
autoimmune screen 262
automatism 275
autonomic neuropathies 286
AV (atrioventricular) block 167
azathioprine 230, 231, 232, 252, 280, 320, 322,
      323, 325, 330
azelaic acid 328

B
B cell lymphonas 348
B symptoms 126, **346**
β-blockers 184
  management of overdose **366**
  and treatment of acute MI 165–6
    secondary prevention 169

and treatment of atrial fibrillation 170
and treatment of chronic cardiac failure
    177–8
and treatment of hypertension 182
    in pregnancy 183
and treatment of hypertrophic
    cardiomyopathy 187
and treatment of IHD 160
and treatment of migraine 267
and treatment of multiple sclerosis 272
and treatment of NSTEMI 162
and treatment of supraventricular and
    ventricular arrhythmias 173
see also intravenous β-blockers; non-
    cardioselective β-blockers; non-selective
    β-blockers
β-interferon 272
β-thalassaemia 339, **340**
Bacillus Calmette-Guérin (BCG) vaccination 204
baclofen 267, 272
bacterial endocarditis **127**
bacterial overgrowth 226–7
bacteriology and PUO 35–6
balloon valvuloplasty 185
balsalazide 230
'bamboo spine' 97, 319
Bamford classification of stroke 122, 261, **262**
barium enemas 47, 153, 229–30, 233, 234,
    235, 418
barium imaging 231
barium meals 32, 38, 43, 153, 222, 418
barium swallow 222, 418
barrel chest 10, 388
Barrett's oesophagus 221, 222
basal cell carcinoma 100, 331
base excess 416
basophils **426**
BCG (Bacillus Calmette-Guérin) vaccination 204
Beau's lines 382
Beck's triad 188
Behçet's disease 330
Bell's palsy 279
below knee DVT 352
Bence-Jones protein 345
benign intracranial hypertension 87, 265
benign MS 272
benign positional vertigo **146**
benign proteinuria 75
benzhexol 270
benzodiazepines 276
  management of overdose **366**
benzoyl peroxide 328

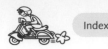

benzylpenicillin 189, 273
Berger's disease 246–7
berry aneurysms 191, 264
bicarbonate concentration 416
biguanides 287
bilateral adrenalectomy 310
bilateral palpable kidneys, causes **392**
bile salt absorption 47
bile salts 243
bilirubin 153, 240, 417
bilirubin metabolism, normal **58**
biopsy
    for sensory and/or motor neurological
        deficits 137
    see also duodenal biopsy; liver biopsy; lung
        biopsy; muscle biopsy; pleural biopsy; renal
        biopsy; temporal artery biopsy
bisoprolol 160, 178
bisphosphonates 294, 295, 296
    see also intravenous bisphosphonate therapy
biventricular pacemakers 178–9
blackouts 105, **106**
    diagnosis in the patient **111**
    examining patients with 108
bladder, and the differential diagnosis of
        haematuria 75
Blalock shunt 192
bleeding and bruising 139–43
    differential diagnosis 139–40
    examining the patient 140–1
    history in the patient 140
    investigating the patient 141–3
    see also GI bleeding; rectal bleeding
bleeding disorders 349–50
bleeding time 143
blind loop syndrome 223
blindness
    and DM 284
    see also vision
blisters **103**, 390
blood cultures for stroke patients 124
blood films 427
    abnormalities in anaemia **152**
    abnormalities in conditions presenting with
        lymphadenopathy and splenomegaly **130**
    for bleeding and bruising 141
blood glucose
    control 166
    see also fasting glucose
blood glucose investigations 288
    for abdominal pain 66

for change in bowel habit 46
    for dyspnoea 12
    for hypertension 83
    for stroke patients 124, 261
    for weight loss 54
blood lipids, and IHD 158
blood pressure
    and examination of the cardiovascular
        system 384
    and examination of the respiratory system 388
    and examining the patient with abdominal
        pain 65
    measurement 83, 179–80
    see also hypertension; hypotension
blood sugar tests 109
blood and systemic lupus erythematosus
    (SLE) 321
blood tests
    for chest pain 4–5
    for the confused patient 115
    for haematuria and proteinuria 80
    for palpitations 18
    for skin diseases 102
blood transfusion 333–4, 335, 337, 338, 339
    complications **334**
blue naevus 99
body habitus, examining 381
boils 101, 286
bone densitometry 294
bone disease
    pattern of biochemical abnormalities **425**
    see also metabolic bone disease; renal
        osteodystrophy
bone marrow aspirate
    for anaemia 152
    for bleeding and bruising 141
    for multiple myeloma 345
bone marrow examination 128, 152, 346–7, 427
bone marrow failure, features **342**
bone marrow transplantation 339, 341,
    343, 348
    see also allogeneic bone marrow
        transplantation
bone marrow trephine 152
bone pain, causes **377**
bone scan 297
Bouchard's nodes 95, 318, 383
Boutonnière deformity 94, **315**
bowel, preventing absorption 364–5
bowel habit, change in 45–9, 63, 373
    differential diagnosis 45

bowel habit, change in (*Continued*)
  examining the patient **48**
    history in the patient 45
    investigating the patient 45–9
bowel sounds 66, 392
Bowen's disease 99
brachial and carotid artery 384–5
bradycardia 17, 109
    rhythm of 12-lead ECG 410–11
    see also sinus bradycardia
bradykinesia 268
brain (B-type) natriuretic peptide 177
brain tumours 265
    origins **277**
breast examination 380
breath, shortness of *see* dyspnoea
Breslow thickness 331
bretylium 174
British National Formulary 158
bromocriptine 241, 270, 302, 303, 304
bronchial breathing 12
bronchiectasis 215, **389**
    radiological findings **414**
Bronchoalveolar cell carcinoma 204, 205
Bronchoalveolar lavage 417
bronchodilators 200–1
bronchoscopy 12, 417
    see also fibre-optic bronchoscopy
bronchospasm **389**
'Bronze Diabetes' 241
Brudzinski's sign 89
bruising
    of the abdomen 391
    see also bleeding and bruising
Budd-Chiari syndrome 351
budesonide 201, 231
bulbar palsy 278
bullae **103**, 390
bullectomy 201
bullous lesions 100
bullous pemphigoid 100
bumetanide 178
Burton's line 335

C
C-reactive protein *see* CRP
CA 19–9 **428**
CA 125 **428**
CA 153 **428**
CABG (coronary artery bypass graft) surgery 161
cachexia 65, 127

café-au-lait spots 330, 380
calcipotriol 327
calcitonin 295, 296, 298
calcitonin secretion 309
calcitriol 297, 299
calcium channel blockers
    and secondary prevention of acute MI 169
    and treatment of hypertension 182
    and treatment of IHD 160–1
calcium homeostasis **423**
calcium metabolism 422–5
calcium profiles 54
calculi **418**
calf swelling 4, 372
caloric tests 147
Candida **360**
candidiasis 100
CAPD (continuous ambulatory peritoneal
    dialysis) 252
capsaicin 329
captopril 177
'captopril renogram' 420
carbamazepine 267, 272, 276, 329
carbimazole 308
carbon tagged breath tests 38
carcinoembryonic antigen (CEA) **428**
carcinoid syndrome 47, 227–8
carcinoid tumours 227
carcinoma of the pancreas 236–7
carcinomatous meningitis 87
cardiac catheterisation 413
    for aortic regurgitation 26
    for aortic stenosis 25
    for atrial septal defect (ASD) 191
    for Fallot's tetralogy 192
    for heart failure 177
    for hypertrophic cardiomyopathy 187
    for mitral stenosis 23
    for patent ductus arteriosus (PDA) 191
    for ventricular septal defect (VSD) 190
cardiac enzymes 5, 176, 409
    and the diagnosis of acute MI 163–4
    elevation post MI **409**
cardiac failure **166**
    evidence 387
cardiac failure and shock 166–7
cardiac ischaemic pain 3
cardiac rehabilitation 178
cardiac rupture **166**, 167
cardiac syncope 107
cardiac transplantation 178, 187

cardiac valves, positions of auscultation 387
cardiogenic heart failure 176
cardiogenic shock 166–7
cardiogenic syncope **106**
cardiomegaly 192
'cardiomemo' 18
cardiomyopathy 186–7
  causes **186**
cardiorespiratory examination 66
cardiovascular disease
    and CRF 252
    and the use of statins 291–3
cardiovascular disease risk prediction charts
        291–4
cardiovascular symptoms 372–3
cardiovascular system 157–93
    examination 384–7
    investigations 409–14
    and systemic lupus erythematosus (SLE) 321
    and systemic sclerosis 324
cardioversion 184
carditis 189
carotenaemia 380
carotid angiography 124
carotid artery
    brachial and 384–5
    dissection of 87
carotid bruits 171
carotid doppler ultrasound 124
carotid dopplers 109
carotid duplex scan 262
carotid endarterectomy 263
carotid pulsation, differences between JVP
        and **385**
carotid sinus hypersensitivity 105, 109
carotid sinus massage 109, 167, 171
carvedilol 162, 178
cataract formation 285
catechol-O-methyltransferase (COMT)
        inhibitors 270
CCF (congestive cardiac failure) 176
CD4+ cell counts 356, 358
CEA (carcinoembryonic antigen) **428**
cefotaxime 330
cellulitis 100
central abdomen, causes of pain in **64**
central chest pain 3
central cyanosis 10, 379, 385, 388
central lesions **146**
central nervous system 261–82
    and systemic lupus erythematosus (SLE) 321
central sleep apnoea 216

centriacinar emphysema 198
cephalosporins 254
    see also third generation cephalosporin
cerebellar disease 399
cerebellar signs in multiple sclerosis 271
cerebral abscess 87, 119
cerebral angiography 90
cerebral haemorrhage 261
cerebral infarction 119, 261
cerebral lymphoma **358**
cerebral tumours 87, 277
cerebrospinal fluid examination see CSF
        examination
cerebrovascular disease 261–5
cervical carcinoma **358**
cervical lymphadenopathy 127
CF (cystic fibrosis) 213–14
Charcot-Marie-Tooth disease 400
chemoprophylaxis 361
chemotherapy 207, 222, 233, 255, 345, 347,
        348, 358
    for acute lymphoblastic leukaemia (ALL) 341
    see also cytotoxic chemotherapy;
        photochemotherapy; preventative
        chemotherapy
chest
    expansion 388
    inspection 388
chest pain 3–7, 161
    as a cardiovascular symptom 372
    differential diagnosis 3
    and dyspepsia 37
    examining the patient 4, **5**
    history in the patient 3–4
    investigating the patient 4–7
    as a respiratory symptom 373
chest radiography see CXR
chest wall tenderness 3
chest X-ray see CXR
Cheyne-Stokes respiration 11
Chlamydia pneumoniae 159
chlorambucil 322, 343, 348
chloramphenicol 227
chloroquine 317, 360, 361
chlorpheniramine 252
chlorpromazine 322
chlorpropamide 287
cholangitis 236
cholecystectomy 236
cholestasis screen 60
cholesterol 290
cholesterol stones 235

cholestyramine 231, 240, 243, 291
chondrocalcinosis in the joints 241, 242
chondroitin 318
CHOP (cyclophosphamide, doxorubicin,
　　vincristine and prednisolone) 348
Christmas disease 349
chronic arthritis 94
chronic asthma 197
　stepped-care plan for the management **197**
chronic bronchitis 198
　aetiology 198–9
　pathophysiology 198
　radiological findings **414**
chronic cardiac failure 177–9
　drug treatment 177–8
　non drug treatment 178–9
chronic cholecystitis 236
chronic encephalopathy 241
chronic fibrotic lung disease **213**
chronic gastritis 222
chronic headache/facial pain **88**, 89, 267–8
chronic hepatitis 240–1
chronic hyponatraemia 256
chronic intestinal ischaemia 234
chronic leukaemias 341
chronic liver disease 58, 115, 240–4
　management 240
chronic lymphocytic leukaemia (CLL) 343–4
chronic myeloid leukaemia (CML) 344
chronic obstructive pulmonary disease *see* COPD
chronic pancreatitis 225, 238
　radiological abdominal abnormalities **418**
chronic plaque psoriasis 327
chronic pyelonephritis 253
chronic renal failure *see* CRF
chronic stable angina 3, 160, 161
chronic tophaceous gout 95, 300
Chvostek's sign 299
chylomicrons 290
cigarette smoking *see* smoking
ciprofloxacin 203
cirrhosis 243–4
CJD (Creutzfeldt-Jakob disease) 114, 115
CK 97, 136, 163, 409
　and the diagnosis of acute MI 163
CK-MB 409
clarithromycin 203
'clasp-knife' phenomenon 399
claudication 372–3
　see also jaw claudication
clerking 405–8
click 390

clindamycin 234, 328
CLL (chronic lymphocytic leukaemia) 343–4
clonazepam 267
clonus 402
clopidogrel 160, 162, 165
Clostridium difficile 234
　culture and detection 46
clotting pathway, modulation 350
clotting screen
　for patients with haematemesis and melaena 43
　for stroke patients 124, 261
clotting tests **143**
clubbing 382, 384
　and abdominal pain 65, 390
　causes **384**
　and jaundice 65
　and patients with weight loss 52
　respiratory causes 10, 387
cluster headache 88–9, 267
CML (chronic myeloid leukaemia) 344
co-amoxiclav 254
coagulation assessment 427
coagulation pathway **141**
coagulopathies 139
　effect 140
coal tar 327, 328
coarctation of the aorta 191–2
coarse crackles 390
cocaine use 5
Cockcroft-Gault equation 251, 419
codeine phosphate 231
coeliac disease 46, 153, 225–6
　skin manifestations 330
'cogwheel' rigidity 268, 399
'coin' lesion, causes on a CXR 196
colchicine 243, 300, 330
colectomy 231
colectomy with ileorectal anastamosis 232
　see also subtotal colectomy with ileorectal
　　anastamosis
colestipol 291
colicky pain 63, 77
collapse and commom respiratory diseases 389
'collapse?cause' patients 105
collapsing pulse, causes **385**
colonic adenocarcinoma 232
colonic carcinomas 228, 232
colonic Crohn's disease 231
colonic polyps 232
colonic transit study 47
colonoscopy 47, 153, 231, 233, 234, **419**
　see also CT colonoscopy

colorectal carcinoma, modified Duke's classification **233**
colorectal disease 232–4
colorectal neoplasia 232–3
coma 105, **106**
  diagnosis in the patient **110**
  examining the patient 107–8
  see also diabetic coma; myxoedema coma
common investigations *see* investigations
'common migraine' 266
community acquired pneumonia 208–9
complete heart block *see* third degree heart block
complex partial seizures **106**, 275
computed tomography *see* CT
COMT (catechol-O-methyltransferase) inhibitors 270
confusional states 113–17
  differential diagnosis 113
  examining the patient 114–15
  history in the patient 113–14
  investigating the patient 115–17
congenital heart disease 21, 190–2
congenital hypothyroidism 305
congestive cardiac failure (CCF) 176
conjugate gaze, assessment 395
Conn's syndrome 313
consciousness, loss of *see* loss of consciousness
consolidation **389**
constipation 45, 63, 65
  causes **47**
constrictive pericarditis 188
contact dermatitis 327–8
continuous ambulatory peritoneal dialysis (CAPD) 252
continuous murmurs 21
Coombs' test 154
coordination
  in the lower limbs 402
  in the upper limbs 399
COPD 198–201
  acute exacerbation 201
  clinical features 200
  definitions 198
  investigations 200
  long term treatment 200–1
  management 200
  pathophysiology 198
  prognosis 201
coronary angiography 7, 159
coronary arteriography 187
coronary artery bypass graft (CABG) surgery 161
coronary artery disease, major risk factors **157**

coronary artery stenting 7, 161
Corrigan's sign 25, 385
corticosteroids
  for minimal change nephropathy 247
  and treatment of allergic bronchopulmonary aspergillosis 215
  and treatment of carditis 190
  and treatment of COPD 201
  and treatment of Crohn's disease 231
  and treatment of eczema 328
  and treatment of herpes (varicella) zoster 329
  and treatment of multiple sclerosis 272
  and treatment of OA 318
  and treatment of polymyalgia rheumatica (PMR) 323
  and treatment of psoriasis 327
  and treatment of RA 317
cortisol 310
cortisol deficiency, tests for 422
cortisol excess, tests for 421–2
cough 4, 9, 29–32
  breathlessness associated with 9
  differential diagnosis 29
  examining the patient 30–1
  history in the patient 29–30
  important details for diagnosis **30**
  investigating the patient 32
  as a respiratory symptom 373
Courvoisier's law 235
COX-1 (cyclo-oxygenase 1) inhibitors 317
COX-2 (cyclo-oxygenase 2) antagonists 223
COX-2 (cyclo-oxygenase 2) inhibitors 317
crackles 12, 390
cranial arteritis 265–6
cranial diabetes insipidus **70**, 304
  treatment 305
cranial nerves 393–8
cranial root 398
creatine kinase *see* CK
creatinine 248, 251, 419
crepitations 12
'crescendo TIAs' 263
crescentic GN 247
CREST syndrome 324
Creutzfeldt-Jakob disease (CJD) 114, 115
CRF **70**, 250–2
  aetiology 250
  clinical features 250
  investigations 250–1
  management 251
  prevention of complications 252

Crohn's disease 228, **229**, 231–2, 391
  skin manifestations 330
croup **30**
CRP 35, 427
  effects of elevated 158
  in joint disease 96
  in lymphadenopathy and splenomegaly 128
  in pneumonia 209
  in stroke patients 124
  see also serum CRP
crust **103**
cryoprecipitate 350
cryotherapy 358
cryptococcal meningitis **360**
crystal arthropathy 299–300
CSF changes in meningitis **274**
CSF examination
  for confusional states 117
  for encephalitis 274
  for Guillain-Barré syndrome 279
  for headache/facial pain 90
  for multiple sclerosis 271
  for sensory and/or motor neurological deficits **137**
CT brain scan 124
CT colonoscopy 418
CT head scan
  for lung cancer 207
  for patients with loss of consciousness 109
  for stroke patients 124
CT pulmonary angiography 7
  see also spiral CT pulmonary angiography
CT scanning 253, 416–17
  for breathlessness 12
  for carcinoma of the pancreas 237
  for change in bowel habit 47
  for chest pain 7
  for chronic pancreatitis 238
  for colorectal neoplasia 233
  for confusional states 115, 117
  for dyspnoea 12
  for epilepsy 275–6
  for gastric carcinoma 225
  for gastrointestinal disease 418
  for haematemesis and melaena 43
  for headache/facial pain 90, 265
  for jaundice 60
  for joint disease 97
  for lung cancer 206, 207
  for lymphadenopathy and splenomegaly 128
  for meningitis 273
  for oesophageal cancer 222

for polyuria and polydipsia 73
for sensory and/or motor neurological deficits 136
for stroke patients 261–2
for subarachnoid haemorrhage 264
for subdural haematoma 264, 265
for the urinary system 420
for UTIs 253
for vertigo 148
  see also abdominal CT scan
Cullen's sign 65, 237
culture-negative endocarditis 189
cushingoid appearance 141
Cushing's syndrome 310–11, 420–1
CXR
  for acute MI 164
  for acute pancreatitis 237
  for aortic regurgitation 26
  for aortic stenosis 25
  for atrial septal defect (ASD) 191
  for bronchiectasis 215
  causes of a 'coin' lesion 196
  for chest pain 7
  for confusional states 115
  for cough and haemoptysis 32
  features of pulmonary oedema **414**
  for glomerular disease 246
  for heart failure 176
  for hyperparathyroidism 299
  for infective endocarditis 188
  for investigating the cardiovascular system 413
  for investigating the respiratory system 414
  for joint disease 97
  for loss of consciousness 109
  for lung cancer 206
  for lymphadenopathy and splenomegaly 128
  for mitral regurgitation 24
  for mitral stenosis 23
  for patent ductus arteriosus 192
  for patients with loss of consciousness 109
  for PE 212
  for pericarditis 188
  for pneumonia 209
  for pneumothorax 212
  for polyuria and polydipsia 73
  for pulmonary oedema **414**
  for PUO 36
  for secondary hypertension 181
  for stroke patients 261
  for TB 203
  for tricuspid regurgitation 26

CXR (*Continued*)
   for ventricular septal defect (VSD) 190
   for weight loss 54
   see also erect chest X-ray
cyanosis 10, 114, 379, 384, 387
cyclo-oxygenase 1 (COX-1) inhibitors 317
cyclo-oxygenase 2 (COX-2) antagonists 223
cyclo-oxygenase 2 (COX-2) inhibitors 317
cyclophosphamide 247, 322, 348
cycloserine 203
cyclosporin 230, 252, 327, 328, 329
cyproheptadine 228, 267
cyproterone acetate 255
cystectomy 255
cystic fibrosis (CF) 213–14
cystitis 253
cystoscopy 80, 255, 420
cysts **103**
cytogenetic analysis 348
cytology 128
   diagnostic yield in lung cancer **206**
   see also fine-needle aspiration cytology
cytomegalovirus **360**
cytotoxic chemotherapy 341, 343, 344, 345, 348
cytotoxic drugs 327, 330

D
D2 biopsy 47
D-dimers 427
   and patients with bleeding and bruising 143
   and PE 212
dantrolene 272
dapsone 330
DC (direct current) cardioversion 167, 170, 171, 179, 184
DC shock 171
DCCT (Diabetes Control and Complications Trial) 286
DDAVP (desmopressin) 305, 349, 350
de Musset's sign 25, 385
de Quervain's (subacute) thyroiditis 309
deafness
   causes **398**
   see also hearing
decubiti 101
deep vein thrombosis *see* DVT
defibrillators, implantable 168, 187
dehydration 380
déjà vu 275
delirium
   development 114
   differential diagnosis 113

delirium tremens 114
dementia
   development 114
   differential diagnosis 113
depression 114
dermatitis 99, 102, 327–8
   see also acute-contact allergic dermatitis
dermatitis herpetiformis 99, 330
dermatological lesions, terms and characteristics **103**
dermatomyositis 324–5
dermatome testing **402**
dermatophytid 99
desmopressin (DDAVP) 305, 349, 350
destructive arthropathy 383
dexamethasone 278, 281, 345
diabetes, symptoms 51
Diabetes Control and Complications Trial (DCCT) 286
diabetes insipidus 304–5
diabetes mellitus *see* DM
diabetic amyotrophy 286
diabetic coma 287–9
diabetic feet 286
diabetic ketoacidosis (DKA) 283, 288–9
diabetic nephropathy 251, 285
diabetic neuropathy 285–6
diabetic retinopathy 284
   stages **395**
diagnostic endoscopy 38
diagnostic paracentesis 241
dialysis 252, 254
   for drug overdose 365
   indications in end-stage renal failure (ESRF) 252
   indications for 249
diamorphine 164, 179
diarrhoea 45, 63
   causes **46**
diastolic hypertension and IHD 158
diastolic murmurs 21
diazepam 190
diazoxide 227
DIC (disseminated intravascular coagulation) 350–1
diclofenac 317
didanosine 358
DIDMOAD syndrome 304
diet
   and the management of diabetes 286–7
   and secondary prevention of acute MI 168
dietary potassium, effect on blood pressure 180

dietary sodium intake, effect on blood pressure 180
dietary vitamin D deficiency 297
differential protein clearance 80
differential white cell count 34
DiGeorge syndrome 299
digital rectal examinations 233
digoxin 167, 170, 171, 178, 179, 186
   management of overdose **366**
dihydropyridines 160, 182
dilated cardiomyopathy 187
diltiazem 160, 162, 169, 182
diplopia 271, 396
dipstick testing of urine 66, 78, 83, 245, 248,
      253, 419
dipyridamole MR 263
direct antigen test 154
direct current (DC) cardioversion 167, 170, 171,
      179, 184
disability 134, 136, 375
   and joint examination 404
discharge, vaginal or penile 375
discoid lupus erythematosus 99, 321
disease-modifying antirheumatic drugs
      (DMARDS) 316, 317
dissecting aortic aneurysm 3
disseminated intravascular coagulation (DIC)
      350–1
disseminated sclerosis see multiple sclerosis (MS)
distension of the abdomen 66
dithranol 327
diuretics 185, 186
   see also loop diuretics; potassium-sparing
      diuretics; thiazide diuretics
diverticular disease 233
diverticulosis 233
diving reflex 171
dizziness 145–8, 375
   differential diagnosis **146**
DKA (diabetic ketoacidosis) 283, 288–9
DM 283–9, 420
   classification 283
   clinical presentation 283
   complications 283–6
   diagnosis 420
   and IHD 158
   management 286–7
   monitoring response to diet or treatment 420
   skin manifestations 330, **404**
   and surgery 287
   symptoms **377**
DMARDS (disease-modifying antirheumatic
      drugs) 316, 317

dobutamine 167, 178, 179, 249
domicillary oxygen therapy 201
domperidone 266, 270
dopamine 249
dopamine agonists 269–70, 302, 304
Doppler studies 190, 191
Down's syndrome 384
doxapram 211
doxycycline 361
Dressler's syndrome **166**, 168
driving and epilepsy 276
drug eruptions 102
drug overdose 363–6
   aetiology 363
   complications **364**
   epidemiology 363
   investigations 364
   management 364–6
   presentation 363–4
   psychiatric and social assessment 365
drug resistant TB 203
drug-induced lupus 322
drugs, elimination of 365
dual chamber pacemakers 172, 187
Duchene muscular dystrophy 280
dumping syndrome 223
duodenal biopsy 153
duodenal ulcers see DUs
Dupuytren's contractures 383, 390
dural venous sinus thrombosis 87
Duroziez's sign 25, 387
DUs 37, 222
   bleeds from 224
   management 223
DVT 168, 351
   see also above knee DVT; below knee DVT
dysarthria 375, **376**
dysdiadochokinesis 399
dyspepsia 37–9, 222, 373
   causes 37
   history and examination in the
      patient 37–8
   investigating the patient 38–9
   prevalence 37
   see also non-ulcer dyspepsia
dysphagia 42
   causes **374**
   as a symptom of gastrointestinal
      disease 373
dysphasia 375, **376**
dysphonia 375, **376**
dysplastic naevus 99

dyspnoea 3, 4, 9–13
  as a cardiovascular symptom 372
  examining the patient 10–12
  history in the patient 9–10
  investigating the patient 12–13
  as a respiratory symptom 373
dysuria 77, 374

E
early crackles 390
ears
  and examining the patient with vertigo 147
  see also hearing
EBV (Epstein-Barr virus) 346
ecchymoses 141
ECG
  for acute MI 164, 168
  for acute pancreatitis 237
  for acute renal failure 249
  for aortic regurgitation 26
  for aortic stenosis 25
  for arrhythmias 169
  for atrial fibrillation 169–70
  for atrial flutter 170
  for atrial septal defect (ASD) 191
  for breathlessness 12
  causes of ST elevation **6**
  for chest pain 5–7
  for coarctation of the aorta 192
  of complete heart block **174**
  for dyspepsia 38
  for dyspnoea 12
  effect of hyperkalaemia and hypokalaemia 258
  for encephalitis 274
  for epilepsy 275
  for Fallot's tetralogy 192
  of first degree heart block **172**
  for heart failure 176
  for hypertension 83
  for hypertrophic cardiomyopathy 187
  for IHD 159
  for infective endocarditis 188
  for loss of consciousness 109
  for mitral regurgitation 24
  for mitral stenosis 23
  for mitral valve prolapse 185
  of Mobitz type II heart block **173**
  for NSTEMI 161
  for patent ductus arteriosus (PDA) 191, 192
  for patients with chest pain 5
  for PE **7**, 212

for pericarditis 187, 188
for stroke patients 124
for tricuspid regurgitation 26
of ventricular fibrillation **172**
for ventricular septal defect (VSD) 190
of Wenckebach heart block **173**
see also 24-hour ECG; 12-lead ECG; exercise
  ECG
ECG treadmill exercise testing, contraindications
  412
echocardiography
  for aortic regurgitation 26
  for aortic stenosis 25
  for atrial septal defect (ASD) 191
  for chest pain 7
  for dilated cardiomyopathy 187
  for Fallot's tetralogy 192
  for heart failure 176
  for hypertrophic cardiomyopathy 187
  for IHD 159
  for infective endocarditis 188–9
  for investigating the cardiovascular
    system 413
  for mitral regurgitation 24
  for mitral stenosis 23
  for palpitations 18
  for patent ductus arteriosus (PDA) 191
  for PE 212
  for secondary hypertension 181
  for stroke patients 124, 262
  for tricuspid regurgitation 26
ectopic ACTH syndrome 311
eczema 99, 327–8
efavirenz 358
Ehlers-Danlos syndrome 140, 141
eighth cranial nerve (vestibulocochlear) 397
Eisenmenger's syndrome 190
ejection systolic murmurs 21
elbows 384
electrocardiography *see* ECG
electroencephalography
  for confusional states 117
  for headache/facial pain 90
  for patients with loss of consciousness 109
  for sensory and/or motor neurological
    deficits 136
electrolyte balance, fluid and 256–9
electrolytes
  and stroke patients 261
  see also urea and electrolytes (U&Es)
electromyograms 136

electronystagmography 147
electrophysiological studies
    of arrhythmias 169
    of palpitations 19
elemental diets 232
eleventh cranial nerve (accessory) 398
elimination of drugs 265
embolism 119, 188
embolus, sources **119**
emphysema 10, 198
    aetiology 198–9
    management 200
    pathophysiology 198
    radiological findings **414**
emptying stomach 364
encephalitis 274
encephalopathy
    evidence of 57–8
    see also chronic encephalopathy; hepatic
        encephalopathy; Wernicke's encephalopathy
encrusted lesions 100
end-stage renal failure (ESRF) 250, 252
endobronchial growth of primary tumours in lung
        cancer 205
endocarditis prophylaxis 185
endocrine disorders *see* metabolic and endocrine
        disorders
endocrine symptoms, metabolic and 375
endocrine tumours of the gut 227–8
endocrinopathies, symptoms 51
endoscopic retrograde cholangiopancreatography
        (ERCP) 47, 57, 60, 235, 237, 238
endoscopic ultrasound (EUS) 47, 60, 236, 237
endoscopy 418–19
    for bleeding oesophageal varices 224
    for Crohn's disease 231
    for dyspepsia 38
    for gastro-oesophageal reflux disease
        (GORD) 221
    for upper GI bleeding 224
    for vitamin B_{12} deficiency 153
    see also fibre-optic endoscopy; upper GI
        endoscopy
endotracheal intubation 201
enfuvirtide 358
enoxaparin 162
entacapone 270
enteropathic arthropathies 320
enteroscopy 43, 47, 234
enzyme assays 154
enzyme inducers 243, 313

eosinophilia 34
eosinophilic inclusion bodies 268
eosinophils **426**
ephelides 99
epigastric pain 37
    causes **64**
epigastric tenderness 43
epigastrium, venous hum 392
epilepsia partialis continuans 275
epilepsy 105, **106**, 107, 119, 274–7
    aetiology 275
    classification 274–5
    differential diagnosis 275
    and driving 276
    investigations 275–6
    precipitants 275
    and pregnancy 277
    treatment 276–7
episodic headache/facial pain 88–9, 266–7
EPO (recombinant erythropoietin) 334, 335
Epstein-Barr virus (EBV) 346
eptifibatide 162
Erb's syndrome 280
ERCP (endoscopic retrograde
        cholangiopancreatography) 47, 57, 60,
        235, 237, 238
erect chest X-ray 43, 417
ergocalciferol 297
ergotamine 266–7
erosive duodenitis 222
erosive gastritis **41**
erosive lesions 101
eruptive xanthomata 330
erysipelas 100
erysipeloid 100
erythema **103**
    see also figurate erythema; palmar erythema
erythema chronicum migrans 330
erythema gyratum repens 330
erythema marginatum 190, 329
erythema migrams 100
erythema multiforme 100, 329
erythema nodosum 101, 329, 330
erythrocyte sedimentation rate *see* ESR
erythromycin 328
erythropoietin 334
ESR 427
    and anaemia 152
    and confusional states 115
    and cranial (giant cell) arteritis 265
    and headache/facial pain 89

ESR (*Continued*)
  and joint disease 96
  and lymphadenopathy and
    splenomegaly 128
  and polymyositis and dermatomyositis 325
  and PUO 34–5
  and sensory and/or motor neurological
    deficits 136
  and stroke patients 124, 261
ESRF (end-stage renal failure) 250, 252
essential hypertension 81, 180
etanercept 317
ethambutol 203
ethinyloestradiol 328
ethosuximide 276
EUS (endoscopic ultrasound) 47, 60, 236, 237
examining the patient 379–404
  the abdomen 390–3
  the cardiovascular system 384–7
  the face and body habitus 381
  general inspection 379–81
  the hands 382–4
  the joints 402–4
  the neck 381–2
  the nervous system 393–402
  the respiratory system 387–90
  the skin 404
exercise ECG 159, 412
exercise echocardiography 159
exercise testing
  for chest pain 7
  for heart failure 176
  for palpitations 18
  see also ECG treadmill exercise testing
exercise tolerance and dyspnoea 9
exertional dyspnoea 372
exertional syncope 105
exfoliative dermatitis 99
expansion of the chest 388
expiratory stridor 9
extracerebral haemorrhage 264–5
extradural haematoma 265
extramammary Paget's disease 99
extrapulmonary TB 203
eye pressure 171
eyes
  and complications of DM 284–5
  examination in the coma patient **108**
  and examining the patient with vertigo 147
  and systemic sclerosis 324
  see also vision

F
FAB classification
  of acute lymphoblastic leukaemia (ALL) **341**
  of acute myeloid leukaemia (AML) **342**
face
  and examination of the abdomen 390
  and examination of the cardiovascular
    system 385
  and examination of the respiratory system 388
  examining 381
facial nerve palsies, causes **397**
facial pain *see* headache/facial pain
facial (seventh facial nerve) 397
factitious fever 36
factor deficiency 139
factor IX concentrates 349
factor VIII 349, 350
faecal clearance of alpha 1 antitrypsin 47
faecal fat estimation 47
faecal occult blood 235
faecal stercobilinogen 154
faeculent vomiting 63
Fallot's tetralogy 192
familial adenomatous polyposis (FAP) 232
familial combined hyperlipidaemia 290
familial cranial diabetes insipidus 304
familial hypercholesterolaemia 157, 290, 330
familial hypertriglyceridaemia 290
family history 371
  and IHD 157
fansidar 360
FAP (familial adenomatous polyposis) 232
fasciculation 398, 399
fascioscapulohumeral dystrophy 280
fast atrial fibrillation 19
  treatment 179
fast heart beats, bursts 15
fast heart rate 15
fast irregular heart beats 16
fasting glucose 168–9, 181, 246, 420
fasting lipids 124, 168, 181
fatigue 371
feet, diabetic problems 286
Felty's syndrome 95
ferritin 153, 154
fever *see* pyrexia
FEVI (forced expiratory volume in 1 second)
  196, 415
fibrates 291
fibre-optic bronchoscopy 205, 209, 417
fibre-optic endoscopy 43

fibrin degradation products 143
fibrosing alveolitis 218
fibrosis **389**
   radiological findings **414**
fibrotic lung disease 215
fifth cranial nerve (trigeminal) 396
figurate erythema 100
fine crackles 390
fine tremor 388
fine-needle aspiration cytology 309
first cranial nerve (olfactory) 393–4
first degree heart block 172
   rhythm of 12-lead ECG 410
fish oils 291
fissures **103**
flecainide 174
   see also intravenous flecainide
flexible sigmoidoscopy 47, **419**
flexural psoriasis 327
flucloxacillin 189
fludrocortisone 310, 313
fluid and electrolyte balance 256–9
fluticasone 201
focal motor attacks 275
focal neurological deficit 89
focal segmental glomerulosclerosis (FSGS) 247
focal sensory attacks 275
folate deficiency
   causes **150**
   investigations 153–4
folate replacement for anaemia 333
folic acid 227
follicle-stimulating hormone (FSH) 301
follicular thyroid carcinoma 310
folliculitis 100
forced alkaline diuresis 365
forced expiratory volume in 1 second (FEVI)
   196, 415
formoterol 201
fourth cranial nerve palsy 396
fourth cranial nerve (trochlear) 395–6
frank haematuria 80
freckles 99
French-American-British classification see FAB
   classification
frequency of micturition 77, 374
friction rubs 12, 392
Friedrich's sign 385
frusemide 178, 179, 241, 252, 265, 298
   see also intravenous frusemide
FSGS (focal segmental glomerulosclerosis) 247

FSH (follicle-stimulating hormone) 301
full blood count (FBC) 425–7
   for abdominal pain 66
   for anaemia 152
   for coeliac disease 226
   for confusional states 115
   for the CREST syndrome 324
   for dyspepsia 38
   for dyspnoea 12
   for gastric carcinoma 225
   for haematemesis and melaena 43
   for haematuria and proteinuria 80
   for headache/facial pain 89
   for joint disease 96
   and loss of consciousness 109
   for lymphadenopathy and splenomegaly 128
   for pneumonia 209
   for polyuria and polydipsia 72
   for PUO 34
   for sensory and/or motor neurological
      deficits 136
   for stroke patients 123, 261
   for weight loss 54
fulminant hepatitis 240
functional proteinuria 75
fundoscopy 83, 114–15, 181, 395
furuncle 101, 286
fusion inhibitors 358

G
G6PD (glucose-6-phosphate dehydrogenate
   deficiency) 336–7
gabapentin 276, 329
gait 400
   abnormalities **136**
gallbladder, diseases 235–6
gallstones 235–6
gastrectomy 223
gastric carcinoma 222, 225
gastric emptying 364
gastric lavage 364
gastric neoplasm **41**
gastric parietal antibodies 153
gastric transection with reanastamosis 225
gastric ulcers see GUs
gastro-duodenitis 222–3
gastro-oesophageal reflux disease
   (GORD) 221
gastroduodenal disorders 222–5
gastrointestinal absorption, prevention 364–5
gastrointestinal bleeding see GI bleeding

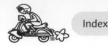

gastrointestinal disease 373–4
  liver and 221–44
  radiological abdominal abnormalities associated
    with **418**
gastrointestinal system
  investigations 417–19
  and systemic sclerosis 324
gastrointestinal tract, 'scopes' used to
    examine **419**
gastroscopy 32, 222, 225, **419**
Gaucher's disease **127**
gay bowel syndrome 45
gene therapy 339
general symptoms 371–2
generalised itching **102**
generalised lymphadenopathy 356
  differential diagnosis 125
  evidence of an underlying cause 127
  history in the patient 126
generalised seizure **106**
generalised wasting 383
genetic testing 242
genitourinary disease 245–59
genitourinary symptoms 374–5
gentamicin 189
GFR 80, 250, 419
  relationship between creatinine and 251
GH 301, 302
GH-secreting tumours 301, 302
GI bleeding 41
  adverse prognostic factors **224**
  see also lower GI bleeding; upper GI bleeding
giant cell arteritis 265–6
gingival hypertrophy **391**
Glasgow coma scale **108**, 122
glatiramer acetate 272
glaucoma 267–8, 285
glibenclamide 287
glomerular disease 245–7
  general principles of management 246
  histological classification 246
  history 245
  investigations 245–6
  primary and secondary diseases 246–7
glomerular filtration rate see GFR
glomerulus, systemic disorders that involve **245**
glossitis 390
glossopharyngeal neuralgia 267
glossopharyngeal (ninth cranial nerve) 397
glossopharyngeal palsies, causes **398**
glucagon 288

glucagonomas 227
glucosamine 318
glucose-6-phosphate dehydrogenase deficiency
    (G6PD) 336–7
gluten-free diet 225, 226
glycated haemoglobin (HBA1c) 420
glyceryl trinitrate 179
glycoprotein IIb/IIIa receptor antagonists 162
glycosuria 420
goitre cancer 309
gold 317
Goodpasture's syndrome 246
GORD (gastro-oesophageal reflux disease) 221
goserelin 255
gout 299–300
  examining the patient 95
  X-ray of affected joints 97
grand mal fits 274
granuloma annulare 330
Graves' disease 306, **383**
  investigations 308
Grey Turner's sign 65, 237
growth hormone see GH
GTN 3, 183
Guillan-Barré syndrome 279
GUs 37, 223
  bleeds from 224
'gut claudication' 234
guttate psoriasis 327
gynaecomastia 391

H
H₂ receptor antagonists 221, 223, 324
HAART (anti-retroviral therapy) 358
haematemesis 41–4
  differential diagnosis 41
  examining the patient 42–3
  history in the patient 41–2
  investigating the patient 43–4
haematinics 427
haematological disorders 333–53
  investigations 425–7
haematological symptoms 376
haematomas 265
haematuria 75–80, 188
  differential diagnosis 75
  examining the patient 77–8
  history in the patient 77
  investigating the patient 78–80
haemochromatosis 241–2
  interpretation of iron storage results **153**

haemofiltration, indications for 249
haemoglobin 223, 244, 425
   see also normal haemoglobin synthesis
haemoglobin electrophoresis 154
haemolysis
   changes on blood film **152**
   investigations 154
haemolysis screen 236
haemolytic anaemia, causes **149**
haemolytic sickle cell anaemia crisis 338
haemolytic uraemic syndrome 254
haemophilia A 349
haemophilia B 349
Haemophilus 209
haemoptysis 9, 29–32
   differential diagnosis 29
   examining the patient 30–1
   history in the patient 29–30
   investigating the patient 32
haemorrhagic strokes **119**, 120
haemorrhagic telangiectasia 141
haemostasis 139
   investigating abnormality 141
half-and-half nails 383, 390
Hallpike's manoeuvre 147
halofantrine 360
Hamman's sign 390
Ham's test 154
hand X-ray 299, 302, 324
handicap 136
hands examination 382–4
   and the abdomen 390
   and the cardiovascular system 384
   and OA 95
   and the respiratory system 387
   and weight loss 52–3
Harrison's sulci 388
Hashimoto's thyroiditis 305
HAV (hepatitis A virus) 238
HBA1c (glycated haemoglobin) 420
HBV (hepatitis B virus) 238–9, 240
HCM (hypertrophic cardiomyopathy) 22, 186–7
HCV (hepatitis C virus) 239
HD (Hodgkin's disease) 346–8, **358**
HDL (high density lipoprotein) cholesterol
      158, 290
HDLs (high density lipoproteins) 290
HDV (hepatitis D virus) 239
headache/facial pain 87–91, 375
   differential diagnosis **88**
   examining the patient 89, **90**

history in the patient 87–9
investigating the patient 89–91
management of conditions causing 265–8
Heaf test 203
hearing
   assessment 397
   disturbed 375
   see also deafness
heart block 167–8, 172–3
heart block with anterior MI 167–8
heart failure 174–9
   causes 175–6
   clinical features 176
   investigation **175**, 176–7
   management **175**, 177–9
heart murmurs 21–7, 192
   consequences 22
   describing 27
   differential diagnosis 21
   examining the patient 22–7
   history in the patient 22
heart-lung transplantation 214
heartburn 37, 373
heat rash 100
heavy heart beats 15
Heberden's nodes 95, 318, 383
Helicobacter pylori 159, 221, 222, 223,
      225, 235
helicobacter pylori testing 38
hemiplegic migraine 119, 266
Henle, Loop of 69
Henoch-Schönlein purpura 246, 247
heparin 247
   management of overdose **366**
   and prevention of deep vein thrombosis (DVT)
      and PE 168
   and treatment of acute MI 166
   and treatment of NSTEMI 162
   and treatment of PE 213
   and treatment of thrombotic disorders 351–2
   see also prophylactic subcutaneous heparin
heparin induced thrombocytopenia (HIT) 139
hepatic decompensation 244
hepatic encephalopathy 58, 115, 224, 241
hepatic iminodiacetic acid scintigraphy 236
'hepatic' jaundice 57, **59**
hepatitis A virus (HAV) 238
hepatitis B virus (HBV) 238–9, 240
hepatitis C virus (HCV) 239
hepatitis D virus (HDV) 239

hepatitis E virus 239–40
hepatocellular dysfunction 240
hepatocellular screen 60
hepatolenticular degeneration 243
hepatomegaly 127, 387
  causes **392**
hepatorenal syndrome (HRS) 254
hepatosplenomegaly 127, 393
hereditary elliptocytosis 336
hereditary haemochromatosis *see* primary
    haemochromatosis
hereditary haemorrhagic telangiectasia 139, 141
hereditary non-polyposis colon cancer 232
hereditary spherocytosis 336
hernial orifices 66
herpes simplex *see* HSV
herpes (varicella) zoster 4, 99, 328–9, **360**
hesitancy in micturition 375
hiatus hernia 221
high density lipoprotein (HDL) cholesterol
    158, 290
high density lipoproteins (HDLs) 290
high output heart failure 175–6
high resolution CT (HRCT) 32, 215, 216, 417
high-dose dexamethasone suppression test
    421, 422
high-grade NHL 348
Hirschsprung's disease 46
history, taking a *see* taking a history
history of presenting complaint 370, 405
HIT (heparin induced thrombocytopenia) 139
HIV 355–9
  aetiology 355
  epidemiology 355
  investigations 356, **358**
  opportunistic infections **360**
  pathology 355
  patients infected with TB and 202
  phases 355–6
  prevention 358
  prognosis 358
  transmission routes 355
  treatment 356, 358
HIV antibody tests 356
HIV associated nephropathy 247
HIV drugs 358
  site of action **359**
HIV genes and the proteins they encode **356**
HIV RNA detection 356
HIV-1 355
HIV-2 355
HMG CoA reductase inhibitors *see* statins

hoarse voice 373
Hodgkin's disease (HD) 346–8, **358**
Holmes-Adie pupil 394
Holter monitoring 185
HONK (hyperosmolar non-ketotic coma) 283
hormone replacement 301
hormone replacement therapy (HRT) 295
Horner's syndrome 88, 205, 278, 388
hospital-acquired pneumonia 208
  drug choice **210**
HRCT (high resolution CT) 32, 215, 216, 417
HRS (hepatorenal syndrome) 254
HRT (hormone replacement therapy) 295
HSV 99, 328, **360**
HSV encephalitis 274
human immunodeficiency virus *see* HIV
hydralazine 178, 183, 322
hydration 380
hydrocephalus 114
hydrocortisone 301, 312–13
  see also intravenous hydrocortisone
hydroxychloroquine 317, 322, 325
hydroxycobalamin 333
hyperbilirubinaemia 417
hypercalcaemia 66, 69, 297–8
  causes **424**
hypercholesterolaemia 124, 252, 290
hyperfibrinogenaemia 158
hyperglycaemia 66, 69
hyperglycaemic hyperosmolar non-ketotic
    coma 289
hyperhomocysteinaemia 158
hyperkalaemia 258
  causes **259**
  treatment 249
hyperlipidaemia 290
  skin manifestations **404**
hypernatraemia 256, **258**
hypernephroma 33, 255
hyperosmolar non-ketotic coma (HONK) 283
hyperparathyroidism 298–9
hyperprolactinaemia 302, 303
  causes **304**
hypersensitivity pneumonitis **213**
hypersplenism 126
hypertension 81–5, 114, 122, 179–84
  and age 183
  clinical evaluation **181**
  differential diagnosis 81
  examining the patient 82–3
  follow up 183
  history in the patient 81–2

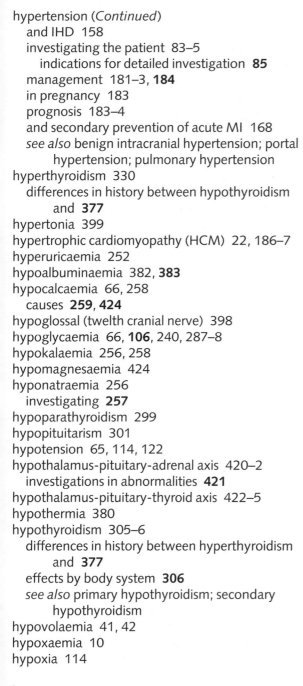

hypertension (*Continued*)
  and IHD 158
  investigating the patient 83–5
    indications for detailed investigation **85**
  management 181–3, **184**
  in pregnancy 183
  prognosis 183–4
  and secondary prevention of acute MI 168
  see also benign intracranial hypertension; portal
      hypertension; pulmonary hypertension
hyperthyroidism 330
  differences in history between hypothyroidism
      and **377**
hypertonia 399
hypertrophic cardiomyopathy (HCM) 22, 186–7
hyperuricaemia 252
hypoalbuminaemia 382, **383**
hypocalcaemia 66, 258
  causes **259, 424**
hypoglossal (twelfth cranial nerve) 398
hypoglycaemia 66, **106**, 240, 287–8
hypokalaemia 256, 258
hypomagnesaemia 424
hyponatraemia 256
  investigating **257**
hypoparathyroidism 299
hypopituitarism 301
hypotension 65, 114, 122
hypothalamus-pituitary-adrenal axis 420–2
  investigations in abnormalities **421**
hypothalamus-pituitary-thyroid axis 422–5
hypothermia 380
hypothyroidism 305–6
  differences in history between hyperthyroidism
      and **377**
  effects by body system **306**
  see also primary hypothyroidism; secondary
      hypothyroidism
hypovolaemia 41, 42
hypoxaemia 10
hypoxia 114

I
iatrogenic hypothyroidism 305
iatrogenic pneumothoraces 217
IBD 228–32
  aetiology 228
  extraintestinal complications 228–9
  extraintestinal manifestations 228
  skin manifestations 330
ibuprofen 300, 317
icterus *see* jaundice

IDDM *see* type I DM
idiopathic atrophic hypothyroidism 305
idiopathic generalised epilepsies 274–5
  first-line drugs 276
idiopathic hypoparathyroidism 299
idiosyncratic asthma 195
IDL (intermediate density lipoprotein) 290
IgA nephropathy 246–7
IHD 157–62
  acute coronary syndromes 161
  incidence 157
  investigations 159
  pathology 158–9
  risk factors 4, 157–8
  treatment 160–1
ileostomy 230
ileus, causes **393**
imaging
  for lung cancer 206–7
  for lymphadenopathy and splenomegaly 128
  for vertigo 148
  see also barium imaging; CT scanning; MRI;
      nuclear imaging; radionuclide imaging;
      ultrasound examinations; X-ray
imatinib 344
immunoglobulin G serological tests 38
immunoglobulins 136
immunohistochemistry 348
immunological tests **326**
immunosuppressive therapy 232, 243, 246, 247,
      280, 320, 322, 325, 353
immunotherapy 343, 345
impairment 134
impetigo 100
implantable defibrillators 168, 187
incontinence 375
indigestion 373
indinavir 358
indomethacin 191, 305
induced emesis 364
infarction **119**
infectious diseases 355–62
infectious mononucleosis **127**
infective endocarditis 188–9
infective meningitis 87
inflammatory bowel disease *see* IBD
inflammatory markers
  and investigating infective endocarditis 188
  and investigating PUO 34–5
  and investigating weight loss 54
infliximab 232, 317
inhaled steroid 197

inotropes 249
  see also intravenous inotropic agents
INR (international normalized ratio) 352
inspiratory stridor 9
insulin 287
  examples of different regimens **288**
insulinomas 227, 288
integrase inhibitors 358
intention tremor in the hands 384
interferon 331, 345, 358
  see also α-interferon
interleukin-1 receptor antagonists 317
intermediate density lipoprotein (IDL) 290
intermittent claudication 372
international normalized ratio (INR) 352
internuclear ophthalmoplegia 395
interstitial lung diseases 215–16
intertrigo 99
intestinal obstruction **418**
intra-aortic balloon counterpulsation 179
intra-articular corticosteroids 318
intracerebral haemorrhage 119
intracorporeal papaverine 272
intracranial pressure, raised see raised intracranial
        pressure
intracranial tumours 277–8
intramuscular opiates 237
intramuscular penicillin G 190
intravenous aciclovir 273, 274, 328, 329
intravenous adenosine 171
intravenous ampicillin 273
intravenous antibiotics for endocarditis 189
intravenous β-blockers 171
intravenous bisphosphonate therapy 298
intravenous calcium gluconate 299
intravenous ceftriaxone 273
intravenous edrophonium 279
intravenous flecainide 170
intravenous fludarabine 343
intravenous frusemide 249
intravenous hydrocortisone 230, 312
intravenous inotropic agents 179
intravenous magnesium chloride 299
intravenous naloxone 164
intravenous opiates 237
intravenous pyelogram 80
intravenous therapy for chronic cardiac
        failure 178
intravenous thiamine 241
intravenous urography (IVU) 253, 420
intravenous venodilators 179

intravenous verapamil 171
intraventricular thrombus 168
intrinsic asthma 195
intrinsic factor antibodies 153
investigations 409–28
  of the cardiovascular system 409–14
  of the gastrointestinal system 417–19
  haematological disorders 425–7
  metabolic and endocrine disorders 420–5
  musculoskeletal and skin disease 425
  the nervous system 420
  of the respiratory system 414–17
  of the urinary system 419–20
involuntary weight loss 51
involutional osteoporosis 294
iodine 308
iodine-deficient hypothyroidism 305
ion exchange resin 231
ipratropium 201
irbesartan 183
iridectomy 268
iron, management of overdose **366**
iron replacement for anaemia 333
iron storage results, interpretation **153**
iron-deficiency anaemia 152
  causes **149**
  investigations 153
irregular palpitations 15–16
irregularly irregular pulse 18
irritable bowel syndrome 234–5
irritant contact dermatitis 327
ischaemic colitis 234
ischaemic heart disease see IHD
ischaemic strokes 261
ISDN (isosorbide dinitrate) 160
ISMN (isosorbide mononitrate) 160
isoniazid 203, 204, 272, 322
isoprenaline infusion 172
isosorbide dinitrate (ISDN) 160
isosorbide mononitrate (ISMN) 160
isotope labelled red blood cell studies 234
isotope scanning 253
isotope studies 43
isotretinoin 328
ispaghula 291
itching
  causes of generalized and localized **102**
  as a general symptom 372
  see also pruritus
itraconazole 215
IVU (intravenous urogram) 253, 420

J

Jacksonian seizure 275
jamais vu 275
Janeway's lesions 384
jaundice 57–61, 127, 379–80, 385
    as an underlying cause of abdominal pain 65
    biochemical abnormalities in different types 61
    differential diagnosis 57, **59**
    examining the patient 57–9
    history in the patient 57
    investigating the patient 59–61
jaw claudication 87
jejunal biopsy 154, 226
joint aspiration 97, 300
joint disease 93–7
    differential diagnosis 93, **94**
    examining the patient 94–6
    history in the patient 93–4
    investigating the patient 96–7
joints
    chondrocalcinosis 241, 242
    examining 402–4
        the hands 383
    swelling 375
Jones' criteria for guidance in diagnosis of
        rheumatic fever 189–90
jugular venous pressure *see* JVP
jugulovenous waveform, abnormalities **386**
juvenile myoclonic epilepsy 277
JVP
    causes of raised **386**
    differences between carotid pulsation and **385**
    and examination of the respiratory system
        388
    examining 385

K

Kallmann's syndrome 394
Kaposi's sarcoma 100, 358
Kayser-Fleischer rings 243, 390
Keith-Wagner classification of retinopathy **181**
keratoderma blenorrhagica 95
Kernig's sign 89, 264, 273
ketoconazole 310
ketonuria 419
kidneys
    causes of unilateral and bilateral palpable **392**
    and complications of DM 285
    and the differential diagnosis of haematuria 75
    see also adult polycystic kidney disease; left
        kidney

Killip classification **167**
Kimmelstiel-Wilson lesion 285
Klebsiella 209
Köebner's phenomenon **103**, 329
koilonychia 53, 382, 390
'KUB' film 419
Kussmaul respiration 12, 289
Kussmaul's sign 188, 385
kyphoscoliosis 10

L

labetalol 183
LACI (lacunar infarct) **262**
lactate dehydrogenase *see* LDH
lactose hydrogen breath test 47
lacunar infarct (LACI) **262**
lacunar strokes 261
lamotrigine 276
Landouzy-Dejerine syndrome 280
laparoscopic cholecystectomy 236
laparotomy 44
large cell carcinoma 204
large a waves 388
lariam 360
'late dumping' 223
late ventricular arrhythmias 168
lateral tarsorrhaphy 279
LDH 409
    and the anaemic patient 153, 154
    and chest pain 4
    and lymphadenopathy and splenomegaly 128
    use to assess MI 163
LDL (low density lipoprotein) cholesterol 158
'lead pipe' rigidity 268, 399
lead poisoning 335–6
leather-bottle type adenocarcinomas 225
left heart failure 176
left hypochondrium, causes of pain in **64**
left iliac fossa, causes of pain in **64**
left kidney, distinguishing between the spleen
    and **127**
left supraclavicular lymphadenopathy 391
left ventricular angiography 190
left ventricular failure (LVF) 166
left ventricular hypertrophy 412
left-sided heart murmurs 26
lentigo 99
leptospirosis 57
leuconychia 53, 382, 390
leucopenia 34, 126
leucophoresis 344

leukaemias 341–4
leukotriene modifiers 197
levodopa 269
levosimendan 178
Lewy bodies 268
LFTs 417
   for abdominal pain 66
   for confusional states 115
   for gallstones 235
   for gastric carcinoma 225
   for heart failure 176
   for joint disease 97
   for loss of consciousness 109
   for lymphadenopathy and splenomegaly 128
   for primary biliary cirrhosis (PBC) 243
   for PUO 35
   for sensory and/or motor neurological
      deficits 136
   for weight loss 54
LH (luteinising hormone) 301
Lhermitte's sign 271
lichen planus 100, 328, 329
lichen simplex chronicus 99
lichenification **103**
lidocaine 167, 171, 174
limb girdle dystrophy 280
limb weakness 375
linezolid 362
linitis plastica 225
lipid disorders 290–3
   management 291–3
lipid profile 83
lipid-lowering agents 169
   see also statins
lipids
   and stroke prevention 263
   see also blood lipids; fasting lipids
lipoatrophy 286
liposomal doxorubicin 358
lisinopril 177
liver, palpable 390
liver biopsy 60, 242, 419
liver disease
   changes on blood film **152**
   gastrointestinal and *see* gastrointestinal and
      liver disease
   skin manifestations **404**
   see also chronic liver disease
liver enzymes 240
liver function tests *see* LFTs
liver transplantation 241, 243

LMWH (low molecular weight heparin) 162
lobectomy 207
localized itching **102**
localized lymphadenopathy
   differential diagnosis 125
   evidence of an underlying cause 127
   history in the patient 125–6
localized scleroderma 324
localized wasting 383
loin pain **64**, 77, 375
long acting β$_2$-agonists 197, 201
long Synacthen stimulation test **421**, 422
loop diuretics 178
loop of Henle, water and electrolyte balance 69
Looser's zones 297
loperamide 231, 235
losartan 183
loss of consciousness 105–11
   differential diagnosis 105, **106**
   examining the patient 107–8
   history in the patient 105, 107
   investigating the patient 109–11
low density lipoprotein (LDL) cholesterol 158
low molecular weight heparin (LMWH) 162
low-grade NHL 348
low-renin hypertension 182
lower GI bleeding 234
lower limb oedema, causes **393**
lower limbs, examining 399–402
lower motor neurone lesions 397, 398
lower UTIs 253
lumbar puncture
   for confusional states 117
   for headache/facial pain 90, 265
   for loss of consciousness 109
   for lymphadenopathy and splenomegaly 128
   for meningitis 273
   for patients with loss of consciousness 109
   for sensory and/or motor neurological deficits
      136
   for subarachnoid haemorrhage 264
lung biopsy 216, 417
lung cancer 204–8, **213**
   aetiology 204
   clinical findings 204–5
   extent of disease and tumour-node-metastasis
      (TNM) staging 207
   investigations 205–7
   prognosis 207–8
   treatment 207, **208**
lung function tests 414–15

lung transplantation 201
lung volume reduction surgery 201
lung volumes 415
lupus nephritis 247
lupus pernio 330
luteinising hormone (LH) 301
luteinising hormone-releasing hormone
        analogues 255
LVF (left ventricular failure) 166
lyme disease 330
lymph node biopsy 205, 348
lymphadenopathy 65, 125–30
    differential diagnosis 125
    examining the patient 126–7, 380–1
    history in the patient 125–6
    and HIV 356
    investigating the patient 128–30
    see also left supraclavicular lymphadenopathy
lymphatic systems and systemic lupus
        erythematosus (SLE) 321
lymphocytes **426**
lymphoma 33, 126, 310
    see also malignant lymphonas

M
macrocytic red blood cells 149–50
macrolides 203
macrovascular disease 283, 284
macule **103**
maculopapular lesions 101
magnetic resonance angiography 83, 262, 420
magnetic resonance cholangiopancreatography
        (MRCP) 47, 60, 236, 237
magnetic resonance imaging see MRI
Major Jones' criteria for rheumatic fever 189–90
malabsorption 46, 225–7
malabsorption in diarrhoea, investigations 46
malabsorptive surgery 290
maladie de Roger 190
Malar flush 385
malaria 359–62
    aetiology 359
    epidemiology 359
    investigations 360
    life cycle **361**
    pathology 359
    presentation 359–60
    prevention 361–2
    prognosis 362
    treatment 360–1
malarone 360, 361

malignant lymphomas 346–8
malignant melanoma 331
malignant skin tumours 331
Mallory-Weiss tear **41**
manometry 38
Mantoux test 203
MAO B (monoamine oxidase) inhibitors 270
Marcus-Gunn pupil 394
Marfan's syndrome 191, 384
Marjolin's ulcer 331
mass, features of any **382**
massive splenomegaly 125
MCTD 325
    immunological tests **326**
mean corpuscular volume 425
mebeverine 235
mediastinoscopy 205
medical sample clerking 406–8
medications, recording 370
medium crackles 390
medullary thyroid carcinoma 47, 310
mefloquine 360, 361
melaena 41–4
    differential diagnosis 41
    examining the patient 42 3
    history in the patient 41–2
    investigating the patient 43–4
melanoma 99
    see also malignant melanoma
melphalan 345
Ménière's disease **146**
meningiomas 278
meningism, signs 89, 273
meningitis 87, 272–4
    causative organisms 272
    clinical features 273
    differential diagnosis 273
    investigations 273
    pathophysiology 272
    predisposing factors 272–3
    treatment 273–4
        of suspected 91
    see also cryptococcal meningitis
menstruation 375
mesalazine 230
mesenteric angiography 43, 153
metabolic acidosis 12
metabolic bone disease 294–7
metabolic coma **106**
metabolic and endocrine disorders 283–314
    investigations 420–5

metabolic and endocrine symptoms 375
metastases **425**
metastatic ocular melanoma 331
metformin 287
methicillin resistant *Staphylococcus aureus* (MRSA) 362
methotrexate 317, 325, 327
methylprednisolone 218
methysergide 228
metoclopramide 221, 266
metolazone 178
metoprolol 160, 162, 178
metronidazole 227, 231, 234
metyrapone 310
MI 3, 4, 162
    elevation of cardiac enzymes post **409**
    see also acute MI
microalbuminuria 285
microangiopathic haemolytic anaemia 353
microcytic red blood cells 149
micrographia 268
microscopic polyangiitis 246
microvascular disease 283, 284
micturating cystogram 253
micturition
    discomfort during or after 374
    frequency 77, 374
    hesitancy 375
    see also polyuria
migraine 88, 266–7
'migraine sine cephalgia' 266
migrainous neuralgia 88–9, 267
mild splenomegaly 125
miliaria 100
milrinone 178
mini-mental state examination (MMSE) 114
minimal change nephropathy 247
minoxidil 183
miotics 268
misoprostol 223
missed heart beats 15
mitral incompetence **166**
mitral regurgitation 22, 23–4, 167, 185, 192
    management 185
mitral stenosis 22–3, 184–5
mitral valve prolapse 185
mitral valve replacement 185
mitral valvotomy scar 386
mixed apnoeas 217
mixed connective tissue disease *see* MCTD
mixed stones 235

MMSE (mini-mental state examination) 114
Mobitz type I and II heart blocks 172, **173**
moderate splenomegaly 125
modified Duke's classification of colorectal carcinoma **233**
mofetil 252
molluscum contagiosum 100
monoamine oxidase B (MAO B) inhibitors 270
monoclonal gammopathy 346
monocytes **426**
monocytosis 34
mononeuritis 286
mononuclear cells, abnormal 34
MOPP (mustine, oncovin, procarbazine and prednisolone) 347
Moraxella 209
morphoea 324
mosquito bites, avoidance 361–2
motor neurological deficits 131–7
    differential diagnosis 131, **132–3**
    examining the patient 133–6
    history in the patient 131
    investigating the patient 136–7
motor neurone disease 278
motor weakness in multiple sclerosis 271
mouth
    and examination of the abdomen 390–1
    and examination of the cardiovascular system 385
MRCP (magnetic resonance cholangiopancreatography) 47, 60, 236, 237
MRI
    for Crohn's disease 231
    for gastrointestinal disease 418
    for joint disease 97
    for lung cancer 206
    for multiple sclerosis 271
    for sensory and/or motor neurological deficits 136
    for vertigo 148
MRI of the brain 73, 207
MRI of the head
    for confusional states 115, 117
    for headache/facial pain 90
MRSA (methicillin resistant *Staphylococcus aureus*) 362
multi-infarct dementia 114
multiple endocrine neoplasia 313–14
multiple myeloma 344–6
    causes of renal failure **345**

multiple sclerosis (MS) 131, 270–2
  aetiology 270
  clinical features 270–1
  diagnosis and differential diagnosis 271
  investigations 271
  management 272
  pathology 270
  prognosis 272
mural thrombus **166**
Murphy's sign 66, 236
muscle biopsy 325
muscle disorders 279–80
  see also polymyositis
muscle group movement, nerve roots for **400**
muscle power, grading **399**
muscle wasting 402
muscular dystrophies 280
musculoskeletal and skin disorders 315–31
  investigations 425
musculoskeletal symptoms 375
musculoskeletal system
  and systemic lupus erythematosus
    (SLE) 321
  and systemic sclerosis 324
myasthenia gravis 279–80
Mycobacterium avium intracellulare 360
Mycobacterium bovis 201
Mycobacterium tuberculosis 201, 202, 203
mycophenolate 252
myelography 136–7
myocardial infarction see MI
myocardial necrosis 409
myoclonic epilepsy 275
myotomy 187
myotonia 383
myotonic dystrophy (myotonia dystrophica) 280
myotonic pupil 394
myxoedema 16
myxoedema coma 306

N
naevus 99
nails
  examining 382–3
  and examining the patient with polyuria or
    polydipsia 71
naloxone 243
  see also intravenous naloxone
naproxen 300
nausea and CRF 252
neck, examining 381–2, 391
necrobiosis lipoidica diabeticorum 286, 330

Nelson's syndrome 310
neomycin 241
neoplasia 330
neoplastic polyps 232
neostigmine 280
nephrectomy 255
nephritic syndrome 80, 245, 247
nephrogenic diabetes insipidus 70, 304, 305
nephrotic syndrome 245, 247
  causes **76**
nerve conduction studies 136
nerve roots for each muscle group
    movement **400**
nervous system
  examining 393–402
  investigations 420
neurocardiogenic syncope **106**
neurofibromatosis 330, 380
  skin manifestations **404**
neurological coma **106**
neurological examination, for polyuria and
    polydipsia 72
neurological symptoms 375
  of vertigo 146–7
neuromuscular examination of the hands 383
neuropathies
  and complications of DM 285–6
  see also peripheral neuropathies
neutrophil leucocytosis 34
neutrophils **426**
nevirapine 358
New York Heart Association classification of heart
    failure **174**
NHL (Non-Hodgkin's lymphomas) 348, **358**
nicorandil 161
nicotinic acid group 291
NIDDM see type II DM
nifedipine 160, 324
  see also sublingual nifedipine
Nikolsky's sign 100
nimodipine 264
ninth cranial nerve (glossopharyngeal) 397
nitrates 3, 160, 161, 164, 178, 179
nitroprusside 183
NIV
  for COPD 201
  for respiratory failure 211
nocturia 375
nodules **103**
non Q wave myocardial infarctions see NSTEMI
non ST segment elevation myocardial infarction
    see NSTEMI

non-cardioselective β-blockers 10
Non-Hodgkin's lymphomas (NHL) 348, **358**
non-invasive ventilation *see* NIV
non-neoplastic polyps 232
non-nucleoside analogue reverse transcriptase
    inhibitors 358
non-oliguric renal failure 247, 250
non-selective β-blockers 225
non-small cell lung cancer 204
    treatment 207, **208**
non-steroidal anti-inflammatory drugs *see*
    NSAIDS
non-ulcer dyspepsia 235
non-valvular causes of heart murmurs 21
noradrenaline 249
normal coagulation pathway **141**
normal haemoglobin synthesis 338
normocytic red blood cells 149
nosocomial pneumonia 209
NSAIDS 168, 222, 223, 309, 318, 319, 320, 322
    and treatment of gout 300
    and treatment of RA 316, 317
NSTEMI 161–2
    diagnosis 161
    management 161–2
    symptoms 161
nuclear imaging 159
nuclear techniques for investigating heart failure
    177
nucleoside analogue reverse transcriptase
    inhibitors 358
nystagmus 147, 395

O
OA 93, 317–18
    clinical features 318
    examining the patient 95
    investigations 318
    management 318
    X-ray of affected joints 97
oat cell carcinoma *see* small cell carcinoma
obesity 289–90
    relationship between blood pressure and 180
obstructive airways disorders **213**
obstructive sleep apnoea 180, 217, 373
    and IHD 158
obstructive uropathy 81
occupation
    and asthma 196
    and COPD 199
    and jaundice 57

occupational history and dyspnoea 10
occupational lung diseases 10, **213**, 216
octreotide 224, 227, 228, 302
oculomotor (third cranial nerve) 395–6
odynophagia 42, 222
oesophageal cancer 222
oesophageal disorders 3–4, 221–2
oesophageal dysmotility 383
oesophageal manometry 222
oesophageal motility disorders 222
oesophageal motility studies 38
oesophageal transection with anastamosis 225
oesophageal varices, management of bleeding
    224–5
oesophagitis **41**, 221
oesophagogastroduodenoscopy *see* OGD
oestrogen 301
ofloxacin 203
OGD
    for change in bowel habit 47
    for dyspepsia 38
OGTT (oral glucose tolerance test) 283, 420
olfactory (first cranial nerve) 393–4
oliguria 77
omeprazole 227
onycholysis 382
open lung biopsy via thoracotomy 205
ophthalmoplegia 147
opiate antagonists 243
opiates 162, 164, 278
    management of overdose 364, **366**
    see also intravenous opiates
opioids 235
optic atrophy 147
    causes **395**
optic neuritis 270–1
optic (second cranial nerve) 394–5
oral contraceptive efficacy 276
oral folic acid 333
oral glucose tolerance test (OGTT) 283, 420
oral hypoglycaemic agents 287
oral iron replacement therapy 333
oral laxatives 241
oral methyldopa 183
oral prednisolone 230
oral steroids 197, 201
oral vancomycin 234
oral warfarin 213, 352
orchidectomy 255
orlistat 290
orthopnoea 9, 372

orthostatic (postural) hypotension 105, **106**, 109
orthostatic proteinuria 75
Ortner's syndrome 22
Osler-Weber-Rendu syndrome 43, 139
Osler's nodes 384
osmolality, calculation of 289
osmotic diuresis **70**
osmotic fragility 154
osteoarthritis *see* OA
osteomalacia 296–7
    biochemical abnormalities **425**
osteopenia 294
osteoporosis 294–5
    biochemical abnormalities **425**
ostium primum 191
ostium secundum 191
otoscopy 147
overdiuresis 241
overdose, drug *see* drug overdose
overflow proteinuria 76
overhydration 380
overnight dexamethasone suppression test
        421, 422
oxybutynin 272
oxygen therapy 210–11
    see also domicillary oxygen therapy
oxytetracycline 227

P
P wave of the 12-lead ECG 411
pacemakers 173
    see also biventricular pacemakers; dual
        chamber pacemakers
PACI (partial anterior circulation infarct) **262**
pacing wires 172
Paget's disease 89, 268, 295–6
    biochemical abnormalities **425**
    see also extramammary Paget's disease
pain 375
    see also abdominal pain; bone pain; chest pain;
        headache/facial pain; loin pain
painful sickle cell anaemia crisis 338
pallor 380
palmar erythema 53, 390
    causes **383**
palpatation
    of the abdomen 391–2
    and examination of the cardiovascular system
        386–7
    and examining the patient with
        breathlessness 11

palpitations 4, 15–19, 372
    as a cardiovascular symptom 372
    consequences 16–17
    differential diagnosis 15–16
    examining the patient 17–19
    history 16
    investigating the patient 18–19
panacinar emphysema 198
Pancoast's tumour 205, 387
pancrealauryl test 47
pancreas, diseases of 236–8
pancreatectomy 238
pancreatic carcinoma 236–7
pancreatic endocrine tumours 227
pancreatic pain 63
pancreatitis 236
    causes 237
    see also chronic pancreatitis
panhypopituitarism, symptoms 51
panproctocolectomy with ileoanal pouch 230
pansystolic murmurs 21
papaverine 272
papillary thyroid carcinoma 309–10
papilloedema 147
    causes **395**
papular lesions 100–1
papules **103**
para-oesophageal hiatus hernia 221
paracentesis 241
paracetamol, management of overdose **366**
paraesthesiae 375
paraneoplastic syndromes associated with lung
        cancer 205, **206**
parasternal heave 386
parathyroid hormone (PTH) 295, 424–5
parathyroidectomy 252, 297, 299
parenteral chelation therapy with
        desferrioxamine 242
parkinsonism 115, 268–70
    causes 268, 269
    clinical features 268–9
    management 269–70
'parkinsonism plus' syndromes 269
Parkinson's disease 268
paroxysmal nocturnal dyspnoea 9, 372
paroxysmal supraventricular tachycardias 170–1
partial anterior circulation infarct (PACI) **262**
partial epilepsies 275
    first-line drugs 276
partial gastrectomy 223
passive smoking 204

past medical history 370–1
patches **103**
patent ductus arteriosus (PDA) 191
Paterson-Brown-Kelly syndrome 150
pathological proteinuria 75–6
patient, examining *see* examining the patient
PBC (primary biliary cirrhosis) 242–3
pCO$_2$ 416
PDA (patent ductus arteriosus) 191
PE 3, 4, **166**, 212–13, 216, 351
   after acute MI 168
   clinical features 212
   ECG changes associated with **7**
   investigations 212
   radiological findings **414**
   risk factors 4
   treatment 213
     length of 352
peak expiratory flow rate (PEFR) 12, 196,
     197, 414
peak expiratory flow rate (PEFR) diary 196, 197
pectus carinatum 388
Pel-Ebstein fever 346
pelvic examinations 66
pemphigus 100
penicillamine 243, 317
penicillin 190, 330
penile discharge 375
pentazocine 237
peptic stricture 221
peptic ulcer disease (PUD) 37, **41**, 222–3
percussion
   of the abdomen 392
   and examining the patient with
     breathlessness 12
   and the respiratory system 388, 389
percutaneous coronary intervention 7
percutaneous needle aspiration 205
percutaneous transhepatic cholangiography 60
perforation 223
pergolide 270
pericardial effusion 187–8
pericardial tamponade 188
pericardiectomy 188
pericardiocentesis 188
pericarditis 3, **166**, 187–8
   after acute MI 168
   causes 165, **187**
   investigations 187–8
   management 188
perilymphatic fistula **146**

perindopril 177
peripheral cyanosis 10, 379
peripheral neuropathies 252, 279, 286
peripheral pulses 387
peripheral tumour growth in lung cancer 205
peritonism 65
Perl's stain 427
permanent ileostomy 230
pernicious anaemia 339–40
pes cavus 400
petechiae **103**, 141
pethidine 237
petit mal 275
pets 10
Peutz-Jeghers' syndrome 43, 232, 380
pH 416
phaeochromocytoma 51, 313
pharmacological stress echocardiography 159
pharyngoscopy 32
phenobarbitone 243
phenytoin 267, 276, 313
'Philadelphia chromosome' 344
phosphate 424–5
photochemotherapy 327
photodermatoses 101
physiological anisocoria 394
'pigeon fanciers' lung' 10
pigment stones 235
pigmentation 380, 390
pigmented lesions 99
pistol shots 387
pitting oedema 387, 390
pituitary disorders 301–3
pituitary function tests 422
pituitary tumours 301–2
pityriasis rosea 99
pizotifen 267
plain abdominal X-ray 417
plain X-ray 419
plantar response 402
plaque **103**
plasma ACTH **421**, 422
plasma calcium 422
plasma cortisol 421
plasma glucose 238
plasmapheresis 280, 353
Plasmodium falciparum 359, 360, 362
   complications of infection with **361**
Plasmodium malariae 359, 360, 362
Plasmodium ovale 359, 360, 361, 362
Plasmodium vivax 359, 360, 361, 362

platelet abnormalities 139
  effect 140
platelet count 141, 152, 426
platelet dysfunction 139
plethoric facies 388
pleural biopsy, diagnostic yield in lung
        cancer **206**
pleural diseases **213**
pleural effusion 209
  findings on examination **10**, **389**
    radiological findings **414**
pleural fluid, investigating 415–16
pleural rub 390
pleuritic chest pain 3
Plummer-Vinson syndrome 150
PMR (polymyalgia rheumatica) 322–3
Pneumocystis carinii **360**
pneumonectomy 207
pneumonia 208–10
  classification 208–9
  clinical features 209
  diagnosis 209
  findings on examination **10**
  radiological findings **414**
  severity 209–10
  treatment 210
  see also usual interstitial pneumonia (UIP)
pneumothorax 3, 211–12
  clinical features 212
  findings on examination **10**, **389**
  radiological findings **414**
  risk factors 4
  treatment 212, **214**, **217**
pO₂ 416
POCI (posterior circulation infarct) **262**
polyarteritis nodosa 325–6
polycythaemia 425
  causes **426**
  tumours presenting with 255
polydipsia 69–73
  examining the patient 71–2
  history in the patient 70–1
  investigating the patient 72–3
'polymorphic' VT 171
polymyalgia rheumatica (PMR) 322–3
polymyositis 324–5
polyuria 69–73, 77, 374
  differential diagnosis 69–70
  examining the patient 71–2
  history in the patient 70–1
  investigating the patient 72–3

pompholyx 99
portal hypertension **127**, 240
positron electron tomography 207
post primary pulmonary TB 202
post-traumatic headache 89
postcricoid oesophageal web 150
posterior circulation infarct (POCI) **262**
'posthepatic' jaundice 57, **59**
postherpetic neuralgia 89, 267
postrenal failure **248**, 250
postsyncope 107
postural hypotension 105, **106**, 109
potassium channel activators 161
potassium permanganate 328
potassium-sparing diuretics 182
power
  in the lower limbs 402
  in the upper limbs 399
PPIs (proton pump inhibitors) 221, 223, 324
PR interval of the 12-lead ECG 411
praecordium 385–6
prednisolone 231, 252, 265–6, 279, 280, 298,
        309, 317, 323, 345
  see also oral prednisolone
pregnancy
  and epilepsy 277
  hypertension in 183
'prehepatic' jaundice 57, **59**
prerenal failure **248**, 250
presyncope 105
pretibial myxoedema 306, 330
preventive chemotherapy for TB 204
primaquine 361
primary angioplasty 165
primary biliary cirrhosis (PBC) 242–3
primary haemochromatosis 241
  course and prognosis 242
primary hyperaldosteronism 313
primary hyperlipidaemia 290
primary hyperparathyroidism 298
  biochemical abnormalities **425**
primary hyperthyroidism 306
primary hypoparathyroidism 299
  biochemical abnormalities **425**
primary hypothyroidism, biochemical
        abnormalities **423**
primary osteoporosis 294
primary pneumothorax, treatment **214**
primary progressive MS 272
primary pulmonary TB 202
primary skin diseases 326–9

primary spontaneous pneumothorax 212
  treatment 212, **214**
primary thyrotoxicosis **423**
PRL 301
PRL disorders 303–4
PRL-secreting tumours 301, 302
pro-kinetics 221
probenecid 300
'problem list' 405
procainamide 171, 174, 322
prochlorperazine 237
procyclidine 270
progressive bulbar palsy 278
progressive headache 87–8, 265–6
progressive muscular atrophy 278
progressive primary TB 202
progressive supranuclear palsy 269
proguanil 360
projectile vomiting 373
prolactin see PRL
pronator drift in the upper limbs 398–9
propanolol 225, 267, 308
prophylactic antibiotics 192, 224, 334
  for COPD 201
  for endocarditis 189
  for mitral stenosis 185
prophylactic drugs for migraine 267
prophylactic subcutaneous heparin 230
propofol 243
propylthiouracil (PTU) 308
prostate, and the differential diagnosis of
        haematuria 75
prostate-specific antigen (PSA) 255, 256, **428**
prostatectomy 255
prostatic carcinoma 255–6
prosthetic valve endocarditis 188
protease inhibitors 358
protein to creatinine ratio 80
proteinuria 75–80, 188
  differential diagnosis 75–6
  examining the patient 77–8
  history in the patient 77
  investigating the patient 78–80
  levels **76**
prothrombin time 59, 60, 143, 226, 240, 244
prothrombin time prolongation 235
proton pump inhibitors (PPIs) 221, 223, 324
proctoscopes **419**
pruritus 252, 372
  see also itching
PSA (prostate-specific antigen) 255, 256, **428**

pseudo-Cushing's syndrome 421
pseudobulbar palsy 279
'pseudodementia' 113
pseudogout 97
pseudohyponatraemia 256
pseudohypoparathyroidism 299
  biochemical abnormalities **425**
pseudomembranous colitis 234
Pseudomonas 209
pseudopseudohypoparathyroidism 299
pseudoseizure **106**
pseudotumour cerebri 87, 265
pseudoxanthoma elasticum 141
psoriasis 99, 326–7
psoriatic arthritis 96, 320
psychogenic polydipsia **70**
psychosocial factors and IHD 158
PTH (parathyroid hormone) 295, 424–5
PTU (propylthiouracil) 308
PUD (peptic ulcer disease) 37, **41**, 222–3
pulmonary angiography 7, 212
    see also spiral CT pulmonary angiography
pulmonary disease 3
pulmonary embolism see PE
pulmonary fibrosis, findings on examination **10**
pulmonary function tests 216
pulmonary hypertension 31
pulmonary oedema, CXR features **414**
pulmonary rehabilitation 201
pulmonary TB 202–3
'pulmonary-renal syndromes' 246
pulse
  in aortic regurgitation 25
  and examination of the respiratory system 388
  and examining the patient with abdominal
      pain 65
  and examining the patient with palpitations
      17, 18
  see also collapsing pulse; peripheral pulses;
      radial pulse
pulsus paradoxus 384, 388
PUO 33–6
  causes 33
  examining the patient 33, **34**
  history in the patient 33
  investigating the patient 33–6
pupillary reflexes 394
purpura **103**, 141
pustular lesions 100
pustular psoriasis 327
pustules **103**

pyloric stenosis 223
pyloroplasty 223
pyoderma gangrenosum 329, 330
pyrazinamide 203
pyrexia 65, 380
pyrexia of unknown origin *see* PUO
pyridostigmine 280
pyridoxine 203, 272, 293
pyruvate kinase deficiency 337

Q
QRS complex of the 12-lead ECG 411
QT interval of the 12-lead ECG 412
Quincke's sign 25, 382, 384
quinine 360
quinolones 203, 254

R
RA 93, 315–17
    causes of anaemia in 95, **333**
    drug treatment 316–17
    examining the patient with 94–5, 316
    management 316
    organ systems affected **316**
    pathological features 316
    X ray of affected joints 97
race and IHD 158
radial pulse 384
radiofrequency ablations 169
radioiodine 308
radioisotope studies 420
radiological investigations
    for confusional states 115, 117
    for haematuria and proteinuria 80
    for hypertension 83
    for sensory and/or motor neurological
        deficits 136
radionuclide imaging 309
radiotherapy 207, 222, 233, 255, 278, 281, 331,
        345, 347, 348
    for acromegaly 302
raised intracranial pressure 273
    symptoms **88**, 89, 278
raloxifene 294–5
ramipril 177
Ramsay Hunt syndrome 397
RAPD (relative afferent pupillary defect) 394
rapidly progressive glomerulonephritis (RPGN) 247
rash 376
Raynaud's phenomenon 323, 324, 380
reactivation TB 202

reactive arthritis 320
'reactive' blood picture 427
REAL (Revised European American Lymphoma)
        classification 348
recombinant erythropoietin (EPO) 334, 335
recombinant factor VIII concentrates 349, 350
rectal biopsy 229
rectal bleeding 63, 373–4
    causes **374**
rectal examinations 66, 153, 234
    see also digital rectal examinations
rectosigmoid tumours 233
red-coloured urine 75
reflexes
    eliciting **401**
    in the lower limbs 402
    in the upper limbs 399
    see also pupillary reflexes
reflux 37, 38, 221
Refsum's disease 400
regional spread of tumours in the chest 205
regular palpitations 15
Reiter's syndrome 95, 319–20
relapsing-remitting MS 272
relative afferent pupillary defect (RAPD) 394
renal angiography 83, 420
renal artery stenosis 180
renal biopsy 78, 246, 247, 251, 420
renal cell carcinoma 33, 255
renal concentration tests 73
renal disease 81, 180
    skin manifestations **404**
renal failure **248**, 419
    biochemical abnormalities **425**
    in multiple myeloma **345**
    see also ARF; CRF
renal function
    monitoring 251
    prevention of decline 251
renal insufficiency, symptoms 51
renal mass, causes **392**
renal osteodystrophy 252, 297
renal parenchymal disease 81
renal replacement therapy 252
    indications for 249
    for renal osteodystrophy 297
renal scintigraphy 420
renal stones 254–5
renal system
    and systemic lupus erythematosus (SLE) 321
    and systemic sclerosis 324

renal transplantation 252
renal ultrasound 80, 246, 249, 419–20
renin-dependent hypertension 182
renovascular hypertension 181
respiratory abnormalities, patterns of **389**
respiratory disease 195–218
    findings on examination **10, 389**
    radiological findings 414–17
respiratory failure 210–12
respiratory symptoms 373
respiratory system
    examination of 387–90
    investigations 414–17
    and systemic lupus erythematosus (SLE) 321
    and systemic sclerosis 324
resting tremor in the hands 384
restrictive cardiomyopathy 187
restrictive surgery 290
reticulocyte count 152, 154
reticulocytes 152, 426
retinopathy
    Keith-Wagner classification 181
    see also diabetic retinopathy
retrograde pyelogram 80
retrosternal pain 3
    and dyspepsia 37
Revised European American Lymphona (REAL)
        classification 348
Revised Jones' criteria for guidance in diagnosis of
        rheumatic fever 189–90
rheumatoid arthritis *see* RA
rheumatoid factor 96
rhonchi 12
rickets 296, 297
rifampicin 203, 218, 313
right heart failure 176
right hypochondrium, causes of pain in **64**
right iliac fossa, causes of pain in **64**
right ventricular failure 388, 390
right-sided heart murmurs 26
rigid sigmoidoscopy 47, **419**
rigidity 268, 399
rigors 4, 63
riluzole 278
ring sideroblasts 335
Rinne's test 397
risk stratification and secondary prevention of
        acute MI 168
rituximab 348
rolling hiatus hernia 221
ropinirole 270

Roth's spots in the retina 385
Rovsing's sign 66
RPGN (rapidly progressive
        glomerulonephritis) 247
rubeosis iridis 285
ruptured oesophageal varices **41**
Rye classification of Hodgkin's disease 346

S
sacral oedema 387
sacroiliitis 319
SAH (subarachnoid haemorrhage) 87, 89, 264
salbutamol 200
salicylic acid 327
salmeterol 201
salt intake, effect on blood pressure 180
salt and water balance 256
saquinavir 358
sarcoidosis 330, **404**
scabies 100
scales **103**
scaly lesions 99
scars **103**
Schilling test 153
Schirmer's test 325
sclerodactyly 383
scleroderma 323, 323–4
'scopes' used to examine the gastrointestinal tract
        419
scurvy 141
seborrhoeic dermatitis 328
seborrhoeic keratosis 99
second cranial nerve (optic) 394–5
second degree heart block 172
    rhythm of 12-lead ECG 410–11
secondary DM 283
secondary haemochromatosis 241
secondary hyperaldosteronism 313
secondary hyperlipidaemia 290
secondary hyperparathyroidism 298
    investigations 299
secondary hypertension 81, 180–1
    causes 180
    coarctation of the aorta as a cause 191
    examination 180–1
    history 180
    investigation policy 181
    management 181
secondary hyperthyroidism 307
secondary hypothyroidism **423**
secondary meningitis 272–3

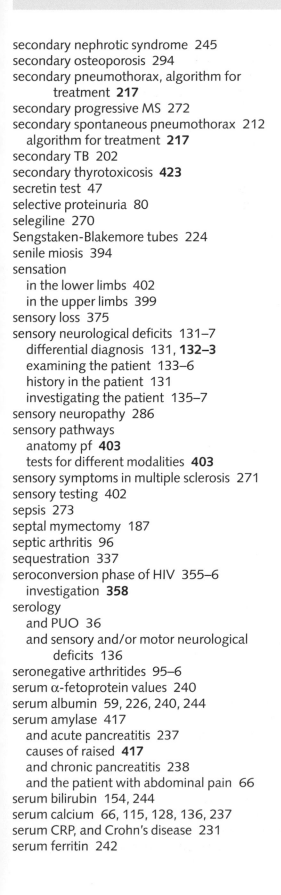

secondary nephrotic syndrome 245
secondary osteoporosis 294
secondary pneumothorax, algorithm for treatment **217**
secondary progressive MS 272
secondary spontaneous pneumothorax 212
  algorithm for treatment **217**
secondary TB 202
secondary thyrotoxicosis **423**
secretin test 47
selective proteinuria 80
selegiline 270
Sengstaken-Blakemore tubes 224
senile miosis 394
sensation
  in the lower limbs 402
  in the upper limbs 399
sensory loss 375
sensory neurological deficits 131–7
  differential diagnosis 131, **132–3**
  examining the patient 133–6
  history in the patient 131
  investigating the patient 135–7
sensory neuropathy 286
sensory pathways
  anatomy pf **403**
  tests for different modalities **403**
sensory symptoms in multiple sclerosis 271
sensory testing 402
sepsis 273
septal mymectomy 187
septic arthritis 96
sequestration 337
seroconversion phase of HIV 355–6
  investigation **358**
serology
  and PUO 36
  and sensory and/or motor neurological deficits 136
seronegative arthritides 95–6
serum α-fetoprotein values 240
serum albumin 59, 226, 240, 244
serum amylase 417
  and acute pancreatitis 237
  causes of raised **417**
  and chronic pancreatitis 238
  and the patient with abdominal pain 66
serum bilirubin 154, 244
serum calcium 66, 115, 128, 136, 237
serum CRP, and Crohn's disease 231
serum ferritin 242

serum glucose 115, 136, 237
serum haptoglobins 154
serum immunoelectrophoresis 246
serum iron 242
serum total cholesterol 158
serum urate 97
serum uric acid 128
seventh cranial nerve (facial) 397
sex and IHD 157
sexual hair loss 391
Sheffield risk tables 158
shingles 4, 99, 328–9, **360**
shockwave lithotripsy 236
short acting β$_2$-agonists 197, 200
short Synacthen stimulation test 288, 301, **421**, 422
shortness of breath see dyspnoea
Shy-Drager syndrome 269
SIADH 256
  causes **257**
sibutramine 290
sick euthyroid syndrome **423**
sick sinus syndrome 172
sickle cell anaemia 151, 337–8
  changes on blood film **152**
sideroblastic anaemia 335
  interpretation of iron storage results **153**
sigmoid volvulus **418**
sigmoidoscopy 153, 229, 233, 234, 235, 418
  see also flexible sigmoidoscopy; rigid sigmoidoscopy
simple partial seizures 275
sinus bradycardia 167
  causes **16, 410**
sinus tachycardia
  causes **16, 410**
  rhythm of 12-lead ECG 410
situational syncope **106**
sixth cranial nerve (abducens) 395–6
Sjögren's syndrome 95, 324, 325
skeletal deformities and examination of the cardiovascular system 386
skin
  and complications of DM 286
  examining 404
  and systemic lupus erythematosus (SLE) 321
  and systemic sclerosis 323–4
  see also uraemic skin
skin diseases 99–103
  differential diagnosis by appearance 99–101
  examining the patient 101–2
  history in the patient 101

skin diseases (*Continued*)
  investigating the patient 102
  see also primary skin diseases
skin disorders
  associated with underlying systemic disease
    329–30, **404**
  musculoskeletal and 315–31
skin symptoms 375–6
skin tumours, malignant 331
skip lesions 231, 265
skull X-ray 299
SLE (systemic lupus erythematosus) 246, 247,
    263, 320–2
sleep apnoea 216–17, 372
  see also obstructive sleep apnoea
sleep apnoea syndrome 216
sleep disordered breathing 373
sleep patterns 372
sliding hiatus hernia 221
slow heart rate 15
small bowel contrast studies 418
small bowel disorders 225–8
small bowel follow-through 234, 418
small bowel meal/enema 47, 418
small cell carcinoma 204
  treatment 207, **208**
smell
  disturbed 375
  sense of 393
smoking
  and COPD 198, 200
  and Crohn's disease 232
  effect on blood pressure 180
  and IHD 157
  and lung cancer 204, **205**
  and secondary prevention of acute MI 168
social history 371
sodium valproate 276
solitary acute headache *see* acute headache
somatic neuropathies 286
'somatization' 131
somatosensory evoked potentials 137
somatostatin analogues 302
sotalol 170, 173
spade hands 383
spasticity 399
speech
  altered 375
  causes and features of abnormalities **376**
sphincterotomy via ERCP 236
spider naevi 391

spinal claudication 373
spinal cord, disorders 280–1
spinal cord compression 281
spinal root 398
spiral CT 417
spiral CT pulmonary angiography 212
spirometry 12, 200, 415
spironolactone 178, 241, 313
spleen
  distinguishing between the left kidney and **127**
  palpitating 128, 130
splenectomy 334, 336, 337, 339, 344
splenic sequestration 337
splenomegaly 125–30, 141
  differential diagnosis 125
  examining the patient 126–7
  history in the patient 126
  investigating the patient 128–30
splinter haemorrhages 382, 384
spondyloarthropathies 318–20
spontaneous pneumothorax 211
'spot diagnoses' 381
sputum 373
sputum microscopy and culture 209
sputum pots 11
squamous cell carcinoma 204, 331
ST segment of the 12-lead ECG 411–12
  causes of elevation **6**
stable angina
  and coronary angiography 159
  see also chronic stable angina
Staphylococcus aureus 188, 189, 209
Staphylococcus epidermidis 188
statins
  and treatment of acute MI 166
  and treatment of lipid disorders 291
  and treatment of NSTEMI 162
  use for IHD 161
  use of 263, 291–3
status epilepticus 277
STEMI (acute myocardial infarction with ST
    elevation) 161
stenting, angioplasty and 161
stepped-care plan for the management of chronic
    asthma **197**
stereotactic surgery 270
sterile pyuria, causes 255
sternotomy scar 385
steroids 168, 222, 230, 300, 322, 325, 328, 330
  see also corticosteroids; inhaled steroid; oral
    steroids; systemic steroids

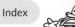

Stevens-Johnson syndrome 329
stiffness 375
Stokes-Adams attacks 105
stomach emptying 364
stool appearance 45
strangury 77
streptococcal infection, diagnosis 190
streptococcus faecalis 188
Streptococcus pneumoniae 208–9
Streptococcus viridans 188
streptokinase 164–5
stress 222
  and IHD 158
stress incontinence 375
stricturoplasty 232
stridor 9
stroke 119, 261–3
  clinical features 261
  complications 122–3
  differential diagnosis 119
  examining the patient 121–3
  history in the patient 120–1
  incidence 261
  investigations 123–4, 261–2
  management 262–3
    acute 123
  prognosis 263
  risk factors **121, 261**
  symptoms and signs associated with **120**
  types **119**
subacute combined degeneration of the spinal
    cord 281
subacute (de Quervain's) thyroiditis 309
subarachnoid haemorrhage (SAH) 87,
    89, 264
subcutaneous nodules 102, 190
subdural haematoma 119, 264–5
subendocardial myocardial infarctions *see*
    NSTEMI
sublingual nifedipine 183
subtotal colectomy with ileorectal
    anastamosis 230
subtotal thyroidectomy 308
succussion splash 392
suicide risk, assessment 363
sulphasalazine 230, 317, 319, 320
sulphinpyrazone 300
sulphonylureas 287
sumatriptan 266, 267
superior vena caval obstruction 388
suprapubic pain, causes **64**

supraventricular arrhythmias 167, 169–71
  drugs for 173–4
supraventricular tachycardia
  distinguishing between VT and 172
  see also paroxysmal supraventricular
    tachycardias
swan neck deformity 94, **315**
sweats 372
swelling
  abdominal 391
  ankle 372
  calf 4, 372
  of the joints 403
Sydenham's chorea 190
symptomatic HIV infection 356, **357**
  investigation at **358**
syncope 105, **106**, 107
  as a cardiovascular symptom 372
syndrome of inappropriate antidiuretic hormone
    production *see* SIADH
syndrome X 157
synovial fluid 300
syphilis serology 124
syringobulbia 281
syringomyelia 280
systemic acidosis 252
systemic disease, skin manifestations
    329–30, **404**
systemic emboli 168
systemic lupus erythematosus (SLE) 246, 247,
    263, 320–2
systemic sclerosis 323–4
systemic steroids 329
systolic hypertension and IHD 158

T
T_3 (total tri-iodothyronine) 422, **423**
T_4 (total thyroxine) 422, **423**
T cell lymphomas 348
T wave of the 12-lead ECG 412
tachycardia 17, 42, 65, 388
  rhythm of 12-lead ECG 410
  see also sinus tachycardia; supraventricular
    tachycardia; ventricular tachycardia (VT)
TACI (total anterior circulation infarct) **262**
taking a history 369–77
  at the start 369
  family history 371
  general principles 369
  past medical history 370–1
    allergies 371

taking a history (*Continued*)
    medications 370
   presenting complaint 369–70
    history of 370
   social history 371
   systems review 371–7
    cardiovascular symptoms 372–3
    gastrointestinal disease 373–4
    general symptoms 371–2
    genitourinary symptoms 374–5
    haematological symptoms 376
    metabolic and endocrine symptoms 375
    musculoskeletal symptoms 375
    neurological symptoms 375
    respiratory symptoms 373
    skin symptoms 375–6
taste 397
tazarotene 327
TB 31, 201–4, 286
  clinical manifestations 202–3
  control 204
  diagnostic tests 203
  and HIV 358
  notification in the UK **202**
  radiological findings **414**
  treatment 203
   monitoring 203
teeth 385
teicoplanin 362
telangiectasia 391
  see also hereditary haemorrhagic telangiectasia
temperature 380
temporal arteritis 87–8, 89, **266**
temporal artery biopsy 89–90
temporal lobe epilepsy 275
tenderness of the abdomen 66
tendon xanthomata 330
tendons of the hands, examining 383
tenecteplase **165**
tenesmus 374
tension headache 89, 267
tension pneumothorax 212
tenth cranial nerve (vagus) 397, 398
terbutaline 200
terlipressin 224
terminal ileal disease 231
tertiary hyperparathyroidism 297, 298
testosterone 255, 301
tetracycline 227, 328, 330
thalassaemia 151, 338–9
  changes on blood film **152**
  interpretation of iron storage results **153**

thalidomide 345
thallium perfusion scan 413
theophyllines 197, 201
thiamine deficiency, red cell transketolase for 117
thiazide diuretics 265, 305
  and treatment of chronic cardiac failure 178
  and treatment of hypertension 182, 265
  and treatment of stroke patients 263
thiazolidinediones 287
thick and thin blood films 117, 288, 360
third cranial nerve (oculomotor) 395–6
third degree heart block 172–3, **174**
  rhythm of 12-lead ECG 411
third generation cephalosporin 330
thrill 386
thrombin time 143
thrombocytopenia 126, 139, 141
thrombocytosis, causes **427**
thrombolytic treatment 5
  for acute MI 164–5
  contraindications **165**
  for NSTEMI 162
  see also acute thrombolysis
thrombophilia screen 262
thrombophlebitis migrans 330
thrombosis 119
thrombotic disorders 351–2
thrombotic thrombocytopenic purpura (TTP)
  352–3
'thumps' 15
thymectomy 280
thyroid acropachy 306
thyroid cancer 309
thyroid disorders 305–10
  biochemical abnormalities **423**
thyroid function tests
  for change in bowel habit 46
  for confusional states 115
  for loss of consciousness 109
  for lymphadenopathy and splenomegaly 128
  for sensory and/or motor neurological
   deficits 136
thyroid gland enlargement, causes **382**
thyroid malignancy 309–10
thyroid status, examination of **383**
thyroid stimulating hormone (TSH) 301,
  422, **423**
thyrotoxic crisis (thyroid 'storm') 308–9
thyrotoxicosis 16, 306–9
  aetiology 306–7
  clinical presentation 51, 307–8
  investigations 308

thyrotoxicosis (*Continued*)
  treatment 308
  see also primary thyrotoxicosis; secondary
     thyrotosicosis
thyrotoxicosis without hyperthyroidism 307
thyroxine 301, 308
thyroxine sodium 306
TIA/vertebrobasilar insufficiency **106**
TIAs (transient ischaemic attacks) 107, 119, 263–4
tic douloureux 89, 267
tilt table testing 109
tinea corporis 99
tinea versicolor 99
tiotropium 201
tirofiban 162
tissue-type plasminogen activator (tPA) 164, 165
TLCO (transfer factor) 415
TNF 317
TNF inhibition 319
TNM (tumour-node-metastasis) classification for
    lung cancer 207
Todd's paresis 107, 275
tone
  in the lower limbs 400, 402
  in the upper limbs 399
tonic-clonic fits 274
tonometry 267
topical antibiotics 328
torsade de pointes 171
total anterior circulation infarct (TACI) **262**
total thyroxine (T4) 422, **423**
total tri-iodothyronine (T3) 422, **423**
toxic epidermal necrolysis 100
toxic lung injury **213**
toxoplasmosis **360**
tPA (tissue-type plasminogen activator) 164, 165
trachea, examination of 388
tracheal deviation, causes 388
tranexamic acid 350, 351
trans-sphenoidal surgery 304, 310
transbronchial spread in lung cancer 205
transfer factor (TLCO) 415
transient ischaemic attacks (TIAs) 107, 119, 263–4
transitional cell carcinoma 255
transjugular intrahepatic portosystemic shunts
    224–5
transmural MIs 162–3
transplantation
  bone marrow *see* bone marrow transplantation
  cardiac 178, 187
  heart-lung 214

  liver 241, 243
  lung 201
  renal 252
transthoracic transoesophageal ligation of
    varices 225
Traube's sign 25
traumatic pneumothorax 212
tremor 268, 398
  causes **399**
  see also fine tremor
Trendelenburg's sign 95
tricuspid endocarditis 188
tricuspid regurgitation 26–7, 186
tricyclic antidepressant drugs
  and gastric emptying 364
  and treatment of atypical facial pain 267
  and treatment of irritable bowel syndrome 235
  and treatment of migraine 267
  and treatment of multiple sclerosis 272
trigeminal (fifth cranial nerve) 396
trigeminal nerve lesions, causes **396**
trigeminal neuralgia 89, 267
triglycerides 158
trimethoprim 253, 254
triple stimulation test 301
trochlear (fourth cranial nerve) 395–6
Troisier's sign 42, 391
Tropheryma whippelii 227
tropical sprue 227
troponin measurement 4, 5, 162, 176, 409
  and myocardial damage 163–4
Trousseau's sign 299
trunk, examination of 391
TSH (thyroid stimulating hormone) 301,
    422, **423**
TTP (thrombotic thrombocytopenic purpura)
    352–3
tuberculosis *see* TB
tuberculous meningitis 87, 272, 273
tubular proteinuria 76
tumour markers 427–8
tumour necrosis factor *see* TNF
tumour-node-metastasis (TNM) classification for
    lung cancer 207
tumours
  radiological findings **414**
  see also adrenocortical tumours; brain tumours;
    cerebral tumours; endocrine tumours of
    the gut; pituitary tumours; skin tumours
Turner's syndrome 191, 384
twelfth cranial nerve (hypoglossal) 398

'twisting of the points' 171
type I DM 283, 420
    and blindness 284
    differences in presentation between type II
        and **284**
type I respiratory failure 210–11
type II DM 283, 420
    differences in presentation between type I
        and **284**
type II respiratory failure 211, 213

U
U&Es *see* urea and electrolytes
U wave of the 12-lead ECG 412
UC 228–31
    clinical features 228
    complications 228–9
    investigations 229–30
    management 230
    prognosis 230–1
    skin manifestations 330
UIP (usual interstitial pneumonia) 216
UK, notification of TB **202**
UK Prospective Diabetes Study (UKPDS)
        286, 287
ulcerated lesions 101
ulcerative colitis *see* UC
ulcers **103**, 222
ultrasound examinations 43, 206, 233, 235, 236,
        237, 244, 253, 309, 418
    see also abdominal ultrasound; carotid doppler
        ultrasound; endoscopic ultrasound (EUS);
        renal ultrasound
ultrasound of the liver 243
ultraviolet B radiation therapy 327
unilateral palpable kidneys, causes **392**
units of alcohol **371**
unstable angina 3
upper GI bleeding (gastrointestinal haemorrhage)
        41, 43, 223–5, 419
upper GI endoscopy 7, 153, 234
upper limbs, examination 398–9
upper motor neurone lesions 397, 398
upper UTIs 253
uraemic skin 250
urea 419
    raised 43, 44, 209
urea and electrolytes (U&Es)
    and abdominal pain 66
    and acute renal failure 248
    and chronic renal failure 250–1

    and colorectal neoplasia 233
    and confusional states 115
    and dyspnoea 12
    and heart failure 176
    and hypertension 83
    and joint disease 97
    and loss of consciousness 109
    and palpitations 18
    and PUO 35
    and sensory and/or motor neurological
        deficits 136
    and stroke patients 124
    and weight loss 54
urease tests 38
ureteric pain 63
ureteroscopy 80
ureters, and the differential diagnosis of
        haematuria 75
urethra, and the differential diagnosis of
        haematuria 75
urge incontinence 375
uric acid-lowering drug therapy 300
urinalysis 72
urinary cortisol 421
urinary system, investigations 419–20
urinary tract infections *see* UTIs
urinary tract malignancies 255–6
urinary urobilinogen 154
urination *see* micturition
urine, appearance 77, 374
urine dipstick testing 66, 78, 83, 245, 248,
        253, 419
urine microscopy 245, 248, 250, 419
urine testing 419
    for haematuria and proteinuria 78, 80
ursodeoxycholic acid 236, 243
urticaria 100
usual interstitial pneumonia (UIP) 216
Uthoff's phenomenon 271
UTIs 252–4
    clinical features 253
    investigations 253
    management 253–4
    precipitating causes **253**
uvulopalatopharyngoplasty 217

V
V/Q scan 12, 416
    for PE 7, 212
vaccination for TB 204
vagal stimulation 171

vaginal discharge 375
vagotomy 223
vagus palsies, causes **398**
vagus (tenth cranial nerve) 397, 398
valsalva manoeuvre 171
valvotomy 185
valvular heart disease 184–6
vancomycin 189, 362
    see also oral vancomycin
variceal bleeds, management 224
vascular abnormalities **41**
vasoconstrictor therapy 224
vasodilators 185
vasopressors 249
vasovagal syndrome 109
Vaughan Williams classification of anti-arrhythmic
        drugs 173, **174**
venesection 242
venous hum in the epigastrium 392
venous thrombosis see VTE
ventilation-perfusion scan see V/Q scan
ventricular aneurysm **166**
ventricular arrhythmias 167
    drugs for 173–4
    see also late ventricular arrhythmias
ventricular ectopics 167, 169
ventricular fibrillation 167, 171–2
ventricular septal defect (VSD) **166**, 167, 190–1
ventricular tachycardia see VT
ventriculoperitoneal CSF shunt 265
verapamil 160, 169, 170, 173, 182, 184, 267
    see also intravenous verapamil
vertebral artery, dissection of 87
vertebral collapse 3, 4
vertebrobasilar insufficiency 105, **146**
vertical nystagmus 147
vertigo 145–8
    differential diagnosis 145
    examining the patient 147
    features of diseases causing **146**
    history in the patient 145–7
    investigating the patient 147–8
vesicles **103**
vesicular lesions 99–100
vessel wall abnormalities 139–40
    effect 140
vestibular neuronitis **146**
vestibulocochlear (eighth cranial nerve) 397
vigabatrin 272, 276
vincristine 345
vipomas 47, 227

viral meningitis 272
Virchow's node 42, 391
Virchow's triad 351
viscus, perforation **418**
vision
    disturbed 375
    see also eyes;
visual acuity 394
visual evoked potentials 137
visual field assessment 90, 302
visual fields 394–5
    defects **394**
vitamin B_{12} deficiency
    causes 150
    changes on blood film **152**
    investigations 153
vitamin B_{12} replacement for anaemia 333, 340
vitamin D
    metabolism **295**
    see also dietary vitamin D deficiency
vitamin K deficiency 139
vitiligo 329
vocal fremitus 388
vocal resonance, assessment 12
voice, hoarse 373, 387
vomiting 63
    and CRF 252
    as a symptom of gastrointestinal disease 373
von Willebrand's disease (VWD) 349–50
von Willebrand's factor (VWF) 350
voriconazole 215
VSD (ventricular septal defect) **166**, 167, 190–1
VT 17, 167, 171
    distinguishing between supraventricular
        tachycardias and 172
VTE 351
    risk factors **352**
VWD (von Willebrand's disease) 349–50
VWF (von Willebrand's factor) 350

W
walking, abnormalities **136**
warfarin 170, 178, 216, 352
    management of overdose **366**
    and treatment of stroke patients 262–3
    see also oral warfarin
wasting 398, 399
    see also muscle wasting
water balance, salt and 256
water deprivation test 301
'waterbrash' 37

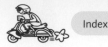
Waterhouse-Friderichsen syndrome 311
weakness 375
Weber's test 397
weeping eczema 328
weepy lesions 100
Wegener's granulomatosis 246
weight
   changes in 372
   and IHD 158
weight gain 372
  see also obesity
weight loss 51–5, 372
   differential diagnosis 51, **52**
   examining the patient 52–4
   history in the patient 51–2
   investigating the patient 54–5
   and polyuria and polydipsia 70
Wenckebach heart block 172, **173**
Wernicke's encephalopathy 241
wheals **103**
wheezing 9, 12, 31, 373, 390
Whipple's disease 227
white cell count 152, 237, 426
  see also differential white cell count
Wickham's striae 329
Wilson's disease 243
Wolff-Parkinson-White syndrome 18
   PR interval of the 12-lead ECG 411

X
X-ray
   for ankylosing spondylitis 319
   of bones 207, 296, 297
   of the chest and hands 151, 251
   of diseased joints 97
   for gout 300
   of the hands 299, 302, 324
   for hyperparathyroidism 299
   of the skull 299
   for the urinary system 419
   see also abdominal X-ray; CXR; plain X-ray
xanthelasmata 330, 385, 390
xanthomata 383, 384
xanthomatosis 330
xerosis 99
ximelagatran 352
xylose absorption test 47

Y
yellow nails 382

Z
zidovudine 358
Zollinger-Ellison syndrome 47, 222, 227
zoonoses 33